Handbook of
Experimental Pharmacology

Volume 110

Pharmacokinetics of Drugs

Contributors

G.L. Amidon, J.P.F. Bai, L.P. Balant, C.M. Barksdale, I.A. Blair
D.D. Breimer, M. Chiba, J. Delforge, M. Eichelbaum
B.L. Ferraiolo, A.J. Fischman, M. Gex-Fabry, N. Holford
J. Kantrowitz, H.K. Kroemer, T.M. Ludden, J.M. Mayer
B. Mazière, C. McMartin, G. Mikus, M.A. Mohler
G.D. Nordblom, R. O'Neill, K.S. Pang, O. Pelkonen
A. Racine-Poon, R.H. Rubin, J.-L. Steimer, B.H. Stewart
H.W. Strauss, B. Testa, S. Vozeh, P.G. Welling, R.J. Wills
A. Yacobi

Editors
Peter G. Welling and Luc P. Balant

With a Foreword by J.G. Wagner

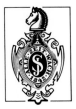

Springer-Verlag
Berlin Heidelberg New York London Paris
Tokyo Hong Kong Barcelona Budapest

Peter G. Welling, Ph.D., D.Sc.
Vice President
Pharmacokinetics/Drug Metabolism
Parke-Davis Pharmaceutical Research Division
Warner-Lambert Company
2800 Plymouth Road
Ann Arbor, MI 48105-1047
USA

Luc P. Balant, Ph.D.
Reader
Clinical Research Unit
Department of Psychiatry
47, Rue du XXXI Décembre
CH-1207 Geneva
Switzerland

With 69 Figures and 51 Tables

ISBN 3-540-57506-5 Springer-Verlag Berlin Heidelberg New York
ISBN 0-387-57506-5 Springer-Verlag New York Berlin Heidelberg

Library of Congress Cataloging-in-Publication Data. Pharmacokinetics of drugs / contributors, Amidon, G.L. ...[et al.]; editors, Peter G. Welling and Luc P. Balant. p. cm. – (Handbook of experimental pharmacology; v. 110) Includes bibliographical references and index. ISBN 3-540-57506-5. – ISBN 0-387-57506-5 1. Pharmacokinetics. I. Welling, Peter G. II. Balant, Luc P., 1941– . III. Series. QP905.H3 vol. 110 [RM301.5] 615′.1 s–dc20 [615′.7] 93-43145

© Springer-Verlag Berlin Heidelberg 1994
Printed in Germany

The use of general descriptive names, registered names, trademarks, etc. in this publication does not imply, even in the absence of a specific statement, that such names are exempt from the relevant protective laws and regulations and therefore free for general use.

Product liability: The publishers cannot guarantee the accuracy of any information about dosage and application contained in this book. In every individual case the user must check such information by consulting the relevant literature.

Typesetting: Best-set Typesetter Ltd., Hong Kong

SPIN: 10040028   27/3130/SPS – 5 4 3 2 1 0 – Printed on acid-free paper

List of Contributors

AMIDON, G.L., University of Michigan, College of Pharmacy, Ann Arbor, MI 48109-1065, USA

BAI, J.P.F., University of Minnesota, College of Pharmacy, 308 Harvard Street SE, Minneapolis, MN 55455, USA

BALANT, L.P., Clinical Research Unit, Department of Psychiatry, 47, Rue du XXXI Décembre, CH-1207 Geneva, Switzerland

BARKSDALE, C.M., Department of Pharmacokinetics and Drug Metabolism, Parke-Davis Pharmaceutical Research Division, Warner-Lambert Company, 2800 Plymouth Road, Ann Arbor, MI 48105, USA

BLAIR, I.A., Department of Pharmacology and Chemistry, Vanderbilt University, 804 MRB, 23rd Avenue South at Pierce Avenue, Nashville, TN 37232-6602, USA

BREIMER, D.D., Center for Bio-Pharmaceutical Sciences, University of Leiden, P.O. Box 9503, NL-2300 RA Leiden, The Netherlands

CHIBA, M., Merck Sharp and Dohme Research Laboratories, West Point, PA 19486, USA

DELFORGE, J., SHFJ, Commissariat a l'Energie Atomique, Direction des Sciences du Vivant, Département de Recherche en Imagerie, Pharmacologie et Physiologie, 4, Place du Général-Leclerc, F-91406 Orsay, France

EICHELBAUM, M., Dr. Margarete Fischer-Bosch-Institut, Auerbachstr. 112, D-70376 Stuttgart, Germany

FERRAIOLO, B.L., Drug Metabolism, R.W. Johnson Pharmaceutical Research Institute, Welsh and McKean Rds., Spring-House, PA 19477, USA

FISCHMAN, A.J., Division of Nuclear Medicine of the Department of Radiology, Massachusetts General Hospital, Harvard Medical School, Fruit Street, Boston, MA 02114, USA

GEX-FABRY, M., Unité de Recherche Clinique, Institutions Universitaires de Psychiatrie, 47, Rue du XXXI Décembre, CH-1207 Geneva, Switzerland

HOLFORD, N., Department of Pharmacology and Clinical Pharmacology, University of Auckland Medical School, Private Bag, Auckland, New Zealand

KANTROWITZ, J., American Cyanamid Company, Medical Research Division, Pharmacodynamics Research, Lederle Laboratories, Pearl River, NY 10965-1299, USA

KROEMER, H.K., Dr. Margarete Fischer-Bosch-Institut für Klinische Pharmakologie, Auerbachstr. 112, D-70376 Stuttgart, Germany

LUDDEN, T.M., Division of Biopharmaceutics, Office of Research Resources, Food and Drug Administration, Rockville, MD 20857, USA

MAYER, J.M., School of Pharmacy, B.E.P., University of Lausanne, CH-1015 Lausanne, Switzerland

MAZIÈRE, B., SHFJ, Commissariat a l'Energie Atomique, Direction des Sciences du Vivant, Département de Recherche en Imagerie, Pharmacologie et Physiologie, 4, Place du Général-Leclerc, F-91406 Orsay, France

MCMARTIN, C., CIBA-GEIGY Corporation, Pharmaceuticals Division, 556 Morris Avenue, Summit, NJ 07901, USA

MIKUS, G., Dr. Margarete Fischer-Bosch-Institut, Auerbachstr. 112, D-70376 Stuttgart, Germany

MOHLER, M.A., Preclinical Development, Prizm Pharmaceuticals 10655 Sorrento Valley Rd. Suit 200, San Diego, CA 92121, USA

NORDBLOM, G.D., Department of Pharmacokinetics and Drug Metabolism, Parke-Davis Pharmaceutical Research Division, Warner-Lambert Company, 2800 Plymouth Road, Ann Arbor, MI 48105, USA

O'NEILL, R., Food and Drug Administration, Center for Drug Evaluation and Research, Division of Biometrics, 5600 Fishers Lane, Rockville, MD 20857, USA

PANG, K.S., Faculty of Pharmacy and Department of Pharmacology, Faculty of Medicine, University of Toronto, 19 Russel Street, Toronto, Ontario M5S 1A1, Canada

PELKONEN, O., Department of Pharmacology and Toxicology, University of Oulu, FIN-90220 Oulu, Finland

RACINE-POON, A., CIBA-GEIGY AG, Biometrics, Pharma-Division, CH-4002 Basel, Switzerland

RUBIN, R.H., The Clinical Investigation Program of the Medical Service, Massachusetts General Hospital, Harvard Medical School, Fruit Street, Boston, MA 02114, USA

STEIMER, J.-L., Pharmacometrics, Drug Safety, 751/306, Sandoz Pharma AG, CH-4002 Basel, Switzerland

STEWART, B.H., Parke-Davis Pharmaceutical Research Division, Warner-Lambert Company, 2800 Plymouth Road, Ann Arbor, MI 48105-1047, USA

STRAUSS, H.W., Division of Nuclear Medicine of the Department of Radiology, Massachusetts General Hospital, Harvard Medical School, Fruit Street, Boston, MA 02114, USA

TESTA, B., School of Pharmacy, B.E.P., University of Lausanne, CH-1015 Lausanne, Switzerland

VOZEH, S., Intercantonal Office for the Control of Medicines, Erlachstr. 8, CH-3012 Bern 9, Switzerland

WELLING, P.G., Department of Pharmacokinetics and Drug Metabolism, Parke-Davis Pharmaceutical Research Division, Warner-Lambert Company, 2800 Plymouth Road, Ann Arbor, MI 48105-1047, USA

WILLS, R.J., Drug Metabolism, R.W. Johnson Pharmaceutical Research Institute, Route 202, P.O.Box 300, Raritan, NJ 08869, USA

YACOBI, A., American Cyanamid Company, Medical Research Division, Pharmacodynamics Research, Lederle Laboratories, Pearl River, NY 10965-1299, USA

Foreword

The author of this Foreword has recently retired after spending 25 years in academia and 15 years in the pharmaceutical industry. Most of this time has been spent following and, hopefully in some instances, contributing to advancement of the discipline of pharmacokinetics.

During the last 40 years, pharmacokinetics has grown from a fledgling in the 1950s to an adult in the 1990s. The late development of the discipline of pharmacokinetics, relative to other disciplines such as chemistry, biochemistry, and pharmacology, probably stems both from general ignorance of the importance of the time course of concentration–effect relationships in drug therapy and from our technical inability to do anything about it had we been more enlightened. Just as the end of the historical dark ages had to await the beginning of the Carolingian revival, so the end of the pharmacokinetic dark age had to await the discovery of adequate analytical methods and also an intellectual leap of faith to accept that drug action is in some way dependent on receptor site occupancy, and therefore on drug concentration.

The recent evolution of pharmacokinetics has occurred in three phases which may be identified as those of discovery, stabilization, and rationalization. The discovery phase, which occurred in the 1950s and 1960s, established the mathematics and concepts of "modern" pharmacokinetics and sought areas of application, ranging from model-independent methods, through compartment approaches, to complex physiological models. The stabilization period, which occurred mainly during the 1970s, was one of maturation. Concepts were examined and the proliferation of complex equations gave way to realistic approaches to drug disposition and its relationship to drug use in therapy. Pharmacokinetics was becoming useful!

The third, rationalization period is still with us. This is the period during which the potential of pharmacokinetics is being tested and realized, in both drug development and therapy. Pharmacokinetics is no longer considered to be a stand-alone discipline, but rather has become an integral factor contributing to understanding of the complex interaction between foreign molecules and biological systems, compound activity, toxicity, and therapy. The importance of pharmacokinetics, and more recently of pharmacokinetic–pharmacodynamic relationships and the concept of population kinetics (with all its controversies), is now accepted and these approaches are being actively pursued by the drug industry. This has been due, in no small part, to the demands of regulatory agencies worldwide, who have developed a keen appreciation of the importance of the very simple drug concentration–effect concept.

Of equal importance to, and in fact an integral part of, pharmacokinetics is the closely related discipline of drug metabolism. This discipline languished for many years waiting for appreciation of its importance and also for evolution of analytical technology. Drug metabolism surprisingly developed more slowly than pharmacokinetics. While pharmacokinetic education pro-liferated through schools of pharmacy in the United States, Europe, and elsewhere, drug metabolism struggled to established itself. Only during the last decade has drug metabolism become established as a major discipline, predominantly in schools of pharmacy, and become recognized as a critical component in drug discovery, development, and therapy. The rate of advancement in metabolism technology and the explosion of knowledge in xenobiotic metabolism during the last few years have been awesome, and are yet likely to continue as in vitro systems become more sophisticated and rapid screens become standardized in drug discovery and development.

The last 40 years have thus witnessed the birth, growth, and maturation of many disciplines associated with drug discovery, development, and also therapy. One cannot help but feel that, with all the technical advances that have already been made and the increased awareness of our own potential, we are at the threshold of rapid advances in sophistication in all these areas, particularly in in vitro and in vivo screening in both pharmacokinetics and metabolism so that these disciplines will play roles of ever-increasing importance in pharmaceutical research and development and in therapy. It has been rewarding and gratifying to witness and share in the development of these disciplines. It is even more rewarding to appreciate, and speculate perhaps, where they will take us in the future.

Ann Arbor, Michigan   J.G. WAGNER
February 1994

Preface

The last book on the kinetics of drug action in this series was published in 1977. During the intervening period a number of books and reviews have been published on pharmacokinetics and related topics. On being invited to edit a book on pharmacokinetics for this series, we felt the need to examine the topic from a different perspective.

As stated in the Foreword to this book, the sciences of pharmacokinetics and drug metabolism have evolved, and continue to do so, at a rapid pace consistent with advancing technology and also appreciation of the fundamental importance of drug disposition to the nature, intensity, and duration of drug action. In this book we have attempted to capture and describe the dynamic evolution that is occurring in pharmacokinetics and the closely related disciplines of drug metabolism and analytical methodology. We have moved our focus away from description of classical pharmacokinetics, on which enough has perhaps already been said. We have, instead, sought the help of those who are leading in new and exciting fields that portend the future of these disciplines and will continue to increase in importance in the discipline loosely defined as pharmacokinetics.

Topics for this book have thus been selected to address a wide spectrum of issues including the changing role of pharmacokinetics in drug discovery and development, the critical analytical areas of immunoassay, mass spectrometry, and analysis of biotechnology products, and the emerging technologies of positron emission tomography and imaging. Other sections address the clinical relevance of pharmacogenetics and environmental factors, and the time course of drug action. The increasing importance of drug metabolism, particularly in drug discovery, is acknowledged by inclusion of sections on in vitro methods to examine drug metabolism and transport, stereoselective metabolism and pharmacokinetics of chiral compounds, and interethnic and genetic factors. Other sections of the book specifically addressing future trends are devoted to the new discipline of toxicokinetics and to observational and investigational approaches to population pharmacokinetics. The book concludes with an appendix that critically reviews available and developing pharmacokinetic computer program software.

We appreciate that no single book can provide complete coverage of these rapidly expanding fields. All are important and all contribute to the kaleidoscope that we call pharmacokinetics. However, in combining these topics into a single book we hope to capture the essence of change that is occurring in the various disciplines, and also to demonstrate the power of the sum of all these parts in investigating, describing, and using drug disposition concepts in drug discovery, development, and therapeutic management.

We hope that the contents of this book will reflect the perspectives of change that we feel is happening, and that many will find it not only informative but sufficiently provocative to generate further advances in this exciting area of research.

We thank all the experts worldwide whose contributions have enhanced this book and also our secretaries Theresa Davis, Evelyne Gueblez, and Jacqueline Vouga, without whose help it would not have come to fruition.

Ann Arbor, MI, USA   P.G. WELLING
Geneva, Switzerland   LUC P. BALANT
February 1994

Contents

CHAPTER 3

Mass Spectrometry in Drug Disposition and Pharmacokinetics

CHAPTER 6

Gastrointestinal Transport of Peptide and Protein Drugs and Prodrugs
J.P.F. BAI, B.H. STEWART, and G.L. AMIDON. With 7 Figures   189

CHAPTER 9

Clinical Relevance of Pharmacogenetics
H.K. KROEMER, G. MIKUS, and M. EICHELBAUM 265

CHAPTER 15

**The Population Approach: Rationale, Methods, and Applications in
Clinical Pharmacology and Drug Development**
J.-L. STEIMER, S. VOZEH, A. RACINE-POON, N. HOLFORD, and
R. O'NEILL. With 8 Figures

F. Impact of New Methods on Pharmacokinetics

CHAPTER 16

**Contribution of Positron Emission Tomography
to Pharmacokinetic Studies**
B. MAZIÈRE and J. DELFORGE. With 7 Figures 455

CHAPTER 17

In Vivo Imaging in Drug Discovery and Design
A.J. FISCHMAN, R.H. RUBIN, and H.W. STRAUSS. With 8 Figures 481

G. Appendix

CHAPTER 18

**Considerations on Data Analysis Using Computer Methods and
Currently Available Software for Personal Computers**
M. Gex-Fabry and L.P. Balant 507

A. Introduction

CHAPTER 1

Role of Pharmacokinetics in Drug Discovery and Development

P.G. WELLING

A. Historical Background

Compared to other disciplines involved in drug discovery and development, with the possible exception of biotechnology, pharmacokinetics is a relative newcomer. If one delves into the literature one can find early articles that relate to the subject matter. For example, in 1847 Buchanan related depth of narcosis to brain content and arterial concentrations of anesthetics, while in the same year, SNOW (1847) commented on the need to regulate the strength of medicinal compounds. However, these were early days, and preceded the introduction of analytical technology and the intellectual maturation necessary for the study of pharmacokinetics in its present form.

The birth of pharmacokinetics really occurred in the 1920s and 1930s, being marked by the classical papers of HAGGARD (1924) on the disposition of ethyl ether, WIDMARK (1932) on ethyl alcohol elimination, and TEORELL (1937a,b) on the mathematics associated with pharmacokinetic modeling. Teorell's papers were among the first to describe physiologically based pharmacokinetic models based on oral and intravenous administration of compounds using one- and two-compartment pharmacokinetic models.

During the 1950s and 1960s the discipline of pharmacokinetics was landmarked by major contributions from GOLDSTEIN (1949), DOST (1953), NELSON (1961), WAGNER (1968), and others. During the 1970s there was rapid growth in pharmacokinetics which essentially paralleled advances in analytical instrumentation and technology, particularly high-pressure liquid chromatography (HPLC). The rapid growth in pharmacokinetics was accompanied by similar, although somewhat slower, growth in metabolism technology. At the present time, the three disciplines of pharmacokinetics, analytical technology, and drug metabolism have all reached an advanced level of sophistication.

The study of pharmacokinetics as an end in itself is now essentially redundant. The present and future challenges are in the areas of pharmacokinetic/pharmacodynamic modeling, population kinetics, and toxicokinetics. Metabolism studies are now focusing on rapid in vitro methods using organ tissues, purified cell lines, and enzyme systems. Analytical technology is advancing in several areas, particularly nuclear magnetic resonance, positron emission tomography, and autoradiography. In addition to advances in conventional techniques such as radioimmunoassay, HPLC, and mass spectroscopy, further advances are necessary in analytical technology in order to address the increasing use of highly potent compounds and also biologically based materials, which are notoriously difficult to analyze and may rapidly degrade in biological matrices and systems.

B. Regulatory Submissions

Prior to 1960, pharmacokinetic and drug metabolism information accounted for a very small proportion of regulatory submissions. Not only was there little appreciation of the importance of this type of information to the understanding of drug activity, but there were also only limited means to provide the information, even if it were required.

Times have changed! Current submissions for drug marketing approval contain a large proportion of pharmacokinetics and metabolism data. In the New Drug Application (NDA) in the United States, three complete sections are devoted to this topic: Section 5, Preclinical Pharmacokinetics; Section 6, Clinical Pharmacokinetics; and Section 8, Clinical Pharmacology. In fact, pharmacokinetic information is used in almost every section of the NDA, or equivalent international documents, as it draws together concepts in pharmacology, toxicology, and clinical pharmacology. In particular, it links preclinical and clinical experiences, validates (or otherwise) species used in toxicology, and provides a rational basis for therapy based on drug concentration–effect relationships.

Thus, pharmacokinetics and drug metabolism activities relate to virtually every aspect of the drug discovery and development process and have become pivotal components not only of regulatory submission documents but also of the armamentarium of knowledge that can be used to optimize drug therapy (BALANT et al. 1990).

In order to incorporate pharmacokinetic concepts during drug discovery and development, pharmacokinetic and drug metabolism disciplines are required to interact on an almost continuous basis with other disciplines involved in the process. The remainder of this chapter will describe the interactive nature of pharmacokinetic and drug metabolism programs.

C. The Process

The process of discovery and development for new drug candidates is summarized diagrammatically in Fig. 1.

Different organizations subdivide the entire discovery and development process in different ways. For ease of discussion it will be considered here as comprising three components: discovery, preclinical development, and clinical development. As a compound progresses through the process it draws on different resources and disciplines. However, unlike other dis-

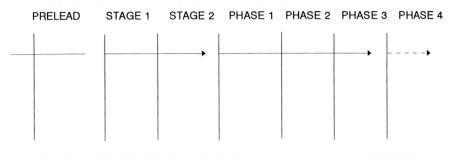

Fig. 1. Drug discovery and development process. *IND/CSA*, Investigation New Drug/Clinical Study Agreement; *NDA/MAA*, New Drug Application/Marketing Authorization Application

ciplines, pharmacokinetics plays a major and pivotal role throughout the entire process, from initial discovery to filing the final application for marketing approval, and beyond.

D. Discovery

The discovery period is generally recognized as the period from investigation of chemical leads to declaration of a development candidate, or lead compound. The disciplines most involved during this time are chemistry and the many branches of biology. Historically, pharmacokinetics had not played a significant role. However, this has changed dramatically in recent years. Metabolism expertise now plays a major role, in collaboration with both chemistry and biology, in molecular design to reduce, enhance, or redirect the metabolic profiles and activity of drug candidates. This involves a high level of interaction between synthetic chemistry, computer-assisted molecular design, and drug metabolism sciences. This level of interaction continues to increase as the sophistication of in vitro metabolism technology, using pure cell lines and enzyme systems, increases. The actual metabolic pathway that a chemical lead follows in vivo may, in many cases, be predicted in vitro using purified systems from test animal species or man.

It is no longer sufficient for a compound to exhibit pharmacological activity in vivo and/or in vitro to be elevated to lead status. Most organizations now require some pharmacokinetic characteristics, particularly absorption, elimination, and binding characteristics, before putting a drug into development. Thus, before a drug candidate enters the preclinical component of a development program it has likely been at least partially characterized in terms of pharmacokinetics and metabolism.

It is generally not until a compound reaches lead status that radiosynthesis is considered. Attempts to prepare radioactively labeled compound earlier in the process would be costly, in terms of both the uncertain status of the compound at that stage and the preliminary nature of synthetic methods. Thus, analytical work during the prelead discovery period is generally done with "cold" compound. This presents a considerable challenge to the analytical branch of a pharmacokinetics department in requiring development of sensitive and specific assays for a large number of novel compounds, most of which will not survive beyond early preclinical development.

On many occasions pharmacokinetic and systemic availability information is requested to provide an initial screen in order to determine the suitability of compounds for advancement. This is an incorrect approach and is generally a gross misuse of resources. If a series of compounds is being screened for advancement to lead status then it is far more economical to use some form of pharmacological screen which examines activity than to use a pharmacokinetic screen for which analytical procedures have to be developed and validated for individual compounds. There may be some exceptions to this rule, but not many.

E. Preclinical Development

Referring to Fig. 1, preclinical development refers to the period from declaration of lead compound status to submission of the Investigation New Drug (IND) application, or its equivalent outside the United States. At this stage, a drug candidate enters a period of formal development, a period during which input from several disciplines is necessary. The spectrum of studies that may comprise a preclinical pharmacokinetic and metabolism development program, and their approximate chronological sequence, is shown in Fig. 2. In this figure, studies are confined to the rat and dog. However, other species may be used depending on the compound, the compound class, and the questions being asked.

The duration of stages 1 and 2 of the preclinical development may range from a few months to 2 or 3 years, depending on the compound. The term "analytical development" is repeated a number of times throughout development. This reflects the need to continuously modify and revalidate analytical methods as knowledge of the compounds increases and as drug disposition is investigated in additional species and biological matrices.

A biopharmaceutical profile may be prepared at an early stage in order to provide preliminary information on the physical properties, stability, protein binding, bioavailability, and pharmacokinetics of the compound. This is typically followed by more extensive bioavailability and pharmacokinetic studies in appropriate species in order to gain insight as to how the compound behaves in these preclinical species, and possible prediction to humans. Radioactively labeled compound is prepared at this stage, so that mass balance, autoradiography, and preliminary metabolism studies may be conducted.

PRELEAD	Stage 1	Stage 2	IND	Phase 1	Phase 2	Phase 3	NDA

Analytical development
Bioavailability
    Biopharmaceutical profile
    Dog bioavailability and pharmacokinetics
    Analytical development
        Rat bioavailability and pharmacokinetics
        Dog multiple-dose pharmacokinetics
        Rat mass balance
        Analytical development
            Dog mass balance
                Autoradiography
                Toxicology dose ranging
                2-week toxicology
                    Rat single-dose toxicokinetics
                    Rat multiple-dose toxicokinetics
                    Dog single-dose toxicokinetics
                    Dog multiple-dose toxicokinetics
                    Rat, dog preliminary metabolism
                        13-week toxicology dog/rat
                        Dog major metabolites
                        Rat major metabolites
                            Regulatory submission documentation
                            Rat tissue distribution
                                Toxicology, 52-week definitive
                                Placental transfer
                                Enzyme induction

Fig. 2. Preclinical pharmacokinetic studies

Autoradiography has recently moved to a central and pivotal position in the preclinical development program as a means to characterize disposition in the body. While many autoradiography studies, which are performed predominantly in the rat and mouse, are conducted after administration of single doses of radiolabeled drug, there is a compelling argument for them to be conducted routinely after repeated dosing, using radiolabeled drug for all doses. In some instances both single and repeated doses may be desirable. This consumes a considerable quantity of time, and of radiolabeled drug, but may be necessary in order to adequately characterize disposition and tissue accumulation of radiolabel after single and repeated doses. Autoradiographic data obtained in animals are important for extrapolation to humans since physicochemical properties of tissues are similar across mammalian species.

Inclusion of extensive metabolism work at this stage may be controversial, but this writer is convinced that metabolic characterization of a drug candidate early in a development program is at least as important as, if not more so than, the pharmacokinetic component. The pattern and speed of compound degradation, the possible creation of active metabolites, and the nature of metabolite disposition are critical components of the overall body of knowledge vital to intelligent, and hopefully successful, further compound development.

I. Toxicology and Toxicokinetics

A major portion of a preclinical development program is associated with toxicology and toxicokinetics. The nature of toxicology studies is generally well established and has steadily evolved to its current level of sophistication. The principal objective of these studies is to establish an appropriate safety margin for a drug candidate in species that are relevant and may be predictive of the situation in humans.

Toxicokinetic studies, on the other hand, are of more recent interest – so recent, in fact, that the term "toxicokinetics" is not accepted by many and is not understood by most. Toxicokinetics is in its infancy now, but is maturing and expanding rapidly as the relatively distant disciplines of pharmacokinetics (and metabolism studies) and pathology and toxicology come to grips with each other and come to terms with their common destiny. The subject of toxicokinetics is discussed in detail in Chap. 14.

Just as regulatory agencies are demanding more information on pharmacokinetics and on pharmacokinetic/pharmacodynamic relationships, so it is inevitable that more information will be required on toxicokinetics and toxicokinetic/toxicodynamic relationships. It is no longer sufficient to conduct toxicology on a dose–response basis. The science has matured, albeit belatedly, to recognize that it must be conducted on a toxicokinetic–response relationship (DE LA IGLESIA and GREAVES 1989; LEMBERGER 1989).

Having established the concept, it may be useful to pause for a moment and compare the disciplines of toxicokinetics and pharmacokinetics. The major difference, of course, is that toxicokinetic doses are generally much higher than pharmacokinetic doses. The latter are restricted, for the most part, to doses in the therapeutic or pharmacological range. At the high doses used in toxicokinetics, on the other hand, the ability of animal species to cope with the drug is tested to the absolute limit, to the point of toxicity. It would be unrealistic to assume that the body could handle drugs in similar ways from such different dose ranges. The following are some examples of differences that must be expected from pharmacokinetic and toxicokinetic studies:

1. *Solubility*. Doses used in toxicokinetics often given rise to solubility problems, both in dosage form preparation and in terms of drug solubility in the GI tract and in the blood stream, urine, or other biological fluids.
2. *Dosage*. Dosage forms may vary in toxicokinetics relative to pharmacokinetics and this is a serious issue that impacts on interpretation of toxicokinetic studies. Traditionally drugs are often administered with diet in long-term toxicology studies. This is quite realistic in terms of resources. Dosing compounds in large toxicology studies by gavage doses is labor intensive and expensive. However, plasma drug profiles from the two methods of administration are quite different and are likely to give rise to different dose–effect and concentration–effect relationships.

3. *Stability*. Compound stability may be different at the concentrations and amounts of substances used in toxicokinetics compared to pharmacokinetics. Drug stability in feed may be quite different to that in an encapsulated dosage form.

4. *Absorption*. While most orally administered drugs are absorbed by passive processes, so that the quantity administered should not influence intrinsic absorption, the amounts of drug used in toxicology studies are almost certain to introduce changes in absorption. This may be due to limited solubility of the compound in the GI tract or to pharmacological/toxicological effects of the compound on the GI absorption and feedback mechanisms.

5. *First-pass effect*. First-pass effect, the hepatic or gastrointestinal clearance of drugs during absorption, is generally enzyme dependent and is therefore saturable. It is inevitable that first-pass clearance will saturate during toxicology studies, giving rise to changes in absorption efficiency.

6. *Bioavailability*. Bioavailability of compounds may be markedly influenced by dose size for reasons described above. It cannot be assumed that bioavailability in toxicokinetic studies is the same or even similar to that in pharmacokinetic studies.

7. *Protein binding*. Protein binding is saturable and considerable changes may occur in this phenomenon at toxicological doses. This can in turn influence compound pharmacokinetics, distribution, and penetration into tissues.

8. *Metabolism rate and pathways*. As with other enzyme-dependent systems, the metabolism of compounds is notoriously concentration dependent, and metabolic pathways may differ, both quantitatively and qualitatively, in toxicokinetics compared to those at therapeutic or pharmacological dose levels. This is important because differences in metabolism, even small differences in some cases, may invalidate a toxicity species relative to man.

9. *Renal excretion*. Renal excretion comprises both saturable and non-saturable mechanisms and can be markedly influenced by drug concentration.

10. *Physiological feedback*. High concentrations of drug in toxicology studies are, by definition, likely to be toxic to the host, thus having pathological influences and affecting physiological feedback. This type of phenomenon can affect compound absorption, distribution, metabolism, and excretion.

11. *Interactions*. Drug interactions are frequently concentration dependent and different interactions may occur in toxicity studies compared to pharmacokinetic studies. This is particularly relevant to toxicokinetic studies of drug combinations and of enantiomeric compounds.

12. *Saturable processes*. As described above, most processes in the body, even those that involve passive drug transport, may be affected by saturable processes in some way or another. These may influence the

toxicokinetics and toxicokinetic/toxicodynamic relationships of a drug candidate.

Thus, from many perspectives, toxicokinetics cannot be considered to be the same as pharmacokinetics, but is rather an extension of this discipline to examine the behavior of compounds administered at higher doses. In view of these factors, and of the great body of knowledge that is now being produced on concentration–effect relationships, it is important that detailed toxicokinetics be established at an early (initial) stage in a toxicology program.

Acute, single rising dose toxicology studies in all species should include toxicokinetics, probably in satellite animal groups. These early studies will provide an important data base for dose adjustment and toxicological interpretation during longer term toxicology studies.

Autoradiography might be conducted at toxicological doses as well as at pharmacological doses in appropriate species. These studies are important to establish radiolabel distribution and the relationship between compound concentration and/or persistence in organs relative to observed toxicity.

In summary, early toxicokinetic data will:

1. Provide complete toxicokinetic profiles
2. Guide subsequent toxicology dosing regimens
3. Establish early concentration–effect relationships
4. Establish bioavailability at toxicokinetic dose levels
5. Characterize saturable processes

Drug metabolism profiles also need to be established at toxicological doses in relevant toxicity species. These studies are critical because of the need to establish the relevance of toxicity data to the human situation and to validate the predictability of toxicity species. Once short-term drug toxicity/ toxicokinetic studies are conducted, then drug concentration monitoring (which may include detailed toxicokinetics) should be conducted in satellite animal groups in all chronic toxicity and genotoxicity studies. The need for toxicokinetic and metabolism profiling is independent of therapeutic class and route of administration.

II. Pharmacokinetic–Pharmacodynamic Relationships

Studies of pharmacokinetic–pharmacodynamic relationships are an important component of clinical development programs. However, they are also playing an important role in preclinical development. This is particularly true for cardiovascular agents for which measurable pharmacodynamic parameters are available in order to determine concentration–effect relationships. However, pharmacokinetic–pharmacodynamic relationships also need to be investigated wherever possible in other therapeutic areas in order to generate information which is useful for subsequent phase 1 and phase 2 studies in man, and to obtain accurate prediction of the therapeutic dosage range and margin of safety.

Note, from Fig. 2, that preclinical studies extend beyond the time of IND submission and may extend into mid or late phase 2 of the clinical program. In many instances they may extend well into phase 3, or beyond. This occurs particularly when observations made during clinical studies require additional preclinical work for clarification or resolution of problems.

The overall pharmacokinetic and metabolism support for a drug development program is thus a continuum between preclinical and clinical phases and should not be divided, as has mistakenly been done by some, into rigidly defined preclinical and clinical responsibilities.

III. Interactions

During preclinical discovery and development, pharmacokinetics departments interact with almost every other discipline. During early discovery, interaction is primarily with chemistry and biology. As a drug candidate moves into the preclinical development pipeline, interactions with chemistry and biology continue but more intensive interactions occur with product development, toxicology, and clinical pharmacology. As described earlier, toxicokinetic data and also drug monitoring data from longer term toxicology studies now provide critical concentration–effect information that helps to establish dose ranges in initial clinical dose studies and a realistic safety margin.

As will be demonstrated in the next section, interactions between pharmacokinetics and other disciplines continue to increase during clinical development, culminating in the multidisciplinary strategies that are required for successful submission of regulatory documents for marketing.

F. Clinical Development

The spectrum of clinical pharmacokinetic and metabolism studies that may be conducted, and their approximate chronological sequence, is described in Fig. 3. Referring to Fig. 1, the entire clinical development program is conveniently subdivided into phases 1, 2, and 3.

I. Phase 1

The major objective during phase 1 clinical studies is to examine the safety of a drug candidate in a small population of individuals. These studies are generally conducted in healthy adult volunteers. However, for some drug classes, e.g., anticancer agents and some cardiovascular compounds, these studies may be conducted in an appropriate patient population. Initial doses administered at this early stage in the clinical development program are well

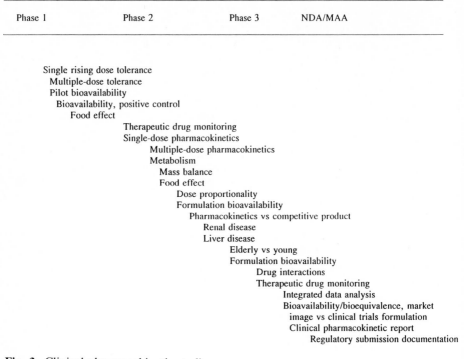

Phase 1	Phase 2	Phase 3	NDA/MAA

Single rising dose tolerance
　Multiple-dose tolerance
　Pilot bioavailability
　　Bioavailability, positive control
　　　Food effect
　　　　Therapeutic drug monitoring
　　　　Single-dose pharmacokinetics
　　　　　Multiple-dose pharmacokinetics
　　　　　Metabolism
　　　　　　Mass balance
　　　　　Food effect
　　　　　　Dose proportionality
　　　　　　Formulation bioavailability
　　　　　　　Pharmacokinetics vs competitive product
　　　　　　　Renal disease
　　　　　　Liver disease
　　　　　　　Elderly vs young
　　　　　　　Formulation bioavailability
　　　　　　　　Drug interactions
　　　　　　　Therapeutic drug monitoring
　　　　　　　　Integrated data analysis
　　　　　　　　Bioavailability/bioequivalence, market
　　　　　　　　　image vs clinical trials formulation
　　　　　　　　Clinical pharmacokinetic report
　　　　　　　　　Regulatory submission documentation

Fig. 3. Clinical pharmacokinetic studies

below the anticipated therapeutic dosage range, and subjects or patients are carefully monitored for tolerance and possible side-effects. The pharmacokinetic component of these studies is extensive, and rapid analytical turnaround is routinely required, consistent with increasing emphasis on concentration-based dose escalation and study termination.

Typical collaborative studies conducted during phase 1 are described in Table 1. The initial single rising dose tolerance study and the subsequent repeated dose tolerance study both contain a substantial pharmacokinetic component. In addition to the tolerance component, these studies provide preliminary information on compound pharmacokinetics following single and repeated doses, accumulation, and any pharmacokinetic changes that may arise from the repeated dose regimen. Other studies conducted during

Table 1. Phase 1 studies involving pharmacokinetics

Single rising dose tolerance
Repeated dose tolerance
Bioavailability
Food effect
Bioavailability, positive control

phase 1, or early phase 2, while continuing to address tolerance studies, are predominantly pharmacokinetic in nature. They may include absolute systemic bioavailability relative to parental dosage or relative bioavailability relative to another enteral dosage form, dose proportionality, and relative bioavailability of any reformulated compound that may be used as positive control during subsequent phase 2 or 3 efficacy studies.

Ingestion of food is now recognized as being a key factor influencing drug absorption (WELLING 1977; TOOTHAKER and WELLING 1980), and a food–drug interaction study is virtually mandatory during phase 1. As the final "market image" has not yet been developed, additional food-effect studies will be required later in the development program. However, the nature of this interaction should be examined early using a formulation which is hopefully similar or identical to that used in clinical trials in order to guide dosage regimens in later studies.

Thus, while the main interest during phase 1 clinical studies has historically been that of examining safety, much of the focus is now pharmacokinetic in nature and by far the greatest resource commitment involves pharmacokinetic expertise. This trend of placing ever-increasing emphasis on bioavailability and pharmacokinetic disposition of drug candidates and their metabolites, so evident during phase 1 clinical trials, continues throughout the clinical development program and represents the recognition, albeit belated, of the critical relationship that so often exists between circulating levels of medicinal agents, be they parent compounds or active metabolites, and pharmacological activity.

During phase 1 there is generally no attempt to formally examine pharmacokinetic–pharmacodynamic relationships. However, much spadework is done indirectly in order to initiate these studies during early phase 2.

II. Phase 2

During phase 2 a drug candidate is typically tested in small, well-defined patient populations. Although a measure of efficacy may be derived from phase 1 studies for some drug classes, formal determination of efficacy is not usually achieved until phase 2. It is during this phase that many drug

Table 2. Phase 2 studies involving pharmacokinetics

Therapeutic monitoring, small-scale clinical efficacy and tolerance trials
Single-dose pharmacokinetics
Repeated-dose pharmacokinetics
Pharmacokinetics versus competitive product
Food effect
Dose proportionality
Mass balance
Metabolism

candidates fail owing to lack of efficacy or unacceptable side-effects, and are withdrawn from development. Typical collaborative studies conducted during phase 2 are described in Table 2.

Pharmacokinetics of the drug candidate are often characterized after single and repeated doses in patients or in healthy individuals and comparison may be made between the drug candidate and competitive products. In the competitive pharmaceutical environment, a modest pharmacokinetic advantage of one product over another may be critical to its success. Additional food-effect studies may be conducted in order to refine observations made during phase 1, and to better define the labeling. The interplay of food effects in terms of opposing influences of food affecting absorption and possible protection by food against adverse GI effects may dictate how a drug is administered in clinical practice.

Apart from continuing pharmacokinetic studies, three additional components are introduced during phase 2: mass balance, metabolism, and therapeutic drug monitoring. Mass balance and metabolism studies traditionally use radioactively labeled compound and are generally conducted in volunteers. Mass balance studies are designed to examine recovery of total radioactivity following oral and/or intravenous administration of labeled compound and may identify drug sequestration or covalent binding to tissue in the event of incomplete mass balance. Metabolism studies are essential at this stage, not only to better understand the pathways and rate of formation of biologically active or inactive metabolites, but also to validate the animal species used in toxicity studies.

If humans generate metabolites that are qualitatively, or in some cases quantitatively, different from those observed in toxicity species, then the question of toxicity species validity must arise. In these cases the question is invariably raised of whether a metabolite formed in man, or formed in man to a greater extent than in the toxicity species, should be reexamined in that toxicity species. If so, then by what route should it be administered? If given intravenously, it may give rise to specific toxic effects that might not occur in the case of in situ generation from parent drug. If given orally, the same argument may apply, but in this case it is confounded by concerns regarding metabolite bioavailability. There are no rules in these circumstances and they must be considered on a compound by compound basis.

One of the most important activities that starts during phase 2, and continues throughout the clinical development program, is that of therapeutic drug monitoring during efficacy trials. Careful and accurate plasma sampling and/or urine collection during appropriate segments of efficacy and tolerance protocols can provide a wealth of information regarding dose concentration–effect relationships for a drug candidate. This is probably one of the most important pharmacokinetic activities and pharmacokinetic–clinical collaborations in the entire clinical development program, and one that has hitherto been sadly neglected. Pharmacokineticists have been literally hammering at the door for many years to become more involved in clinical protocol design, study monitoring, and data interpretation. In some cases, they have been successful, and exciting and productive collaborations have resulted. In most cases, however, such efforts have met with only moderate success or have been completely rejected so that the potential to derive useful additional information from clinical trials has been lost. This situation may have continued had not regulatory agencies taken the initiative and started to demand more concentration–effect information. This has provided the necessary incentive for closer collaboration in the conception, design, conduct, and interpretation of clinical efficacy and tolerance studies. Such collaboration will not only provide more information on dose concentration–effect relationships for particular new drug candidates but will also advance understanding of the determinants of drug activity on a broad front. Strategic incorporation of the population approach during clinical evaluation of drug candidates was the subject of a recent major symposium (ROWLAND and AARONS 1992).

III. Phase 3

The major focus during phase 3 is on the "make or break" pivotal efficacy trials. These trials, conducted in large patient populations, provide efficacy data to support the marketing application. As in the phase 2 efficacy studies, collaborative use should be made of these studies to employ integrated data analysis techniques in order to learn as much as possible regarding the pharmacokinetic–pharmacodynamic characteristics of the drug candidate in a large, heterogeneous patient population. It would probably be unrealistic to attempt to conduct this level of investigation on all participating patients at all investigative sites. However, use of a large representative sample of patients from a number of sites will provide valuable information. Typical collaborative studies conducted during phase 3 are described in Table 3.

Regardless of the above population screen approach, other more traditional studies in special populations still constitute a major part of a phase 3 development program. Studies in elderly versus young patients, patients with hepatic or renal impairment, and perhaps other special populations and required in order to characterize drug disposition under these special

Table 3. Phase 3 studies involving pharmacokinetics

Therapeutic monitoring, pivotal efficacy trials
Renal failure
Hepatic failure
Elderly versus young
Other special patient populations
Drug interactions
Bioavailability/bioequivalence of market image versus clinical trial formulations
Regulatory submission documentation

---

conditions. Drug interaction studies are also mandatory. In this case the investigator has to decide how many studies to conduct and how best to conduct them in order to obtain the most information for a considerable capital and resource outlay. As many as six to eight interaction studies may be required, with appropriate focus on drugs that may be given concomitantly and/or drugs that are likely to interact mechanistically and whose interaction may be therapeutically important. Clearly, compounds that are highly protein bound or are extensively metabolized, and have narrow therapeutic indices, are candidates for these studies.

Market image formulations for a drug candidate are seldom finalized before the compound enters phase 3. Thus most clinical studies, including the pivotal multicenter efficacy trials, are conducted on clinical samples that may differ in form or composition from the final market image. Once the market image formulation is prepared, bioequivalent studies must be conducted comparing the market image and clinical trial formulations. Bioinequivalence is seldom encountered in these studies. But if it is, it can profoundly disrupt a clinical development program. This circumstance can be avoided if market image formulations are prepared early during a clinical development program, preferably before the small-scale efficacy and safety studies in phase 2. The decision-making process in the pharmaceutical industry is usually such that this is impractical, but it would be a worthwhile goal to have all clinical efficacy studies conducted using the market image formulation. This might cause stress in some disciplines associated with drug development but it would certainly relieve considerable stress in others.

Pharmacokinetics and drug metabolism studies are thus a major component of a phase 3 clinical development program. Not only are a considerable number of discrete pharmacokinetic studies conducted in order to characterize drug disposition under a variety of conditions and thus guide doses in patient populations, but also there is a growing pharmacokinetic component to the large, multicenter efficacy studies.

IV. Interactions

During phase 3, pharmacokinetic departments interact with clinical pharmacology, clinical development, and also regulatory authorities to provide the bulk of the pivotal data to support drug labeling. Interaction during the multicenter trials is often difficult, and in some instances may be costly, but the ultimate value added by an integrated approach is substantial and fully justifies commitment of additional resources.

V. Regulatory Submissions

The pharmacokinetic contribution to the final marketing submission document was briefly described earlier in this chapter. Suffice it to reflect here on the highly interactive nature of this documentation. Preparation of Sections

5, 6, and 8 of the United States NDA, and equivalent sections of international filings, has become a multidisciplinary exercise. Section 5 requires
integration of pharmacokinetics, metabolism, and toxicology information,
with increasing emphasis on toxicokinetics. Input is also required from
chemistry and pharmacology. Sections 6 and 8 require close collaboration
between pharmacokinetics, clinical pharmacology, clinical development, and
product development, with input from other disciplines. Prudent integration
of relevant information will result in a submission document that relates the
disciplines to each other and thus provides a meaningful characterization of
safety and efficacy that will support marketing approval with the requested
labeling.

The increased emphasis on drug/metabolite concentration effects is also
reflected in the labeling. In the past, pharmacokinetic data have been minor
and have largely been submerged within clinical pharmacology material.
Preclinical data have been minimal. With the change of focus within the
United States Food and Drug Administration, the pharmacokinetics section
of the labeling has greatly increased and often includes appropriate figures
and tables which provide detailed characteristics of drug disposition including bioavailability, dose proportionality, and pharmacokinetics in patient
populations.

G. Postsubmission and Postmarketing Studies

The period between submission for marketing and eventual approval is
often one of intensive negotiation between the company and regulatory
authorities. Issues have to be clarified, claims have to be substantiated, and
labeling has to be justified and finally agreed upon. While many disciplines
are called upon during this period, it is this writer's experience that pharmacokinetics is frequently involved and is often central to the process. As
a result of the shift in regulatory emphasis toward concentration–effect
and pharmacokinetic–pharmacodynamic relationships, many questions are
raised that involve collaborative response or even additional collaborative
studies to clearly define drug behavior.

Once regulatory approval is obtained, an intense program is initiated by
the company to support the marketed product, to explore new dosage forms
and indications, to respond to international issues, and, as the patent ex-
piration date approaches, to defend the product against generic erosion.
During this period, pharmacokinetics departments work in close collaboration with clinical development, marketing, and product development to
provide appropriate support for these different areas. In particular, investigations of modified dosage forms, sustained release, transdermal preparations, and other alternative drug delivery forms require extensive
pharmacokinetic input to negotiate approvability of a new product, hopefully
without the need for additional clinical trials.

H. Summary

The discipline of pharmacokinetics, and the closely related discipline of drug metabolism, have evolved rapidly from being minor, almost insignificant contributors to the drug discovery and development process, to the present situation where they play a major, pivotal role in all phases from early discovery through development, and beyond. The increasing role of pharmacokinetics in drug discovery and development has emerged as a result of maturation of scientific awareness of its importance and also advances in analytical and computer technology. Analytical methodology will continue to be a major challenge as the pharmacological potency of new molecules increases, driving doses down to microgram levels, and as the proportion of biotechnology-derived molecules entering the development pipeline increases. One can anticipate major advances in mass spectrometric and immunoanalytic methodology as biotechnology-derived materials account for a larger proportion of new drug molecules.

Pharmacokinetics now plays a vital and central role in drug discovery and in all phases of drug development. By necessity, it is a highly interactive discipline. These interactions reflect the ultimate purpose of pharmacokinetics, which is not merely to mathematically describe the time course of drug disposition, but to provide one of the critical scientific components that contribute to understanding of drug efficacy and safety. It is interesting to note that much of the impetus that has recently driven pharmacokinetics into this central role has come from regulatory authorities.

Through its continuous involvement during the entire process of discovery, development, and postmarketing, pharmacokinetics is unique among disciplines in the pharmaceutical industry. The extensive collaborations that are demanded with other disciplines are very gratifying for those who "practice the art." However, this role brings with it responsibilities that must be discharged in a rapidly changing research environment. This is the challenge that pharmacokinetics has to meet in the future. Current signs are that, with its maturity of perspective, strength of identity, and burgeoning technology, it is well equipped to do this.

References

Balant LP, Roseboom H, Gundert-Remy UM (1990) Pharmacokinetic criteria for drug research and development. Adv Drug Res 19:6–139

Buchanan A (1847) Physiologic effects of the inhalation of ether. Lond Med Gaz 39:715–717

De la Iglesia FA, Greaves P (1989) Role of toxicokinetics in drug safety evaluations. In: Yacobi A, Skelly JP, Batra VK (eds) Toxicokinetics and new drug development. Pergamon, New York, pp 21–32

Dost FH (1953) Die Blutspiegelkinetik der Konzentrationsabläufe in der Kreislaufflüssigkeit. Thieme, Leipzig

Goldstein A (1949) The interaction of drugs and plasma proteins. Pharmacol Rev 1:102–165

Haggard HW (1924) The absorption, distribution and elimination of ethyl ether. I. The amount of ether absorbed in relation to the concentration inhaled and its fate in the body. J Biol Chem 59:737–751

Lemberger L (1989) Pharmacokinetics and adverse reactions: an overview. In: Yacobi A, Skelly JP, Batra VK (eds) Toxicokinetics and new drug development. Pergamon, New York, pp 114–123

Nelson E (1961) Kinetics of drug absorption, distribution, metabolism, and excretion. J Pharm Sci 50:181–192

Rowland E, Aarons L (eds) (1992) New strategies in drug development and clinical evaluation: the population approach. Conference, Manchester, UK, September 21–23, 1991. Office for Official Publications of the European Communities, Luxembourg

Snow J (1847) On the inhalation of the vapour of ether. Lond Med Gaz 39:498–502

Teorell T (1937a) Kinetic of distribution of substances administered to the body. I. The extravascular modes of administration. Arch Int Pharmacodyn 57:205–225

Teorell T (1937b) Kinetics of distribution of substances administered to the body. II. The intravascular modes of administration. Arch Int Pharmacodyn 57:226–240

Toothaker RD, Welling PG (1980) The effect of food on drug bioavailability. Annu Rev Pharmacol Toxicol 20:173–199

Wagner JG (1968) Pharmacokinetics. Annu Rev Pharmacol 8:67–94

Welling PG (1977) Influence of food and diet on gastrointestinal drug absorption: a review. J Pharmacokinet Biopharm 5:291–334

Widmark EMP (1932) Die theoretischen Grundlagen und die praktische Verwendbarkeit der gerichtlichmedizinischen Alkoholbestimmung. Urban and Schwarzenberg, Berlin

B. Analytical Methods

CHAPTER 2

Contemporary Aspects of Radioimmunoassay Development for Drug Analysis

G.D. NORDBLOM and C.M. BARKSDALE

A. Introduction

The application of radioimmunoassay (RIA) for quantitation of pharmaceutical drug concentration in biological matrices has increased in recent years due to several factors. The first reason has been the development of more efficacious drugs, resulting in lower effective doses and subsequent lower concentrations in matrices such as plasma or urine. Although traditional chromatographic analytical procedures such as high-performance liquid chromatography (HPLC) or gas chromatography (GC) have demonstrated improved sensitivity, compounds continue to be developed that cannot be measured by HPLC or GC. A second factor involved in the increased use of RIA is an enhanced awareness and willingness to develop the complex synthetic chemistry necessary to produce the requisite immunological and radiochemical reagents for RIA. Lastly, with the advent of radioactivity counters that can rapidly count large numbers of assay samples and perform the required data reduction, RIA has become more time efficient than chromatographic methods.

FINDLAY (1987) recently provided an excellent general review of the use of immunoassays for drug disposition studies. This chapter will be more specific in covering several aspects of increasing importance relative to developing and implementing RIA for drug analysis. These include: (a) the complex synthetic chemistry needed to prepare the required drug derivatives for immunogen preparation, (b) preparation of drug–protein immunogens (conjugates), (c) immunization considerations, (d) methods for identifying and eliminating biological matrix interferences, and (e) assay suitability and validity considerations relative to recent regulatory concerns and guidelines.

Throughout this discussion we will concentrate on radioisotopic immunoassay methodologies although nonisotopic immunoanalytical procedures are also used for drug analysis. Most of the synthetic aspects together with the immunological, matrix, and assay acceptability considerations are equally applicable to these nonisotopic methods.

B. Synthesis of Drug Derivatives for Immunogen Preparation

The development of an RIA requires an antibody, almost exclusively raised in animals, that will bind the drug or analyte of interest. However, extensive research has demonstrated that substances, such as most ethical pharmaceuticals, with molecular weights less than approximately 2 kDa are generally not antigenic. Nevertheless, antibodies to these small molecules or haptens (i.e., low-molecular-weight substances) can frequently be produced by immunization with conjugates of the hapten covalently coupled to carrier proteins or polypeptides (Youngblood and Kizer 1983).

I. Coupling of Hapten Carboxyl Group to Carrier Protein

The most common method for producing the hapten–protein conjugate involves reacting a carboxyl group on the hapten with a protein amine to form an amide bond. This is usually accomplished with a water-soluble carbodiimide to activate the carboxyl group, although the procedure of generating an activated mixed anhydride is also occasionally used. If a $[^{125}I]$ radiolabel is required for the assay, the same chemistry is employed by reacting the $-CO_2H$ moiety with either histamine or tyramine followed by radioiodination with $Na[^{125}I]$ and a mild oxidant such as chloramine-T (Greenwood et al. 1963). With the increased use of RIA, the chemistry needed to prepare haptens with the requisite carboxyl groups has become necessarily more complex. Figure 1 illustrates, with increasing complexity, the general synthetic schemes that have been used. Scheme 1 is the simple formation of an amide using an existing carboxylic acid on the hapten.

II. Addition of Carboxyl to Existing Functional Group

Scheme 2 employs an existing functional group as a bridge or attachment point for the required carboxylic acid. A common example of this procedure is the reaction of an amine on the hapten with succinic anhydride to yield a hemisuccinamide. Walker et al. (1991) reacted an aniline analog of the antidysrhythmic drug UK-68,798 with succinic anhydride and coupled the resulting acid to ovalbumin to produce an antigen. Nordblom et al. (1989) used an existing secondary aliphatic amine on the cancer chemotherapy agent CI-937 with succinic anhydride followed by conjugation to porcine thyroglobulin to successfully generate a CI-937 immunogen.

Alcohol moieties can also be used in the anhydride reaction although the reactions are not as energetically favorable, and the resulting ester hemisuccinates are not as stable as hemisuccinamides. Nordblom et al. (1981, 1984) used this type of ester linkage with either primary or secondary alcohols while developing RIAs for the sex steroid hormone androstenedione. The authors also used ethyl diazoacetate with the same alcohols to obtain carboxymethylethers that were not susceptible to ester hydrolysis, yet re-

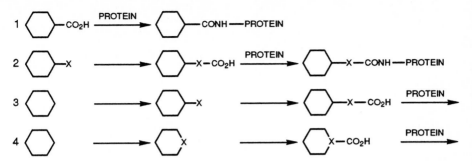

Fig. 1. Schematic representation of general synthetic routes to hapten–carrier protein immunogens: *1*, coupling of existing carboxyl group to protein; *2*, addition of carboxyl to existing functional group; *3*, addition of bridging functional group for carboxyl; *4*, alteration of hapten structure to provide attachment of carboxyl

sulted in antibody-producing antigens. The formation of a secondary hemisuccinate from an existing alcohol was successfully employed to prepare antisera for haloperidol (OIDA et al. 1989) along with several other synthetic methods.

III. Addition of a Functional Group for Bridge to Carboxylic Acid

When no reactive functional moiety exists, a hapten must be altered, as in scheme 3, prior to the addition of an acid for coupling. A common procedure is the addition of a thiol to an existing carbon–carbon double bond. BEALE (1991) added an α,ω-dithiol to a gibberellic acid analog, in a free radical reaction, to yield a free thiol. This was then reacted with maleic anhydride, producing a substituted succinic anhydride which is in effect an activated carboxyl group. Reaction with keyhole limpet hemocyanin or bovine serum albumin produced a very effective gibberellic acid antigen. An interesting application of the use of thiols is the free radical addition of $HS-CH_2CH_2-CO_2H$ to a 15,16-dihydro derivative of testosterone to form the 15β-thiopropanoic acid of testosterone (WHITE et al. 1985). This method is particularly appealing because the bridging group and the carboxyl group are added simultaneously.

When an aromatic ring system exists in the hapten, diazotized *p*-aminobenzoic acid may be added to yield a hapten–N_2–*p*-phenyl–CO_2H derivative. Recent examples of this synthetic approach have been used to prepare antigens for the anticholinergic agent trospiumchloride (LEHTOLA et al. 1988) and the reversible anticholinesterase inhibitor physostigmine (MILLER and VERMA 1989). A drawback to this procedure is the lack of control of the site specificity of the reaction. This could be critical if the location of the attachment site must be synthetically directed relative to metabolite considerations.

We recently developed an RIA for the analgesic κ opioid receptor agonist CI-977 (NORDBLOM et al. 1990a). Because of metabolite considerations, it was necessary to attach the carrier protein specifically at the 7-position of the benzofuran portion of the drug. To accomplish this, 7-hydroxy-4-benzofuran acetic acid was prepared in a very extensive, nine-step synthesis (KESTEN et al. 1989) and coupled to the appropriate diamine, resulting in 7-hydroxy-CI-977. The hydroxyl compound was then reacted with ethyl bromoacetate in the presence of Cs_2CO_3 catalyst to yield the desired acid, protected as an ethyl ester. Hydrolysis of the ester and coupling of the resultant acid to porcine thyroglobulin (pTG) produced a very effective immunogen.

IV. Altering the Basic Structure of the Hapten

In some cases, the integral structure of the hapten precludes adding a bridging functional group and subsequent carboxyl group. As seen in scheme 4 of Fig. 1, the basic structure of the hapten must be altered to facilitate antigen formation. An example of this was our recent development of an RIA for the renin inhibitor PD132002 (Fig. 2). It was necessary to attach the drug to the carrier protein at the morpholine portion of the molecule. A piperazine analog of PD132002 (I) was prepared and reacted with succinic anhydride to form the hemisuccinamide (II). This material was easily coupled to porcine thyroglobulin to yield the desired antigen (III). Antibody obtained from immunization with III bound PD132002, resulting in a very efficient RIA.

There are two points to consider: (a) although we did not know whether antibody raised against the piperazine analog would result in an RIA for PD132002, we attempted the method because there was no alternative analytical procedure with the required sensitivity, and (b) as one might expect, the piperazine derivative, I, cross-reacted to approximately 100% in the PD132002 RIA, but since it was never dosed nor could arise as a metabolite the cross-reactivity was not important.

In conclusion, we have attempted to show with a limited number of examples a variety of synthetic routes that may be used to obtain drug antigens that have proven successful for the development of RIAs. This is not meant to be an inclusive survey, rather it is hoped that the reader will obtain a feeling for the complexity of the required chemistry. It is also hoped that the reader will better appreciate that the ability to develop RIAs is dependent on the synthetic competency of our chemists.

C. Immunogen Preparation

I. Hapten–Carrier Protein Ratios

The essential prerequisite for a sensitive RIA is the availability of a high-affinity, specific antibody for the substance being investigated. While molecular weight is not the only determinant of intrinsic antigenicity, research

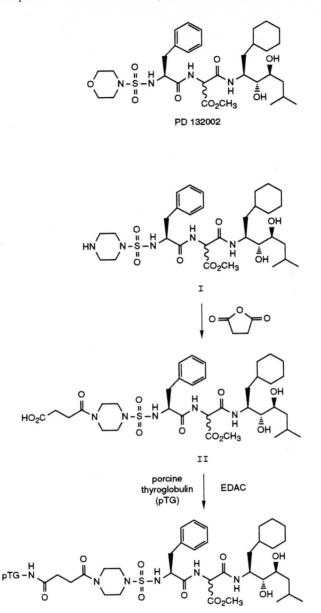

Fig. 2. Structure of renin inhibitor PD132002. Synthesis of PD132002 immunogen III by reaction of piperazine analog I with succinic anhydride followed by coupling to pTG. *EDAC*, 1-ethyl-3-(3-dimethylaminopropyl)carbodiimide

has shown that molecules of less than 2 kDa will usually not elicit an immunological response (Yalow 1978; Erlanger 1980). To produce antibodies to small molecules (haptens) they must be attached to large immunogenic carrier proteins.

Historically, the original research into the immunochemical characterizations of such low-molecular-weight substances was done by Landsteiner (1945). Using organic acids such as the various enantiomers of tartaric acid conjugated to serum albumin, he found that ten hapten groups was the optimal number for the production of the most efficacious antibody response.

Carrier proteins in general use today for conjugation to haptens include globulin fractions, serum albumins of various animals, hemocyanin, ovalbumin, and thyroglobulin. Optimal epitope density (i.e., hapten to carrier protein ratio) has been examined for several model systems. Work on steroid–protein conjugates with bovine serum albumin (BSA) suggests that at least 20 steroid groups must be conjugated (Niswender and Midgley 1970). Studies with dinitrophenol–BSA (DNP-BSA) conjugates indicated good responses with as few as five DNP groups, and nearly comparable responses are obtained with 19 DNP groups. However, $DNP_{50}BSA$ and $DNP_{60}BSA$ elicit only an IgM response (Klause and Cross 1974). Erlanger (1980) found that good antibody titers could usually be obtained with epitope densities of 8–25, while even conjugates with only two hapten groups ultimately gave responses, although their use necessitated a longer period for adequate titer and sensitivity development.

II. Carrier Protein Characteristics

We have used pTG with consistent success to produce drug–protein conjugates for the immunization of rabbits and sheep. Following the procedure of Skowsky and Fisher (1972), we generally use drug–thyroglobulin–carbodiimide coupling reagent ratios of 150:1:200 for the conjugate preparation. Drug–thyroglobulin conjugates with molar incorporation ratios of 40:1 to 80:1 have resulted in the successful production of antibody titers and RIA sensitivities in rabbits and sheep in the shortest immunization period.

Although hapten–protein conjugates of serum albumins are generally soluble in aqueous systems, we have found that conjugates with thyroglobulin, γ-globulin, or ovalbumin frequently precipitate during preparation and cannot be redissolved even during dialysis. Furthermore, conjugate precipitation is often a pH-related phenomenon, with steroid–protein conjugates prepared from bovine, rabbit, and human albumins generally being soluble above pH 5.5, while thyroglobulin and hemocyanin conjugates are notoriously insoluble even at physiological pH values (Rittenberg and Amkraut 1966). Because of this observation, we customarily dialyze all of our conjugates against phosphate-buffered normal saline solutions at pH 7.40 over a 3- to 4-day period at room temperature. In cases where the conjugate is not totally soluble, we do not separate the precipitate. The resulting suspension is used and generally results in adequate antisera. Whether the choice of carrier significantly influences the antihapten response remains a controversial subject, and according to ERLANGER (1980) no definitive study has been reported.

D. Immunization Considerations

During the past several decades there has been a significant increase in the investigation of the factors involved in the production, stimulation, and modulation of the classical immune response. Subjects of concern have included: (a) appropriate animal species for immunization; (b) adjuvant and immunostimulant effects; (c) variable immunization routes; and (d) immunization, boosting, and bleeding schedules (STEWART-TULL 1989; JOHNSTON et al. 1991).

I. Species Effects

Historically, rabbits have been the species of choice for the production of polyclonal antisera. While the older strains of outbred rabbits normally produced a wide range of humoral immune responses, the development of the newer inbred New Zealand rabbit species has led to a more predictable immunological response. Although rabbits have been adopted as the laboratory animal of greatest general immunological utility, other species are being utilized. Guinea pigs are now generally used for the production of antibodies to human HBO blood group antigens and coagulation factors; chickens for parathyroid, calcitonin, and calmodulin: chicken eggs for bacterial and viral agents; sheep for steroids, nephelometric grade antisera for nonisotopic assays and precipitating antibodies; burros and donkeys for antibodies to hepatitis agents; horses for tetanus toxoid antibodies and antilymphocyte γ-globulin fractions for organ transplant rejection inhibition; and mice for the production of monoclonal antibodies of all types. Researchers most commonly use the species described in publications on the production of antibodies to the same or similar antigens, unless space or expense considerations preclude the larger animal model.

II. Use of Adjuvants

While the potential exists to produce completely synthetic antibody molecules, it has become apparent that immunological research will also continue into adjuvant substances that have minimally adverse toxic side-effects. Adjuvants are able to enhance the immunogenicity of antigens in two different ways: first, by producing an emulsion reservoir which protects the antigen from metabolism, most adjuvants allow prolonged exposure to the host animal's immune system; secondly, the majority of adjuvants contain agents that stimulate the host animal's antibody-producing system by directly initiating and activating the immune system's antibody-producing cells (Warren et al. 1986). The most commonly used adjuvants contain significant amounts of mineral oils, which often cause intense localized inflammation or sterile abscesses at the immunization site (Broderson 1989). Mitogenic and lymphocytic activating substances are frequently a component of the mineral oil-based adjuvants: well-known examples include heat-deactivated bacteria of the genus *Mycobacterium* in Freund's complete adjuvant (FCA), trehalose dimycolate (TDM), monophosphoryl lipid A (MPL), cell wall skeletons (CWS), 6-bromoguanisine, and *N*-acetyl-muramyl-L-alanyl-isoglutamine (adjuvant peptide).

The choice of adjuvant should depend on the chemical characteristics of the antigen molecules, there being no advantage in the use of FCA or Freund's incomplete adjuvant (FIA) if the antigen molecules are devoid of a hydrophobic sequence, because such a requirement is essential for sequestering the molecules in the mineral oil at the oil–water interface (Freund et al. 1937).

Recently, an independent comparison of four well-characterized adjuvants was released as a technical note by CytRx Corporation (Check et al. 1990). Rabbits and mice were immunized with a peptide–protein conjugate of luteinizing hormone-releasing hormone–bovine serum albumin (LHRH-BSA) reconstituted in: (a) FCA or FIA, (b) CytRx TiterMax #R-1 adjuvant, (c) Ribi Adjuvant System (MPL + TDM + CWS emulsion), and (d) Adjuvax. In the protocol, four rabbits and four mice were immunized according to the manufacturer's specifications for reconstitution, dosing, immunization site, and immunization schedule. After 8 weeks, with boosting every 2 weeks, it was found that TiterMax produced anti-LHRH IgG titers in rabbits and mice superior to the Ribi and Adjuvax adjuvants, with the additional benefits of an equivalent titer, smaller injection volume, and less toxicity than FCA.

For generating an immune response we have found that the use of Adjuvax, following an initial immunization with FCA, was superior to use of FCA alone or the Ribi system. In addition, we are currently evaluating TiterMax but have not completed the study.

III. Immunization Sites and Schedules

Over the years many immunization sites have been evaluated: subcutaneous (SC), intradermal (ID), intramuscular (IM), footpads, and lymph nodes. Recently, Grumstrup-Scott and Greenhouse (1988) at the National Institutes of Health (NIH) recommended the use of FCA and ID injections in rabbits. The other inoculation sites were felt to be too stressful and were associated with a greater incidence of inflammation and apparent tissue abscesses with no increase in desirable immunological response. In addition,

JOHNSTON et al. (1991) suggested: (a) a 1.5-ml total inoculum with 1.0 ml delivered in four 0.25-ml boluses in the subcutaneous tissue at intrascapular locations with an additional 0.5 ml to be delivered by either IM or ID injection; (b) inoculation at only one or the other (IM or ID) site for a given injection alternating between sites if necessary due to ulceration, localized abscess formation, or apparent distress; (c) 21 days between boosts, for inflammation to resolve and to allow sufficient recovery time between hand-ling, bleeding, or sedation; and (d) immunization not be permitted during periods of fever, injury, or loss of appetite. These guidelines were thought to be "effective, practical, and humane."

Our experience, in conjunction with the recommendations of AMYX (1987) and the NIH (GRUMSTRUP-SCOTT and GREENHOUSE 1988) for the minimization of stress to our animals, has demonstrated that the most efficacious method for the generation of polyclonal antisera in the shortest period of time incorporates the following procedures: (a) 200–500 μg of hapten–protein immunogen is prepared in 1.0 ml FCA (normal saline–FCA; 50/50; v/v) for each rabbit or sheep; (b) only the first immunization is made with FCA, and this is injected in five or more ID or SC sites; (c) 14 days later another dose of 200–500 μg immunogen in 1.0 ml FIA with synthetic adjuvant (Ribi, Adjuvax, or TiterMax) is injected ID or SC as before; (d) step c is repeated one or more times before initial bleeding; (e) 10–14 days after last immunization, a test bleeding is obtained, and titers and sensitivities are determined; and (f) steps c through e are repeated until antisera with adequate titer and sensitivity are obtained or a new immun-ization program is begun.

E. Matrix Effects of Biological Fluids

Once antibody and radiolabeled reagents are obtained and characterized in a buffer system, the next and often most critical step in developing an RIA is eliminating or reducing the nonspecific matrix effect of the biological fluid being quantitated. WOOD (1991) defines matrix effect as "the sum of all components (both qualitative and quantitative) in a system, with the excep-tion of the analyte to be measured." These components include the sample, buffer, label, antibodies, and separation reagents. This section will deal only with the sample matrix component and experimental methods for eliminating or reducing its deleterious contribution.

Individual components of the sample matrix that could potentially inter-fere with an RIA include binding proteins, lipids, heterophilic antibodies, complement factors, and any other material that would interact with the various dynamic processes in an RIA (antibody–antigen binding, nonspecific binding, bound/free label separation). The general methods for removal of interferants from sample matrices are: (a) protein precipitation or filtration,

(b) solvent extraction of analyte, and (c) specific chromatographic separation of analyte.

I. Methods for Sample Matrix Effect Elimination

1. Filtration/Precipitation of Protein

Filtration is not widely used due to potential loss of drug on the filtration media and because the procedure is labor intensive relative to other methods. Protein precipitation, by either solvents or organic acid, is also used but requires recovery studies to ensure that the material being quantitated is not lost with the precipitated protein.

In an assay we recently developed for the β_2 agonist bronchodilator procaterol, predose plasma samples from study subjects showed highly variable effects on antibody binding (Nordblom et al. 1992). After trying several methods to eliminate this variability, it was found that plasma protein precipitation with trifluoroacetic acid resulted in an RIA that was very reproducible and sensitive to about 15 pg/ml. However, this procedure worked only because the drug was not tightly bound to plasma protein. The RIA was also applied to urine samples where drug concentrations were higher than in plasma and 10 μl of sample was sufficient for analysis. This reduction in sample size is an introduction to the best procedure for eliminating matrix interference, namely, diminishing sample size until the interference is negligible (see Sect. E.II).

An interesting alternative to protein precipitation was described recently for an RIA for the α_2-adrenoreceptor antagonist idazoxan (Lynn et al. 1990). The assay employed pepsin digestion of protein to eliminate interference. In this case the resulting sample digest was used directly without the removal of the precipitate.

2. Solvent Extraction

Extraction procedures are widely used, especially for nonpolar analytes that can be removed from aqueous matrices with organic solvents. The resulting organic phase must be separated, evaporated to dryness, and reconstituted, usually in assay buffer. Solvent extraction also allows the concentration of analyte relative to the original sample; i.e., 2 ml of sample extracted and reconstituted to 0.5 ml effectively increases the assay sensitivity fourfold. Numerous examples of extraction-based RIAs have been published, varying from the phosphodiesterase inhibitor rolipram (Krause and Kühne 1988) to the bronchodilator albuterol (Loo et al. 1987) to chlorpromazine N-oxide (Yeung et al. 1987). Extraction procedures have also been developed that employ an initial protein precipitation, as in the case of the dihydropyridine calcium antagonist benidipine (Akinaga et al. 1988). Methods have also been devised where the extraction procedure selectively removes cross-reacting metabolites (Ho et al. 1985). In our laboratories we have adapted the assay for the opioid agonist CI-977 described above for $10\,\mu l$ of dog or rat plasma (NORDBLOM et al. 1990) to human plasma using a methylene chloride/pentane extraction procedure. The result was the elimination of matrix interferences and a sensitivity of 2.8 pg/ml.

3. Solid Phase Chromatographic Extraction

For drugs that are not efficiently removed from aqueous samples by traditional liquid/liquid extraction, an effective alternative is the use of C_{18} reversed-phase cartridges. ANGWIN and BARCHAS (1982) devised such a method for preparing enkephalin and endorphin samples for RIA. Plasma was added directly to preconditioned C_{18} columns. Interfering materials were washed off with 4% acetic acid followed by 0.2 N HCl elution of the desired peptides. The eluate was evaporated and reconstituted in assay buffer. GASPAR and MAGHUIN-ROGISTER (1985) employed the same technique for a diethylstilbestrol assay in bovine urine using ethyl acetate to elute the analyte.

4. High-Performance Liquid Chromatographic Sample Preparation

The evolution of chromatographic complexity prior to RIA eventually led to HPLC treatment of biological samples. The most important aspect of the method is the tremendous gain in assay selectivity. The analyte of choice can be separated from all interferences and closely related cross-reactants prior to the assay. The RIA essentially becomes an off-line detection method for the HPLC. Since the levels of analyte in the samples are usually too low for normal ultraviolet or fluorescent detectors, elution times for the analytes must be determined at high concentrations and the eluant collected at those times for sample purification.

Several HPLC/RIA methods have been reported for digoxin and metabolites (GAULT et al. 1985; PLUM and DALDRUP 1986). STRETCHER et al. (1991) developed a method for analyzing the metabolites of the anti-HIV drug zidovudine in extracts of peripheral blood mononuclear cells by purifying the metabolites with HPLC and quantitating them with commercially available RIA kits. LEE et al. (1987) were able to measure both of the active steroids in an oral contraceptive, ethinyl estradiol and norethindrone, from a single sample by HPLC separation followed by the two respective RIAs. This procedure was especially important because until recently antisera for ethinyl estradiol cross-reacted with naturally occurring estradiol. EIBS and SCHÖNESHÖFER (1984) took the multiple analyte concept to an extreme when they developed an HPLC/RIA procedure that measured 15 different steroids from a single small-volume plasma sample.

The utility of any sample purification/RIA procedure is dependent on the ability to determine the recovery efficiency of the purification procedure. The most common method is accomplished using radiolabeled drug, usually

[^{3}H]-drug, and the preferred procedure entails adding a small amount of recovery tracer to each individual sample during analysis. However, if a tritium label is also used in the RIA, extreme care must be taken to ensure correction for the recovery label. A potential alternative would be to determine the recovery prior to assay validation using a large number of replicates and then applying the recovery factor to each value determined for individual samples. However, this has the drawback that the individual values do not reflect any abnormal distribution in sample variation. Lastly, recovery could be determined by measuring a known quantity of spiked analyte during validation, although this technique will not account for sample-to-sample variability and is not method independent.

II. Elimination of Sample Matrix Effect by Sample Size

The use of a diminished sample size to reduce or eliminate matrix effect was discussed briefly above. Basically, as the volume of sample used in an RIA is reduced, at some volume the matrix effect becomes negligible. However, if the sensitivity of the assay or concentration of drug is such that the levels can still be measured, an assay may be developed that eliminates preassay purification. We would like to discuss a second application of the usage of small sample size, which is the development of a "generic" RIA (NORDBLOM et al. 1990b).

The usual series of events leading to the development of a new assay includes preparation of standards and quality control materials followed by validation. This section will focus on an unusual scenario we encountered while generating quality control samples for a particular assay in development.

A study was conducted to evaluate transplacental effects of the antihypertensive compound quinapril (CI-906) in rats. The protocol was designed to obtain plasma and milk samples from the dams, and plasma from the fetuses and postnatal pups. These samples were then to be analyzed using a previously described RIA for the active metabolite, quinaprilat (CI-928) (MICHNIEWICZ et al. 1987).

According to our standard operating procedures (SOPs), we must prepare a supply of quality control samples in the biological matrix of interest. This is usually not a difficult task when the matrix of interest is plasma or urine from humans or other large species. However, what does one do when asked to measure an analyte in fetal rat plasma, rat pup plasma, or rat milk? This problem could also be clinically significant when considering pediatric samples, cerebrospinal fluid, synovial fluid, intraocular fluid, or biopsy samples.

The normal validation of an assay to measure CI-928 would have required enough adult rat plasma, fetal rat plasma, rat pup plasma, and rat milk for use in the preparation of at least three different levels of quality control (QC) sample, and for generation of a standard curve [i.e., the addition of matrix to the zero standard (B_0), nonspecific binding (NSB), and standard tubes (ST)] for each assay. While sufficient normal rat plasma was available to validate an assay for this matrix, a method was still required for the pre- and postnatal plasma and milk samples.

The concentration of drug was sufficiently elevated in all of the matrices to enable us to use only $10 \mu l$ of the sample for analysis. Consequently, because we could obtain at most $1-2$ ml of control material for each matrix (no small endeavor for fetal rat plasma), we could generate the standard curves but not prepare the required QCs. The solution to this dilemma was pragmatically simple: QCs were prepared in assay buffer. The method was then validated according to our SOPs; the QC levels were measured, the mean and standard deviation were determined, and a range of the mean $\pm$ two standard deviations was calculated.

When the need arose to assay actual experimental samples, the assay was run identically to the validation, except that $10 \mu l$ of control matrix (fetal and postnatal plasma or milk) was added to all assay tubes (i.e., NSB, B_0, ST, and QC). Thus all tubes, including the unknowns, had $10 \mu l$ of matrix present during the incubation. An assay was acceptably "in control" if two out of the three QC values were within the range determined in assay buffer alone. When actual rat milk and fetal rat or rat pup plasma samples were quantitated, all QCs were in the validated buffer range and the analyses were judged as acceptable.

An important point to consider when developing a generic procedure is that although the conditions are the same in all assay tubes during equilibrium, this method does not take into account possible stability differences that may arise from long-term storage since the QCs are in buffer while the samples are in matrix. Nevertheless, it has been our experience that when we are called upon to perform analyses in these unusual biological fluids, the number of samples is small and they can be processed without undue delay.

One must ask whether it is not worth the effort to use this procedure to obtain results, as opposed to any other method, since this is closest to the normal procedure. The key is that the ultimate recipients of the resulting data, whether they be clinicians or pharmaceutical researchers, must be made aware of the situation so that they understand that although the assay is not exactly as it should be, it is as close to normal as is realistically possible.

F. The Suitability of Radioimmunoassay for Drug Analysis

Within the last 2 years several conferences consisting of regulatory, pharmaceutical, and academic scientists have been convened to discuss, among other things, the suitability of RIA as an analytical method for measuring drug concentrations in biological fluids. We will briefly present the consensus that was reached at these conferences.

In June 1990 the Health Protection Branch of Health and Welfare Canada held a workshop in Ottawa, Ontario on the bioavailability of oral contraceptives (GALLICANO et al. 1991). Among the issues discussed were several pertaining to the use of RIA since until recently it has been the only available method sensitive enough to quantitate the estrogen component, ethinyl estradiol, in most formulations. The issues included: (a) the specificity and sensitivity that can be expected using RIA; (b) whether a direct (no preassay sample preparation) RIA alone can be used to generate data for new drug submissions or whether a chromatographic procedure should be used in conjunction with the RIA; and (c) what new techniques are being developed and whether they can be used for analysis or validation of RIA.

After many presentations and a vigorous discussion, several conclusions were reached. It was felt that until recently RIAs were sensitive enough (approximately 5 pg/ml) to measure ethinyl estradiol although the specificity of the antibodies used was questionable. To alleviate this problem it was concluded that a chromatographic sample preparation such as HPLC (LEE et al. 1987) should be used. Other chromatographic procedures should be used with care. For instance, Celite removes most endogenous steroids but not estradiol, which cross-reacts with ethinyl estradiol for most available antibody.

It became clear from the presentations and discussion that newer analytical procedures such as gas chromatography/mass spectrometry (GC/MS) are beginning to approach acceptable quantitation levels and specificity for use to analyze actual samples. However, due to current cost and time constraints, GC/MS may be best used now for RIA cross-validation.

In December 1990, well over 400 representatives of pharmaceutical manufacturers, contract laboratories, academic facilities, and regulatory agencies met in Arlington, Virginia to discuss "Analytical Method Validation: Bioequivalence, Bioavailability and Pharmacokinetics" (SHAH et al. 1992). Since the scope of the discussion covered pharmaceutics in general, compared to only oral contraceptives at the Ottawa meeting, the majority of the topics dealt with HPLC methods. However, one main session was dedicated to immunoassays and the objectives of the conference: (a) to reach a consensus on requirements of analytical method validation, (b) application of validation procedures, and (c) to develop guidelines for method validation that apply equally as well to RIA. Most of the suggested guidelines would seem to be obvious, but since they were debated we will discuss several of the more salient points below.

In immunoassays the system response must be shown to relate to the concentration of the analyte; that is, it must demonstrate specificity. To do this, it was emphasized that an alternative established method should be used for comparison. For RIA this may prove to be unattainable since RIAs are usually used when other methods are not sensitive enough. One approach would be to analyze samples with both procedures at higher concentrations and assume that the immunoassay will be equally selective at lower concentrations. With the recent emergence of GC/MS techniques there is now a method with equal sensitivity and greater specificity for comparison. If the RIA agrees well with GC/MS one could be assured that the RIA is an acceptable analytical tool. Unfortunately, due to availability and cost, GC/MS currently is not a viable solution for routine analysis. Other selectivity suggestions included ensuring parallelism of the assay by studying sample dilutions and comparing analyte standards in both buffer and sample matrix.

The precision and accuracy of the assay, as defined by the standard curve, should both be within ±15% CV and relative error except at the lower limit of quantitation (LOQ) where ±20% is acceptable. The LOQ *must* be determined by the low standard since sample concentrations should not be extrapolated from the curve. This point was vigorously defended by representatives of the Food and Drug Authority. These points really illustrate one of the most important considerations in developing an analytical method; that is, serious thought must be given to the question of the need for sensitivity versus the precision of the assay. This can only be accomplished by a good interaction between the study director and the analyst.

The best possible curve-fitting model must be found during the validation and then used for sample analysis. Other topics included the used of "spiked" QC samples to determine the accuracy and precision of the assay during validation followed by the use of the same QCs during sample analysis to determine assay acceptability. Once the first study has been completed, it was suggested that pools of samples ("dosed" QCs) be made and followed in subsequent studies. Analyte stability during sampling, handling, and storage should be determined with both spiked and dosed QCs. The effect of several thaw-freeze cycles on the QCs should be determined.

For RIAs that require sample purification prior to analysis to remove matrix interferences, it is necessary to establish recovery, much like that described in Sect. E. Finally, an interesting suggestion, which is not commonly used, was to prepare standards in sample matrix to reduce matrix effects.

References

Akinaga S, Kobayashi H, Kobayashi S, Inoue A, Nakamizo N, Oka T (1988) Determination of the calcium antagonist benodipine hydrochloride in plasma by sensitive radioimmunoassay. Arzneimittelforschung 38:1738–1741

Amyx HL (1987) Control of animal pain and distress in antibody production and infectious disease studies. J Am Vet Med Assoc 91:1287–1289

Angwin P, Barchas JD (1982) Analysis of peptides in tissues. Use of silisic acid extraction and reversed-phase columns for rapid purification prior to radioimmunoassay. J Chromatogr 231:173–177

Beale MH (1991) The preparation of gibberellin hapten-protein conjugates. II. Conjugates and gibberellin probes formed via the addition of α,ω-dithiols to C-16-enes. J Chem Soc Perkins Trans 1:2559–2563

Broderson JR (1989) A retrospective review of lesions associated with the use of Freund's adjuvant. Lab Anim Sci 39:400–405

Check IR, Bennett B, Hunter RL (1990) Hunter's Titer Max™: research adjuvant. Technical note. CytRx Corporation, Norcross, Georgia

Eibs G, Schöneshöfer M (1984) Simultaneous determination of fifteen steroid hormones from a single serum sample by high-performance liquid chromatography and radioimmunoassay. J Chromatogr 310:386–389

Erlanger BF (1980) The preparation of antigenic hapten-carrier conjugates: a survey. Methods Enzymol 70:85

Findlay JWA (1987) Applications of immunoassay methods to drug disposition studies. Drug Metab Rev 18:83–129

Freund J, Casals J, Hismer EP (1937) Sensitization and antibody formation after injection of tubercle bacilli and paraffin oil. Proc Soc Exp Biol Med 37:509–517

Gallicano KD, McGilvery IJ, Qureshi S, Nitchuk W, Chakraborty B, Boyd C (1991) Situation paper: comparative bioavailability of oral contraceptive products. Clin Biochem 24:107–111

Gaspar P, Maghuin-Rogister G (1985) Rapid extraction and purification of diethylstilboestrol in bovine urine hydrolysates using reversed-phase C_{18} columns before determination by radioimmunoassay. J Chromatogr 328:423–426

Gault MH, Longerich L, Dawe M, Vasdev SC (1985) Combined liquid chromatography/radioimmunoassay with improved specificity for serum digoxin. Clin Chem 31:1272–1277

Greenwood FC, Hunter WH, Glover JS (1963) The preparation of ^{131}I-labelled human growth hormone to a high specific radioactivity. Biochem J 89:114–123

Grumstrup-Scott J, Greenhouse DD (1988) NIH intramural recommendations for the research use of complete Freund's adjuvant. Int Lab Anim Res News 30(2):9–22

Ho DH, Kanellopoulos KS, Brown NS, Issell BF, Bodey GP (1985) Radioimmunoassay for etoposide and teniposide. J Immunol Methods 85:5–15

Johnston BA, Eisen H, Fry D (1991) An evaluation of several adjuvant emulsion regimens for the production of polyclonal antisera in rabbits. Lab Anim Sci 41:15–21

Kesten SJ, Pattison IC, Goel OP (1989) Synthesis of 7-hydroxy-4-benzofuran acetic acid. Organ Prep Proc Int 21:763–770

Klause GGB, Cross AM (1974) The influence of epitope density on the immunological properties of hapten-protein conjugates. I. Characteristics of the immune response to hapten-coupled albumen with varying epitope density. Cell Immunol 14:226–233

Krause W, Kühne G (1988) Pharmacokinetics of rolipram in the rhesus and cynomolgus monkeys, the rat and the rabbit. Studies on species differences. Xenobiotica 18:561–571

Landsteiner K (1945) The specificity of serological reactions. Harvard University Press, Cambridge

Lee GJ-L, Oyang M-H, Bautista J, Kushinsky S (1987) Determination of ethinyl estradiol and norethindrone in a single specimen of plasma by automated high-performance liquid chromatography and subsequent radioimmunoassay. J Liquid Chromatogr 10:2305–2318

Lehtola T, Lavikainen O, Huhtikangas A (1988) Radioimmunoassay of trospiumchloride, a quaternary tropane derivative. J Immunoassay 9:297–307

Loo JCK, Beaulieu N, Jordan N, Brien R, McGilerary IJ (1987) A specific radioimmunoassay (RIA) for salbutamol (albuterol) in human plasma. Res Commun Clin Pathol Pharmacol 55:283–286

Lynn AG, Coxon RE, Gallacher G, Landon J (1990) Development of a radioimmunoassay for idazoxan hydrochloride. J Pharm Biomed Anal 8:685–689

Michniewicz BM, Hodges JC, England BG, Chang T, Blankley CJ, Nordblom GD (1987) A radioimmunoassay for the diacid metabolite of CI-906, a potent angiotensin-I converting enzyme inhibitor. J Clin Immunoassay 10:111–115

Miller RL, Verma PS (1989) A radioimmunoassay for physostigmine in biological fluids and tissues. J Pharm Biomed Anal 7:955–963

Niswender GD, Midgley AR (1970) Hapten-radioimmunoassay for steroid hormones. In: Peron FG, Caldwell BF (eds) Immunological methods in steroid determination. Appleton, New York, pp 149–173

Nordblom GD, Webb R, Counsell RE, England BG (1981) A chemical approach to solving bridging phenomena in steroid radioimmunoassays. Steroids 38:161–173

Nordblom GD, Counsell RE, England BG (1984) A specific radioimmunoassay for androstenedione with reduced bridge-binding. Steroids 44:275–282

Nordblom GD, Pachla LA, Chang T, Whitfield LR, Showalter HDH (1989) Development of a radioimmunoassay for the anthrapyrazole chemotherapy agent CI-937 and the pharmacokinetics of CI-937 in rats. Cancer Res 49:5345–5451

Nordblom GD, Barksdale CM, Coon MJ, Kesten SJ, Pattison IC, Goel OP, Pachla LA, Wright DS (1990a) Development of a radioimmunoassay for the novel analgesic kappa opioid receptor agonist CI-977. J Clin Immunoassay 13:132–139

Nordblom GD, Coon MJ, Barksdale CM (1990b) Development of a radioimmunoassay when there is insufficient control matrix. J Clin Immunoassay 13:89–90

Nordblom GD, Coon MJ, Suto MJ, Pachla LA, Colburn WA (1992) Development of radioimmunoassays for the measurement of the beta-2 specific bronchodilator, procaterol in human plasma and urine. J Clin Immunoassay 15:258–264

Oida T, Terauchi Y, Yoshida K, Kagemoto A, Sekine Y (1989) Use of antisera in the isolation of human specific conjugates of haloperidol. Xenobiotica 19:781–793

Plum J, Daldrup T (1986) Detection of digoxin, digitoxin, their cardioactive metabolites and derivatives by high-performance liquid chromatography and high-performance liquid chromatography-radioimmunoassay. J Chromatogr 377:221–231

Rittenberg MB, Amkraut AA (1966) Immunogenicity of trinitrophenyl-hemocyanin: production of primary and secondary anti-hapten precipitins. J Immunol 97:421–429

Shah VP, Midah KK, Dighe S, McGilvery IJ, Skelly JP, Yacobi A, Layloff T, Viswanathan CT, Cook CE, McDowall RD, Pittman KA, Spector S (1992) Analytical method validation: bioavailability, bioequivalence and pharmacokinetic studies. J Pharm Sci 81:309–312

Skowsky WR, Fisher DA (1972) The use of thyroglobulin to induce antigenicity to small molecules. J Lab Clin Med 80:131–141

Stewart-Tull DES (1989) Recommendations for the assessment of adjuvants (immunopotentiators). NATO Adv Study Inst Ser [A] 179:213–226

Stretcher BN, Pesce AJ, Geisler BA, Vine WH (1991) A coupled HPLC/radioimmunoassay for analysis of zidovudine metabolites in mononuclear cells. J Liquid Chromatogr 14:2261–2272

Walker DK, Aherne GW, Arrowsmith JE, Cross PE, Kaye B, Smith DA, Stopher DA, Wild W (1991) Measurement of the class III antidysrhythmic drug, UK-68,798 in plasma by radioimmunoassay. J Pharm Biomed Anal 9:141–149

Warren HS, Vogel FR, Chedid LA (1986) Current status of immunological adjuvants. Annu Rev Immunol 4:369–388

White A, Gray C, Corrie JET (1985) Monoclonal antibodies to testosterone: the effect of immunogen structure on specificity. J Steroid Biochem 22:169–175

Wood WG (1991) "Matrix effects" in immunoassays. Scand J Clin Lab Invest 51 Suppl 205:105–112

Yalow RS (1978) Radioimmunoassay: a probe for the fine structure of biological systems. Science 200:1236–1243

Yeung PFK, Hubbard JW, Korchinski ED, Midah KK (1987) Radioimmunoassay for the N-oxide metabolite of Chlorpromazine in human plasma and its application to a pharmacokinetic study in healthy humans. J Pharm Sci 76:803–808

Youngblood WW, Kizer JS (1983) Strategies for the preparation of haptens for conjugation and substrates for iodination for use in radioimmunoassay of small oligopeptides. Methods Enzymol 103:435

CHAPTER 3
Mass Spectrometry in Drug Disposition and Pharmacokinetics

I.A. Blair

A. Introduction

An examination of the recent literature suggests that the role of mass spectrometry (MS) in the fields of drug disposition and pharmacokinetics is expanding. This is most likely a consequence of the availability of new instrumentation and ionization techniques that can be used to help solve difficult bioanalytical problems associated with these fields (Burlingame et al. 1990, 1992). This can perhaps be best illustrated in the development of electrospray (ESI) and related atmospheric pressure ionization (API) techniques such as ionspray and atmospheric pressure chemical ionization (APCI) for studies in drug disposition. Over the last 2 years there has been an unprecedented explosion in the use of instrumentation dedicated to APIMS (Smith et al. 1990; Fenn et al. 1990; Hamdan and Curcuruto 1991; Huang et al. 1990; Huang and Henion 1991; Bruins 1991; Wachs et al. 1991). Perusal of the literature would suggest that thermospray (TSP) is still the most popular liquid chromatography (LC)/MS technique for structural and quantitative studies (Arpino 1990). However, this is to some extent a reflection of the fact that many APIMS studies have not been reported in full and remain only in abstract form (predominantly in Proceedings of 39th and 40th ASMS Conferences on Mass Spectrometry). With time there is no doubt that the full papers derived from these initial reports will eventually appear. Perhaps another major factor slowing publication is that many studies have been carried out with proprietary compounds and it will take several years for patent clearance to be obtained for the full release of all the findings to take place. The pharmaceutical industry has certainly been at the forefront of implementing API-based methodology and this perhaps reflects the utility of these techniques for studies on drug disposition. Several reviews have appeared recently on the use of MS in drug disposition (Baillie 1992; Garland and Vandenheuvel 1992), pharmacology (Abramson 1990; Fenselau 1992), and biology (Burlingame and McCloskey 1990; Suelter and Watson 1990; McEwen and Larsen 1990; McCloskey 1991; Gross 1992; Stroh and Rinehart 1992).

Stable isotope analogs have increasingly assumed importance in studies on drug disposition (Vandenheuvel 1987; Baillie and Jones 1989; Lee et al. 1991; Barbalas and Garland 1991). Of particular utility is the isotope cluster technique, which allows the recognition of metabolites in complex biological matrices such as urine and plasma (KASUYA et al. 1991; WEIDOLF and COVEY 1992). Several methods have been developed for the deconvolution of isotope clusters from stable isotope analogs so that mass spectral identification is facilitated (VANDENHEUVEL 1987; KORZEKWA et al. 1990; BARBALAS and GARLAND 1991). In the field of pharmacokinetics, stable isotope analogs are used as internal standards for quantitative purposes, to determine bioequivalence and in chiral drug disposition (PENG and CHIOU 1990). In studies on chiral drugs, the use of a pseudoracemate where one enantiomer is labeled and the other is unlabeled, provides the basis for a robust method that can be used to determine pharmacokinetic parameters of individual enantiomers and their metabolites (MIKUS et al. 1990; PRAKASH et al. 1991; ERIKSSON et al. 1991; SHINOHARA et al. 1990, 1991). An exciting innovative approach to the use of stable isotopes comes from ABRAMSON and his co-workers (CHACE and ABRAMSON 1990; MOINI et al. 1990; MOINI and ABRAMSON 1991), who have introduced the chemical reaction interface (CRI) mass spectrometer for quantitative studies on drug metabolism. Ultimately this type of approach will provide an alternative to the use of radioisotopes for drug disposition studies. There is a real need for this type of methodology in view of the increasing cost of disposal of radioactive waste, the questionable ethics in dosing normal subjects with radioactivity, and the inability to dose women and children with radioactivity. The enormous literature that has accrued over the last decade illustrates the importance of MS in the fields of drug disposition and pharmacokinetics. The present review will focus on literature published since 1988 and will use selected examples rather than attempting to cite all the references that have accrued in the field. This should provide the reader with sufficient information to allow consultation of all the relevant background sources.

B. Ionization Techniques

I. Electron Ionization

Electron ionization (EI) is the oldest available technique in MS (BEYNON and MORGAN 1978) and is still extremely useful, particularly when compounds can be derivatized to improve their EI characteristics. Although there are numerous soft ionization techniques for the analysis of drug conjugates, in some suitable cases derivatization can be carried out to facilitate their analysis by EIMS (HOFFMANN and BAILLIE 1988; BRASHEAR et al. 1990). The advantage of EI is that extensive fragmentation can occur in the source of the mass spectrometer and this can provide a wealth of structural information. Further, the fragmentation processes that occur are very reproducible and so it is relatively easy to reproduce spectra obtained in other laboratories. Soft ionization techniques provide enhanced molecular species with less fragmentation so that collision-induced dissociation (CID) and MS/MS techniques are required to obtain structurally relevant fragment ions. There are numerous examples in the literature of how useful EI can be for structure determinations of drug metabolites. Pertinent examples include those for the anxiolytic buspirone (JAJOO et al. 1989a,b), the antiarrhythmic encainide (JAJOO et al. 1990c), the antiepileptic stiripentol (ZHANG et al. 1990), the methadone analog recipavrin (SLATTER et al. 1990), the anti-depressant trimipramine (COUTTS et al. 1990), and the anti-infective imuthiol (SCAPPATICCI et al. 1990). In many cases it is necessary to carry out deri-vatization prior to analysis, particularly when gas chromatography (GC) is carried out (KNAPP 1979). This can facilitate analysis on relatively cheap instrumentation such as mass selective detectors or bench top mass spectrometers.

II. Positive Chemical Ionization

Positive chemical ionization is often used to complement data obtained with EI because it is a relatively soft ionization technique. Fragmentation pro-cesses are normally much reduced compared with EI and protonated mole-cular or adduct ions are detected depending on the type of gas that is used (MURRAY et al. 1983). This can be extremely useful both in structural studies and in quantitative studies where inadequate specificity is obtained with EI. Desorption PCI can be particularly useful when trace amounts of material are available and there are a number of recent reports on the use of this technique in structural studies. The analysis of taxol metabolites from rat bile by PCI (MONSARRAT et al. 1990) has been given special prominence because the drug has stimulated so much interest with the general public. An interesting use of PCI was in the study of the metabolism of the anti-psychotic agent tiospirone, where sulfone and sulfoxide metabolites could be desorbed without reduction (JAJOO et al. 1990a; MAYOL et al. 1991). Several other reports have appeared on the use of PCI in structural analysis, including identification of metabolites of methapyriline (KELLY et al. 1990) and zonisamide (STIFF and ZEMAITIS 1990). A number of reports have appeared on the use of PCI in combination with GC/MS for quantitative studies.

III. Electron Capture Negative Chemical Ionization

The exquisite sensitivity of electron capture negative chemical ionization (EC NcI) MS has facilitated quantitative determinations of drugs (DAWSON et al. 1990; FISCHER et al. 1990; GIRAULT et al. 1990a,b; KASSAHUN 1990; KAYGANICH et al. 1990; LEIS et al. 1990; CHANGCHIT et al. 1991; KOMATSU et al. 1991; LEIS and MALLE 1991; PRAKASH et al. 1991; ROBINSON et al.

1991) and endogenous autocoids (BLAIR 1990) at femtomole concentrations. A recent report has described the analysis of DNA adducts at sub-attamole concentrations using NCIMS (ABDEL-BAKY and GIESE 1991). EC NCIMS is probably the method of choice where pharmacokinetic determinations require a very high level of sensitivity. The method normally requires that analyte molecules are derivatized so that they can capture thermal electrons generated in the source of the mass spectrometer. The pentafluorobenzyl (PFB) derivative has found the widest applicability because it is relatively easy to prepare in high yield under very mild conditions (BLAIR 1990). The derivative is extremely efficient in capturing gas phase thermal electrons but paradoxically it is lost during ionization through a homolytic cleavage to give the molecular negative ion (M)-PFB. This process, known as dissociative electron capture, occurs with almost all PFB derivatives independent of whether they are attached to oxygen or nitrogen. Dissociative electron capture provides an anion that contains the intact analyte molecule and very little fragmentation is observed. Thus, assays using this technique have high specificity in addition to high sensitivity.

The sensitivity of EC NCIMS is exemplified in a study of valproic acid metabolism where this ionization technique was used to identify 14 urinary metabolites after dosing a human subject with 20 mg/day of the drug (KASSAHUN et al. 1989). Highly polar glucuronide metabolites were analyzed with high sensitivity by GC/EC NCIMS as their trimethylsilyl (TMS), PFB derivatives (BROWN et al. 1990a). Intense ions corresponding to [M-PFB]$^-$ were observed and it was even possible to analyze the carbamoyl glucuronide of rimantidine by this technique. An interesting application of GC/EC NCIMS to chiral drug metabolism was reported in the analysis of the barbiturate drug hexobarbital and its metabolites (PRAKASH et al. 1991). EC NCI has continued to be used in studies that require debrisoquine phenotyping of human subjects (ZHOU et al. 1989; SHAHEEN et al. 1989; MAY et al. 1990). Most studies have employed single analyzer mass spectrometers although here are some examples where tandem MS was used to provide additional specificity. For example, analysis of the nonsteroidal anti-inflammatory drug (NSAID) indomethacin was carried out using selected reaction monitoring (SRM) in combination with GC/EC NCIMS (DAWSON et al. 1990)

IV. Liquid Secondary Ion/Fast Atom Bombardment

Liquid secondary ion (LSI) MS has the highest sensitivity when using Cs$^+$ ionization but more studies have been carried out using fast atom bombardment (FAB) with Xe atoms, probably because of the wider availability of this technique (IWABUCHI et al. 1987; STRAUB et al. 1987). Most studies have employed the use of off-line LC purification of metabolites followed by LSI analysis usually by FAB. An interesting application for the analysis of drugs and their metabolites is the use of scanning thin-layer chromatography–LSIMS (NAKAGAWA and IWATANI 1991). Although this technique has not found wide acceptance, its inherent simplicity suggests that it could play a useful role in drug metabolism studies. One problem that is often encountered in LSIMS is the interference from material present in organic solvents used to extract drugs and their metabolites from biological fluids. Even HPLC grade solvents contain significant amounts of impurities. A recent study has advocated the use of reversed-phase extraction cartridges in the final stage of sample purification to remove such impurities (KAJBAF et al. 1992).

FABMS was employed in the analysis of metabolites derived from the HMG-CoA reductase inhibitors lovastatin (VYAS et al. 1990) and provastatin (EVERETT et al. 1991), the analysis of peptides related to cyclosporin A (MEIER et al. 1990; CHRISTIANS et al. 1991b,c), the synthetic decapeptide RS-26306, an LHRH antagonist (CHAN et al. 1991), the H_2 antagonist etintidine (WONG FA et al. 1990), the NSAID diflunisal (MACDONALD et al. 1991), and adducts of the anticancer agent cisplatin with oligonucleotides (MARTIN et al. 1991). An unusual metabolite of the antiepileptic drug valproic acid from rat liver mitochondrial preparations was characterized by the use of Cs^+ LSIMS (MAO et al. 1992). From CID analysis it was possible to show that the compound was an acyl adenylate derivative of the parent drug. This was thought to be formed as an intermediate in the conversion of valproate to a CoA thioester derivative. A study by (LAURIAULT and O'BRIEN 1991) employed FABMS to characterize the adduct formed between diethyldithiocarbamate and the reactive metabolite responsible for acetaminophen toxicity. From this study it was shown that diethyldithiocarbamate and thiols such as dithiothreitol exerted their protective effects by quite different mechanisms. In a similar study (LAURIAULT et al. 1990) showed that benzoquinone toxicity was ameliorated by the formation of an adduct with diethyldithiocarbamate. (STAHL et al. 1992) used FABMS to show that the glutathione conjugate of the antineoplastic agent 1,3-bis(2-chloroethyl)-N-nitrosourea (BCNU) transferred an aminoethyl group to N-7 of guanosine. The resulting adduct then readily underwent depurination, suggesting that BCNU exerts its antineoplastic effects through an alkylation mechanism. Several other reports have appeared on the use of FABMS for the identification of DNA base adducts derived from anticancer agents (KOSEVICH and ZHILKOVA 1988; ANDRIEVSKY et al. 1991; MARTIN et al. 1991).

Without doubt FABMS has made an enormous contribution to the structural characterization of drug conjugates. This technique has been responsible for the characterization of structures that would have previously required a formidable effort. Conjugates tend to show prominent ions from the protonated molecule in the positive mode or ions from molecules that have lost a proton in the negative ion mode (JACOBS et al. 1987). Polar metabolites that have been identified by FAB and LSIMS include sulfates (STRAUB et al. 1987; LAUWERS et al. 1988; JACKSON et al. 1991b), glutathione adducts (HAROLDSON et al. 1988; HOFFMANN and BAILLIE 1988; LAUWERS et al. 1988; BAILLIE et al. 1989; DULIK et al. 1990), ether (HANDE et al. 1988; GOOD et al. 1990; HAUMONT et al. 1990; SHU et al. 1990b; CRETTON et al. 1990; JACKSON et al. 1991a; MAYS et al. 1991), ester (TANAKA et al. 1990), and N-linked and quaternary glucuronides (LUO et al. 1991; SINZ and REMMEL 1991; MACRAE et al. 1990). An interesting use of FAB was in the identification of the aglycone of the anticancer agent etoposide in the plasma of patients undergoing treatment with the drug (GOUYETTE 1987). The aglycone inhibits topoisomerase II (a similar mode of action to the parent drug) and is cytotoxic. Autologous bone marrow transplantation was delayed for 72 h in these patients to ensure that the cytotoxic aglycone was excreted.

Significant improvements in sensitivity have also been obtained by the use of flow techniques (CAPRIOLI 1990a,b; KENNY and ORLANDO 1992). However, there are few reports on the use of flow LSIMS for trace analysis, presumably because of the reluctance to use fused silica capillary columns. Most reports on the use of flow techniques either employ direct infusions or sample splitting from a conventional column. Using this type of methodology, it is necessary to have significant amounts (nmol) available in the first place. Continuous flow FAB was used to identify the major metabolites of the decapeptide anticoagulant dug, MDL 28,050 (KNADLER et al. 1992). The major urinary metabolites were formed through hydrolysis at four peptide bonds. Two initial sites of hydrolysis were identified as 4I-5P and 6E-7E, which resulted in the formation of four peptide fragments. Further metabolism of these fragments resulted in the N-terminal pentapeptide and the C-terminal dipeptide. This example illustrates the power of continuous flow FAB for characterization of peptide drugs.

Exciting developments in multichannel array detectors (COTTRELL and EVANS 1987; HILL et al. 1991) should permit LSI analysis to be carried out on significantly smaller amounts of material than has been possible to date. It is anticipated that this methodology will be extremely powerful for the analysis of trace amounts of material in the future, particularly when scanning array detectors become available for use in combination with chromatography.

V. Thermospray

The enormous current interest in techniques based on API tends to obscure the important role that TSP has played in drug metabolism studies over the last 5 years (BURLINGAME et al. 1990, 1992). In TSP analysis, the effluent from an LC column is sprayed directly into the source by means of differentially heated probe (ARPINO 1990). A fine mist of solution droplets is produced and as this enters into the heated source of the mass spectrometer the solvent rapidly evaporates (ANDEREGG 1990). The exact mechanism by which ions are formed remains controversial but it appears that a combination of liquid and gas phase reactions ultimately leads to the production of ions (ARPINO 1990). TSP provided the first practical method for obtaining reproducible LC/MS data on a routine basis (BLAKE 1987; SCHELLENBERG et al. 1987; BEATTIE and BLAKE 1989). Researchers from the field of drug disposition have been at the forefront in applying TSP methodology to bioanalytical problems (BLAKE 1987; SCHELLENBERG et al. 1987; STRAUB et al. 1988). A recent report described the application of a continuous flow dialysis system, consisting of a membrane dialyzer and a trace enrichment column on-line with a mass spectrometer via a TSP interface (VANBAKERGEM et al. 1992). This technique was used to monitor drug concentrations in plasma subsequent to treatment of patients with the anticancer drug rogletimide. Interestingly, TSP also proved to be particularly useful for the identification of metabolites of rogletimide (POON et al. 1991b). The soft ionization possible with TSP allowed the characterization of an N-oxide derivative in addition to more conventional oxidation products. Other unusual metabolites identified by TSP include: S-(N-methylcarbamoyl)-glutathiones as further conjugates derived from monomethylcarbamate metabolites of the bronchodilator bambuterol (RASHED et al. 1989), the N-glucuronide of the antiepileptic lamotrigine (MAGDALOU et al. 1992), an N-glucuronide of lamotrigine that was resistant to cleavage in vitro by a crude β-glucuronidase preparation from *Helix pomatia* (DOIG and CLARE 1991), a sulfate conjugate of the investigational gastrointestinal drug cisapride (LAUWERS et al. 1988), and glutathione conjugates of the bifunctional alkylating anticancer agent chlorambucil (DULIK et al. 1990). In this latter study, no molecular ions were observed but ions derived from the glutathione moiety were useful in identifying the structures. A particularly impressive use of TSP for metabolite identification can be found in a study on metabolism of the calcium antagonist amlodipine (BERESFORD et al. 1989). Eighteen metabolites were identified and their structures confirmed by comparison with authentic standards. TSP was used to identify the oxidized and glucuronidated metabolites of retinol (ECKHOFF et al. 1990), a new heptobarbital derivative (HEEREMANS et al. 1991), and two previously unidentified metabolites of the antihistamine, terfenidine (CHEN et al. 1991).

VI. Atmospheric Pressure Ionization

Without doubt, API is the most rapidly evolving technique being applied to studies in drug disposition. The recent interest in API stems from the recognition that ESI and pneumatically assisted ESI (ionspray) are incredibly useful techniques for structural and quantitative analyses of drugs and their metabolites (HUANG et al. 1990; HAMDAN and CURCURUTOTO 1991; WACHS et al. 1991; CARR et al. 1991). Flow rates for ESI are in the low μl/min range whereas for ionspray they are in the $50\,\mu$l/min range. The ionspray technique is more rugged because of the higher flow rates that are used (BRUINS 1991). Sensitivity is related to concentration and so ESI is inherently more sensitive than ionspray (FENN et al. 1990). However, LC has to be carried out with capillary columns (320 μm diameter), which places constraints on the amount of material that can be injected (<1 μl) on column. Alternatively, injections have to be made in solvents with a high aqueous content and gradient chromatography has to be carried out. This can be rather tedious and is really suited to structural studies when the analyte is only available in trace amounts. If sufficient quantities of material are available it is possible to split the LC effluent from a microbore column (1 mm diameter) into the ESI source (usually split of 1:20) so that more conventional chromatography can be carried out. The effluent that does not pass into the ESI source can be collected and used again. The mechanism by which API results in the conversion of charged droplets to ions in the gas phase is not completely understood (DOLE et al. 1968; HUANG et al. 1990). However, it is known that the charged droplets contain both positive and negative ions and the predominant charge is dependent on the plarity of the induced potential. Heat exchange with a countercurrent flow of gas causes rapid size reduction of the droplets until the coulombic forces overcome attractive forces and the droplets explode into smaller droplets. These droplets undergo further ion evaporation so that ions are transferred from the condensed phase to the gaseous phase and are then analyzed by the mass spectrometer (FENN et al. 1990).

Ionization of compounds using API-based techniques appears to be much less sample dependent than TSP ionization. The interface is not heated and so the thermal degradation of samples often seen with TSP is eliminated. ESI has been particularly useful in the analysis of platinum-containing drugs and their metabolites (POON et al. 1991c). Quantification and identification of platinum drugs and their metabolites in biological samples has always been difficult because the compounds are thermally labile, nonvolatile, and insoluble. ESI provided molecular ions and a series of structurally informative fragment ions with samples of approximately 10 pmol. This improved sensitivity should be useful for monitoring metabolites in patients being treated with platinum anticancer agents. An impressive study on the metabolism of the HMG-CoA reductase inhibitor provastatin used ESI (EVERETT et al. 1991). Biotransformation pathways that were elucidated include: isomerization, ring hydroxylation, ω-1 oxidation of the ester side chain, β-oxidation of the carboxy side chain, ring oxidation followed by aromatization, oxidation of a hydroxyl group, and conjugation. Structural assignments were confirmed by ^{1}H-NMR spectroscopy. ESI has been used in the analysis of sulfonamides (PERKINS et al. 1992) and a series of β-agonists (DEBRAUWER and BORIES 1992). Several other thermally labile drugs and their metabolites have been analyzed by API-based techniques including a potentially neurotoxic pyridinium metabolite of the antipsychotic agent haloperidol (SUBRAMANYAM et al. 1991), the polyether antibiotic semduramicin (SCHNEIDER et al. 1991), and the anabolic steroid stanozolol in human urine (MUCK and HENION 1990). Ionspray MS has been used to identify the presence of more than 40 metabolites of the antiulcer agent omeprazole (WEIDOLF and COVEY 1992).

VII. Collision-Induced Dissociation

Collision-induced dissociation requires the tandem pairing of two mass analyzers (tandem mass spectrometers). An ion of one particular mass is allowed to pass through the first analyzer into a field free region where it is allowed to collide with an inert gas, whereupon it forms fragment (or daughter) ions. The daughter ions are then separated in the second analyzer, which in turn transmits them to the detector (FENSELAU 1992). The type of instrumentation used in these studies can be a triple quadrupole, a four-sector instrument, or a hybrid of sector and quadrupoles. In the triple quadrupole the first and third set of quadrupole rods act as the first and second analyzers, respectively. CID is carried out inside the second set of quadrupoles where only the Rf can be varied. The tandem four-sector instruments employ an electrostatic and magnetic sector as the first analyzer and an electrostatic and magnetic sector as the second analyzer; a collision cell is located between the two analyzers. Quadrupole-based instruments employ collision energies of approximately 50 V whereas tandem four-sector instruments use 4 kV. The higher collision energy of the four-sector instrument usually induces more C–C cleavage reactions than is observed with quadrupoles. Neutral loss scans can be carried out with both quadrupole and sector instruments. In this mode of operation, the first analyzer is scanned through the desired mass range and the second analyzer is scanned at a constant mass lower than the first analyzer. This constant mass scan corresponds to the neutral molecule lost during fragmentation. It is possible to use structurally diagnostic ions to screen for particular metabolites that may be present in a complex biological matrix. Metabolites can then be identified based on their full CID spectra (LEE and YOST 1988).

Tandem four-sector mass spectrometers can be extremely powerful for metabolite identification because of the high collision energies that can be used to induce structurally significant fragmentations. However, the triple-quadrupole instruments do have some significant advantages. First, they can be readily interfaced on-line with LC. Second, they can readily carry out scans for parents of selected daughter ions. In this mode, the second mass analyzer is fixed to transmit the daughter ions of interest and the first mass analyzer is scanned over a wide mass range to detect the parent ions for this daughter ion. A signal is obtained on the detector when a true parent ion is allowed to pass through the first mass analyzer and the appropriate daughter ion is transmitted through the second mass analyzer. This can be particularly useful when it is difficult to detect the molecular ions because of interfering peaks from the biological matrix. A combination of neutral loss and parent ion scans can be used to classify the number and type of primary metabolites and polar drug conjugates that are present in a complex sample matrix (STRAUB et al. 1987; LEE and YOST 1988). The resulting information can be used to assess the overall biotransformation routes that are available to a drug or other xenobiotic substance. These techniques in combination with CI MS/MS were used in the identification of an astonishing number of hydroxylated metabolites of the antischistosomal drug praziquantel (ALI et al. 1990a,b) and the identification of urinary metabolites of a new bronchodilator, MDL 257 (COUTANT et al. 1987).

When used in combination with CID, FABMS is a particularly powerful structural tool. FAB MS/MS was used in the characterization of oligo-nucleotide adducts of the antitumor drug cisplatin (MARTIN et al. 1991), to show that an impurity in the oxytocin antagonist atosiban contained 5-aminovaleric acid instead of a proline (BURINSKY et al. 1992), the identifi-cation of DNA adducts of phosphoramide mustard from the anticancer drug cyclophosphamide (CUSHNIR et al. 1990), the analysis of glutathione- and related S-linked conjugates of N-methylformamide (BAILLIE et al. 1989), the characterization of metabolites of the H_2-receptor antagonist mifentidine (KAJBAF et al. 1991), the analysis of metabolites from the antimuscarinic agent cimetropium bromide (KAJBAF et al. 1992; NAYLOR et al. 1992), and the identification of S-oxidized metabolites of the investigative calcium channel blocker AJ-2615 in rat plasma (KURONO et al. 1992). These reports illustrate the diverse applications of CID in combination with FAB and tandem MS that have appeared over the last 5 years. It is anticipated that ESI and ionspray techniques will make an equally valuable contribution to the field of drug disposition over the next 5 years.

An interesting application of CID involves the use of on-line continuous flow dialysis TSP coupled with tandem MS for quantitative screening of drugs in plasma (VAN BAKERGEM et al. 1992). The potential utility of the method was demonstrated by the quantitative analysis of the anticancer drug rogletimide in the plasma of patients after treatment. In vivo micro-dialysis and TSP tandem MS of the dopamine uptake blocker 1-[2-[bis(4-fluorophenyl)methoxy]ethyl]-4-(3-phenylpropyl)-piperazine (GBR-12909) was carried out in the rat (MENACHERRY and JUSTICE 1990). The maximum concentration of GBR-12909 in the brain for a dose of 100 mg/kg i.p. was determined to be 250 nmol/l with the maximal concentration occurring approximately 2 h post injection. This represents a 40-fold lower concentra-tion of GBR-12909 in the brain as compared to cocaine concentrations obtained at a dose of 30 mg/kg. The authors suggested that this could explain the discrepancy between relative in vivo and in vitro potencies of the two drugs. A combination of microdialysis and tandem FABMS was used to follow the pharmacokinetics of penicillin G directly in the bloodstream of a live rat (CAPRIOLI and LIN 1990). After intramuscular injection of the antibiotic, the blood dialysate was allowed to flow into the mass spectrometer via the continuous flow/FAB interface.

C. Chromatographic Techniques

I. Gas Chromatography/Mass Spectrometry

This mature technique does not generate the same excitement as new developments that involve the coupling of LC with MS. However, it remains a workhorse method that is used for carrying out quantitative determinations on a routine basis. The wide availability of robust fused capillary columns during the 1980s really revolutionized the field. Very complex separations can be carried out on these columns, and in conjunction with an autoinjector it is possible to routinely analyze thousands of samples with a high degree of precision and accuracy. Recent examples of the use of GC/EIMS in quantitative studies include: quantification of plasma and tissue tebufelone, a new anti-inflammatory drug (EICHHOLD and DOYLE 1990), quantification of the antiparkinsonian drug trihexyphenidyl in plasma using a mass-selective detector (DESAGE et al. 1991), and determination of plasma concentrations of the α-adrenoceptor agonist phenylpropanolamine in children (AMARK and BECK 1992).

There are a number of reports of the use of GC/EC NCIMS for the analysis of drugs. The sensitivity of analysis that can be obtained with this technique makes it very attractive for human pharmacokinetic studies, where samples are precious and limited amounts are available. Quantitative analyses of drugs in plasma that have been carried out by this technique include: the α_2-agonist S3341 (UNG et al. 1987), the tranquilizer fluphenazine (JEMAL et al. 1987), the α_2-agonist clonidine (HARING et al. 1988; GIRAULT and FOURTILLAN 1988), the HMG-CoA reductase inhibitor pravastatin (FUNKE et al. 1989), the glucocorticoid dexamethasone (GIRAULT et al. 1990b; KAYGANICH et al. 1990), 3-amino-1-phenylbutane, a metabolite of labetalol (CHANGCHIT et al. 1991), the antianaphylactic carbamazepine (WILDING et al. 1991), identification and determination of the antiarrhythmic agent ketotifen in plasma (LEIS and MALLE 1991), and the anxiolytic clebopride (ROBINSON et al. 1991).

Gas chromatography/EIMS was used in studies on the metabolism of the calcium antagonist felodipine in human subjects (NISHIOKA et al. 1991), studies on pharmacokinetics of the individual felodipine enantiomers in the dog after intravenous infusion of a pseudoracemic mixture (ERIKSSON et al. 1991), determination of plasma drug concentrations after a single oral administration of a suspension of the antiepileptic carbamazepine (WILDING et al. 1991), identification and determination of the antiarrhythmic agent propafenone and its metabolites (LELOUX and MAES 1991), determination of plasma concentrations of the anti-infective drug diethyldithiocarbamate (imuthiol) and its S-methyl metabolite (SCAPPATICCI et al. 1990), and quantification in human plasma of simvastatin, a pro-drug HMG-CoA reductase inhibitor and its active acid metabolite (TAKANO et al. 1990).

An interesting new method of sample preparation prior to GC/MS analysis was described recently (LIU et al. 1992). Supercritical fluid extraction was coupled with solid-phase extraction using octadecylsilane cartridges for the selective isolation of ultratrace levels of a drug metabolite, mebeverine alcohol, from plasma. The plasma was directly applied to the extraction cartridge; the cartridge was washed to remove protein and then extracted under supercritical conditions using $CO_2/5\%$ methanol. This rapid and reproducible extraction procedure allowed GC/MS analysis of the metabolite to be carried out with no interference from the biological matrix. Another efficient method for the purification of analytes prior to GC/MS analysis involves the use of immunoaffinity procedures. A recent report describes the use of this technique for cleanup of the PGI_2 mimetic ciprostene (KOMATSU et al. 1991). The anticiprostene antibody obtained from rabbit serum was coupled to an agarose support matrix. The isolated drug was converted to its PFB, TMS derivatives and analyzed by GC/EC NCIMS. The lower limit of quantitation was 50 pg/ml when 1 ml of human plasma was used.

The specificity that can be obtained with GC/MS makes it useful for structural confirmation of known compounds. For example, the structure of a peptide impurity in atosiban (a synthetic oxytocin antagonist) tentatively identified by FAB MS/MS was confirmed by the use of GC/MS (BURINSKY et al. 1992). GC/MS was also used in the analysis of DNA base modifications induced in isolated human chromatin by NADH dehydrogenase-catalyzed reduction of the anticancer agent doxorubicin (AKMAN et al. 1992). While new methods of MS can be useful in structural studies, GC/MS can also be very powerful. It is particularly useful in the structural characterization of drug metabolites that are not conjugated in vivo or that have been subsequently deconjugated using β-glucuronidase/arylsulfatase. The metabolic fate of the new angiotensin-converting enzyme inhibitor imidapril was determined by GC/MS (YAMADA et al. 1992). Four metabolites were detected in the plasma, bile, and urine of rats, dogs, and monkeys that had been dosed with imidapril. These four metabolites were isolated by LC and characterized by GC/MS. There was no evidence of any glucuronides or sulfates of drug-related compounds.

GC/MS can be extremely useful for quantitative determination of large numbers of metabolites. In a recent report, quantitative determination of valproic acid and 14 metabolites in serum and urine was carried out by GC/MS (FISHER et al. 1992). Metabolites were first of all converted to trimethylsilyl derivatives and then analysis was carried out by selected ion monitoring (SIM) with chromatography on a DB 1701 fused silica capillary column. The method can be used for screening patient serum and urine samples for unusual metabolite patterns. The authors suggest that this may have predictive value for early detection of liver injury. A GC/MS method has been reported for the quantification of debrisoquine (an in vivo marker for P-4502D6) and its metabolites in the urine of healthy individuals and patients with chronic renal failure (DAUMAS et al. 1991). SIM of the drug and the metabolites 4-hydroxydebrisoquine and 8-hydroxydebrisoquine. Ganoxan was used as the internal standard and the limit of detection was 200 ng/ml for each of the compounds. The healthy individuals and patients with chronic renal failure could be divided into two groups of extensive metabolizers and poor metabolizers, respectively. The extensive metabolizers excreted large amounts of 4-hydroxydebrisoquine and minor amounts of 8-hydroxydebrisoquine. Poor metabolizers excreted small amounts of the 4-hydroxy metabolite, and no 8-hydroxydebrisoquine was detected in the urine. Metabolites of the new thiazolidinedione hypoglycemic agent CP-68,722 isolated from rat urine were characterized by GC/MS (FOUDA et al. 1991a). Seven in vivo generated metabolites were isolated by HPLC. Capillary GC/MS analysis of the derivatives indicated that five metabolites result from hydroxylation and one from oxidation to the chromanone. The sites of metabolism were deduced from the EI spectra and authentic standards for five of the metabolites were synthesized. GC/MS was used to examine the effects of polytherapy with phenytoin, carbamazepine, and stiripentol on the formation of 4-enevalproate, a hepatotoxic metabolite of valproic acid (LEVY et al. 1990).

Metabolites of the widely used uricosuric drug benzbromarone (3,5-dibromo-4-hydroxyphenyl)-(2-ethyl-3-benzofuranyl)-ketone) were identified in urine samples from two different patients who attempted suicide with high doses of the drug (MAURER and WOLLENBERG 1990). After cleavage of conjugates and extraction from the urine, metabolites were acetylated and analyzed by GC/MS. Five metabolites were identified suggesting two major metabolic pathways: successive oxidation of the ethyl side chain and mono- and bis-hydroxylation of the benzofuran ring followed by methylation of one of the hydroxyl groups. Debrominated metabolites could not be detected, although the concentrations of benzbromarone and its metabolites were very high in the urine samples studied. GC/EIMS was used to examine deconjugated metabolites of the antianxiety agent buspirone in the rat (JAJOO et al. 1990a) and in human subjects (JAJOO et al. 1990b). An unusual observation was the presence of two metabolites that slowly interconverted in methanol solutions. The metabolites had identical EI mass spectra as TMS derivatives. From ^{1}H-NMR spectroscopy and total synthesis it was shown that the two derivatives arose from hydroxylation α- to the glutarimide carbonyl. The initially formed α-hydroxy metabolite then underwent rearrangement to an oxa-bicyclo lactone derivative.

Studies in enantioselective drug disposition are still being carried out by GC/MS even though chiral LC columns are widely available. This is most likely due to the robust nature of GC/MS assays and the ability to use heavy isotope internal standards. A recent report on the chiral disposition of the NSAID suprofen exemplifies the strategy that can be employed. A pseudo-racemic mixture containing equimolar mixtures of unlabeled-(R)-(−)- and $[^2H_3]$-(S)-(+)-suprofen [or unlabeled-(S)- and $[^2H_3]$-(R)-suprofen] was given to three healthy male subjects (SHINOHARA et al. 1990, 1991). Chiral deri-vatization was carried out with (S)-(−)-1-(naphthyl)ethylamine. Plasma con-centrations of the drug were then determined by GC/MS using $[^2H_7]$suprofen as an internal standard. In another pseudoracemate approach to chiral drug metabolism, analysis of hexobarbital and its enantiomers was carried out (PRAKASH et al. 1991). This method used the high sensitivity of EC NCI to quantify the plasma and urinary metabolites. Another interesting use of the high sensitivity of GC/EC NCIMS in chiral drug disposition has been re-ported in the assay of the chiral labetalol metabolite 3-amino-1-phenylbutane (CHANGCHIT et al. 1991). 3-Amino-1-phenylbutane isolated from the urine of subjects given labetalol was derivatized with the optically active acid chloride prepared from (S)-α-methoxy-α-trifluoromethylphenylacetic acid. The diastereomeric derivatives were separated by capillary GC and detected by EC NCIMS.

Tandem MS has not been used in many GC/MS assays probably because of limited instrument availability. However, there is one particular example where GC/MS/MS has been extremely robust and provided more than 3000 analyses over a 2-year period (DOBSON et al. 1990). The assay was devel-oped for analysis of the exploratory anti-inflammatory/antirheumatic agent tebufelone in plasma and involved the use of a stable isotope internal standard (^{13}C, ^{18}O-tebufelone) and minimal sample preparation. Chromato-graphy was carried out on 15 m fused silica capillary columns and SRM analysis was carried out on $M^{+\cdot}$ (m/z 300) → $[M^+-C_4H_4]$ (m/z 248) for the analyte and $M^{+\cdot}$ (m/z 303) → $[M^+-C_4H_4]$ (m/z 251) for the internal standard. The GC run time was minimized by the use of a high starting column temperature (200°C) and rapid column heating (25°C/min). The limit of quantitation was 1 ng/sample with less than 10% relative standard deviation in the range 1–3000 ng/sample. Tandem MS was also used in the GC/EC NCIMS analysis of the NSAID indomethacin (DAWSON et al. 1990). It was possible to detect down to 100 pg/ml with a high degree of precision using this method.

II. Liquid Chromatography/Mass Spectrometry

Reversed-phase LC has always played an important role in drug disposition studies because of the ease with which polar metabolites can be isolated and quantified using this technique. The need for on-line MS for structural characterization and specific quantification has driven the development of interfaces that can handle the flow of solvent into the mass spectrometer. In the past 10 years, significant progress has been made toward producing a reliable interface for LC. TSP, ESI, and ionspray are now all viable technologies with significant advantages and disadvantages (BOWERS 1989; HUANG et al. 1990; SMITH et al. 1990). Up until 1990 most laboratories involved in studies on drug disposition used TSP methodology. Pertinent published work on LC/TSP MS has been discussed above in the section on ionization techniques. In spite of improvements in continuous flow LSI interfaces there are still very few reports on the use of this technique in combination with LC/MS for drug disposition studies. The sensitivity of detection has not been able to compete with that found for TSP and more recently API-based techniques. For example KOKKONEN et al. (1991) described the use of LC continuous flow FAB/MS for the analysis of erythromycin-2'-ethylsuccinate, where the lowest level quantified was 105 ng/ml plasma.

Compared to TSP, API-based techniques appear to be more universal techniques. They are able to impart a high charge density to proteins and polypeptides, giving them m/z ratios in the range of quadrupole instruments. This has allowed MS analyses of macromolecules to be carried out on relatively low cost quadrupole instrumentation (FENN et al. 1990). Such exciting studies have to some extent overshadowed the potential of LC/API-based techniques for studies of drug disposition. The low flow rates of $1-2 \mu l/min$ that are required for ESI MS make the technique rather tedious when carried out in combination with LC. However, the related technique of ionspray can operate at much higher flow rates and so can be used with conventional microbore chromatography. This methodology is much better suited to the needs of laboratories involved in studies of drug disposition. Reports are now emerging in the literature on the use of LC/ionspray methodology for both quantitative and structural analyses.

Liquid chromatography/ionspray MS was used in quantitative studies on a second-generation HMG-CoA reductase inhibitor SQ 33,600 (WANG-IVERSON et al. 1992). The molecule contains a carboxylic acid, a phosphinic acid, and a hydroxyl group, making analysis by GC/MS a formidable task with at least three derivatization steps. Serum samples were extracted using a reversed-phase C_8 extraction cartridge and an analog with an additional fluorine on the indole ring was used as the internal standard. LC/MS was carried out using a reversed-phase C_{18} microbore column (100 mm $\times$ 1 mm) monitoring $[M-H]^-$ at m/z 442 for SQ 33,600 and m/z 460 for the internal standard. The limit of detection was 0.5 ng/ml and the minimum quantifiable limit was 1.6 ng/ml. The major problem encountered with the assay was occasional plugging of the inlet frit but some 500 injections were made on the microbore column without deterioration in the chromatography. LC ionspray/MS/MS was used to quantify the new NSAID drug tenidap in rat plasma (AVERY et al. 1992). Rats were dosed intravenously with tenidap or 3',4',5'-trideuterotenidap and plasma samples were collected. An analog was used as internal standard and samples were analyzed by SRM. Tenidap and its deuterated analog gave identical serum concentration profiles, demonstrating that there were no isotope effects.

An example of the use of LC/ionspray in the trace analysis of drugs is provided by studies on the polyether antibiotic semduramicin (SCHNEIDER et al. 1991). Sodium acetate was added to the LC mobile phase in order to induce the formation of a single metal adduct ion. SRM was carried out on the decompositions $[MNa]^+$ (m/z 896) → $[MNa-CO_2]^+$ (m/z 852) and $[MNa-CO_2-H_2O]^+$ (m/z 834). This allowed the identification of as little as 50 pg semduramicin. An elegant study using LC ionspray/MS/MS for the analysis of drug metabolites identified some 40 metabolites of omeprazole in rat urine (WEIDOLF and COVEY 1992). Rats were dosed with a 200 μmol/kg of 1:1 mixture of $[^{34}S]/[^{32}S]$omeprazole and the urine was collected. Conventional reversed-phase C_{18} column chromatography (150 mm × 4.6 mm) was carried out with a flow rate of 1 ml/min and 6:1 split into the API instrument. Approximately 8 μg of metabolites was allowed into the mass spectrometer. By analysis of the artificial isotope clusters it was possible to show the presence of more than 40 metabolites. Interestingly, it was possible to detect sulfate conjugates in the positive ion mode whereas most previous studies have employed negative ion techniques. The summed background-subtracted mass spectrum of the entire sample provided a representation of the entire metabolic pattern of pyridine metabolites, reductive demethylation, oxygenation products, sulfoconjugates, and glucuronides. This approach also has potential value in drug development when searching for compounds that are resistant to metabolism.

In APCI a heated nebulizer coupled with a corona discharge is used to cause ionization of analytes eluting in the mobile phase from an LC system (HUANG et al. 1990). Rapid desolvation of the nebulized droplets minimizes fragmentation or thermal decomposition and provides abundant protonated molecular ions. An impressive demonstration of the use of this technique in the quantification of drugs in plasma was reported by FOUDA et al. (1991b). More than 4000 analyses of the experimental renin inhibitor CP-80,794 in serum were carried out. Concentrations as low as 50 pg/ml serum were quantified with a coefficient of variation of 7.7%. The limited linear dynamic range of APCI was overcome by the use of two different standard curves for serum concentrations in the range 0.05–10 ng/ml. Quantitative determinations of L-365,260, a new cholecystokinin receptor antagonist, were carried out in the range 1–200 ng/ml by LC APCI/MS/MS (GILBERT et al. 1992). High specificity of analysis was obtained with run times of only 1 min. Precision below 1 ng/ml was not evaluated but it was possible to detect as little as 1 pg/ml with a signal–noise ratio of 10:1. This level of sensitivity is approaching that observed with EC NCIMS and suggests that APCI methodology will be applied to trace analysis of drugs in the future.

D. Metabolism Studies

I. In Vitro Studies

Polar conjugates of drugs and their metabolites can be prepared by synthesis or from in vitro incubations. The synthesis of glucuronides can be challenging whereas sulfates can be prepared relatively easily (KASPERSEN and VAN BOECKEL 1987). Unusual N-glucuronides of the calcium channel antagonists gallopamil and verapamil were synthesized in an elegant study by MUTLIB and NELSON (1990b). FAB mass spectra of the conjugates were obtained and characteristic ions were found in the FAB mass spectra of glucuronides isolated from the bile of rats dosed with gallopamil and verapamil. Fortunately, glucuronides can also be readily prepared in vitro. For example, glucuronides of the new antiepileptic agent lamotrigine (MAGDALOU et al. 1992), the neuroleptic fluphenazine (JACKSON et al. 1991), the anti-AIDS drug azidodeoxythymidine (AZT) (HAUMONT ET AL. 1990; GOOD et al. 1990), and the combined α-and β-adrenoceptor antagonist labetalol (NIEMEIJER et al. 1991) were prepared by UDPGA-fortified microsomal preparations. The lamotrigine glucuronide was unusual in that glucuronidation occurred at N^2 of the triazine ring, which led to the formation of a quaternary glucuronide. Glutathione conjugates can be prepared either synthetically (PEARSON et al. 1988; RASHED et al. 1989) or by the use of immobilized glutathione transferases (DULIK and FENSELAU 1987; DULIK et al. 1990). The availability of these conjugates has allowed their mass spectral characteristics to be examined so that they can then be identified from in vivo metabolism studies.

In addition to the preparation of conjugates, in vitro studies can be useful for helping to establish the primary routes of metabolism of a particular drug. Perfused rat liver preparations have provided valuable information on the metabolism of the nootropic drug ethimizol (BEZEK et al. 1990) and the antileishmanial drug WR6026 (SHIPLEY et al. 1990). MS was used in metabolite identification. Ethimizol gave some nine metabolites of which seven were characterized by MS, whereas WR6026 gave at least 13 metabolites of which six were identified and two partially identified. Two glucuronide conjugates were identified as a major metabolite of the anticancer drug etoposide by negative FABMS (HANDE et al. 1988).

Hepatocytes and microsomes can also provide information on pathways of metabolism that occur in vivo (JAJOO et al. 1990b). The immunosuppressive agent FK506, a 23-member macrolide, was shown to produce two metabolites when incubated with human microsomes (CHRISTIANS et al. 1991a). However, these were eventually shown to be different conformers with the same structure. The negative FAB mass spectrum of the metabolite showed a molecular ion at m/z 766, indicating that it was simply a demethylation product although it was not possible to determine which of the seven methyl groups had been lost. Rat hepatocytes were used in a study of the metabolism of the NSAID ibuprofen and the contents of the cells and media were analyzed by a stereoselective GC/MS assay (SANINS et al. 1990). When (R)-(−)-ibuprofen was incubated with the hepatocytes its concentration declined in an apparent first-order manner with the concomitant formation of metabolites. It was also shown to undergo a chiral inversion to the (S)-(+)-enantiomer. The (S)-(+)-enantiomer was not converted to the (R)-(−)-enantiomer, indicating that chiral inversion was unidirectional in these cells. Microsomal incubations coupled with mass spectral analysis of products has also been carried out for the anticancer drug etoposide (HAIM et al. 1987), the HMG-CoA reductase inhibitor lovastatin (VYAS et al. 1990), the H$_2$-receptor antagonist mifentidine (KAJBAF et al. 1991), the antipsychotic drug tiospirone (JAJOO et al. 1990), the anthelmintic drug praziquantel (HOGEMANN et al. 1990), the antifertility drug norgestimate (MADDEN and BACK 1991), and the calcium channel blocker gallopamil (MUTLIB and NELSON 1990a). Primary metabolites of the important immunosuppressive drug cyclosporin isolated from human urine were shown to undergo further biotransformations when incubated with human liver microsomes (CHRISTIANS et al. 1991b). Five of the 14 new metabolites were characterized by FABMS.

In vitro studies have also been carried out in order to provide mechanistic support for proposed pathways of metabolism. Valproic acid metabolism has been extensively studied because of the wide use of the drug and its potential for causing fatal liver toxicity in a small number of cases. The metabolism of 2-n-propyl-4-pentenoic acid enantiomers, hepatotoxic metabolites of valproic acid, was studied in rat hepatocytes (PORUBEK et al. 1988). Striking differences were observed in biotransformations of the two enantiomers, indicating that they may have different hepatotoxic potential. Three recent studies have examined the metabolism of valproate by rat liver mitochondria. In two of these studies it was demonstrated that valproic acid undergoes metabolism through β-oxidation (LI et al. 1991; BJORGE and BAILLIE 1991). An unidentified metabolite observed in these studies was later shown by LSI MS/MS to be valproyl-AMP formed during the activation of valproic acid in rat liver (MAO et al. 1992). Aldehyde oxidase isolated from mouse liver cytosol was shown by in vitro studies to be involved in the oxidative metabolism of the antischistosomal agent niridazole (TRACY et al. 1991). The metabolic conversion of pentamidine, a drug effective against Pneumocystis carnii pneumonia in AIDS patients, was found to undergo N-hydroxylation in the supernatant of rat liver homogenate (BERGER et al. 1990). The glucuronide metabolite of AZT was isolated from rat and human liver microsomal incubations (CRETTON et al. 1990) and the formation of a toxic metabolite of AZT was demonstrated in rat hepatocytes and liver microsomes (CRETTON et al. 1991).

In vitro studies have also used MS to examine potential drug–drug interactions. For example, KHARASCH et al. (1991) demonstrated that the α$_2$-agonist dexmedetomidine inhibited metabolism of the anesthetic alfentanil whereas clonidine had no effect. There are few reports on the use of tissues other than those from the liver in drug metabolism studies that have employed MS. However, MADDEN et al. (1989) used intestinal mucosa from normal ileum or colon of patients undergoing resections to study the metabolism of the contraceptive steroid desogerol. It was shown using EIMS that the active 3-keto metabolite was actually formed in the mucosa. Glutathione conjugation of the secretory inhibitor methazolamide was shown to occur in the homogenate of bovine ciliary bodies (KISHIDA et al. 1990).

II. In Vivo Studies in Animal Models

Drug metabolism studies in animal models provide important information on the structures of metabolites prior to embarking on costly human studies. MS is used to provide confirmatory information if synthetic metabolites are available and to help in the structural characterization of novel metabolites. Most studies have employed off-line HPLC purification of urinary metabolites followed by mass spectral analysis. Surprisingly, in view of the recognized utility of soft ionization techniques, a majority of studies published over the last 5 years have employed EI for the structural characterization of metabolites. This probably reflects the availability of EI instrumentation coupled with the ease of operation in this mode. Seven plasma and urine metabolites of indeloxazine, a drug with antiamnesic and antihypoxic activity, were identified by EIMS in rats dosed with the drug (KAMIMURA et al. 1987). Some of the metabolites were excreted as glucuronide or glucose conjugates but no mass spectral data were obtained on these compounds. GC/MS analysis of the urinary metabolites of the cytoprotective drug arbaprostil allowed the identification of 96% of the urinary metabolites from the dog after intravenous administration of the drug (THORNBURGH et al. 1988). Major routes of metabolism were similar to those observed with endogenous eicosanoids. Two metabolites of MOTP, a platelet activating factor antagonist, were identified in rat and dog urine after dosing with the drug (KOBAYASHI et al. 1988). Seven deconjugated metabolites of the antianxiety glutarimide drug, buspirone, were identified in the urine and bile of rats dosed with the drug and ten minor metabolites were qualitatively identified (JAJOO et al. 1989a). More than 90% of the urinary metabolites of the anticlaudication agent pentoxifylline were identified by EIMS (BRYCE et al. 1989). Two urinary metabolites of the anticancer drug DTIC were identified in sarcoma-bearing mice (BENFENATI et al. 1989). Stable isotope ion cluster techniques were used to identify 12 urinary metabolites of cocaine in the rat (JINDAL and LUTZ 1989). The artificially created isotope cluster of "twin ions" greatly facilitated metabolite identification.

Metabolites of the methadone analog recipavrin were identified after deconjugation of urine from rats dosed with the drug (SLATTER et al. 1990). Mass spectral data are reported for some 17 metabolites. The difficulties associated with identification of an N-hydroxy metabolite subsequent to β-glucuronidase treatment are discussed in some detail. Workup conditions used in the assay would most likely have resulted in oxidation to a nitrone which could then undergo a Beckman rearrangement to give the identified formamide metabolite isolated from the deconjugated rat urine. This problem illustrates the need to analyze the intact glucuronides in a complex metabolic study such as this. Fifteen metabolites of the anticonvulsant drug stiripentol were identified in the urine of rats treated with the drug (ZHANG et al. 1990). The major pathway of metabolism involved hydroxylation of the methylenedioxy ring. The tricyclic antidepressant trimipramine was shown to undergo extensive metabolism in the rat (COUTTS et al. 1990). In this extremely thorough study, 20 metabolites were identified in the urine after hydrolysis with β-glucuronidase. Four major routes of metabolism were identified: aliphatic and aromatic hydroxylation and two different kinds of N-demethylation. Four new rat urinary metabolites of the potent anti-histamines tripelennamine and pyrilamine were identified by YEH (1990). The metabolites arose by N-dealkylation pathways most likely as a con-sequence of oxidation α- to the nitrogen atom undergoing N-dealkylation. An interesting mechanism for the depyridination of tripelennamine and pyrilamine is proposed that involves the formation of an oxazine inter-mediate. A new urinary hydroxylated metabolite of aprophen was identified in the rat (BROWN et al. 1991). The antiarrhythmic agent bucromarone was shown to undergo both O- and N-dealkylation in rats and mice (MAURIZIS et al. 1991).

A new thiazolidinedione hypoglycemic agent, CP-68,722, was shown to undergo biotransformation to seven metabolites in the rat (FOUDA et al. 1991a). Five of the metabolites arose by hydroxylation and one by oxidation of the chromone. Chlorpheniramine, a potent antihistamine, underwent extensive metabolism in the rat and was shown to form primarily hydroxy-lated metabolites (KASUYA et al. 1991). The new antiatherosclerotic agent CI-976 was shown to undergo both β- and ω-oxidation in the rat in a manner analogous to long chain fatty acids (WOOLF et al. 1991). A new *meta*-hydroxylated metabolite of the antiarrhythmic drug mexilitine was identified in the hydrolyzed urine of rats dosed with the drug (GRECH-BELANGER et al. 1991). Three metabolites of the new anticonvulsant drug felbamate that arose through oxidation and hydrolysis were identified in the rat, rabbit, and dog (YANG et al. 1991). Unchanged drug and metabolites were excreted mainly in the urine. In an extension of earlier in vitro studies, stable isotope methodology was used to investigate the mechanism by which (R)-$(-)$-ibuprofen undergoes chiral inversion in vivo in the rat (SANINS et al. 1991). The data were consistent with stereoselective formation of a CoA thioester of (R)-$(-)$-ibuprofen, conversion of this metabolite to an enolate tautomer which afforded a symmetrical intermediate through which racemization of ibuprofen occurred in vivo. Two novel N-oxide metabolites of metyrapone, a diagnostic drug used to test pituitary function, were identified in the urine of rats dosed with the drug (USANSKY and DAMANI 1992). The N-oxides were surprisingly stable under EI conditions and it was possible to observe molecular ions for both of the metabolites. A combination of EI and PCIMS was used in the identification of urinary metabolites of the calcium antagonists nisoldipine and diltiazem (SCHERLING et al. 1988; YEUNG et al. 1990) and imidapril, a new ACE inhibitor (YAMADA et al. 1992), in several animal models.

Thermospray analyses have been used predominantly in combination with on-line LC separations. These studies have allowed the identification of polar conjugates in urine, bile, and plasma without recourse to β-glucuronidase/arylsulfatase treatment. Multiple metabolites were observed in the urine and bile of rats treated with the anticancer agent trimetrexate (WONG BK et al. 1990). Pathways of metabolism that were identified using stable isotope labeled drug included N-dealkylation, O-dealkylation, hydroxylation, oxidation, glucuronidation, and sulfation. Urinary metabolites of the antihistamine pyrilamine were identified in the rat (KORFMACHER et al. 1990). TSP was used to confirm the structures of metabolites in rat and dog urine and bile after dosing with the anxiolytic enciprazine (SCATINA et al. 1991). Metabolites, excreted mainly in the bile, were formed by hydroxylation, O-dealkylation, and glucuronidation. The novel antiepileptic drug lamotrigine was shown to form two different N-glucuronides, one of which was resistant to β-glucuronidase from *Helix pomatia* (DOIG and CLARE 1991). The glucuronides were excreted in the urine of a number of animal species dosed with the drug. Carbovir, a carbocyclic guanosine derivative with in vitro activity against the AIDS virus, was shown to form a glucuronide, an acid derivative, and a small amount of a glucose conjugate (PATANELLA et al. 1990; WALSH et al. 1990). TSP was used in the analysis of metabolites of the analgesic pentamorphone (KESWANI et al. 1990). In an impressive metabolism study, 12 metabolites of the antimalarial arteether were identified in the plasma of rats dosed intravenously with the drug (CHI et al. 1991). The availability of 16 potential metabolites conferred a level of sophistication on this study rarely seen in the field. Metabolites arose through a complex multistep process but could be readily rationalized through standard metabolic processes. TSP was used to confirm the structure of retinoic acid metabolites in the monkey (KRAFT et al. 1991). It was possible to identify 13-*cis*- and all-*trans*-retinoyl glucuronide based on their protonated molecular ions and fragment ions. A combination of TSP and FAB was used in the identification of urinary metabolites of the benzazepine SKF 86466 in the dog (STRAUB et al. 1988). TSP and PCIMS were used in the identification of urinary metabolites of the anticonvulsant zonisamide in the rat (STIFF and ZEMAITIS 1990). A combination of TSP and GC/MS was used in the identification of metabolites from α-methylacetohydroxamic acids, potential antiasthmatic agents (WOOLLARD et al. 1991).

Liquid secondary ion methodology has been applied to the important emerging field of peptide drugs. An early example of the use of FAB was in establishing the molecular weights of 13 metabolites of the cyclic peptide cyclosporine in the rabbit (HARTMAN and JARDINE 1987). Three truncated peptide metabolites of the synthetic decapeptide RS-26306 were characterized by FAB/MS (CHAN et al. 1991). Initial FAB analyses were unsuccessful due to interfering substances derived from the biological matrix. However, hexyl ester formation allowed protonated molecular ions to be detected. The synthetic anticoagulant decapeptide MDL 28,050 underwent hydrolysis at four peptide bonds when administered to rats and metabolites were excreted in the urine (KNADLER et al. 1992). Six resulting peptides and a des-A impurity present in the drug, together with a metabolite derived from this impurity, were identified by continuous flow LSI/MS. An ether glucuronide of AZT was identified in monkey urine (GOOD et al. 1990). Urinary metabolites of the H_1-antagonist methapyrilene were identified in the rat (KELLY et al. 1990). Two biliary metabolites of irinotecan, a new antitumor agent, were identified in the rat (ATSUMI et al. 1991). The first characterization of intact sulfate and glucuronide metabolites of the neuroleptic fluphenazine was carried out by FAB/MS (JACKSON et al. 1991a). An interesting study on the metabolism of chlorpromazine N-oxide revealed that it could be reduced and excreted as an ether glucuronide in the bile of rats dosed with the drug (JAWORSKI et al. 1991). This is the first systematic study of N-oxide disposition that has been carried out with modern techniques of structural characterization. A combination of LSI and EIMS was used in metabolism studies on the anticancer agent crisnatol (PATEL et al. 1991) and the identification of urinary metabolites of the pro-drug (+)-chloro-5-(2,3-dihydrobenzofuran-7-yl)-7-methoxymethyloxy-3-methyl-2,3,4,5-tetrahydro-1H-3-benzapine, a D_1-antagonist in the rat (NORDHOLM et al. 1992). A combination of FAB and PCIMS was used in a study of the metabolism of taxol in the rat (MONSARRAT et al. 1990). Three major metabolites were identified in the bile. Two arose through hydroxylation of the aromatic residue and the other arose through saponification.

Although PCI has been used primarily in quantitative studies and in combination with other ionization techniques, there are two recent reports on its use in combination with tandem MS. Using this technique it was possible to identify 17 hydroxylated urinary metabolites of praziquantel in the rat (ALI et al. 1990a). The relative abundance of ten of these metabolites was then compared in the urine of normal and infected mice (ALI et al. 1990b). As noted above, reports of ionspray techniques for drug metabolism studies are just starting to appear in the literature (MUCK and HENION 1990; WEIDOLF and COVEY 1992). A combination of ionspray MS/MS and FAB/MS/MS was used to identify the major metabolites of the anticancer agent mitoxantrone in pig urine (BLANZ et al. 1991a).

III. In Vivo Studies in Humans

Human drug metabolism studies have made extensive use of EI methodology. Major metabolites of the anti-inflammatory toxicortol pivalate were identified in human urine (CHANOINE et al. 1987), as were metabolites of the antibacterial rifabutin (COCCHIARA et al. 1989), valproic acid (RETTENMEIER et al. 1989), the β_2-agonist ritodrine (BRASHEAR et al. 1990), benzbromarone (DE VRIES et al. 1989; MAURER and WOLLENBERG 1990), encainide (JAJOO et al. 1990c), the cognition enhancer DMPPA (FUJIMAKI et al. 1990), the β-antagonist 4'-methylthiopropranolol (WALLE et al. 1990), the anxiolytic difebarbamate (VACHTA et al. 1990), and the respiratory stimulant doxepram (COUTTS et al. 1991). Compared with animal model studiies there have been relatively few reports on the use of TSP for structural characterization. TSP was used in the identification of metabolites of dideoxycytidine (RUBIO et al. 1988), doxepin (SHU et al. 1990a), and rogletimide (POON et al. 1991b). Metabolites of the steroidal aromatase inhibitor 4-hydroxyandrost-4-ene-3,17-dione were identified in the urine of women dosed with the drug (POON et al. 1991a). The major routes of metabolism were through dehydrogenation, ketone reduction, reduction of the C-4, C-5 double bond, and hydroxylation at C-5.

LSI was used in a large number of studies that were focused on the identification of polar conjugates (SWEENY et al. 1987; MACRAE et al. 1990; LUO et al. 1991; KWOK et al. 1990; KASSAHUN et al. 1991; TANAKA et al. 1990; SHU et al. 1990b; SINZ and REMMEL 1991). FABMS provided fascinating data on 12 new cyclosporin metabolites present in human bile from liver-grafted patients being treated with cyclosporine (CHRISTIANS et al. 1991c). One of the metabolites was a glucuronide conjugate and the others arose primarily through oxidative metabolism. The monohydroxylated, carboxylated metabolite was found to be elevated in patients with cholestasis. An unusual reduced and hydroxylated metabolite of cyclosporine was identified in the urine of patients undergoing cyclosporine therapy (MEIER et al. 1990). FAB was also used to identify a new hydroxylated metabolite of diflunisal in human urine (MACDONALD et al. 1991). A combination of FAB and EI was used in the identification of metabolites of the H_2-antagonist etintidine (WONG FA et al. 1990) and the hypolipidimic drug fenofibrate (WEIL et al. 1990).

A majority of the published studies on human metabolism have used either EI or LSI techniques. However, as with animal studies, PCI has made a contribution in selected cases. In the metabolism of tiospirone it was found that sulfoxide and sulfone metabolites could be readily detected by PCI (JAJOO et al. 1990a). Evidence for oxidative activation of the anticancer agent mitoxantrone was obtained by PCI MS/MS (BLANZ et al. 1991b). GC/PCIMS provided an efficient method for profiling metabolites derived from phenobarbitone, primidone, and their N-methyl and N-ethyl derivatives (TRESTON and HOOPER 1992). PCI was used in combination with EI to examine the metabolism of alfentanil (MEULDERMANS et al. 1988) and to screen β-blockers and their metabolites in human urine (LELOUX and MAES 1990).

The difficulty often encountered in obtaining sufficient quantities of metabolites for profiling studies in human subjects has stimulated a number of studies using highly sensitive EC NCIMS methodology. Oxidative urinary metabolites of the antihypertensive agent labetalol were identified in human urine (GAL et al. 1988). Metabolites of rimantidine were identified (HOFFMAN et al. 1988). Valproic acid and 14 of its metabolites were quantified using four internal standards in human urine (KASSAHUN et al. 1989, 1990). A carbomylglucuronide of the antiviral agent ramantadine was identified in human urine (BROWN et al. 1990b). In an important study, HOFMANN et al. (1991) used GC/EC NCIMS to show that the mucolytic agent S-carboxymethyl-L-cysteine (CMC) was metabolized to thiodoglycolic acid, its sulfoxide, and (3-carboxymethylthio)lactic acid. Thus, CMC is not excreted as the sulfoxide or as its decarboxylation product. This careful study has provided compelling evidence that CMC does not undergo polymorphic sulfoxidation, as had been suggested previously.

There are several reports on the use of API-based techniques in human metabolism studies. The major metabolites of stanozolol in human urine were identified using LC APCI and ionspray/MS/MS (MUCK and HENION 1990). Conjugated metabolites were identified using the ionspray technique. The biotransformation of pravastatin in humans was studied using ESI MS (EVERETT et al. 1991). The parent drug was the major drug-related material found in the urine and at least 15 metabolites were also detected. None of the metabolites accounted for more than 6% of the dose but by careful use of ESI MS and NMR spectroscopy it was possible to provide structures for nearly all of them.

E. Pharmacokinetic Studies

I. Introduction

An enormous number of studies have employed MS to determine pharmacokinetic parameters and so it is possible to highlight only selected examples. Recent review articles have described the contribution of MS to pharmacokinetic studies in general (BAILLIE 1992) and to endocrine agents in particular (LONNING et al. 1992). PENG and CHIOU (1990) have provided detailed information on the requirements and pitfalls of MS in pharmacokinetic studies. The advantages and disadvantages of use of stable isotopes in pharmacokinetic investigations have been discussed by BROWNE (1990) and the use of stable isotope methodology in human pharmacokinetic studies of androgenic steroids has been discussed by SHINOHARA and BABA (1990). MS has also played a role in assessing phenotypic differences in drug metabolism. Two studies have described the use of MS for in vivo assessment of P-450 status (BAUMANN and JONZIER-PEREY 1988; GUILLUY et al. 1991). There is increasing interest in the use of microdialysis systems for obtaining pharmacokinetic information (LUNTE and SCOTT 1991) and MS is starting to make a contribution to this interesting field (CAPRIOLI and LIN 1990; MENACHERRY and JUSTICE 1990; CHANG et al. 1991; CELARDO et al. 1991).

II. Animal Models

Most pharmacokinetic studies on animal models have been carried out using HPLC analysis of radiolabeled or unlabeled drug. MS was used only in selected studies that generally involved stable isotope methodology. A sensitive and specific assay for imipramine and desipramine and their [^{2}H$_4$]analogs in rat plasma was developed using [^{2}H$_8$]analogs as internal standards (SASAKI and BABA 1988). The bioequivalence of labeled and unlabeled material was established so that more extensive pharmacokinetic studies could be carried out. A stable isotope dilution GC/MS assay was developed for the antihypertensive agent IP/66 using GC/EIMS (AGOSTINI et al. 1989). The assay was used to validate a less expensive and time-consuming HPLC assay. The quantitative significance of the N-demethylation pathway for ketamine in rats was assessed by intravenous administration of aromatic ring labeled [^{2}H$_2$]ketamine oral administration of unlabeled drug (LEUNG and BAILLIE 1989). Plasma ketamine and norketamine concentrations were determined by GC/EIMS and the fraction of drug subjected to N-demethylation was then calculated as 38.6% of the dose. The decrease in hepatic clearance of metoprolol caused by verapamil coadministration was investigated in dogs using a pseudoracemic approach (MURTHY et al. 1991). The greater inhibition of metabolic clearance by verapamil observed with (S)-metoprolol compared with (R)-metoprolol was ascribed to preferential inhibition of demethylation of the (S)-enantiomer. A study on the interaction of probenicid with AZT was carried out in a rat model (MAYS et al. 1991). Using FAB/MS it was demonstrated that the glucuronidation of AZT was inhibited by probenecid.

III. Humans

Most of the studies reported over the last 5 years have used a rather conservative approach to analysis. The two main techniques employed were GC/EIMS and GC/EC NCIMS. It will be interesting to see whether this trend will continue over the next 5 years now that access to reliable LC/MS techniques is available in most laboratories carrying out pharmacokinetic studies. In keeping with this conservative approach, most studies have examined normal volunteers. However, there are several reports on the use of MS for studies on patient populations undergoing drug therapy. The pharmacokinetics of 5-fluorouracil were examined in patients on a dose-escalation schedule (VAN GROENINGEN et al. 1988). The use of a logistic regression showed that clinical toxicity correlated with the plasma concentration–time curve for the parent drug. The penetration of valproate and its active metabolites into the CSF of children with epilepsy was determined by GC/MS (LOSCHER et al. 1988). CSF concentrations of valproate and its metabolites were correlated with total and free plasma concentrations but were always significantly lower than free plasma concentrations. A study on the neurotoxicity of high-dose busulfan in children with cancer employed stable isotope dilution methodology in combination with GC/EIMS to obtain concentrations of the drug in plasma and CSF (VASSEL et al. 1990). The observed dose-dependent toxicity (seizures) was prevented by co-administration of clonazepam. The clinical pharmacokinetic characteristics of prednisolone and of chlorambucil and its β-oxidized metabolite phenyl-acetic mustard (PAM) were studied in the plasma of 12 cancer patients (BASTHOLT et al. 1991). Prednimustone (a pro-drug for prednisolone and chlorambucil) or a regimen of prednisolone plus chlorambucil was given orally to the patients. Chlorambucil and PAM concentrations were determined by GC/MS whereas the prednisolone concentrations were determined by radioimmunoassay. It was found that chlorambucil and PAM persisted in the plasma much longer after prednimustone administration when compared with the combination of chlorambucil plus prednisolone. This may explain why the cytotoxic profile of prednimustone is different from that of the individual components. The clinical pharmacology of deoxyspergualin was examined in cancer patients (MUINDI et al. 1991) and all-*trans* retinoic acid in patients with acute promyelocytic leukemia (MUINDI et al. 1992). A successive decrease in peak plasma concentration was observed with retinoic acid together with a decrease in the area under the plasma concentration–time curve during continuous dosing. This phenomenon was observed previously with animal models and suggested that a discontinuous dosing regimen or the use of P-450 inhibitors may improve the clinical efficacy of the drug.

Three studies have examined the effect of liver or renal dysfunction on pharmacokinetic parameters of drugs. Patients with liver cirrhosis had increased plasma concentrations of the antidepressant amineptine compared with normal volunteers and decreased plasma concentrations of the major metabolite (TSACONAS et al. 1989). Nifedipine pharmacokinetics were examined in patients with hypertensive renal failure (ODAR-CEDERLOF et al. 1990). The plasma half-life and clearance of nifedipine were similar to those observed in normal subjects. Eight of nine patients became normotensive during treatment with normal doses of the drug. The bioavailability and kinetics of the new antiarrhythmic agent cibenzoline were examined in patients with normal and impaired renal function using ^{15}N-labeled drug (ARONOFF et al. 1991). A substantial decrease in clearance of the drug was observed in patients with renal failure.

Mass spectrometry methods have been used in a number of studies that examined variability in drug disposition. GC/MS was used to determine plasma and urine terbutaline concentrations in a study that showed there was no pharmacokinetic interaction between theophylline and terbutaline (JONKMAN et al. 1988). Intersubject variations in the pharmacokinetics of chlorpromazine were determined using a GC/MS assay (MIDHA et al. 1989). The increased formation of 4-ene-valproate, a hepatotoxic metabolite of valproic acid, during polytherapy phenytoin, carbamazepine, and stiripentol was demonstrated using a GC/MS assay (Levy et al. 1990). The systemic availability of carbamazepine when given by an osmotic pump was assessed using ^{15}N-labeled drug coupled with GC/MS analysis of plasma samples (Wilding et al. 1991). A pharmacokinetic interaction between propranolol and lovastatin was demonstrated using GC/EC NCIMS (Pan et al. 1991). Nonlinear pharmacokinetics of phenytoin were examined in detail by giving intravenous doses of ^{13}C^{15}N-phenytoin (Browne et al. 1992).

Stereoselective pharmacokinetics of several drugs have been examined using pseudoracemates in which one enantiomer is labeled with a stable isotope and the other is unlabeled. The parent enantiomers and their metabolites can then be detected based on their different masses. The pharmacokinetics and metabolism of a pseudoracemate of verapamil were evaluated after coadministration of cimetidine (Mikus et al. 1990). It was found that cimetidine interacted with both hepatic and renal elimination in a stereoselective manner. The increased plasma concentration of the more active verapamil enantiomer resulted in a more pronounced pharmacological effect. The inversion of suprofen enantiomers was studied by means of a pseudoracemate methodology in which an equal mixture of unlabelled (R)-(−) and [^{2}H$_3$]-(S)-(+)-suprofen was fed to normal volunteers (Shinohara et al. 1990, 1991). Plasma concentrations of (R)-(−)-suprofen were consistently higher than those of the (S)-(+)-enantiomer. (R)-(−)-suprofen was stereoselectively converted to the (S)-(+)-enantiomer. Enantioselective hexobarbital metabolism was studied using a pseudoracemic approach (Prakash et al. 1991). The pseudoracemate was fed to normal volunteers and plasma and urine were analyzed for the hexobarbital enantiomers and their metabolites as PFB derivatives by CC/EC NCIMS. Stereoselective disposition has also been examined by oral dosing of a racemic drug (methylphenidate) followed by chiral derivatization and GC/MS analysis (Aoyama et al. 1990). A similar approach was employed with the antiarrhythmic agent flecainide, except that analysis was carried out by a highly sensitive GC/EC NCIMS assay (Fischer et al. 1990).

A number of routine pharmacokinetic studies have been carried out using GC/EIMS analysis usually combined with stable isotope dilution methodology. Recent examples include: nitecapone, an inhibitor of catechol-O-methyl transferase (Ottoila et al. 1991), the calcium channel antagonist prenylamine (Paar et al. 1990), the anticancer agent imuthiol (Scappaticci et al. 1990), the antischistosomal agents metrifonate and dichlorovos (Villen et al. 1990), the antidepressant levoprotiline (Ackermann et al. 1991), and the NSAID diclofenac (Puppo et al. 1991). GC/PCIMS was used in the analysis of MK-287, a new platelet activating factor antagonist (Fisher et al. 1991), and in studies on the geometric isomerization of doxepin (Ghabrial et al. 1991). GC/EC NCIMS has been used in studies where high sensitivity is required. Recent examples include: clenbuterol, a bronchiolytic agent with β_2-selectivity (Girault et al. 1990a), the bronchodilators terbutaline and orciprenaline (Leis et al. 1990), the antianaphylactic agent ketotifen

(LEIS and MALLE 1991), the PGI$_2$ analog ciprostene (KOMATSU et al. 1991), and the α_2-agonist moxonidine (THEODOR et al. 1991). GC/NCIMS with N$_2$O as the reagent gas was used in the analysis of CGS 16617, a new angiotensin-converting enzyme inhibitor (GAUDRY et al. 1991).

F. Summary

It is evident from the enormous number of publications that have appeared over the last 5 years that MS plays a critical role in studies of drug disposition and pharmacokinetics. Particular emphasis appears to be given to the use of this technique with human studies. GC/EI and GC/EC NCI have been used in the majority of studies that require extensive quantitative analysis but there is a perceptible trend towards the introduction of LC-based techniques. TSP has never really reached the point where it is used as a routine tool. However, it appears that the two API techniques of ionspray and APCI have the sensitivity and stability for routine quantitative determinations. Reports are starting to appear in the literature on the use of these techniques in quantitative studies and so it is anticipated that pharmacokinetic studies will follow in the near future. The API-based techniques will probably take over from TSP as the LC method of choice for metabolism studies. There have been several reports on the coupling of capillary electrophoresis with APIMS for drug analysis (JOHANSSON et al. 1991). Whether this technique has practical utility for drug disposition studies remains to be fully tested. The power of tandem MS in combination with API ionization techniques has been aptly illustrated in the exciting study of WEIDOLF and COVEY (1992), where more than 40 metabolites were detected. However, a note of caution is probably required at this point: It is one thing to demonstrate that a metabolite is present, but to elucidate is exact structure and to determine what percentage of the dose is represented by this metabolite requires a considerable amount of additional work most likely requiring NMR spectroscopy and total synthesis.

Quantitative aspects of drug metabolism tend to get clouded in the rush to identify new structures. There is as yet no good way to quantify how much of an unknown metabolite is present from either GC/MS or LC/MS analysis. Metabolites may have quite different ionization characteristics so that very minor metabolites can be detected. The ground-breaking studies of ABRAMSON and his co-workers (CHACE and ABRAMSON 1990) on CRI/MS should go a long way towards helping to solve this problem. Finally, the introduction of matrix-assisted laser desorption/ionization time-of-flight MS (HILLENKAMP and KARAS 1991; CHAIT and KENT 1992) should impact significantly on our ability to detect macromolecular drugs such as proteins and targeted monoclonal antibodies (SIEGEL et al. 1991).

Acknowledgements. The support of Bristol-Myers Squibb and NIH grants GM31304 and ES00267 is gratefully acknowledged.

References

Abdel-Baky S, Giese RW (1991) Gas chromatography/electron capture negative-ion mass spectrometry at the zeptomole level. Anal Chem 63:2986–2989

Abramson FP (1990) Mass spectrometry in pharmacology. Methods Biochem Anal 34:289–347

Ackermann R, Kaiser G, Schueller F, Dieterle W (1991) Determination of the antidepressant levoprotiline and its N-desmethyl metabolite in biological fluids by gas chromatography/mass spectrometry. Biol Mass Spectrom 20:709–716

Agostini O, Moneti G, Bonacchi G, Fedi M, Manzini S (1989) Determination of the antihypertensive drug 1-[2-ethoxy-2-(3'-pyridyl)ethyl]-4-(2'-methoxyphenyl) piperazine (IP/66) in rat and human plasma by high-performance liquid chromatography and isotope dilution mass spectrometry. J Chromatogr 487:331–340

Akman SA, Doroshow JH, Burk TG, Dizdaroglu M (1992) DNA base modifications induced in human chromatin by NADH dehydrogenase-catalyzed reduction of doxorubicin. Biochemistry 31:3500–3506

Ali MH, Abramson FP, Ferrerolf DD, Cohn VH (1990a) Metabolism studies of the antischistosomal drug praziquantel using tandem mass spectrometry: distribution of parent drug and ten metabolites obtained from control and schistosome-infected mouse urine. Biomed Environ Mass Spectrom 19:186–190

Ali MH, Ferrerolf DD, Abramson FP, Cohn VH (1990b) Metabolism studies of the antischistosomal drug praziquantel using tandem mass spectrometry: qualitative identification of 17 hydroxylated metabolites from mouse urine. Biomed Environ Mass Spectrom 19:179–185

Amark P, Beck O (1992) Effect of phenylpropanolamine on incontinence in children with neurogenic bladders. A double-blind crossover study. Acta Paediatr 81:345–350

Anderegg RJ (1990) Mass spectrometry: an introduction. Methods Biochem Anal 34:1–89

Andrievsky GV, Sukhodub LF, Pyatigorskaya L, Boryak A, Limanskaya OY, Shelkovsky VS (1991) Direct observation of the alkylation products of deoxy-guanosine and DNA by fast atom bombardment mass spectrometry. Biol Mass Spectrom 20:665–668

Aoyama T, Kotaki H, Honda Y, Nakagawa F (1990) Kinetic analysis of enantiomers of threo-methylphenidate and its metabolite in two healthy subjects after oral administration as determined by a gas chromatographic-mass spectrometric method. J Pharm Sci 79:465–469

Aronoff G, Brier M, Mayer ML, Barbalas M, Aogaichi K, Sloan R, Brazzell R, Massarella J (1991) Bioavailability and kinetics of cibenzoline in patients with normal and impaired renal function. J Clin Pharmacol 31:38–44

Arpino P (1990) Combined liquid-chromatography mass spectrometry. Techniques and mechanisms of thermospray. Mass Spectrom Rev 9:631–669

Atsumi R, Suzuki W, Hakusui H (1991) Identification of the metabolites of irinotecan, a new derivative of camptothecin, in rat bile and its biliary excretion. Xenobiotica 9:1159–1169

Avery MJ, Mitchell DY, Falkner FC, Fouda HG (1992) Simultaneous determination of tenidap and its stable isotope analog in serum by high-performance liquid chromatography/atmospheric pressure chemical ionization tandem mass spectrometry. Biol Mass Spectrom 21:353–357

Baillie TA (1992) Advances in the application of mass spectrometry to studies of drug metabolism, pharmacokinetics and toxicology. Int J Mass Spectrom Ion Processes 118:289–314

Baillie TA, Jones JR (eds) (1989) Synthesis and applications of isotopically labelled compounds 1988. Elsevier, Amsterdam

Baillie TA, Adams WJ, Kaiser DG, Olanoff LS, Halsted GW, Harpootlian H, Van Giessen GJ (1989) Mechanistic studies of the metabolic chiral inversion of (R)-ibuprofen in humans. J Pharmacol Exp Ther 249:517–523

Barbalas MP, Garland WA (1991) A computer program for the deconvolution of mass spectral peak abundance data from experiments using stable isotopes. J Pharm Sci 80:922–927

Bastholt L, Johansson C-J, Pfeiffer P, Svensson L, Johansson S-A, Gunnarsson PO, Mouridsen H (1991) A pharmacokinetic study of prednimustine as compared with prednisolone plus chlorambucil in cancer patients. Cancer Chem Pharmacol 28:205–210

Baumann P, Jonzier-Perey M (1988) GC and GC-MS procedures for simultaneous phenotyping with dextromethorphan and mephenytoin. Clin Chim Acta 171:211–222

Beattie IG, Blake TJA (1978) The structural identification of drug metabolites using thermospray liquid chromatography/mass spectrometry. Biomed Environ Mass Spectrom 18:872–877

Benfenati E, Farina P, Colombo T, DeBellis G, Capodiferro MV, D'Incalci M (1989) Metabolism and pharmacokinetics of p-(3,3-dimethyl-1-triazeno)benzoic acid in M5076 sarcoma-bearing mice. Cancer Chemother Pharmacol 24:354–358

Beresford AP, Macrae PV, Alker D, Kobylecki RJ (1989) Biotransformation of amlodipine. Identification and synthesis of metabolites found in rat, dog and human urine/confirmation of structures by gas chromatography-mass spectrometry and liquid chromatography-mass spectrometry. Arzneimittelforschung 39:201–209

Berger BJ, Lombardy RJ, Marbury GD, Bell CA, Dykstra CC, Hall JE, Tidwell RR (1990) Metabolic N-hydroxylation of pentamidine in vitro. Antimicrob Agents Chemother 34:1678–1684

Beynon JH, Morgan RP (1978) The development of mass spectroscopy: an historical account. Int J Mass Spectrom Ion Physics 27:1–30

Bezek S, Kukan M, Kallay Z, Trnovec T, Stefek M, Piotrovskiy LB (1990) Disposition of ethimizol, a xanthine-related nootropic drug, in perfused rat liver and isolated hepatocytes. Drug Metab Dispos 18:88–95

Bjorge SM, Baillie TA (1991) Studies on the β-oxidation of valproic acid in rat liver mitochondrial preparations. Drug Metab Dispos 19:823–829

Blair IA (1990) Electron-capture negative-ion chemical ionization mass spectrometry of lipid mediators. Methods Enzymol 187:13–23

Blake TJ (1987) Structure elucidation of drug metabolites using thermospray liquid chromatography-mass spectrometry. J Chromatogr 394:171–181

Blanz J, Mewes K, Ehninger G, Proksch B, Greger B, Waidelich D, Zeller K-P (1991a) Isolation and structure elucidation of urinary metabolites of mitoxantrone. Cancer Res 51:3427–3433

Blanz J, Mewes K, Ehninger G, Proksch B, Waidelich D, Greger B, Zeller K-P (1991b) Evidence for oxidative activation of mitoxantrone in human, pig, and rat. Drug Metab Dispos 19:871–880

Bowers LD (1989) High-performance liquid chromatography/mass spectrometry: state of the art for the analysis laboratory. Clin Chem 35:1282–1287

Brashear WT, Kuhnert BR, Wei R (1990) Structural determination of the conjugated metabolites of ritodrine. Drug Metab Dispos 18:488–493

Brown ND, Phillips LR, Leader H, Chiang PK (1991) Isolation and identification of β-hydroxyethylaprophen: a urinary metabolite of aprophen in rats. J Chromatogr 563:466–471

Brown SY, Garland WA, Fukuda EK (1990a) Gas chromatography/negative chemical ionization mass spectrometry of intact glucuronides. Biomed Environ Mass Spectrom 19:32–36

Brown SY, Garland WA, Fukuda EK (1990b) Isolation and characterization of an unusual glucuronide conjugate of ramantadine. Drug Metab Dispos 18:546–547

Browne TR (1990) Stable isotopes in clinical pharmacokinetic investigations. Advantages and disadvantages. Clin Pharmacokinet 18:423–433

Browne TR, Szabo GK, Schumacher GE, Greenblatt DJ, Evans JE, Evans BA (1992) Bioavailability studies of drugs with nonlinear pharmacokinetics. I. Tracer dose AUC varies directly with serum concentration. J Clin Pharmacol 32:1141–1145

Bruins AP (1991) Mass spectrometry with ion sources operating at atmospheric-pressure. Mass Spectrom Rev 10:53–77

Bryce TA, Chamberlain J, Hillbeck D, Macdonald CM (1989) Metabolism and pharmacokinetics of ^{14}C-pentoxifylline in healthy volunteers. Arzneimittelforschung 39:512–517

Burinsky DJ, Dunphy R, Oyler AR, Shaw CJ, Cotter ML (1992) Characterization of a synthetic peptide impurity by fast-atom bombardment-tandem mass spectrometry and gas chromatography-mass spectrometry. J Pharm Sci 81:597–600

Burlingame AL, McCloskey JA (eds) (1990) Biological mass spectrometry. Elsevier, Amsterdam

Burlingame AL, Millington DS, Norwood DL, Russell DH (1990) Mass spectrometry. Anal Chem 62:268R–303R

Burlingame AL, Baillie TA, Russell DH (1992) Mass spectrometry. Anal Chem 64:467R–502R

Caprioli RM (1990a) Continuous-flow fast atom bombardment mass spectrometry. Anal Chem 62:477A–485A

Caprioli RM (ed) (1990b) Continuous-flow fast atom bombardment mass spectrometry. Wiley, New York

Caprioli RM, Lin S-N (1990) On-line analysis of penicillin blood levels in the live rat by combined microdialysis/fast-atom bombardment mass spectrometry. Proc Natl Acad Sci USA 87:240–243

Carr SA, Hemling ME, Bean MF, Roberts GD (1991) Integration of mass spectrometry in analytical biotechnology. Anal Chem 63:2802–2824

Celardo A, Dell'Elba G, Frassanito R (1991) Simultaneous determination of isbufylline and its major metabolites in rabbit blood and urine by reversed-phase high-performance liquid chromatography. J Chromatogr 568:407–418

Chace DH, Abramson FP (1990) Isotope dilution studies: determination of carbon-13, nitrogen-15 and deuterium-enriched compounds using capillary gas chromatography-chemical reaction interface/mass spectrometry. Biomed Environ Mass Spectrom 19:117–122

Chait BT, Kent SBH (1992) Weighing naked proteins: practical, high-accuracy mass measurement of peptides and proteins. Science 257:1885–1894

Chan RL, Hsieh SC, Haroldsen PE, Ho W, Nestor JJ Jr (1991) Disposition of RS-26306, a potent luteinizing hormone-releasing hormone antagonist, in monkeys and rats after single intravenous and subcutaneous administration. Drug Metab Dispos 19:858–864

Chang SY, Moore TA, Devaud LL, Taylor CE, Hollingsworth EB (1991) Analysis of rat brain microdialysate by gas chromatography-high-resolution selected-ion monitoring mass spectrometry. J Chromatogr 562:111–118

Changchit A, Gal J, Zirrolli JA (1991) Stereospecific gas chromatographic/mass spectrometric assay of the chiral labetalol metabolite 3-amino-1-phenylbutane. Biol Mass Spectrom 20:751–758

Chanoine F, Grenot C, Sellier N, Barrett WE, Thompson RM, Fentiman AF, Nixon JR, Goyer R, Junien JL (1987) Isolation and identification of major metabolites to tixocortol pivalate in human urine. Drug Metab Dispos 15:868–876

Chen T-M, Chan KY, Coutant JE, Okerholm RA (1991) Determination of the metabolites of terfenadine in human urine by thermospray liquid chromatography-mass spectrometry. J Pharm Biomed Anal 9:929–933

Chi HT, Ramu K, Baker JK, Hufford CD, Lee I-S (1991) Identification of the in vivo metabolites of the antimalarial arteether by thermospray high-performance liquid chromatography/mass spectrometry. Biol Mass Spectrom 20:609–628

Christians U, Radeke H, Kownatzki R, Schiebel HM, Schottmann R, Sewing K-F
    (1991a) Isolation of an immunosuppressive metabolite of FK506 generated by
    human microsome preparations. Clin Biochem 24:271–275
Christians U, Strohmeyer S, Kownatzki R, Schiebel H-M, Bleck J, Greipel J,
    Kohlhaw K, Schottmann R, Sewing K-F (1991b) Investigations on the metabolic
    pathways of cyclosporine. I. Excretion of cyclosporine and its metabolites in
    human bile-isolation of 12 new cyclosporine metabolites. Xenobiotica 21:1185–
    1198
Christians U, Strohmeyer S, Kownatzki R, Schiebel H-M, Bleck J, Kohlhaw K,
    Schottmann R, Sewing K-F (1991c) Investigations on the metabolic pathways of
    cyclosporine. II. Elucidation of the metabolic pathways in vitro by human liver
    microsomes. Xenobiotica 21:1199–1210
Cocchiara G, Benedetti MS, Vicario GP, Ballabio M, Gioia B, Vioglio S, Vigevani
    A (1989) Urinary metabolites of rifabutin, a new antimycobacterial agent, in
    human volunteers. Xenobiotica 19:769–780
Cottrell JS, Evans S (1987) Characteristics of a multichannel electrooptical detection
    system and its application to the analysis of large molecules by fast atom
    bombardment mass spectrometry. Anal Chem 59:1990–1995
Coutant JE, Barbuch RJ, Satonin DK, Cregge RJ (1987) Identification in man of
    urinary metabolites of a new bronchodilator, MDL 257, using triple stage
    quadrupole mass spectrometry-mass spectrometry. Biomed Environ Mass
    Spectrom 14:325–330
Coutts RT, Hussain MS, Micetich RG, Daneshtalab M (1990) The metabolism of
    trimipramine in the rat. Biomed Environ Mass Spectrom 19:793–806
Coutts RT, Jamali F, Malek F, Peliowski A, Finer NN (1991) Urinary metabolites of
    doxapram in premature neonates. Xenobiotica 21:1407–1418
Cretton EM, Waterhous DV, Bevan R, Sommadossi J-P (1990) Glucuronidaation of
    3'-azido-3'-deoxythymidine by rat and human liver microsomes. Drug Metab
    Dispos 18:369–372
Cretton EM, Xie M-Y, Bevan RJ, Goudgaon NM, Schinazi RF, Sommadossi J-P
    (1991) Catabolism of 3'-azido-3'-deoxythymidine in hepatocytes and liver micro-
    somes, with evidence of formation of 3'-amino-3'-deoxythymidine, a highly toxic
    catabolite for human bone marrow cells. Mol Pharmacol 39:258–266
Cushnir JR, Naylor S, Lamb JH, Farmer PB, Brown NA, Mirkes PE (1990)
    Identification of phosphoramide mustard/DNA adducts using tandem spectro-
    metry. Rapid Commun Mass Spectrom 4:410–414
Daumas L, Sabot J-F, Vermeulen E, Clapot P, Allegre F, Pinatel H (1991) Deter-
    mination of debrisoquine and metabolites in human urine by gas chromatography-
    mass spectrometry. J Chromatogr 570:89–97
Dawson M, Smith MD, McGee CM (1990) Gas chromatography/negative ion chemi-
    cal ionization/tandem mass spectrometric quantification of indomethacin in
    plasma and synovial fluid. Biomed Environ Mass Spectrom 19:453–458
Debrauwer L, Bories G (1992) Electrospray ionization mass spectrometry of some β-
    agonists. Rapid Commun Mass Spectrom 6:382–387
Desage M, Rousseau-Tsangaris M, Lecompte D, Brazier JL (1991) Quantification of
    trihexyphenidyl from plasma using a mass-selective detector and electron-impact
    ionization. J Chromatogr 571:250–256
De Vries JX, Walter-Sack I, Ittensohn A, Weber E (1989) The isolation, identification
    and structure of a new hydroxylated metabolite of benzbromarone in man.
    Xenobiotica 19:1461–1470
Dobson RLM, Neal DM, DeMark BR, Ward SR (1990) Long-term performance of
    a gas chromatography/tandem mass spectrometry assay for tebufelone in plasma.
    Anal Chem 62:1819–1824
Doig MV, Clare RA (1991) Use of the thermospray liquid chromatography-mass
    spectrometry to aid in the identification of urinary metabolites of a novel
    antiepileptic drug, Lamotrigine. J Chromatogr 554:181–189

Dole M, Mack LL, Hines RL (1968) Molecular beams of macroions. J Chem Phys 49:2240–2249

Dulik DM, Fenselau C (1987) Conversion of melphalan to 4-(glutathionyl)phenylalanine. A novel mechanism for conjugation by glutathione-S-transferases. Drug Metab Dispos 15:195–199

Dulik DM, Colvin OM, Fenselau C (1990) Characterization of glutathione conjugates of chlorambucil by fast atom bombardment and thermospray liquid chromatography/mass spectrometry. Biomed Environ Mass Spectrom 19:248–252

Eckhoff C, Wittfoht W, Nau H, Slikker W Jr (1990) Characterization of oxidized and glucuronidated metabolites of retinol in monkey plasma by thermospray liquid chromatography/mass spectrometry. Biomed Environ Mass Spectrom 19:428–433

Eichhold TH, Doyle MJ (1990) Determination of tebufelone, a new anti-inflammatory drug, in plasma and tissue using capillary gas chromatography-stable isotope dilution mass spectrometry. Biomed Environ Mass Spectrom 19:230–234

Eriksson UG, Hoffmann K-J, Simonsson R, Regardh CG (1991) Pharmacokinetics of the enantiomers of felodipine in the dog after oral and intravenous administration of a pseudoracemic mixture. Xenobiotica 21:75–84

Everett DW, Chando TJ, Didonato GC, Singhvi SM, Pan HY, Weinstein SH (1991) Biotransformation of pravastatin sodium in humans. Drug Metab Dispos 19:740–748

Felder TB, McLean MA, Vestal ML, Lu K, Farquhar D, Legha SS, Shah R, Newman RA (1987) Pharmacokinetics and metabolism of the antitumor drug amonafide (NSC-308847) in humans. Drug Metab Dispos 15:773–778

Fenn JB, Mann M, Meng CK, Wong SF, Whitehou CM (1990) Electrospray ionization – principles and practice. Mass Spectrom Rev 9:37–70

Fenselau C (1992) Tandem mass spectrometry: the competitive edge for pharmacology. Annu Rev Pharmacol Toxicol 32:555–578

Fischer C, Schonberger F, Meese CO, Eichelbaum M (1990) Determination of the enantiomers of flecainide and two major metabolites in man by gas chromatography/mass spectrometry using negative ion chemical ionization and stable isotope labelled internal standards. Biomed Environ Mass Spectrom 19:256–266

Fisher AL, Morris MJ, Gilbert JD (1991) Determination of MK-287, a new platelet-activating factor antagonist, in plasma and serum by gas chromatography chemical ionization mass spectrometry. Biol Mass Spectrom 20:408–414

Fisher E, Wittfoht W, Nau H (1992) Quantitative determination of valproic acid and 14 metabolites in serum and urine by gas chromatography/mass spectrometry. Biomed Chromatogr 6:24–29

Fouda HG, Lukaszewicz J, Clark DA, Hulin B (1991a) Metabolism of a new thiazolidinedione hypoglycemic agent CP-68,722 in rat: metabolite identification by gas chromatography mass spectrometry. Xenobiotica 21:925–934

Fouda HG, Nocerini M, Schneider R, Gedutis C (1991b) Quantitative analysis by high-performance liquid chromatography atmospheric pressure chemical ionization mass spectrometry: the determination of the renin inhibitor CP-80,794 in human serum. J Am Soc Mass Spectrom 2:164–167

Fujimaki Y, Hashimoto K, Sudo K, Tachizawa H (1990) Biotransformation of a new pyrrolidinone cognition-enhancing agent: isolation and identification of metabolites in human urine. Xenobiotica 20:1081–1094

Funke PT, Ivashkiv E, Arnold ME, Cohen AI (1989) Determination of pravastatin sodium and its major metabolites in human serum/plasma by capillary gas chromatography/negative ion chemical ionization mass spectrometry. Biomed Environ Mass Spectrom 18:904–909

Gal J, Zirrolli JA, Lichtenstein PS (1988) Labetalol is metabolized oxidatively in humans. Res Commun Chem Pathol Pharmacol 62:3–17

Garland WA, VandenHeuvel V (eds) (1992) Mass spectrometry in pharmaceutical research: current boundaries and future frontiers. Wiley, New York

Gaudry D, Hayes M, Khemani L, Miotto J, Alkalay D (1991) Determination of CGS 16617 and stable isotope-labeled CGS 16617, an angiotensin-converting enzyme inhibitor, in human plasma by gas chromatography/mass spectrometry. Biol Mass Spectrom 20:26–30

Ghabrial H, Prakash C, Tacke UG, Blair IA, Wilkinson GR (1991) Geometric isomerization of doxepin during its N-demethylation in humans. Drug Metab Dispos 19:596–599

Gilbert JD, Hand EL, Yuan AS, Olah TV, Covey TR (1992) Determination of L-365,260, a new cholecystokinin receptor (CCK-B) antagonist, in plasma by liquid chromatography/atmospheric pressure chemical ionization mass spectrometry. Biol Mass Spectrom 21:63–68

Girault J, Fourtillan JB (1988) Quantitative measurement of clonidine in human plasma by combined gas chromatography/electron capture negative ion chemical ionization mass spectrometry. Biomed Environ Mass Spectrom 17:443–448

Girault J, Gobin P, Fourtillan JB (1990a) Quantitative measurement of clenbuterol at the femtomole level in plasma and urine by combined gas chromatography/negative ion chemical ionization mass spectrometry. Biomed Environ Mass Spectrom 19:80–88

Girault J, Istin B, Fourtillan JB (1990b) A rapid and highly sensitive method for the quantitative determination of dexamethasone in plasma, synovial fluid and tissues by combined gas chromatography/negative ion chemical ionization mass spectrometry. Biomed Environ Mass Spectrom 19:295–302

Good SS, Koble CS, Crouch R, Johnson RL, Rideout JL, Miranda PD (1990) Isolation and characterization of an ether glucuronide of zidovudine, a major metabolite in monkeys and humans. Drug Metab Dispos 18:321–326

Gouyette A, Deniel A, Pico JL, Droz JP, Baume D, Ostronoff M, Bail N-L, Hayat M (1987) Clinical pharmacology of high-dose etoposide associated with cisplatin. Pharmacokinetic and metabolic studies. Eur J Cancer Clin Oncol 23:1627–1632

Grech-Belanger O, Turgeon J, Lalande M, Belanger PM (1991) Meta-hydroxymexiletine, a new metabolite of mexiletine. Isolation, characterization, and species differences in its formation. Drug Metab Dispos 19:458–461

Gross ML (ed) (1992) Mass spectrometry in the biological sciences: a tutorial. Kluwer, Dordrecht

Guilluy R, Billion-Rey F, Brazier JL (1991) On-line measurements of ^{13}C enrichments in rat breath. Non-invasive method for in vivo study of drug enzymatic induction. J Chromatogr 562:341–350

Haim N, Nemec J, Roman J, Sinha BK (1987) In vitro metabolism of etoposide (VP-16-213) by liver microsomes and irreversible binding of reactive intermediates to microsomal proteins. Biochem Pharmacol 36:527–536

Hamdan M, Curcuruto O (1991) Development of the electrospray ionisation technique. Int J Mass Spectrom Ion Processes 108:93–113

Hande K, Anthony L, Hamilton R, Bennett R, Sweetman B, Branch R (1988) Identification of etoposide glucuronide as a major metabolite of etoposide in the rat and rabbit. Cancer Res 48:1829–1834

Haring N, Salama Z, Reif G, Jaeger H (1988) Gas chromatography/mass spectrometric determination of clonidine in body fluids. Arzneimittelforschung 38:404–407

Haroldsen PE, Reilly MH, Hughes H, Gaskell SJ (1988) Characterization of glutathione conjugates by fast atom bombardment/tandem mass spectrometry. Biomed Environ Mass Spectrom 15:615–621

Hartman NR, Jardine I (1987) The in vitro activity, radioimmunoassay cross-reactivity, and molecular weight of thirteen rabbit cyclosporine metabolites. Drug Metab Dispos 15:661–664

Haumont M, Magdalou J, Lafaurie C, Ziegler J-M, Siest G, Colin J-N (1990) Phenobarbital inducible UDP-glucuronosyltransferase is responsible for glucuronidation of 3'-azido-3'-deoxythymidine: characterization of the enzyme in human and rat liver microsomes. Arch Biochem Biophys 281:264–270

Heeremans CEM, Stijnen AM, VanDerHoeven RAM, Niessen WMA, Danhof M, VanDerGreef J (1991) Liquid chromatography-thermospray tandem mass spectrometry for identification of a heptabarbital metabolite and sample work-up artefacts. J Chromatogr 554:205–214

Hill JA, Biller JE, Biemann K (1991) A variable dispersion array detector for a tandem mass spectrometer. Int J Mass Spectrom Ion Processes 111:1–25

Hillenkamp F, Karas M, Beavis RC, Chait BT (1991) Matrix-assisted laser desorption/ ionization mass spectrometry of biopolymers. Anal Chem 63:1193A–1202A

Hoffman HE, Gaylord JC, Blasecki JW, Shalaby LM, Whitney CC Jr (1988) Pharmacokinetics and metabolism of rimantadine hydrochloride in mice and dogs. Antimicrob Agents Chemother 32:1699–1704

Hoffmann K-J, Baillie TA (1988) The use of alkoxycarbonyl derivatives for the mass spectral analysis of drug-thioether metabolites. Studies with the cysteine, mercapturic acid and glutathione conjugates of acetaminophen. Biomed Environ Mass Spectrom 15:637–647

Hofmann U, Eichelbaum M, Seefried S, Meese CO (1991) Identification of thiodiglycolic acid, thiodiglycolic acid sulfoxide, and (3-carboxymethylthio)lactic acid as major human biotransformation products of S-carboxymethyl-L-cysteine. Drug Metab Dispos 19:222–226

Hogemann A, Kiec-Kononowicz K, Westhoff F, Blashke G (1990) Microsomal oxidation of praziquantel. Arzneimittelforschung 40:1159–1162

Huang EC, Henion JD (1991) Packed-capillary liquid chromatography/ion-spray tandem mass spectrometry determination of biomolecules. Anal Chem 63:732–739

Huang EC, Wachs T, Conboy JJ, Henion JD (1990) Atmospheric pressure ionization mass spectrometry. Detection for the separation sciences. Anal Chem 62:713A–725A

Iwabuchi H, Nakagawa A, Nakamura K-I (1987) Application of molecular-secondary-ion mass spectrometry for drug metabolism studies. I. Direct analysis of conjugates by thin-layer chromatography-secondary-ion mass spectrometry. J Chromatogr 414:139–148

Jackson C-JC, Hubbard JW, Midha KK (1991a) Biosynthesis and characterization for glucuronide metabolites of fluphenazine: 7-hydroxyfluphenazine glucuronide and fluphenazine glucuronide. Xenobiotica 21:383–393

Jackson C-JC, Hubbard JW, McKay G, Cooper JK, Hawes EM, Midha KK (1991b) Identification of phase-I and phase-II metabolites of fluphenazine in rat bile. Drug Metab Dispos 19:188–193

Jacobs PL, Delbressine LPC, Kaspersen FM, Schmeits GJH (1987) A mass spectrometric approach to the identification of conjugated drug metabolites. Biomed Environ Mass Spectrom 14:689–697

Jajoo HK, Mayol RF, LaBudde JA, Blair IA (1989a) Metabolism of the antianxiety drug buspirone in the rat. Drug Metab Dispos 17:625–633

Jajoo HK, Mayol RF, LaBudde JA, Blair IA (1989b) Metabolism of the antianxiety drug buspirone in human subjects. Drug Metab Dispos 17:634–640

Jajoo HK, Blair IA, Klunk LJ, Mayol RF (1990a) Characterization of in vitro metabolites of the antipsychotic drug tiospirone by mass spectrometry. Biomed Environ Mass Spectrom 19:281–285

Jajoo HK, Blair IA, Klunk LJ, Mayol RF (1990b) In vitro metabolism of the antianxiety drug buspirone as a predictor of its metabolism in vivo. Xenobiotica 20:779–786

Jajoo HK, Mayol RF, LaBudde JA, Blair IA (1990c) Structural characterization of urinary metabolites of the antiarrhythmic drug encainide in human subjects. Drug Metab Dispos 18:28–35

Jaworski TJ, Hawes EM, Hubbard JW, McKay G, Midha KK (1991) The metabolites of chlorpromazine N-oxide in rat bile. Xenobiotica 21:1451–1459

Jemal M, Ivashkiv E, Both D, Koski R, Cohen AI (1987) Picogram level determination of fluphenazine in human plasma by automated gas chromatography/mass selective detection. Biomed Environ Mass Spectrom 14:699–704

Jindal SP, Lutz T (1989) Mass spectrometric studies of cocaine disposition in animals and humans using stable isotope-labeled analogues. J Pharm Sci 78:1009–1014

Johansson IM, Pavelka R, Henion JD (1991) Determination of small drug molecules by capillary electrophoresis-atmospheric pressure ionization mass spectrometry. J Chromatogr 559:515–528

Jonkman JHG, Borgstrom L, VanDerBoon WJV, DeNoord OE (1988) Theophylline-terbutaline, a steady state study on possible pharmacokinetic interactions with special reference to chronopharmacokinetic aspects. Br J Clin Pharmacol 26:285–293

Kajbaf M, Lamb JH, Naylor S, Pattichis K, Gorrod JW (1991) Identification of metabolites derived from the H_2-receptor antagonist mifentidine using tandem mass spectrometry. Anal Chim Acta 247:151–159

Kajbaf M, Jahanshahi M, Pattichis K, Gorrod JW, Naylor S (1992) Rapid and efficient purification of cimetropium bromide and mifentidine drug metabolite mixtures derived from microsomal incubates for analysis by mass spectrometry. J Chromatogr 575:75–85

Kamimura H, Enjoji Y, Sasaki H, Kawai R, Kaniwa H, Niigata K, Kageyama S (1987) Disposition and metabolism of indeloxazine hydrochloride, a cerebral activator, in rats. Xenobiotica 17:645–658

Kaspersen FM, Van Boeckel CAA (1987) A review of the methods of chemical synthesis of sulphate and glucuronide conjugates. Xenobiotica 17:1451–1471

Kassahun K, Burton R, Abbott FS (1989) Negative ion chemical ionization gas chromatography/mass spectrometry of valproic acid metabolites. Biomed Environ Mass Spectrom 18:918–926

Kassahun K, Farrell K, Zheng J, Abbott F (1990) Metabolic profiling of valproic acid in patients using negative-ion chemical ionization gas chromatography-mass spectrometry. J Chromatogr 527:327–341

Kassahun K, Farrell K, Abbott F (1991) Identification of characterization of the glutathione and N-acetylcysteine conjugates of (E)-2-propyl-2,4-pentadienoic acid, a toxic metabolite of valproic acid, in rats and humans. Drug Metab Dispos 19:525–535

Kasuya F, Igarashi K, Fukui M (1991) Metabolism of chlorpheniramine in rat and human by use of stable isotopes. Xenobiotica 21:97–109

Kayganich K, Watson JT, Kilts C, Ritchie J (1990) Determination of plasma dexamethasone by chemical oxidation and electron capture negative ionization mass spectrometry. Biomed Environ Mass Spectrom 19:341–347

Kelly DW, Holder CL, Korfmacher WA, Slikker W Jr (1990) Plasma elimination and urinary excretion of methapyrilene in the rat. Drug Metab Dispos 18:1018–1024

Kenny PTM, Orlando R (1992) Tandem mass spectrometric analysis of peptides at the femtomole level. Anal Chem 64:957–960

Keswani SR, Edfort MJ, Wilhelm JA, Kvalo LT, Venturella VS (1990) Sensitive method for the determination of pentamorphone is serum by liquid chromatography-mass spectrometry with thermospray interface. J Chromatogr 534:77–86

Kharasch ED, Hill HF, Eddy AC (1991) Influence of dexmedetomidine and clonidine on human liver microsomal alfentanil metabolism. Anesthesiology 75:520–524

Kishida K, Akaki Y, Sasabe T, Yamamoto C, Manabe R (1990) Glutathione conjugation of methazolamide and subsequent reactions in the ciliary body in vitro. J Pharm Sci 79:638–642

Knadler MP, Ackermann BL, Coutant JE, Hurst GH (1992) Metabolism of the anticoagulant peptide, MDL 28,050, in rats. Drug Metab Dispos 20:89–95

Knapp DR (1979) Handbook of analytical derivatization reactions. Wiley, New York

Kobayashi T, Hohnoki H, Esumi Y, Ohtsuki T, Washino T, Tanayama S (1988) Metabolism and disposition of (RS)-2-methoxy-3-(octadecylcarbamoyloxy)propyl 2-(3-thiazolio)ethyl phosphate (MOTP) in rats and dogs. Xenobiotica 18:49–59

Kokkonen PS, Niessen WMA, Tjaden UR, VanDerGreef J (1991) Bioanalysis of erythromycin 2'-ethylsuccinate in plasma using phase-system switching continuous-flow fast atom bombardment liquid chromatography-mass spectrometry. J Chromatogr 565:265–275

Komatsu S, Murata S, Aoyama H, Zenki T, Ozawa N, Tateishi M, Vrbanac JJ (1991) Microquantitative determination of ciprostene in plasma by gas chromatography-mass spectrometry coupled with an antibody extraction. J Chromatogr 568:460–466

Korfmacher WA, Freeman JP, Getek TA, Bloom J, Holder CL (1990) Analysis of rat urine for metabolites of pyrilamine via high-performance liquid chromatography/thermospray mass spectrometry and tandem mass spectrometry. Biomed Environ Mass Spectrom 19:191–201

Korzekwa K, Howard WN, Trager WF (1990) The use of Brauman's least squares approach for the quantification of deuterated chlorophenols. Biomed Environ Mass Spectrom 19:211–217

Kosevich MV, Zhilkova OIU (1988) Use of the method of fast atom bombardment mass spectrometry for identification of products of the interaction of thiophosphamide with DNA. Bioorg Khim 14:1698–1699

Kraft JC, Slikker W Jr, Bailey JR, Roberts LG, Fischer B, Wittfoht W, Nau H (1991) Plasma pharmacokinetics and metabolism of 13-*cis*- and all-*trans*-retinoic acid in the cynomolgus monkey and the identification of 13-*cis*- and all-*trans*-retinoyl-*β*-glucuronides. A comparison to one human case study with isotretinoin. Drug Metab Dispos 19:317–324

Kurono M, Itogawa A, Yoshida K, Naruto S, Rudewicz P, Kanai M (1992) Identification of AJ-2615 and its S-oxidized metabolites in rat plasma by use of tandem-mass spectrometry. Biol Mass Spectrom 21:17–21

Kwok DWK, Pillai G, Vaughan R, Axelson JE, McErlane KM (1990) Preparative high-performance liquid chromatography and preparative thin-layer chromatography isolation of tocainide carbamoyl-*O*-*β*-D-glucuronide: structural characterization by gas chromatography-mass spectrometry and fast atom bombardment-mass spectrometry. J Pharm Sci 79:857–861

Lauriault VVM, O'Brien PJ (1991) Molecular mechanism for prevention of *N*-acetyl-*p*-benzoquinoneimine cytotoxicity by the permeable thiol drugs diethyldithiocarbamate and dithiothreitol. Mol Pharmacol 40:125–134

Lauriault VVM, McGirr LG, Wong WWC, O'Brien PJ (1990) Modulation of benzoquinone-induced cytotoxicity by diethyldithiocarbamate in isolated hepatocytes. Arch Biochem Biophys 282:26–33

Lauwers W, LeJeune L (1988) Identification of a biliary metabolite of cisapride. Biomed Environ Mass Spectrom 15:323–328

Lee MS, Yost RA (1988) Rapid identification of drug metabolites with tandem mass spectrometry. Biomed Environ Mass Spectrom 15:193–204

Lee PW-N, Byerley LO, Bergner EA (1991) Mass isotopomer analysis: theoretical and practical considerations. Biol Mass Spectrom 20:451–458

Leis HJ, Malle E (1991) Deuterium-labelling and quantitative measurement of ketotifen in human plasma by gas chromatography/negative ion chemical ionization mass spectrometry. Biol Mass Spectrom 20:467–470

Leis HJ, Gleispach H, Nitsche V, Malle E (1990) Quantitative determination of terbutaline and orciprenaline in human plasma by gas chromatography/negative ion chemical ionization/mass spectrometry. Biomed Environ Mass Spectrom 19:382–386

Leloux MS, Maes RAA (1990) The use of electron impact and positive chemical ionization mass spectrometry in the screening of beta blockers and their metabolites in human urine. Biomed Environ Mass Spectrom 19:137–142

Leloux MS, Maes RAA (1991) Identification and determination of propafenone and its principal metabolites in human urine using capillary gas chromatography/mass spectrometry. Biol Mass Spectrom 20:382–388

Leung LY, Baillie TA (1989) Studies on the biotransformation of ketamine. II. Quantitative significance of the N-demethylation pathway in rats in vivo determined by a novel stable isotope technique. Biomed Environ Mass Spectrom 18:401–404

Levy RH, Rettenmeier AW, Anderson GD, Wilensky AJ, Friel PN, Baillie TA, Acheampong A, Tor J, Guyot M, Loiseau P (1990) Effects of polytherapy with phenytoin, carbamazepine, and stiripentol on formation of 4-ene-valproate, a hepatotoxic metabolite of valproic acid. Clin Pharmacol Ther 48:225–235

Li J, Norwood DL, Mao L-F, Schulz H (1991) Mitochondrial metabolism of valproic acid. Biochemistry 30:388–394

Liu H, Cooper LM, Raynie DE, Pinkston JD, Wehmeyer KR (1992) Combined super-critical fluid extraction/solid-phase extraction with octadecylsilane cartridges as a sample preparation technique for the ultratrace analysis of a drug metabolite in plasma. Anal Chem 64:802–806

Lonning PE, Lien EA, Lundgren S, Kvinnsland S (1992) Clinical pharmacokinetics of endocrine agents used in advanced breast cancer. Clin Pharmacokinet 22: 327–358

Loscher W, Nau H, Siemes H (1988) Penetration of valproate and its active metabo-lites into cerebrospinal fluid of children with epilepsy. Epilepsia 29:311–316

Lunte CE, Scott DO (1991) Sampling living systems using microdialysis probes. Anal Chem 63:773A–778A

Luo H, Hawes EM, McKay G, Korchinski ED, Midha KK (1991) The quaternary ammonium-linked glucuronide of doxepin: a major metabolite in depressed patients treated with doxepin. Drug Metab Dispos 19:722–724

MacDonald JI, Dickinson RG, Reid RS, Edom RW, King AR, Verbeeck RK (1991) Identification of a hydroxy metabolite of diflunisal in rat and human urine. Xenobiotica 21:1521–1533

Macrae PV, Kinns M, Pullen FS, Tarbit MH (1990) Characterization of a quaternary, N-glucuronide metabolite of the imidazole antifungal, tioconazole. Drug Metab Dispos 18:1100–1102

Madden S, Back DJ (1991) Metabolism of norgestimate by human gastrointestinal mucosa and liver microsomes in vitro. J Steroid Biochem Mol Biol 38:497–503

Madden S, Back DJ, Martin CA, Orme MLE (1989) Metabolism of the contracep-tive steroid desogestrel by the intestinal mucosa. Br J Clin Pharmacol 27:295–299

Magdalou J, Herber R, Bidfault R, Siest G (1992) In vitro N-glucuronidation of a novel antiepileptic drug, lamotrigine, by human liver microsomes. J Pharmacol Exp Ther 260:1166–1173

Mao L-F, Millington DS, Schulz H (1992) Formation of a free acyl adenylate during the activation of 2-propylpentanoic acid. J Biol Chem 267:3143–3146

Martin LB III, Schreiner AF, VanBreemen RB (1991) Characterization of cisplatin adducts of oligonucleotides by fast atom bombardment mass spectrometry. Anal Biochem 193:6–15

Maurer H, Wollenberg P (1990) Urinary metabolites of benzbromarone in man. Arzneimittelforschung 40:460–462

Maurizis JC, Nicolas C, Verny M, Ollier M, Faurie M, Payard M, Veyre A (1991) Biodistribution and metabolism in rats and mice of bucromarone. Drug Metab Dispos 19:94–99

May DG, Black CM, Olsen NJ, Cuska ME, Tanner SB, Bellino L, Porter JA, Wilkinson GR, Branch RA (1990) Scleroderma is associated with differences in individual routes of drug metabolism: a study with dapsone, debrisoquin, and mephenytoin. Clin Pharmacol Ther 48:286–295

Mayol RF, Jajoo HK, Klunk LJ, Blair IA (1991) Metabolism of the antipsychotic drug tiospirone in humans. Drug Metab Dispos 19:394–399

Mays DC, Dixon KF, Balboa A, Pawluk LJ, Bauer MR, Nawoot S, Gerber N (1991) A nonprimate animal model applicable to zidovudine pharmacokinetics in humans: inhibition of glucuronidation and renal excretion of zidovudine by probenecid in rats. J Pharmacol Exp Ther 259:1261–1270

McCloskey JA (ed) (1991) Methods in enzymology, vol 193. Academic, New York

McEwan CN, Larsen BS (ed) (1990) Mass spectrometry of biological materials, vol 8. Dekker, New York

Meier GP, Park SB, Yee GC, Gmur DJ (1990) Isolation and identification of a novel human metabolite of cyclosporin A: dihydro-CsA M17. Drug Metab Dispos 18:68–71

Menacherry SD, Justice JB Jr (1990) In vivo microdialysis and thermospray tandem mass spectrometry of the dopamine uptake blocker 1-(2-[bis(4-fluorophenyl)-methoxy]ethyl]-4-(3-phenylpropyl)-piperazine (GBR-12909). Anal Chem 62:597–601

Meuldermans W, Peer AV, Hendrickx J, Woestenborghs R, Lauwers W, Heykants J, Bussche GV, Craeyvelt HV, Der-Aa PV (1988) Alfentanil pharmacokinetics and metabolism in humans. Anesthesiology 69:527–534

Midha KK, Hawes EM, Hubbard JW, Korchinski ED, McKay G (1989) Intersubject variation in the pharmacokinetics of chlorpromazine in healthy men. J Clin Psychopharmacol 9:4–8

Mikus G, Eichelbaum M, Fischer C, Gumulka S, Klotz U, Kroemer HK (1990) Interaction of verapamil and cimetidine: stereochemical aspects of drug metabolism, drug disposition and drug action. J Pharmacol Exp Ther 253:1042–1048

Moini M, Abramson FP (1991) A moving belt device to couple high-performance liquid chromatography and chemical reaction interface mass spectrometry. Biol Mass Spectrom 20:308–312

Moini M, Chace D, Abramson FP (1990) Selective detection of sulfur-containing compounds by gas chromatography/chemical reaction interface mass spectrometry. J Am Soc Mass Spectrom 2:250–255

Monsarrat B, Mariel E, Cros S, Gares M, Guenard D, Gueritte-Voegelein F, Wright M (1990) Taxol metabolism. Isolation and identification of three major metabolites of taxol in rat bile. Drug Metab Dispos 18:895–901

Muck WM, Henion JD (1990) High-performance liquid chromatography/tandem mass spectrometry: its use for the identification of stanozolol and its major metabolites in human and equine urine. Biomed Environ Mass Spectrom 19:37–51

Muindi JRF, Lee S-J, Baltzer L, Jakubowski A, Scher HI, Sprancmanis LA, Riley CM, Velde DV, Young CW (1991) Clinical pharmacology of deoxyspergualin in patients with advanced cancer. Cancer Res 51:3096–3101

Muindi JRF, Frankel SR, Huselton C, DeGrazia F, Garland WA, Young CW, Warrel RP Jr (1992) Clinical pharmacology of oral all-*trans* retinoic acid in patients with acute promyelocytic leukemia. Cancer Res 52:2138–2142

Murray S, Davies DS, Blair IA (1983) Analytical techniques in clinical pharmacology. In: Turner P, Shand DG (ed) Recent advances in clinical pharmacology. Churchill Livingstone, Edinburgh, pp 1–19

Murthy SS, Nelson WL, Shen DD, Power JM, Cahill CM, McLean AJ (1991) Pharmacokinetic interaction between verapamil and metoprolol in the dog: stereochemical aspects. Drug Metab Dispos 19:1093–1100

Mutlib AE, Nelson WL (1990a) Pathways of gallopamil metabolism. Regiochemistry and enantioselectivity of the N-dealkylation processes. Drug Metab Dispos 18:331–337

Mutlib AE, Nelson WL (1990b) Synthesis and identification of the N-glucuronides of norgallopamil and norverapamil, unusual metabolites of gallopamil and verapamil. J Pharmacol Exp Ther 252:593–599

Nakagawa Y, Iwatani K (1991) Scanning thin-layer chromatography-liquid secondary ion mass spectrometry and its application for investigation of drug metabolites. J Chromatogr 562:99–110

Naylor S, Kajbaf M, Lamb JH, Jahanshahi M, Gorrod JW (1992) Rapid identification of cimetropium bromide metabolites using constant neutral loss tandem mass spectrometry. Biol Mass Spectrom 21:165–175

Niemeijer NR, Gerding TK, DeZeeuw RA (1991) Glucuronidation of labetalol at the two hydroxy positions by bovine liver microsomes. Isolation, purification, and structure elucidation of the glucuronides of labetalol. Drug Metab Dispos 19:20–23

Nishioka R, Umeda I, Oi N (1991) Determination of felodipine and its metabolites in plasma using capillary gas chromatography with electron-capture detection and their identification by gas chromatography-mass spectrometry. J Chromatogr 565:237–246

Nordholm L, Wassmann O, Nielsen PG, Thogersen H, Gronvald F (1992) Identification of the major metabolites of [³H]-(+)-8-chloro-5-(2,3-dihydrobenzofuran-7-yl)-7-methoxymethyloxy-3-methyl-2,3,4,5-tetrahydro-1H-3-benzazepine   in rats. Xenobiotica 22:345–356

Odar-Cederlof I, Anderson P, Bondesson U (1990) Nifedipine as an antihypertensive drug in patients with renal failure – pharmacokinetics and effects. J Intem Med 227:329–337

Ottoila P, Pakkala E, Karlsson C, Taskinen J (1991) Determination of nitecapone and (¹³C₆)nitecapone in human plasma by gas chromatography/mass spectrometry. Biol Mass Spectrom 20:771–776

Paar WD, brockmeier D, Hirzebruch M, Schmidt EK, von Unruh GE, Dengler HJ (1990) Pharmacokinetics of prenylamine racemate and enantiomers in man. Arzneimittelforschung 40:657–661

Pan HY, Triscari J, DeVault AR, Smith SA, Wang-Iverson D, Swanson BN, Willard DA (1991) Pharmacokinetic interaction between propranolol and the HMG-CoA reductase inhibitors pravastatin and lovastatin. Br J Clin Pharmacol 31: 665–670

Patanella JE, Walsh JS, Unger SE, Miwa GT, Parry PS, Daniel MJ, Evans GL (1990) Identification of a glucuronide conjugate of the carbocyclic nucleoside, carbovir, isolated from marmoset urine. Drug Metab Dispos 18:1092–1095

Patel DK, Woolley JL Jr, Shockcor JP, Johnson RL, Taylor LC, Sigel CW (1991) Disposition, metabolism, and excretion of the anticancer agent crisnatol in the rat. Drug Metab Dispos 19:491–497

Pearson PG, Threadgill MD, Howald WN, Baillie TA (1988) Applications of tandem mass spectrometry to the characterization of derivatized glutathione conjugates. Studies with S-(N-methylcarbamoyl)-glutathione, a metabolite of the antineoplastic agent N-methylformamide. Biomed Environ Mass Spectrom 16:51–56

Peng GW, Chiou WL (1990) Analysis of drugs and other toxic substances in biological samples for pharmacokinetic studies. J Chromatogr 531:3–50

Perkins JR, Parker CE, Tomer KB (1992) Nanoscale separations combined with electrospray ionization mass spectrometry: sulfonamide determination. J Am Soc Mass Spectrom 3:139–149

Poon GK, Jarman M, Rowlands MG, Dowsett M, Firth J (1991a) Determination of 4-hydroxyandrost-4-ene-3,17-dione metabolism in breast cancer patients using high-performance liquid chromatography-mass spectrometry. J Chromatogr 565: 75–88

Poon GK, McCague R, Griggs LJ, Jarman M, Lewis IAS (1991b) Characterization of metabolites of 3-ethyl-3-(4-pyridyl)-piperadine-2,6-dione, potential breast cancer drug. J Chromatogr 572:143–157

Poon GK, Mistry P, Lewis S (1991c) Electrospray ionization mass spectrometry of platinum anticancer agents. Biol Mass Spectrom 20:687–692

Porubek DJ, Barnes H, Theodore LJ, Baillie TA (1988) Enantioselective synthesis and preliminary metabolic studies of the optical isomers of 2-n-propyl-4-pentenoic acid, a hepatotoxic metabolite of valproic acid. Chem Res Toxicol 1:343–348

Prakash C, Adedoyin A, Wilkinson GR, Blair IA (1991) Enantiospecific quantification of hexobarbital and its metabolites in biological fluids by gas chromatography/electron capture negative ion chemical ionization mass spectrometry. Biol Mass Spectrom 20:559–564

Puppo MD, Cighetti G, Kienle MG, Paroni R, Borghi C (1991) Determination of diclofenac in human plasma by selected ion monitoring. Biol Mass Spectrom 20:426–430

Rashed MS, Pearson PG, Han D-H, Baillie TA (1989) Application of liquid chromatography/thermospray mass spectrometry to studies on the formation of glutathione and cysteine conjugates from monomethylcarbamate metabolites of bambuterol. Rapid Commun Mass Spectrom 3:360–363

Rettenmeier AW, Howard WN, Levy RH, Witek DJ, Gordon WP, Porubek DJ, Baillie TA (1989) Quantitative metabolic profiling of valproic acid in humans using automated gas chromatographic/mass spectrometric techniques. Biomed Environ Mass Spectrom 18:192–199

Robinson PR, Jones MD, Maddock J, Rees LW (1991) Simultaneous determination of clebopride and a major metabolite N-desbenzylclebopride in plasma by capillary gas chroamtography-negative-ion chemical ionization mass spectrometry. J Chromatogr 564:147–161

Rubio FR, Crews T, Garland WA, Fukuda EK (1988) Quantification of dideoxycytidine in human plasma by gas chromatography/mass spectrometry. Biomed Environ Mass Spectrom 17:399–404

Sanins SM, Adams WJ, Kaiser DG, Halstead GW, Baillie TA (1990) Studies of the metabolism and chiral inversion of ibuprofen in isolated rat hepatocytes. Drug Metab Dispos 18:527–533

Sanins SM, Adams WJ, Kaiser DG, Halstead GW, Hosley J, Barnes H, Baillie TA (1991) Mechanistic studies on the metabolic chiral inversion of R-ibuprofen in the rat. Drug Metab Dispos 19:405–410

Sasaki Y, Baba S (1988) Simultaneous determination for imipramine, despramine and their deuterium-labeled analogues in biological fluids by capillary gas chromatography-mass spectrometry. J Chromatogr 426:93–101

Scappaticci B, Souveyrand J, Rousseau-Tsangaris M, Desage M, Brazier JL, Coquet B (1990) Determination of sodium diethyldithiocarbamate (imuthiol) and its S-methyl metabolite by gas chromatography-mass spectrometry. J Chromatogr 534:57–66

Scatina JA, Lockhead SR, Cayen MN, Sisenwine SF (1991) Metabolic disposition of enciprazine, a non-benzodiazepine anxiolytic drug, in rat, dog and man. Xenobiotica 21:1591–1604

Schellenberg KH, Linder M, Groeppelin A, Erni F (1987) Experience with routine applications of liquid chromatography-mass spectrometry in the pharmaceutical industry. J Chromatogr 394:239–251

Scherling D, Karl W, Ahr G, Ahr HJ, Wehinger E (1988) Pharmacokinetics of nisoldipine. III. Biotransformation of nisoldipine in rat, dog, monkey, and man. Arzneimittelforschung 38:1105–1110

Schneider RP, Lynch MJ, Ericson JF, Fouda HG (1991) Electrospray ionization mass spectrometry of semduramicin and other polyether ionophores. Anal Chem 63:1789–1794

Shaheen O, Biollaz J, Koshakji RP, Wilkinson GR, Wood AJJ (1989) Influence of debrisoquin phenotype on the inducibility of propranolol metabolism. Clin Pharmacol Ther 45:439–443

Shinohara Y, Baba S (1990) Stable isotope methodology in the pharmacokinetic studies of androgenic steroids in humans. Steroids 55:170–176

Shinohara Y, Kirii N, Tamaoki H, Magara H, Baba S (1990) Determination of the enantiomers of suprofen and [²H₃]suprofen in plasma by capillary gas chromatography-mass spectrometry. J Chromatogr 525:93–104

Shinohara Y, Magara H, Baba S (1991) Stereoselective pharmacokinetics and inversion of suprofen enantiomers in humans. J Pharm Sci 80:1075–1078

Shipley LA, Coleman MD, Brewer TG, Ashmore RW, Theoharides AD (1990) The disposition of an antileishmanial 8-aminoquinoline drug in the isolated perfused rat liver; thermospray liquid chromatography-mass spectrometry identification of metabolites. Xenobiotica 20:31–44

Shu Y-Z, Hubbard JW, Cooper JK, McKay G, Korchinski ED, Kumar R, Midha KK (1990a) The identification of urinary metabolites of doxepin in patients. Drug Metab Dispos 18:735–741

Shu Y-Z, Hubbard JW, McKay G, Midha KK (1990b) Identification of phenolic doxepin glucuronides from patient urine and rat bile. Drug Metab Dispos 18:1096–1099

Siegel MM, Hollander IJ, Hamann PR, James JP, Hinman L, Smith BJ, Farnsworth APH, Phipps A, King DJ, Karas M, Ingendoh A, Hillenkamp F (1991) Matrix-assisted UV-laser desorption/ionization mass spectrometric analysis of monoclonal antibodies for the determination of carbohydrate, conjugated chelator, and conjugated drug content. Anal Chem 63:2470–2481

Sinz MW, Remmel RP (1991) Isolation and characterization of a novel quaternary ammonium-linked glucuronide of lamotrigine. Drug Metab Dispos 19:149–153

Slatter JG, Abbott FS, Burton R (1990) Identification of the biliary metabolites of (±)-3-dimethylamino-1,1-diphenylbutane HCl (recipavrin) in rats. Xenobiotica 20:999–1024

Smith RD, Loo JA, Edmonds CG, Barinaga CJ, Udseth HR (1990) New developments in biochemical mass spectrometry: electrospray ionization. Anal Chem 62:882–899

Stahl W, Lenhardt S, Przybylski M, Eisenbrand G (1992) Mechanism of glutathione-mediated DNA damage by the antineoplastic agent 1,3-bis(2-chloroethyl)-N-nitrosourea. Chem Res Toxicol 5:106–109

Stiff DD, Zemaitis MA (1990) Metabolism of the anticonvulsant agent zonisamide in the rat. Drug Metab Dispos 18:888–894

Straub KM, Rudewicz P, Garvie C (1987) "Metaboloic mapping" of drugs: rapid screening techniques for xenobiotic metabolites with m.s./m.s. techniques. Xenobiotica 17:413–422

Straub K, Davis M, Hwang B (1988) Benzazepine metabolism revisited. Evidence for the formation of novel amine conjugates. Drug Metab Dispos 16:359–366

Stroh JG, Rinehart KL (1992) Liquid chromatography/fast atom bombardment mass spectrometry. In: Russell DH (ed) Experimental mass spectrometry. Plenum, New York

Subramanyam B, Pond SM, Eyles DW, Whiteford HA, Fouda HG, Castagnoli N Jr (1991) Identification of potentially neurotoxic pyridinium metabolite in the urine of schizophrenic patients treated with haloperidol. Biochem Biophys Res Commun 181:573–578

Suelter CH, Watson JT (eds) (1990) Biomedical applications of mass spectrometry. Wiley, Chichester

Sweeny DJ, Barnes S, Heggie GD, Diasio RB (1987) Metabolism of 5-fluorouracil to an N-cholyl-2-fluoro-β-alanine conjugate: previously unrecognized role for bile acids in drug conjugation. Proc Natl Acad Sci USA 84:5439–5443

Takano T, Abe S, Hata S (1990) A selected ion monitoring method for quantifying simvastatin and its acid form in human plasma, using the ferroceneboronate derivate. Biomed Environ Mass Spectrom 19:577–581

Tanaka M, Ono K, Hakusui H, Takegoshi T, Watanabe Y, Kanao M (1990) Identification of DP-1904 and its ester glucuronide in human urine and determination of their enantiomeric compositions by high-performance liquid chromatography with optical activity and ultraviolet detection. Drug Metab Dispos 18:698–703

Theodor R, Weimann H-J, Weber W, Michaelis K (1991) Absolute bioavailability of moxonidine. Eur J Drug Metab Pharmacokinet 16:153–159

Thornburgh BA, Shaw SR, Bronson GE, Sinha AJW (1988) Isolation and characterization of the urinary metabolites of arbaprostil in the male dog after intravenous administration. Eur J Drug Metab Pharmacokinet 13:113–121

Tracy JW, Catto BA, Webster LT Jr (1991) Formation of N-(5-nitro-2-thiazolyl)-N'-carboxymethylurea from 5-hydroxyniridazole. Role of aldehyde dehydrogenase in the oxidative metabolism of niridazole. Drug Metab Dispos 19:508–515

Treston AM, Hooper WD (1992) Urinary metabolites of phenobarbitone, primidone, and their N-methyl and N-ethyl derivatives in humans. Xenobiotica 22:385–394

Tsaconas C, Padieu P, d'Athis P, Mocaer E, Bromet N (1989) Gas chromatographic-mass spectrometric assessment of the pharmacokinetics of amineptine and its main metabolite in volunteers with liver impairment. J Chromatogr 487:313–329

Ung HL, Girault J, Lefebvre MA, Mignot A, Fourtillan JB (1987) Quantitative analysis of S2241 in human plasma and urine by combined gas chromatography-negative ion chemical ionization mass spectrometry: 15 month inter-day precision and accuracy validation. Biomed Environ Mass Spectrom 14:289–293

Usansky JI, Damani LA (1992) The urinary metabolic profile of metyrapone in the rat. Identification of two novel isomeric metyrapol N-oxide metabolites. Drug Metab Dispos 20:64–69

Vachta J, Valter K, Siegfried B (1990) Metabolism of difebarbamate in man. Eur J Drug Metab Pharmacokinet 15:191–198

Van Bakergem E, VanDerHoeven RA, Niessen WM, Tjaden UR, VanDerGreef J, Poon GK, McCague R (1992) On-line continuous-flow dialysis thermospray tandem mass spectrometry for quantitative screening of drugs in plasma: rogletimide. J Chromatogr 598:189–194

Vandenheuvel WJA (1987) Use of stable isotopes in the elucidation of drug biotransformation processes. Xenobiotica 17:397–412

Van Groeningen CJ, Pinedo HM, Heddes J, Kok RM, DeJong APJM, Wattel E, Peters GJ, Lankelma J (1988) Pharmacokinetics of 5-fluorouracil assessed with a sensitive mass spectrometric method in patients on a dose escalation schedule. Cancer Res 48:6956–6961

Vassel G, Deroussent A, Hartmann O, Challine D, Benhamou E, Valteau-Couanet D, Brugieres L, Kalifa C, Gouyette A, Lemerle J (1990) Dose-dependent neurotoxicity of high-dose busulfan in children: a clinical and pharmacological study. Cancer Res 50:6203–6207

Villen T, Abdi YA, Ericsson O, Gustafsson LL, Sjoqvist F (1990) Determination of metrifonate and dichlorvos in whole blood using gas chromatography and gas chromatography-mass spectrometry. J Chromatogr 529:309–317

Vyas KP, Kari PH, Pitzenberger SM, Halpin RA, Ramjit HG, Arison B, Murphy JS, Hoffman WF, Schwartz MS, Ulm EH, Duggan DE (1990) Biotransformation of lovastatin. I. Structure elucidation of in vitro and in vivo metabolites in the rat and mouse. Drug Metab Dispos 18:203–211

Wachs T, Conboy JC, Garcia F, Henion JD (1991) Liquid chromatography-mass spectrometry and related techniques via atmospheric pressure ionization. J Chromatogr Sci 29:357–366

Walle T, Walle UK, Cowart TD, Conrad EC, Gaffney TE (1990) Pharmacokinetics and metabolism of oral doses of a 4'-methylthio derivative of propranolol in man. Xenobiotica 20:321–331

Walsh JS, Patanella JE, Unger SE, Brouwer KR, Miwa GT (1990) The metabolism and excretion of carbovir, a carbocyclic nucleoside, in the rat. Drug Metab Dispos 18:1084–1091

Wang-Iverson D, Arnold ME, Jemal M, Cohen AI (1992) Determination of SQ 33,600, a phosphinic acid containing HMG CoA reductase inhibitor, in human serum by high-performance liquid chromatography combined with ionspray mass spectrometry. Biol Mass Spectrom 21:189–194

Weidolf L, Covey TR (1992) Studies on the metabolism of omeprazole in the rat using liquid chromatography/ionspray mass spectrometry and the isotope cluster technique with [^{34}S]omeprazole. Rapid Commun Mass Spectrom 6:192–196

Weil A, Caldwell J, Strolin-Benedetti M (1990) The metabolism and disposition of ^{14}C-fenofibrate in human volunteers. Drug Metab Dispos 18:115–120

Wilding IR, Davis SS, Hardy JG, Robertson CS, John VA, Powell ML, Leal M, Lloyd P, Walker SM (1991) Relationship between systemic drug absorption and gastrointestinal transit after the simultaneous oral administration of carbamazepine as a controlled-release system and as a suspension of ^{15}N-labelled drug to healthy volunteers. Br J Clin Pharmacol 32:573–579

Wong BK, Woolf TF, Chang T, Whitfield LR (1990) Metabolic disposition of trimetrexate, a nonclassical dihydrofolate reductase inhibitor, in rat and dog. Drug Metab Dispos 18:980–986

Wong FA, Lloyd JR, Graden DW (1990) The metabolism of etintidine in rat, dog, and human. Drug Metab Dispos 18:949–953

Woolf TF, Bjorge SM, Black AE, Holmes A, Chang T (1991) Metabolism of the acyl-CoA: cholesterol acyltransferase inhibitor 2,2-dimethyl-N-(2,4,6-trimethoxyphenyl)dodecanamide in rat and monkey. Drug Metab Dispos 19:696–702

Woollard PM, Salmon JA, Padfield AD (1991) Use of high-performance liquid chromatography-thermospray mass spectrometry and gas chromatography-electron-impact mass spectrometry in the identification of the metabolites of α-methylacetohydroxamic acids, potential antiasthmatic agents. J Chromatogr 562:249–256

Yamada Y, Ohashi R, Sugawara Y, Otsuka M, Takaiti O (1992) Metabolic fate of the new angiotensin-converting enzyme inhibitor imidapril in animals. Arzneim-Forsch Drug Res 42:490–498

Yang JT, Adusumalli VE, Wong KK, Kucharczyk N, Sofia RD (1991) Felbamate metabolism in the rat, rabbit, and dog. Drug Metab Disposition 19:1126–1134

Yeh SY (1990) N-depyridination and n-dedimethylaminoethylation of tripelennamine and pyrilamine in the rat. Drug Metab Disposition 18:453–461

Yeung PKF, Mosher SJ, Quilliam MA, Montague TJ (1990) Species comparison of pharmacokinetics and metabolism of diltiazem in humans, dogs, rabbits, and rats. Drug Metab Disposition 18:1055–1059

Zhang K, Lepage F, Cuvier G, Astoin J, Rashed MS, Baillie TA (1990) The metabolic fate of stiripentol in the rat. Studies on cytochrome P-450-mediated methylenedioxy ring cleavage and side chain isomerism. Drug Metab Disposition 18:794–803

Zhou H-H, Koshakji RP, Silberstein DJ, Wilkinson GR, Wood AJJ (1989) Racial differences in drug response. Altered sensitivity to and clearance of propranolol in men of Chinese descent as compared with American whites. N Engl J Med 320:565–570

CHAPTER 4

Analytical Methods for Biotechnology Products

B.L. Ferraiolo and M.A. Mohler

A. Introduction

For the purposes of this chapter, biotechnology products will be defined as proteins (polypeptides larger than 5 kDa) and antisense oligonucleotides. Analytical methods used in disposition studies for biotechnology products range from the straightforward and familiar to the elaborate and esoteric. Experience dictates that no one method is likely to address all of the potential analytical questions that arise in these studies, e.g., quantitation of bound and free intact parent or metabolite(s), and assessment of bioactivity. These concepts also apply to peptide drugs (McMartin 1992; see also Chap. 13, this volume). The methods highlighted in this chapter are by no means inclusive, but focus on the methods for biotechnology product analysis in biological matrices supported by the largest bodies of literature.

B. Methods

I. Radiolabels

Radiolabeled techniques have been the mainstay of protein chemists and conventional analytical chemists alike in disposition studies. While radiolabeled methods provide significant advantages with respect to detection in complex matrices, there are numerous limitations to these techniques when used in isolation.

1. Selection of Radiolabel

a) Proteins

Iodine is an attractive protein label due to its high specific activity, the relative ease of preparation of the labeled material, and the choice of several isotopes with relatively short radioactive half-lives. Iodination is accomplished by chemical coupling of a radioligand such as ^{125}I via protein tyrosine or lysine residues. The interested reader is referred to previous reviews that describe a variety of iodination methods in detail (Bailey 1984a; Bolton 1985; Mariani et al. 1985; Parker 1990; Regoeczi 1984; Woltanski et al. 1990).

Proteins may also be internally labeled by growing the production cell line in the presence of amino acids labeled with, for example, ^{3}H, ^{14}C, or ^{35}S (Cossum et al. 1992; Ferraiolo et al. 1988b). Other methods used for protein labeling include semisynthesis, e.g., replacement of the B-chain N-terminal phenylalanine of insulin with [^{3}H]phenylalanine (Halban and Offord 1975), and attachment via bifunctional chelating agents (Serafini et al. 1991).

If the protein contains unnatural amino acids (e.g., D-amino acids), selection of these sites for radiolabel incorporation may eliminate concerns about reutilization of the labeled amino acids (vide infra).

b) Oligonucleotides

Phosphorothioate oligonucleotides incorporating ^{35}S at the internucleoside linkages have been used in disposition studies for these antisense therapeutic agents (Iversen 1991; Stein et al. 1990). Previous investigators have also used oligonucleotides incorporating tritium at the 6-methyl group of thymidine (Chused et al. 1972) or labeled with ^{32}P (Hudnik-Plevnik et al. 1959).

2. Whole-Body Autoradiography

A radiolabeled method that is gaining popularity as a protein disposition study is whole-body autoradiography. The use of whole-body gamma cameras connected to digital computers has added a new dimension to localization and identification of regional distribution of radiolabeled proteins (Mariani et al. 1986). Studies with a radioiodinated antitumor monoclonal IgM antibody have provided information regarding whole-body retention, plasma disappearance, and radioactivity accumulation in liver, spleen, thyroid, and bladder (Mariani and Strober 1990). Ideally, a gamma photon energy of 150 keV is desirable for the radionuclide used to label the protein. Energies greater than 150 keV can be imaged, although detectability decreases with higher photon energies (Chilton and Witcofski 1986).

3. Radiolabel Realities

The labeled molecule should be shown to be indistinguishable in physiochemical and biological properties from the unlabeled material (Bennett and McMartin 1979). Its state of aggregation and purity may be determined by gel-filtration chromatography, various high-performance liquid chromatography (HPLC) modalities, electrophoresis, or immunological techniques. Functional aspects of the protein may be evaluated by bioassay or receptor binding assays. The extent of labeling is an important parameter; if labeled molecules are a small proportion of the total population, their deviant behavior may go unrecognized. Conversely, if the number of radionuclide atoms per protein molecule is excessive, metabolic behavior in vivo and

Table 1. Pitfalls of disposition studies with radiolabeled biotechnology products

Altered biological activity
Altered disposition
Lack of specificity
Intact
Degraded
Free
Bound
Aggregated
Unlabeled portions undetectable
Reutilization
Liberated label

immunoreactivity can be compromised (CESKA et al. 1972; VAN DER ABBEELE et al. 1988). In addition, autoradiolysis (BLOOM et al. 1958) and alteration of tertiary structure as a consequence of incorporation of an atomic species such as iodine into a protein can result in protein denaturation.

Some of the pitfalls to avoid in the use of radiolabels in disposition studies are listed in Table 1. It is imperative to establish whether the radioactive species in a given biological sample represent free or bound intact labeled drug, radiolabeled degradation products, or liberated label (FERRAIOLO and MOHLER 1992). Administration of radioiodinated recombinant human growth hormone in clinical studies has shown that free iodine appears in plasma within minutes postdose, presumably through deiodination by ubiquitous deiodinase enzymes. By 60–90 min postdose, free iodine accounts for the majority of the total plasma radioactivity (CAMERON et al. 1969; PARKER et al. 1962). Acid precipitation or immunological techniques may distinguish grossly between protein-associated label (>1–3 kDa) and small fragments or free label. Size-exclusion and other HPLC modalities may also aid in distinguishing among free and bound intact protein, degraded protein, and free label. However, with a nonuniformly labeled protein, any degradation product that does not contain the labeled amino acid will be undetectable.

Proteolysis will liberate labeled amino acids which may circulate, localize in tissues, or be reutilized and incorporated into endogenous proteins (REGOECZI 1984, 1987a; SCHWENK et al. 1985). Internally labeled proteins may be less desirable than iodinated proteins because of the serious potential for reutilization.

Apparent reutilization of labeled amino acids was observed after intravenous administration of internally labeled ($[^3H]$leucine) recombinant human growth hormone to rats (FERRAIOLO et al. 1990a). The initial plasma time course of radioactivity (1–10 min) was similar to that determined by immunoassay. However, within 30 min postdose, the plasma immunoreactivity decline exceeded the plasma radioactivity decline. Size-exclusion

HPLC suggested that between 1 and 20 min postdose, the radioactivity was contained in either intact growth hormone or small peptides. As early as approximately 60 min postdose, when there was very little intact radioactive growth hormone detectable in plasma, other high-molecular-weight radioactive entities were observed. Identification of one of these entities as rat serum albumin (RSA) was implied by its specific precipitation with anti-RSA antibodies and its apparent molecular weight. Supportive results were observed in rats administered semisynthetic ([^{3}H]phenylalanine) insulin. Subtilisin digestion of a radioactive high-molecular-weight fraction isolated from plasma suggested that [^{3}H]phenylalanine was present in sequences other than those expected for insulin (Berger et al. 1978; Davies et al. 1980; Halban et al. 1979). Acid-precipitable radioactivity is often used as a first approximation of intact protein, but this may be compromised if the label is reutilized and incorporated into other proteins, or if large molecular weight (>1–3 kDa) fragments or metabolites are generated.

Free iodide (liberated from an iodinated protein) is known to accumulate in the thyroid, gastrointestinal tract, and skin (Regoeczi 1987b). The gastrointestinal iodide cycle must always be considered in disposition studies with iodinated proteins. Iodide is secreted and concentrated by the salivary glands and stomach, and reabsorbed into the circulation from the intestines (Regoeczi 1987a). The disposition of free radioiodide may affect the interpretation of both plasma and total body radioactivities (Regoeczi 1987b). Pretreatment with sodium iodide may block specific free iodide uptake (e.g., thyroid), but may not have much impact on uptake in skin, stomach, and intestines. Dehalogenase inhibitors may prevent the liberation of free radioactive iodide; however, proteolysis will yield iodine-labeled tyrosine. Administration of the label alone (e.g., sodium iodide) may aid in determining specific distribution by difference.

Because of these limitations, it may not be possible to rely on the results of disposition studies using radiolabeled proteins without additional characterization of the radioactive species (Bier 1989; Jansen 1979; Regoeczi 1987b). Supplemental analysis providing additional identification of the analytes should usually be sought.

II. Immunoassays

Recently, immunoassays have gained acceptance in protein disposition studies as the "method of choice" for the simple reasons that these methods are rapid, sensitive, economical, and suitable for batch processing (Chen et al. 1991). In addition, for many clinically important proteins the alternatives are limited (Gosling 1990). Of the immunoassays, the most frequently used are enzyme-linked immunosorbent assays (ELISA), radioimmunoassays (RIA), and immunoradiometric assays (IRMA). Immunoassays are relatively specific and easy to perform compared to bioassays and have an objective endpoint.

It is beyond the scope of this chapter to review the immunoassay literature. The authors refer the interested reader to several reviews and texts describing immunoassay methods in detail (CHAN and PERLSTEIN 1987; GOSLING 1990; KEMENY and CHANTLER 1988; MAGGIO 1980).

1. Enzyme Immunoassays

The ELISA is the most commonly used immunoassay method, primarily because it is sensitive, nonradioactive, maximally automated, and amenable to batch processing. These double antibody sandwich assays may employ polyclonal or monoclonal antibodies or both. One common format employs an antianalyte antibody bound to a solid support (coat antibody). The matrix containing the analyte is added, followed by a second antianalyte antibody (conjugated antibody) that provides the means for detection (GAASTRA 1984; GOSLING 1990; KEMENY and CHANTLER 1988; MAGGIO 1980).

2. Radiolabel-Based Immunoassays

Radioimmunoassays are also frequently employed in protein disposition studies (PARKER 1976). In these immunoassays, the quantitation is through a radioactive label (BAILEY 1984b). RIAs are competitive assays; the unlabeled antigen competes with the labeled antigen for a limited number of binding sites on the antibody. The results obtained with RIAs, as with other immunoassays, may be highly dependent on the choice of antibodies (VENTURINI et al. 1990). RIAs may present special problems in that their use may not permit immunoassay of radiolabeled proteins. RIAs may also be subject to endogenous interferences which may compromise their specificity (TEMPLE et al. 1990). Binding of the analyte by plasma proteins can interfere with RIA results; the binding protein may bind the tracer and artifactually increase or decrease the final result depending on the separation method. Some of the disadvantages of RIAs relative to ELISAs include short reagent lifetimes, less convenient protocols, less automation, potential health hazards necessitating radiological protection, and generation of radioactive waste and the consequent disposal problems (GOSLING 1990).

3. Immunoassay Limitations

A serious disadvantage of immunoassays is that positive identification (e.g., exact biochemical composition, sequence) of the analyte is not possible (Table 2). Immunoassays may not distinguish bioactive from inactive forms of the protein. Partial degradation of the protein may alter or eliminate its interaction with the antibodies used in the assay, resulting in incomplete characterization of its disposition. In addition, the protein therapeutic and its metabolites cannot, generally, be measured simultaneously. Finally, immunoassays are subject to interference by a variety of endogenous or exogenous substances.

Table 2. Potential immunoassay limitations

No positive identification of analyte
Lack of discrimination re. bioactivity
Lack of discrimination re. parent structure
Lack of discrimination re. aggregation
Single analyte measurable
Numerous interferences
   Binding proteins
   Metabolites
   Antibodies
   Matrix
   Endogenous protein
   Heterophilic antibodies

4. Immunoassay Interferences

a) Binding Proteins

The presence of plasma binding proteins for protein therapeutics can present serious analytical problems. Interference by binding proteins may make a direct immunoassay useless. Low-affinity interferences may be eliminated by dilution (CHEN et al. 1991), although this solution effectively reduces the assay sensitivity. Specific binding proteins may result in poor or variable recoveries in direct immunoassays, and dilutions may not be able to overcome high-affinity interferences. Extraction methods and multistep sample processing may be necessary to eliminate these effects (CELNIKER et al. 1990; CHEN et al. 1991).

b) Metabolites

Immunoassays may be relatively insensitive to small changes in protein primary and secondary structure; partially degraded forms of protein therapeutics may or may not be immunoreactive in the parent assay. Where biologically active partially degraded forms of protein therapeutics exist, it is particularly important to detect and quantitate these metabolites. For example, preclinical and clinical studies with recombinant human interferon-γ have yielded absolute subcutaneous bioavailabilities as determined by ELISA of greater than 100% (CHEN et al. 1990; FERRAIOLO et al. 1988a, 1990b; KURZROCK et al. 1985; REED et al. 1990). It has been suggested that slightly degraded forms of exogenous interferon-γ may circulate after intravenous and subcutaneous administration and that the production of these metabolites may be route dependent (FERRAIOLO et al. 1990b; FERRAIOLO and MOHLER 1992). These degraded forms may have different disposition properties than the parent protein and may cross-react in the parent immunoassay; this could significantly interfere with the determination of bioavailability.

c) Antibodies

Antibody formation in response to therapeutic protein treatment (MARAFINO and KOPPLIN 1993; WORKING and COSSUM 1991; WORKING 1992) is especially troublesome in preclinical studies where the administered human protein is clearly foreign, although antibody interference in clinical studies with growth hormone, insulin, and interferons has been reported (BOLLI 1989; GIANNARELLI et al. 1988; GRAY et al. 1985; PRINGLE et al. 1989; STEIS et al. 1988; VAN HAEFTEN 1989). These antibodies may be neutralizing or non-neutralizing (GLOFF and BENET 1990; WORKING and COSSUM 1991). They may affect clearance (ARQUILLA et al. 1987, 1989; BOLLI 1989; GRAY et al. 1985; ROSENBLUM et al. 1985; VAN HAEFTEN 1989; WORKING and COSSUM 1991) or the pharmacological effect (STEIS et al. 1988; STOLL et al. 1987; WORKING and COSSUM 1991), and they may have a major impact on quantitation of the administered protein (PRINGLE et al. 1989). The presence of antibodies may result in apparent anomalously low protein concentrations in plasma, even when the antibodies are not frankly detectable.

Conversely, the continued presence of the administered protein may adversely affect the ability to quantitate the antibody that has been raised in response to it. In multiple-dose studies, the protein may interfere with the ELISA determination of the antibody titers since the ELISA may capture the antibodies in plasma with the protein bound to a solid support.

d) Miscellany

Immunoassays are matrix specific; biological fluids tend to modify the immunoreactivity of the protein analyte (CHEN et al. 1991). Some matrix effects may be minimized by adding immunoglobulins to serum samples prior to assay (LUCAS et al. 1989), developing the assay standard curve in the relevant biological fluid, or applying a minimum dilution prior to sample analysis (CHEN et al. 1991).

High endogenous protein concentrations or pulsatile secretion of the endogenous protein may be troublesome (CHEN et al. 1991). Heterophilic antibodies may lead to invalid analyte quantitation in two-site immunoassays and RIAs (BOSCATO and STUART 1988). These antibodies bind immunoglobulins from the species employed to generate the reagents used in the immunoassays (DAHLMANN and BIDLINGMAIER 1989; GOSLING 1990).

III. Bioassays

Traditionally, bioassays are in vivo or in vitro tissue- or cell-based assays (QUIRON 1982). In vivo bioassays are expensive and time consuming, sometimes taking days or weeks to perform. They may lack specificity and sensitivity, and they have subjective endpoints and high variability. In addition, they require the use of laboratory animals and often specialized surgical procedures. Cell-based bioassays may be less expensive and time consuming, but they may still be difficult to perform and they are subject to environmental and supply variables. If transformed cells are used, they may not be representative of normal cells. These assays may be based on, for example, proliferation, differentiation, or cytotoxicity. In general, bioassays are subject to interferences similar to those that pertain for immunoassays. Like immunoassays, bioassays may provide no information about degraded products. Species specificity of biological effects may also limit the usefulness of bioassays in particular species (Gloff and Benet 1990). Other in vitro assays that have been proposed as substitutes for in vivo and cell-based bioassays include receptor binding assays (and HPLC-based receptor binding assays), so-called bio-ELISAs (which combine aspects of bioassays and immunoassays), and biomimetic assays.

IV. Other Immunological Techniques

Other immunologically based methodologies that may aid in the isolation and identification of protein therapeutic-related materials in vivo include immunoprecipitation (Firestone and Winguth 1990), immunoaffinity purification (Mayes 1984a), and immunoblotting procedures (vide infra).

V. Chromatography

Chromatography is also applicable to isolation and identification problems for protein therapeutics (Chicz and Regnier 1990; Gavin 1992). Chromatography may offer poorer recoveries and less sensitivity than immunoassays, but good specificity and quantitation may be provided, as well as the ability to measure multiple analytes simultaneously. The selection of a chromatographic method that will preserve the desired properties of the protein drug-related materials is dependent on the objectives of the particular disposition study and the properties of the protein. A brief description of the separation mechanisms of the most commonly used chromatographic modalities is provided in Table 3.

The application of size-exclusion HPLC (Mayes 1984b; Stellwagen 1990) to the identification of protein binding/inhibitor phenomena for protein

Table 3. HPLC methods and characteristics

Mode	Separation
Size exclusion	Molecular size
Reversed phase	Partition: polar mobile phase to nonpolar stationary phase
Affinity	Specific binding to stationary phase component
Ion exchange	Interaction with cationic or anionic stationary phase groups

therapeutics has been described for insulin-like growth factor-I (COOK et al. 1989) and tissue plasminogen activator (HARRIS et al. 1988). A similar approach has been used to characterize the intactness of growth hormone in vivo (FERRAIOLO et al. 1990a). Reversed-phase HPLC (HANCOCK and HARDING 1984) has also been used to characterize radioiodinated insulin in disposition studies (SATO et al. 1990). Ion-exchange (ROSSOMANDO 1990), affinity (OSTROVE 1990), or immunoaffinity (GRANDICS et al. 1990; PHILIPS 1989) chromatography may be useful for isolation of protein products from dilute mixtures containing numerous contaminants that are often present in much higher concentrations than the desired product.

VI. Electrophoretic Techniques

One of the most powerful and widely used techniques for resolution of mixtures of proteins is polyacrylamide gel electrophoresis (PAGE) (GARFIN 1990; LAEMMLI 1970; MACNAMARA and WHICHER 1990; SMITH 1984; WALKER 1984). This method has excellent powers of resolution and sensitivity (GOODERHAM 1984a), especially when combined with radiolabel methods and autoradiography or immunoblotting methods (FISCHER et al. 1989; GOODERHAM 1984b; HEEGAARD and BJERRUM 1988; HOSSENLOPP et al. 1986; TIMMONS and DUNBAR 1990).

Sodium dodecyl sulfate PAGE/autoradiography has been used to examine plasma samples after intravenous and subcutaneous administration of ^{125}I-labeled recombinant human interferon-γ to rhesus monkeys; apparent route-specifically formed degradation products were detected (FERRAIOLO et al. 1990b).

VII. Mass Spectrometry

Mass spectrometry can significantly aid in identification of protein analytes. However, laborious sample preparation and small amounts of the analyte in biological matrices have limited the usefulness and general applicability of this method. Recent innovations in mass spectrometry permit analysis of proteins larger than 100-kDa (GRIFFIN et al. 1992; SUTER et al. 1992), even in complex mixtures (SWIDEREK et al. 1992).

Fast atom bombardment mass spectrometry has been used to characterize exogenous human relaxin isolated from rhesus monkey plasma by monoclonal antibody affinity purification after administration of a large intravenous relaxin dose (0.5–1.0 mg/kg) (FERRAIOLO et al. 1991). Reversed-phase HPLC separated intact relaxin from its degradation products; this method was able to resolve single amino acid differences in primary structure. The column fractions were submitted to fast atom bombardment mass spectrometry for determination of intact relaxin and its oxidation and degradation products.

C. Conclusions

The panel of analytical methods used for the characterization of a protein therapeutic in a biological matrix may need to be determined on a case-by-case basis. The applicable methods depend, in part, on the physiochemical and biological properties of the protein. In general, a battery of analytical approaches will be required; no single approach is likely to provide an unambiguous answer.

References

Arquilla ER, Stenger D, McDougall B, Ulich TR (1987) Effect of IgG subclasses on the in vivo bioavailability and metabolic fate of immune-complexed insulin in Lewis rats. Diabetes 36:144–151

Arquilla ER, McDougall BR, Stenger DP (1989) Effect of isologous and autologous insulin antibodies on the in vivo bioavailability and metabolic fate of immune-complexed insulin in Lou/M rats. Diabetes 38:343–349

Bailey GS (1984a) Radioiodination of proteins. Methods Mol Biol 1:325

Bailey GS (1984b) Radioimmunoassay. Methods Mol Biol 1:335

Bennett HPJ, McMartin C (1979) Peptide hormones and their analogues: distribution, clearance from the circulation and inactivation in vivo. Pharmacol Rev 30:247–292

Berger M, Halban PA, Muller WA, Offord RE, Renold AE, Vranic M (1978) Mobilization of subcutaneously injected tritiated insulin in rats: effects of muscular exercise. Diabetologia 15:133–140

Bier DM (1989) Intrinsically difficult problems: the kinetics of body proteins and amino acids in man. Diabetes Metab Rev 5:111–132

Bloom HG, Crocket DJ, Stewart FS (1958) The effects of radiation on the stability of radioiodinated human serum albumin. Br J Radiol 31:377–383

Bolli GB (1989) The pharmacokinetic basis of insulin therapy in diabetes mellitus. Diabetes Res Clin Pract 6:S3–S16

Bolton AE (1985) Radioiodination techniques. Review 18. Amersham, Arlington Heights, p 1

Boscato LM, Stuart MC (1988) Heterophilic antibodies: a problem for all immunoassays. Clin Chem 34:27–33

Cameron DP, Burger HG, Catt KJ, Dong A (1969) Metabolic clearance rate of radioiodinated human growth hormone in man. J Clin Invest 48:1600–1608

Celniker AC, Chen S, Spanski N, Pocekay J, Perlman AJ (1990) IGFI: assay methods and pharmacokinetics of free IGF-I in the plasma of normal human subjects following intravenous administration. Proc US Endocrine Soc, vol 72, Program and Abstracts, p 310

Ceska RM, Berglund A, Lundkirst V, Grossmuller F (1972) Influence of the degree of iodination and storage time on the immunological activity of ^{125}I-IgE. Immunochemistry 9:565–575

Chan DW, Perlstein MT (1987) Immunoassay – a practical guide. Academic, New York

Chen AB, Baker DL, Ferraiolo BL (1991) Points to consider in correlating bioassays and immunoassays in the quantitation of peptides and proteins. In: Garzone PD, Colburn WA, Mokotoff, WA (eds) Peptides, peptoids and proteins. Harvey Whitney, Cincinnati, p 53

Chen SA, Izu AE, Baughman RA, Ferraiolo BL, Mordenti J, Reed BR, Jaffee HS (1990) Pharmacokinetic disposition of recombinant interferon-gamma following intravenous and subcutaneous administration in normal volunteers. Annual Meeting of the International Society for Interferon Research, San Francisco

Chicz RM, Regnier FE (1990) High-performance liquid chromatography: effective protein purification by various chromatographic modes. In: Deutscher MP (ed) Guide to protein purification. Academic, San Diego, p 393

Chilton HM, Witcofski RL (1986) Nuclear pharmacy an introduction to the clinical application of radiopharmaceuticals. Lea and Febiger, Philadelphia

Chused TM, Steinberg AD, Talal N (1972) The clearance and localization of nucleic acids by New Zealand and normal mice. Clin Exp Immunol 12:465–476

Cook JE, Ferraiolo BL, Mohler MA (1989) The role of binding proteins in the metabolism of IGF-I. Pharm Res 6:S30

Cossum PA, Dwyer KA, Roth M, Chen SA, Moffat B, Vandlen R, Ferraiolo BL (1992) The disposition of a human relaxin (hRIx-2) in pregnant and non-pregnant rats. Pharm Res 9:415–420

Dahlmann N, Bidlingmaier F (1989) Circulating antibodies to mouse monoclonal immunoglobulins caused false-positive results in a two-site assay for alpha-fetoprotein. Clin Chem 35:23–39

Davies JG, Offord RE, Halban PA, Berger M (1980) The chemical characterization of the products of the processing of subcutaneously injected insulin. In: Brandenburg D, Wollmer A (eds) Insulin. Chemistry, structure and function of insulin and related hormones. De Gruyter, New York, p 517

Ferraiolo BL, Mohler M (1992) Goals and analytical methodologies for therapeutic proteins. In: Ferraiolo BL, Mohler MA, Gloff CA (eds) Protein pharmacokinetics and metabolism. Plenum, New York, p 1

Ferraiolo BL, Fuller GB, Burnett B, Chan E (1988a) Pharmacokinetics of recombinant human interferon-gamma in the rhesus monkey after intravenous and subcutaneous administration. J Biol Response Mod 7:115–122

Ferraiolo BL, Moore JA, Crase D, Gribling P, Wilking H, Baughman RA (1988b) Pharmacokinetics and tissue distribution of recombinant human tumor necrosis factor-alpha in mice. Drug Metab Dispos 16:270–275

Ferraiolo BL, Mohler MA, Cossum PA, Moore JA, Reed B, Vandlen R (1990a) Characterization of therapeutic proteins in disposition studies. Society of Toxicology Annual Meeting, Miami

Ferraiolo BL, Mohler M, Cook J, Chen A, Reed B, O'Connor J, Keck R (1990b) The metabolism of recombinant human interferon-gamma (rIFN-gamma) in rhesus monkeys. Pharm Res 7:S-46

Ferraiolo BL, Winslow J, Laramee G, Celniker A, Johnston P (1991) Pharmacokinetics and metabolism of human relaxins in rhesus monkeys. Pharm Res 8:1032–1038

Firestone GL, Winguth SD (1990) Immunoprecipitation of proteins. Methods Enzymol 182:688–699

Fischer WH, Vaughan J, Karr D, McClintock R, Spiess J, Rivier J, Vale W (1989) Recovery of biological activity, blotting and sequence analysis of protein hormones after SDSPAGE. In: Hugli TE (ed) Techniques in protein chemistry. Academic, San Diego, p 36

Gaastra W (1984) Enzyme-linked immunosorbent assay (ELISA). Methods Mol Biol 1:349

Garfin DE (1990) One dimensional gel electrophoresis. In: Deutscher MP (ed) Guide to protein purification. Academic, San Diego, p 425

Gavin JF (1992) Isolation of peptides from biological fluids. In: Introduction to molecular and cellular research. The Endocrine Society, Serono Symposium, p 121

Giannarelli R, Marchetti P, Giannecchini M, De Cianni G, Cecchetti P, Masoni A, Navalesi R (1988) Free insulin concentrations in immediately extracted plasma samples and their relationships to clinical and metabolic parameters in insulin-treated diabetic patients. Acta Diabetol Lat 25:257–262

Gloff CA, Benet LZ (1990) Pharmacokinetics and protein therapeutics. Adv Drug Del Rev 4:359–386

Gooderham K (1984a) High-sensitivity silver staining of proteins following poly-
    acrylamide gel electrophoresis. Methods Mol Biol 1:113
Gooderham K (1984b) Transfer techniques in protein blotting. Methods Mol Biol
    1:165
Gosling JP (1990) A decade of development of immunoassay methodology. Clin
    Chem 36:1408–1427
Grandics P, Szathmary Z, Szathmary S (1990) A novel immunoaffinity system for the
    purification of therapeutic proteins. Ann NY Acad Sci 589:148–156
Gray RS, Cowan P, di Mario U, Elton RA, Clarke BF, Duncan LJP (1985) Influence
    of insulin antibodies on pharmacokinetics and bioavailability of recombinant
    human and highly purified beef insulins in insulin dependent diabetics. Br Med J
    290:1687–1691
Griffin PR, Furer-Jonscher K, Hood LE, Yates JR (1992) Analysis of proteins by
    mass spectrometry. In: Angeletti RH (ed) Techniques in protein chemistry III.
    Academic, San Diego
Halban PA, Offord RE (1975) The preparation of a semisynthetic tritiated insulin
    with a specific radioactivity of up to 20 curies per millimole. Biochem J 151:
    219–225
Halban PA, Berger M, Offord RE (1979) Distribution and metabolism of in-
    travenously injected tritiated insulin in rats. Metabolism 28:1097–1104
Hancock WS, Harding DRK (1984) Review of separation conditions. In: Hancock
    WS (ed) CRC Handbook of HPLC for the separation of amino acids, peptides
    and proteins, vol 2. CRC, Boca Raton, p 303
Harris R, Frade LG, Creighton LJ, Gascoine PS, Alexandroni MM, Poole S,
    Gaffney PJ (1988) Investigation by HPLC of the catabolism of recombinant
    tissue plasminogen activator in the rat. Thromb Haemost 60:107–112
Heegaard NHH, Bjerrum OJ (1988) Immunoblotting – general principles and pro-
    cedures. In: Bjerrum OJ, Heegaard NHH (eds) Handbook of immunoblotting
    of proteins, vol 1. CRC Boca Raton, p 1
Hossenlopp P, Seurin D, Segovia-Quinson B, Hardouin S, Binoux M (1986) Analysis
    of serum insulin-like growth factor binding proteins using Western blotting: use
    of the method for titration of the binding proteins and competitive binding
    studies. Anal Biochem 154:138–143
Hudnik-Plevnik TA, Glisin VR, Simic MM (1959) Fate of the highly polymerized
    spleen deoxyribonucleic acid labeled with phosphorus-32 injected intraperito-
    neally into rats. Nature 184:1818–1819
Jansen ABA (1979) Total radioactivity half-lives. Drug Metab Dispos 7:350
Iversen P (1991) In vivo studies with phosphorothioate oligonucleotides: pharma-
    cokinetics prologue. Anticancer Drug Design 6:531–538
Kemeny DM, Chantler S (1988) An introduction to ELISA. In: Kemeny DM,
    Challacombe SJ (eds) ELISA and other solid phase immunoassays. Wiley, New
    York, p 1
Kurzrock R, Rosenblum MG, Sherwin SA, Rios A, Talpaz M, Quesada JR, Gut-
    terman JU (1985) Pharmacokinetics, single-dose tolerance and biological activity
    of recombinant gamma-interferon in cancer patients. Cancer Res 45:2866–2872
Laemmli UK (1970) Cleavage of structural proteins during the assembly of the head
    of bacteriophage T4. Nature 227:680–685
Lucas C, Bald LN, Martin MC, Jaffe RB, Drolet DW, Mora-Worms M, Bennett G,
    Chen AB, Johnston PD (1989) An enzyme-linked immunosorbent assay to study
    human relaxin in human pregnancy and in pregnant rhesus monkeys. J En-
    docrinol 120:449–457
MacNamara EM, Whicher JT (1990) Electrophoresis and densitometry of serum and
    urine in the investigation and significance of monoclonal immunoglobulins.
    Electrophoresis 11:376–381
Maggio ET (1980) Enzyme-immunoassays. CRC, Boca Raton

Marafino BJ, Kopplin JR (1993) Characterization of the toxicity profile of peptide and protein therapeutics. In: Lee VL (ed) Peptide and protein drug delivery. Dekker, New York (in press)

Mariani G, Strober W (1990) Immunoglobulin metabolism. In: Metzger H (ed) Receptors and the action of antibodies. American Society of Microbiology, Washington, p 94

Mariani G, Mazzucca N, Molea N, Bianchi N, Donato N (1985) Kinetic distribution studies in vivo of radioiodinated monoclonal preparations as a screening procedure for tumour immunoscintigraphy agents. In: Donato L, Britton K (eds) Immunoscintigraphy. Gordon and Breach, New York, p 83

Mariani G, Ferrante L, Rescigno A (1986) Kinetic modeling for the analysis of digital images from tissue distribution studies of tumor radioimmunoscintigraphy agents. In: Hofer R, Bergman H (eds) Radioaktive Isotope in Klinik und Forschung. Egerman, Vienna, p 741

Mayes ELV (1984a) Immunoaffinity purification of protein antigens. Methods Mol Biol 1:13

Mayes ELV (1984b) Determination of molecular weights by gel permeation HPLC. Methods Mol Biol 1:5

McMartin C (1992) Pharmacokinetics of peptides and proteins; opportunities and challenges. Adv Drug Res 22:39–106

Ostrove S (1990) Affinity chromatography: general methods. In: Deutscher MP (ed) Guide to protein purification. Academic, San Diego, p 357

Parker CW (1976) Radioimmunoassay of biologically active compounds. Prentice-Hall, Englewood Cliffs

Parker CW (1990) Radiolabeling of proteins. Methods Enzymol 182:721–737

Parker ML, Utiger RD, Daughaday WH (1962) Studies on human growth hormone. II. The physiological disposition and metabolic fate of human growth hormone in man. J Clin Invest 41:262–268

Philips TM (1989) Isolation and recovery of biologically active proteins by high performance immunoaffinity chromatography. In: Kerlavage AK (ed) The use of HPLC in receptor biochemistry. Liss, New York, p 129

Pringle PJ, Hindmarsh PC, De Silvio L, Teale JD, Kurtz AB, Brook CGD (1989) The measurement and effect of growth hormone in the presence of growth hormone-binding antibodies. J Endocrinol 121:193–199

Quiron R (1982) Bioassays in modern peptide research. Peptides 3:223–230

Reed BR, Chen AB, Gibson UEM, Chen S, Baughman R, Ferraiolo BL, Mordenti J (1990) Parenteral administration of recombinant interferon-gamma: results in route dependent processing in normal human subjects. Annual Meeting of the International Society for Interferon Research, San Francisco

Regoeczi E (1984) Iodine-labeled plasma proteins, vol 1. CRC, Boca Raton, pp 4–5, 35–102

Regoeczi E (1987a) Iodine-labeled plasma proteins, vol 2A. CRC, Boca Raton, pp 6, 112, 116–117

Regoeczi E (1987b) Iodine-labeled plasma proteins, vol 2B. CRC, Boca Raton, pp 43–62

Rosenblum MG, Unger BW, Gutterman JU, Hersh EM, David GS, Frincke JM (1985) Modification of human leukocyte interferon pharmacology with a monoclonal anticody. Cancer Res 45:2421–2424

Rossomando EF (1990) Ion-exchange chromatography. In: Deutscher MP (ed) Guide to protein purification. Academic, San Diego, p 309

Sato H, Tsuji A, Hirai K-I, Kang YS (1990) Application of HPLC in disposition study of A-14-^{125}I-labeled insulin in mice. Diabetes 39:563–569

Schwenk WF, Tsalikain E, Beaufrere B, Haymond MW (1985) Recycling of an amino acid label with prolonged isotope infusion: implications for kinetic studies. Am J Physiol 248:E482–E487

Serafini AN, Garty I, Vargas-Cuba R, Freedman A, Rauh DA, Neptune M, Landess L, Sfakianakis GN (1991) Clinical evaluation of a scintographic method for diagnosing inflammations/infections using indium-111-labeled nonspecific human IgG. J Nucl Med 32:2227–2232

Smith BJ (1984) SDS polyacrylamide electrophoresis of proteins. Methods Mol Biol 1:41

Stein CA, Iversen PL, Subasinghe C, Cohen JS, Stec W, Zorr G (1990) Preparation of ^{35}S-labeled polyphosphorothioate oligonucleotides by use of hydrogen-phosphonate chemistry. Anal Biochem 188:11–16

Steis RG, Smith JW, Urba WJ, Clark JW, Itri LM, Evans LM, Schoenberger C, Longo DL (1988) Resistance to recombinant interferon alpha-2a in hairy-cell leukemia associated with neutralizing anti-interferon antibodies. N Engl J Med 318:1409–1413

Stellwagen E (1990) Gel filtration. In: Deutscher MP (ed) Guide to protein purification. Academic, New York, p 317

Stoll RE, Ball DJ, Burchiel SW, Robison RL, Smith CL (1987) Case history of a biotechnology product: toxicological protocol, design and results. In: Graham CE (ed) Preclinical safety of biotechnology products for human use. Liss, New York, p 173

Suter MJ-F, Moore WT, Farmer TB, Cottrell JS, Caprioli RM (1992) Analysis of protein-protein binding with laser desorption mass spectrometry: can multimeric forms be studied? In: Angeletti RH (ed) Techniques in protein chemistry III. Academic, San Diego, p 447

Swiderek KM, Chen S, Feistner GJ, Shively JE, Lee TD (1992) Applications of liquid chromatography – electrospray mass spectrometry (LC-ES/MS). In: Angelletti RH (ed) Techniques in protein chemistry III. Academic, San Diego, p 457

Temple RC, Clark PMS, Nagi DK, Schneider AE, Yudkin JS, Hales CN (1990) Radioimmunoassay may overestimate insulin in non-insulin dependent diabetes. Clin Endocrinol (Oxf) 32:689–693

Timmons TM, Dunbar BA (1990) Protein blotting and immunodetection. Methods Enzymol 182:679–688

Van der Abbeele AD, Aronson RA, Adelstein SJ, Kassis AI (1988) Does the in vitro testing of the immunoreactivity of an antibody reflect its in vivo behavior? J Nucl Med Allied Sci 32:260–267

Van Haeften TW (1989) Clinical significance of insulin antibodies in insulin-treated diabetic patients. Diabetes Care 12:641–648

Venturini PL, Remorgida V, Aguggia V, De Cecco L (1990) Luteinizing hormone determinations obtained with either a monoclonal or a polyclonal antibody radioimmunoassay and their correlations with clinical findings. J Endocrinol Invest 13:227–234

Walker JM (1984) Gradient SDS polyacrylamide electrophoresis of proteins. Methods Mol Biol 1:57

Woltanski K-P, Besch W, Keilacker H, Ziegler M, Kohnert K-D (1990) Radioiodination of peptide hormone and immunoglobulin preparations: comparison of the chloramine T and Iodogen method. Exp Clin Endocrinol 95:39–46

Working PK (1992) Potential effects of antibody induction by protein drugs. In: Ferraiolo BL, Mohler MA, Gloff CA (eds) Protein pharmacokinetics and metabolism. Plenum, New York, p 73

Working PK, Cossum PA (1991) Clinical and preclinical studies with recombinant human proteins: effect of antibody production. In: Garzone PD, Colburn WA, Mokotoff M (eds) Peptides, peptoids and proteins. Harvey Whitney, Cincinnati, p 157

C. In Vitro Methods –
Protein and Tissue Binding

CHAPTER 5

Metabolism: Scaling-up from In Vitro to Organ and Whole Body

K.S. PANG and M. CHIBA

A. Introduction

Efforts in developmental drug metabolism in vitro with animal models are aimed at obtaining data which have some utility in predicting the clinical efficacy and/or toxicity of drugs. In vitro studies involving purified iso-enzymes, subcellular fragments (nuclear, $9000 \times g$ supernatant, cytosolic and microsomal fractions), slices, and isolated cells can, in many instances, provide invaluable mechanistic insight inasmuch as the system allows for easy control of experimental variables. Expectedly, the nature of the information provided by the various systems differs. Purified isoenzymes yield information that pertains to cofactor requirements and behavior of that single system, whereas when the system becomes more and more hetero-geneous, other components (enzymes and cell types) and membranes add increasing complexity and metabolic interactions to the system.

A comparison of information obtained with in vitro and in vivo systems is inevitable, and this serves as the basis of many biochemical pharmacolo-gical/toxicological investigations. For this reason, integrative research on both metabolic in vitro and in vivo systems is often performed. When data from these various approaches are examined in concert, judicious applica-tion of in vitro data obtained with subcellular and cellular systems may be maximally utilized and extended to explain events at the organ and whole-body level.

Animal data may be scaled-up such that, in certain instances, they may be extrapolated to humans (DEDRICK et al. 1970; BOXENBAUM 1980; BOXENBAUM and RONFELD 1983). Animal scale-up is seldom successful in terms of metabolic studies, in view of the fact that large difference exists among species, and among genera of the same species. The topic of animal scaling is beyond the scope of the present chapter. Instead, we focus pri-marily on how data obtained from in vitro systems may be extended to organ systems and then in vivo. The concepts and approaches involved in the correlations will be examined, and the reasons why such correlations exist will be discussed.

B. Correlation of In Vitro and In Vivo Data

Data with purified isoenzymes, homogenates, and subcellular fragments (microsomal and cytosolic) yield information which characterizes the enzymatic system. Such information may pertain to protein, lipid, ionic, pH, and cofactor requirements, and/or the rate of catalysis or reaction (V_{max}) and binding/debinding of the enzyme–substrate complex (K_m). A common strategy has been used to correlate data obtained in vitro to an eliminating organ, usually the liver, and then ultimately to the whole body.

The simplest form of expressing the velocity (v) of a metabolic reaction for a given substrate, S, is describable by the Michaelis-Menten equation or variations thereof:

$$v = \frac{V_{max}[S]}{K_m + [S]} = CL_{int}[S],\tag{1}$$

where the intrinsic clearance, CL_{int}, as conceived by Gillette (1971) and introduced by Wilkinson and Shand (1975), is

$$CL_{int} = \frac{V_{max}}{K_m + [S]},\tag{2}$$

which dwindles to a constant, V_{max}/K_m at low substrate concentrations ($[S] \ll K_m$).

I. Concept of Organ Clearance

The events dictating drug loss across an organ lead to a drop in concentration across the organ, and often, steady-state approaches are used since transient loss of drug due to tissue binding can be neglected. At steady state, the rate of loss of drug (Fig. 1) according to Fick's principle is governed primarily by the rate of metabolism and excretion. Hence, in the absence of limitation of permeation by the membrane,

$$v = Q(C_{In} - C_{Out}) = \frac{V_{max}[S]}{K_m + [S]} = CL_{int}[S],\tag{3}$$

where Q is the organ blood flow, and C_{In} and C_{Out} respectively denote the steady-state input and output concentrations across the organ. The notion of the intrinsic clearance (Eq. 2) was fortified by Wilkinson and Shand (1975), who employed the term to describe drug elimination, or the volume of hepatocyte water which is cleared of drug per unit time by the liver. Alternately, the rate of loss (v) can be expressed in terms of the rate of presentation, such that the resultant fraction or extraction ratio, E, is

$$E = \frac{Q(C_{In} - C_{Out})}{QC_{In}} = \frac{C_{In} - C_{Out}}{C_{In}}\tag{4}$$

or expressed in terms of the arterial (input) concentration, C_{In}, such that the organ clearance (CL) is

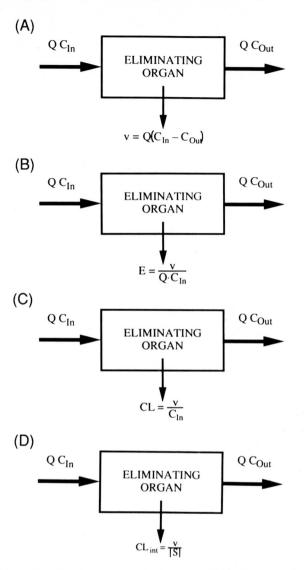

Fig. 1A–D. Schematics for drug removal across an eliminating organ, expressed as the rate of loss, v **(A)**, the extraction ratio, E **(B)**, clearance, CL **(C)**, and intrinsic clearance, CL_{int} **(D)**. [S]denotes the unbound substrate concentration

$$CL = \frac{v}{C_{In}} = \frac{Q(C_{In} - C_{Out})}{C_{In}} = QE \qquad (5)$$

and is the volume of biological fluid (entering the organ) which is cleared of substrate per unit time. Hence, by definition, the intrinsic clearance exceeds or equals the organ clearance ($CL_{int} \geqslant CL$) since the substrate concentration is less than, or at best equals, the input concentration ($[S] \leq C_{In}$). These conceptual frameworks – v, E, CL, and CL_{int} – have been utilized to describe drug removal.

For the whole-organ system, however, additional variables need to be considered, namely binding of substrate to blood components (plasma proteins and red blood cells), membrane permeability (influx, or blood to cell, and efflux, or cell to blood), tissue binding, and excretion mechanisms. The manner in which these variables interrelate in the determination of organ clearance is highly dependent on the inherent assumptions for organ flow in relation to the architecture of the organ.

1. Hepatic Clearance Models

Since the liver is the most important drug-metabolizing organ, models of hepatic drug clearance (Fig. 2) have been introduced to describe the disposition of substrates. Much of the development evolved within the last two decades from basic engineering concepts (Dankwerts 1953; Levenspiel 1970; Himmelblau and Bischoff 1968; Perl and Chinard 1968). In relating to physiological variables such as organ blood flow, vascular binding, permeability, and the enzymatic activity (V_{max}) and affinity (K_m) of intracellular enzyme systems and/or excretory apparatuses, these models serve to provide mechanistic insight into the rate-controlling event that governs the overall disposition of a given compound and to ultimately predict changes in clearance when the physiological status of the liver is altered. The most widely used mathematical descriptions of the models have been for steady-state conditions, wherein drug and metabolite binding to liver tissue is completed and does not contribute to the loss of mass. Accordingly, the liver has been viewed as a well-mixed compartment ("well-mixed" or "well-stirred" model) (Kety 1951; Rowland et al. 1973), as an organ receiving a series of nonsegregated, parallel flows surrounded by identical, single sheets of hepatocytes of uniform enzymatic activity ("parallel tube" model) (Winkler et al. 1973), and as an organ with intercalating sheets of hepatocytes which are perfused with highly branched, heterogeneous flows (Koo et al. 1975; Miller et al. 1979) that result in a dispersion of blood elements flowing through sinusoids of varying dimensions ("dispersion" model) (Roberts and Rowland 1986a,b). Both the parallel tube model and the dispersion model are able to describe the repetitive processes of entry, removal, and efflux of a drug and its metabolites along the length of the sinusoid in a distributed-in-space fashion. Variations thereof have included heterogeneous distributions of drug-metabolizing enzymes and of blood flow (Goresky et al. 1973; Bass et al. 1978, 1987; Pang et al. 1983; Pang and Stillwell 1983; Gray and Tam 1986; Gray et al. 1987; Sawada et al. 1985; Roberts and Rowland 1986a).

The properties of the well-stirred, parallel tube, and dispersion models have been compared in detail for drug and primary and secondary metabo-

CLEARANCE MODEL

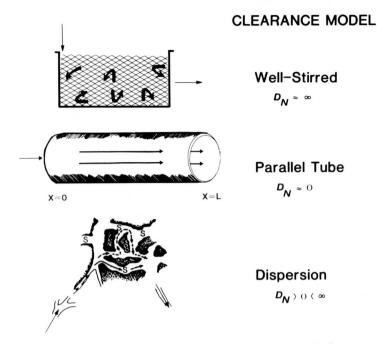

Well–Stirred

$D_N \approx \infty$

Parallel Tube

$D_N \approx 0$

X=0   X=L

Dispersion

$D_N > 0 < \infty$

Fig. 2. Hepatic clearance models that describe drug and metabolite processing. The well-stirred model assumes venous equilibration. The parallel tube model assumes ideal flow through functionally identical sinusoids. The dispersion model describes nonideal flow through circuitous sinusoidal channels. The degree of dispersion of blood elements, shown as the D_N number, is greatest for the well-stirred model and nonexistent for the parallel tube model; the degree of dispersion is intermediate for the dispersion model

lite kinetics (PANG and ROWLAND 1977a,b; PANG and GILLETTE 1978a; COLBURN 1981; AHMAD et al. 1983; KEIDING and CHIARANTINI 1978; KEIDING and STEINESS 1984; ROBERTS and ROWLAND 1986c; JONES et al. 1984; SMALL-WOOD et al. 1988a; ST-PIERRE et al. 1992; ST-PIERRE and PANG, 1993a,b). One feature which distinguishes the models is the degree of mixing achieved with flow within the liver. The well-stirred and parallel tube models represent two extreme flow conditions, well-mixed flow and ideal bulk flow, respectively, whereas for the dispersion model, flow is conceived as flowing through a web of interconnecting sinusoids and is nonideal in nature, in that a variation in the transit times of noneliminated and eliminated substances is assumed to occur (ROBERTS and ROWLAND 1986a,b). This flow behavior is tantamount to a certain degree of geometric dispersion due to the architecture of the liver (GORESKY et al. 1988) and is characterized by the D_N number (or 1/Peclet number) (PERL and CHINARD 1968). There is no dispersion for the parallel tube model ($D_N = 0$), whereas for the well-stirred model, the degree of dispersion is infinite ($D_N = \infty$); for the dispersion model, D_N is intermediate (ROBERTS et al. 1990; ST-PIERRE et al. 1992).

Predictions for the dispersion model hence generally fall between those for the well-stirred model and the parallel tube model.

Due to the different assumptions accompanying the models, differences exist for the estimation of the substrate concentration in liver, $[S]$. The underlying basis of the well-stirred model is that of venous equilibration. In the absence of a transmembrane barrier for drug between the perfusing blood and the intracellular enzyme sites, the concentration of unbound drug in emergent blood is equal to the unbound drug within the hepatic tissue, and the concentration profile across the organ is constant. For the parallel tube model, a concentration gradient develops along the length of the sinusoids due to irreversible drug removal. Equilibration exists at every point x along the length (L) of the sinusoid, and in the presence of perfusion limitation, the substrate concentration is approximated by the logarithmic average of the inlet and outlet concentrations ($\hat{C}$) (Winkler et al. 1974):

$$\hat{C} = \frac{C_{In} - C_{Out}}{\ln(C_{In}/C_{Out})}. \tag{6}$$

When nonlinear protein occurs, the substrate concentration should be approximated by the unbound logarithmic average concentration (Xu et al. 1993):

$$\hat{C}_u = \frac{C_{In,u} - C_{Out,u}}{\ln(C_{In,u}/C_{Out,u})}. \tag{7}$$

No succinct definition of the substrate concentration is presented for the dispersion model, but it can be inferred that the average substrate concentration in liver will fall between those predicted by the well-stirred and parallel tube models.

Due to these presumed concentration terms as an estimate of the substrate concentration in liver, the implied organ enzymatic activity (K_m and V_{max}) will also differ for any given removal rate (v) or extraction of a drug. Whereas very little difference exists for the V_{max}, large differences exist for the projected K_m. The rank order for the K_m is: well-stirred model $<$ dispersion model $<$ parallel tube model, and that for CL_{int} is well-stirred model $>$ dispersion model $>$ parallel tube model.

The following mathematical expressions have been applied to interrelate in vitro data to those in the organ. Membrane-limited transport is assumed to be rapid such that elimination of substrate is perfusion rate limited, that is, the rate-controlling factor is the elimination capacity of the organ.

a) The Well-Stirred Model

Due to venous equilibration, the extraction ratio of precursor drug P, $E\{P\}$, is given by (Rowland et al. 1973; Wilkinson and Shand 1975):

$$E\{P\} = \frac{f_{B(P)}CL_{int(P)}}{Q + f_{B(P)}CL_{int(P)}} \tag{8}$$

where $f_{B(P)}$ is the unbound fraction of precursor in blood, and $CL_{int(P)}$ is the intrinsic clearance for the drug. The hepatic availability of (F), or $(1 - E)$, for P is given as (ROWLAND et al. 1973):

$$F\{P\} = \frac{Q}{Q + f_{B(P)}CL_{int(P)}}. \tag{9}$$

Since formed metabolites are subject to immediate removal within the liver prior to their emergence in the venous circulation, sequential metabolism of the metabolites (PANG and GILLETTE 1979) can be described with respect to the appearance of the metabolite normalized to that formed or the hepatic availability of the formed metabolite. The hepatic availabilities of the primary (M_1) and secondary (M_2) metabolites, when derived from P, are identical to those after administration of M_1 and M_2, respectively (PANG and GILLETTE 1978a; ST-PIERRE et al. 1992):

$$F\{M_1,P\} = F\{M_1\} \tag{10}$$

$$F\{M_2,P\} = F\{M_2\}. \tag{11}$$

The implications of the model are that the handling of a metabolite species is identical regardless of the origin of the metabolite (formed or preformed).

b) The Parallel Tube Model

According to the parallel tube model, the hepatic availability of the parent drug $(F\{P\})$ is related to physiological parameters as follows (WINKLER et al. 1973, 1974; PANG and ROWLAND 1977a):

$$F\{P\} = \frac{C_{(P)Out}}{C_{(P)In}} = e^{-f_{B(P)}CL_{int(P)}/Q}. \tag{12}$$

Hepatic formation and availability of a generated primary metabolite have been derived for flow-limited systems, that is, when an equilibrium exists at any point x along the tube of length L, between the drug or formed primary metabolite(s) in blood and tissue (PANG and GILLETTE 1978a; ST-PIERRE et al. 1992):

$$F\{M_1,P\} = \frac{[F\{M_1\} - F\{P\}]\ln(F\{P\})}{E\{P\}\ln(F\{P\}/F\{M_1\})}. \tag{13}$$

The estimation of $F\{M_1,P\}$ exceeds $F\{M_1\}$ in all cases and is independent of whether competing pathways are absent or present (ST-PIERRE et al. 1992). Conversely, the model predicts that the extent of sequential metabolism of endogenously formed M_1 is less than that of its preformed counterpart $(E\{M_1,P\} < E\{M_1\})$.

   A corresponding expression was derived to predict the hepatic availability of a secondary metabolite (ST-PIERRE et al. 1992):

$$F\{M_2,P\} = \frac{\ln(F\{P\})\ln(F\{M_1\})}{E\{M_1,P\}E\{P\}} \times \left[\frac{F\{P\}}{\ln\left(\frac{F\{P\}}{F\{M_1\}}\right)\ln\left(\frac{F\{P\}}{F\{M_2\}}\right)} \right.$$

$$\left. + \frac{F\{M_1\}}{\ln\left(\frac{F\{P\}}{F\{M_1\}}\right)\ln\left(\frac{F\{M_2\}}{F\{M_1\}}\right)} - \frac{F\{M_2\}}{\ln\left(\frac{F\{P\}}{F\{M_2\}}\right)\ln\left(\frac{F\{M_2\}}{F\{M_1\}}\right)} \right]. \quad (14)$$

c) The Dispersion Model

Two main parameters characterize the model. The axial dispersion number, D_N, is a stochastic measure of the distribution of residence times of blood-borne molecules due to heterogeneous blood flow through the micro-vasculature. The efficiency number, R_N, describes irreversible removal of substrate by the liver under first-order conditions and is given by the general expression:

$$R_{N,i} = \frac{f_{B(i)}CL_{int(i)}P_i}{Q}, \quad (15)$$

where P_i is the permeability coefficient of the plasma membrane to the drug molecules of the i-th species (P, M_1, or M_2), and is calculated from $p_i/(p_i + CL_{int(i)})$, where p_i is the permeability surface area product (trans-membrane clearance) of the ith substrate. The terms: $R_{N,P}$, $R_{N,M1}$, and $R_{N,M2}$ are the efficiency numbers of the preformed substrates P, M_1, and M_2, respectively. Since p_i greatly exceeds $CL_{int(i)}$ for all substrates, P_i is unity and $R_{N,i}$ reduces to $f_{B(i)} \cdot CL_{int(i)}/Q$.

As shown by ROBERTS and ROWLAND (1986a,b), the hepatic availability of any preformed species, is given by:

$$F\{P\} = \frac{C_{(P)Out}}{C_{(P)In}} = \frac{4\alpha}{(1 + \alpha)^2 \cdot e^{(\alpha-1)/2D_N} - (1 - \alpha)^2 \cdot e^{-(\alpha+1)/2D_N}}, \quad (16)$$

where $\alpha = (1 + D_N R_{N,P})^{1/2}$; $C_{(P)Out}$ and $C_{(P)In}$ are input and output drug concentrations, respectively; and the hepatic availability of the formed, primary metabolite $F\{M_1,P\}$ is

---

Fig. 3A,B. The extent of sequential metabolism of a primary ($E\{M_1,P\}$) and secondary ($E\{M_2,P\}$) metabolite according to the well-stirred, parallel tube (**A**), and dispersion (**B**) models, when enzyme systems are evenly distributed. The extraction ratio of the precursor P ($E\{P\}$) was 0.99, 0.95, or 0.1; the extraction ratio of the preformed, primary metabolite ($E\{M_1\}$) was plotted against the predicted extraction ratio of the formed, primary metabolite ($E\{M_1,P\}$) (*upper panels*). The extraction ratios of the precursors P [or ($E\{P\}$)] and M_1 [or $E\{M_1,P\}$] were 0.95 and/or 0.1; the extraction ratio of the preformed, secondary metabolite [$E\{M_2,\}$] was plotted against the predicted extraction ratio of the formed, secondary metabolite [or $E\{M_2,P\}$]. Note that the predictions from the dispersion model fall between those for the well-stirred (----) and parallel tube models. (Data from ST-PIERRE et al. 1992)

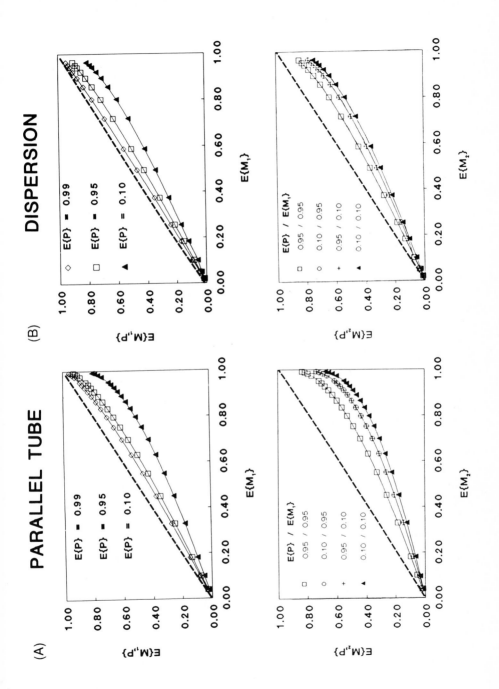

$$F\{M_1,P\} = \frac{C_{(M_1,P)\text{Out}}}{C_{(M_1,P)\text{formed}}} = \frac{R_{N,P}(F\{M_1\} - F\{P\})}{(R_{N,P} - R_{N,M_1})(1 - F\{P\})}, \tag{17}$$

where $C_{(M_1,P)\text{Out}}$ and $C_{(M_1,P)\text{formed}}$ denote the concentrations of primary metabolite detected in venous blood, in the presence and absence of elimination, respectively. The expression for the availability of M_2, arising from a precursor at steady state, is (St-Pierre et al. 1992):

$$F\{M_2,P\} = \frac{R_{N,M_1}R_{N,P}}{E\{P\}E\{M_1,P\}}\left[\frac{F\{P\}}{(R_{N,M_1} - R_{N,P})(R_{N,M_2} - R_{N,P})}\right.$$
$$+ \frac{F\{M_1\}}{(R_{N,P} - R_{N,M_1})(R_{N,M_2} - R_{N,M_1})}$$
$$\left.+ \frac{F\{M_2\}}{(R_{N,M_2} - R_{N,M_1})(R_{N,M_2} - R_{N,P})}\right]. \tag{18}$$

Again, absence or presence of competing pathways will not alter the extent of sequential metabolism of the generated metabolites.

d) Comparison of Hepatic Clearance Models

The predictions of the dispersion model for drug and metabolites are intermediate between those of the well-stirred and parallel tube models (Fig. 3). For the well-stirred model, parent drug behavior fails to exert an influence on the extent of sequential metabolism of the metabolites, whereas for the parallel tube and dispersion models, parameters relating to the precursor (namely $E\{P\}$ or the corresponding intrinsic clearances) exert a strong influence over the extent of sequential metabolism of the primary and secondary metabolites. When $E\{P\}$ is large (with greater values of CL_{int}), the apparent extraction ratios of the formed metabolites, $E\{M_1,P\}$ or $E\{M_2,P\}$, are closer to those of the preformed metabolites, $E\{M_1\}$ and $E\{M_2\}$. When both $E\{P\}$ and $E\{M_1\}$ are high, smaller differences in $E\{M_2,P\}$ versus $E\{M_2\}$ are seen, indicating that rapid consecutive formation steps favor the progression of ensuing metabolism (Fig. 3). An increase in the number of formation steps for a generated metabolite augments the difference between $E\{M_i,P\}$ and $E\{M_i\}$, since $E\{M_1,P\} < E\{M_1\}$ and $E\{M_2,P\} < E\{M_2,M_1\} < E\{M_2\}$ for the parallel tube and dispersion models (St-Pierre et al. 1992).

2. In Vitro–Organ Correlations

In vitro CL_{int} has been used to predict hepatic drug extraction ratios (E) or clearances (CL). In this area of endeavor, correlations have been sought with the well-stirred model, based on the K_m and V_{max} obtained in vitro. On occasion, data obtained in vitro have been used for comparison to the K_m and V_{max} obtained in perfused livers according to equations for the parallel tube model (Keiding et al. 1979). These correlations between the cytochrome P-450s (Table 1), other phase I (Table 2) and phase II reactions (Table 3), and observations and predictions according to models of hepatic clearances are summarized. Correlations of data from isolated liver cells and perfused liver preparations for phase I and phase II reactions (Table 4) have also been performed. Prediction of metabolite date, however, is seldom attempted. This is perhaps because the liver, in particular, possesses mechanisms for further metabolism and excretion of the metabolites. More likely, however, is that interpretation of metabolite data is far more complex than that for the parent substrate, with the added requirements that metabolite levels are assayed with good certainty and sites of further metabolism are identified (PANG and KWAN 1983).

II. Concept of Total Body Clearance

The body is made up of a host of organs and tissues, each used for discrete functions. Each is interconnected by way of the circulation, with the arterial supply bringing oxygenated blood to the organs, and the venous system providing drainage out of organs. When a drug enters an organ/tissue, drug loss ensues due to removal, and the concepts developed above for organs may be applied here, though modifications are often made because of structural variations and the occurrence of different modes of processing. In viewing the body as a whole in carrying out drug metabolism or excretion, organ clearances are usually summed to provide total body clearance (CL_{tot}). This is particularly true when organs are arranged in parallel, that is, an individual organ/tissue receives a separate (parallel) arterial supply arising from the aorta, and the venous return drains into the vena cava for entry to the heart and lung for oxygenation. There are, however, organs arranged in series which deserve consideration, largely because the intestine, liver, and lung constitute a unit involved in the first-pass metabolism of drugs. Clearance relationships between organs in parallel and organs in series do differ, as elaborated in the ensuing section.

  Direct extrapolation of in vitro data to in vivo is often performed, either with compartmental analysis or more rigorously, with physiological modeling. Both approaches take on the assumption of venous equilibration, that is, the compartment is well stirred and venous equilibration occurs. For compartmental analysis, the K_m and V_{max} data for phase I (Table 5) and phase II (Table 6) reactions, mostly from liver subcellular fractions and isolated cells (Table 7), have been utilized to predict either first-pass drug metabolism (availability) or total body clearance in vivo. By contrast for physiological modeling, the K_m and V_{max} but also data on plasma and tissue protein binding (or tissue partitioning characteristics) and physiological volumes and flows are utilized to describe concentration–time profiles. Data of perfused organs, mostly the liver, have been used to predict the first-pass effect or total-body clearance, with the hidden assumption that the liver is the sole organ for drug removal. More recently, combined organ perfusion techniques (YASUHARA et al. 1985; DAUGAARD et al. 1987; HIRAYAMA et al. 1989; XU et al. 1989) have been developed to describe drug and metabolite

Table 1. Scale-up of data from subcellular fractions to organ systems for phase I (cytochrome P-450) reactions in the rat

Drug	In vitro data Preparation[a]	K_m^b (μM)	V_{max}^c (nmol/min/g)	CL_{int}^d (ml/min)	Perfusion data Perfusion conditions[e]	$C(0)$ or CL_{in},ss^f (μM)	f_B^g	Q^h (ml/min)	Predicted E^i WS	DM	PM	Observed E	References
Liver													
Alprenolol	MS*	25	1024	410	0% alb, 0% rbc, R	15	1.00	20	0.953	1.000	1.000	0.980	Börg et al. (1974) Rane et al. (1977)
Antipyrine	MS MS*	22000 3500	1760 272	0.80 0.78	0% alb, 0% rbc, R 0% alb, 0% rbc, R 2% alb, 11.5% rbc, R	1500 6.2 260	1.00 1.00 1.00	20 40 20	0.037 0.019 0.037	0.038 0.019 0.038	0.038 0.019 0.038	0.010 0.009 0.057	Rane et al. (1977) McManus and Ilett (1979) Rane et al. (1977) Øie and Fiori (1985) Chindavijak et al. (1987)
Benzo[a]pyrene	MS* MS (3MC)*	5.5 0.05	41 152	74 28200	3% alb, 20% rbc, R 3% alb, 20% rbc, R	0.2 0.2	NA[j] NA[j]	10 10	0.881 1.000	0.989 1.000	0.999 1.000	0.590 0.670	Wiersma and Roth (1983a) Wiersma and Roth (1983a)
Carbamazepine	S9* MS	60 730	28 80	4.7 1.1	0% alb, 0% rbc, R 1.2% alb, 0% rbc, S	42 35	1.00 0.48	20 10	0.189 0.183	0.202 0.195	0.208 0.200	0.040 0.210	Westenberg (1980) Rane et al. (1977) Chang and Levy (1985)
Diazepam	MS*	1.4	22	156	0% alb, 20% rbc, S 1% alb, 20% rbc, S	0.4 18	0.95[k] 0.23	15 10	0.908 0.783	0.996 0.927	1.000 0.973	0.977 0.956	Igari et al. (1984) Rowland et al. (1984) St-Pierre and Pang (1987)
Hexobarbital	S9 MS*	105 99	168 848	16 86	0% alb, 0% rbc, R	53	1.00	20	0.811	0.950	0.986	0.330	Rane et al. (1977) Igari et al. (1982) Rane et al. (1977)
Imipramine	MS: (N-demethylation)* (2-hydroxylation)*	5.12 0.43	411 63	803 1476	0% alb, 0% rbc, R	11	1.00	20	0.991	1.000	1.000	0.980	Chiba et al. (1990a,b) Chiba et al. (1990a,b) Beaubien and Pakuts (1979)
Lidocaine	MS MS MS: (3-hydroxylation)* (N-deethylation)*	250 58 1.8 595	768 476 15 502	31 82 86 8.4	1% alb, 20% rbc, S 0% alb, 20% rbc, R 20% rat whole blood, R 0% alb, 0% rbc, S 2% alb, 11.5% rbc, R	4 6 12 10 43	0.95 0.95[l] 0.95[l] 1.00 0.95[l]	10 10 20 40 20	0.899 0.899 0.817 0.691 0.817	0.994 0.994 0.955 0.832 0.955	1.000 1.000 0.989 0.893 0.989	0.996 0.991 0.950 0.970 0.855	Nyberg et al. (1977) Roberts and Rowland (1985) Suzuki et al. (1984) Suzuki et al. (1984) Pang and Rowland (1977b) Ahmad et al. (1983) Shand et al. (1975) Tam et al. (1987) Chindavijak et al. (1987)
MEGX	MS*	21	5.7	2.7	1% alb, 20% rbc, R 0% alb, 0% rbc, S	3 2	1.00 1.00	10 40	0.214 0.064	0.231 0.065	0.238 0.066	0.900 0.685	Suzuki et al. (1984) Pang and Rowland (1977c) Saville et al. (1987)

Drug	In vitro data[a]				C_{in}[f]	Binding conditions[e]	f_B[g]	Q[h]	E[i]				Reference
Phenacetin	MS	19											Roberts and Rowland (1985)
					0.1	1% alb, 20% rbc, S	NA[j]	10	0.654	0.787	0.849	0.910	Pang and Gillette (1978a)
					0.4	1% alb, 20% rbc, S	NA[j]	12	0.612	0.734	0.793	0.850	Pang et al. (1988b)
Phenytoin	S9*	31	62	20									Kutt and Fouts (1971)
					20	0% alb, 0% rbc, R	1.00	20	0.499	0.587	0.630	0.530	Rane et al. (1977)
					10	0% alb, 0% rbc, R	1.00	20	0.499	0.587	0.630	0.370	Shand et al. (1975)
Propranolol	MS	5	100	50									Shand and Oates (1971)
	MS	0.16	1247	20									Hori et al. (1985)
	MS: (4-hydroxylation)*[m]	0.17	1156	20									Ishida et al. (1992)
		194	1.5	29									Ishida et al. (1992)
	(5-hydroxylation)*[m]	0.05	434	2									Ishida et al. (1992)
		68	0.43	3									Ishida et al. (1992)
	(7-hydroxylation)*	0.18	599	11									Ishida et al. (1992)
	(N-desisopropylation)*	109	3.1	33									Ishida et al. (1992)
					6	0% alb, 10% rbc, R	0.64	16	1.000	1.000	1.000	0.970	Jones et al. (1984)
					39	0% alb, 20% rbc, R	0.64[n]	20	1.000	1.000	1.000	1.000	Shand et al. (1975)
					15	3% alb, 20% rbc, R	0.29[n]	13	1.000	1.000	1.000	0.945	Keiding and Steiness (1984)
					193	2% alb, 11.5% rbc, R	0.38[a]	20	1.000	1.000	1.000	0.925	Chindavijak et al. (1987)
					6	1% alb, 10% rbc, R	0.46[a]	16	1.000	1.000	1.000	0.993	Smallwood et al. (1988c)
Tolbutamide	MS*	960	116	1.2									Sugita et al. (1981, 1982)
					37	0% alb, 20% rbc, S	1.00	15	0.075	0.077	0.077	0.250	Schary and Rowland (1983)
Lung Benzo[a]pyrene	MS*	0.22	0.11	0.73	0.2	3% alb, 20% rbc, R	NA[j]	45	0.016	0.016	0.016	0.022	Wiersma and Roth (1983a)
	MS (3MC)*	0.23	0.87	5.7	0.2	3% alb, 20% rbc, R	NA[j]	45	0.112	0.116	0.118	0.198	Wiersma and Roth (1983a)

* In vitro data used for prediction

[a] MS, microsomal fraction; S9, 9000 × g supernatant fraction; 3MC, 3-methylcholanthrene treated

[b] Corrected for unbound fraction in the reaction mixture, if binding data were available

[c] V_{max} value obtained in subcellular fraction (nmol/min/mg protein) was converted to that for the intact liver (nmol/min/g liver), after assuming 51.2 mg microsomal protein/g liver (Lin et al. 1980), 96 mg cytosolic protein/g liver, and/or 127 mg S9 protein/g liver (Pang et al. 1985)

[d] Calculated as V_{max}/K_m where the liver and lung had assumed weights of 10 and 1.5 g, respectively

[e] alb, albumin; rbc, blood cells; R, recirculation; S, single pass

[f] Initial or input drug concentration in perfusate

[g] Unbound fraction in perfusate

[h] Perfusate flow rate

[i] E, extraction ratio; WS, well-stirred model; DM, dispersion model (D_N = 0.17 assumed; St-Pierre et al. 1992); PM, parallel tube model

[j] Not available; f_B was assigned as 1.0

[k] Predicted based on C_b/C_p = 1.05 by St. Pierre and Pang (1992b)

[l] Data of Pang and Rowland (1977b)

[m] Biphasic in vitro kinetics (two sets of K_m's and V_{max}'s) have been reported

[n] f_B from Jones et al. (1984)

Table 2. Scale-up of data from subcellular fraction to organ systems for other phase I (non-cytochrome P-450) reactions in the rat

Drug	Major enzymes[a]	Preparation	K_m[b] (μM)	V_{max}[c] (nmol/min/g)	CL_{int}[d] (ml/min)	Perfusion conditions[e]	C(0) or Cln,ss[f] (μM)	fB[g]	Q[h] (ml/min)	Predicted E[i] WS	DM	PT	Observed E	References
Liver: oxidation														
Ethanol	MEOS	Microsomal	20000	420	0.21									Clejan and Cederbaum (1989)
	ADH	Cytosolic	26	14	1344									Messiha and Hughes (1979)
	ADH	4000 × g SUP	285		1724									Ci cero et al. (1980)
	ADH	Homogenate*	480		3667	1% alb, 20% rbc, S	2000	1.00	12	0.997	1.000	1.000	0.925	Lumeng and Crabb (1984)
						2% alb, 30% rbc, S	581	1.00	12	0.997	1.000	1.000	0.932	Pang et al. (1988b); Keiding and Prisholm (1984)
5-Hydroxytryptamine	MAO	600 × g SUP*	70	119	17	4% alb, 20% rbc, R	0.1	0.93	11	0.586	0.701	0.757	0.590	Wiersma and Roth (1980)
Liver: hydrolysis														
Meperidine	Esterase	Microsomal	280	855	31	1% alb, 20% rbc, S	4.0	1.00	10	0.824	0.959	0.991	1.000	Freeman et al. (1977); Yeh (1982)
		Microsomal*	120	563	47	0% alb, 20% rbc, R	6.8	1.00[j]	10	0.824	0.959	0.991	0.976	Babiak et al. (1984)
						1% alb, 20% rbc, S	8.1	1.00[j]	12	0.796	0.938	0.980	0.953	Ahmad et al. (1983); Pang et al. (1988b)
4-Methylumbelliferone glucuronide	β-Glucuronidase	9000 × g SUP	1.8	1.1	6.2	1% alb, 20% rbc, S	150	0.76	12	0.281	0.310	0.323	0.071	Miyauchi et al. (1989); Ratna et al. (1993)
						3% alb, 20% rbc, S	44	0.61[k]	16	0.190	0.203	0.209	0.058	Miyauchi et al. (1989)
4-Methylumbelliferone sulfate	Sulfatase	9000 × g SUP*	309	347	11	1% alb, 20% rbc, S	99	0.18	10	0.168	0.178	0.183	0.100	Miyauchi et al. (1989); Anundi et al. (1986)
		Homogenate	600	833	14	3% alb, 20% rbc, S	41	0.07[k]	16	0.047	0.048	0.054	0.054	Ratna et al. (1993)
						0% alb, 20% rbc, S	122	1.00	10	0.529	0.626	0.674	0.470	Miyauchi et al. (1989); Chiba and Pang (1993)
Lung: oxidation														
5-Hydroxytryptamine	MAO	600 × g SUP*	94	89	1.4	4% alb, 20% rbc, R	0.1	0.93	47	0.027	0.028	0.028	0.426	Wiersma and Roth (1980)

* In vitro data used for predictions

[a] ADH, alcohol dehydrogenase; MEOS, microsomal ethanol oxygenase system; MAO, monoamine oxidase

[b] Corrected for unbound fraction in the reaction mixture, if binding data were available

[c] V_{max} value obtained in subcellular fraction of liver (nmol/min/mg protein) was converted to that in the intact liver (nmol/min/g liver) by assuming that there were 51.2 mg microsomal protein/g liver (Lin et al. 1980), 96 mg cytosolic protein/g liver, and/or 127 mg S9 protein/g liver (Pang et al. 1985)

[d] Calculated as V_{max}/K_m where the liver and the lung had assumed weights of 10 and 1.5 g, respectively

[e] alb, albumin; rbc, blood cells; R, recirculation; S, single pass

[f] Initial or input drug concentration in the perfusate

[g] Unbound fraction in perfusate

[h] Perfusate flow rate

[i] E, extraction ratio; WS, well-stirred model; DM, dispersion model with $D_N = 0.17$ (St-Pierre et al. 1992); PM, parallel tube model

[j] Data of Babiak et al. (1984)　　[k] Predicted based on the binding kinetics reported by Ratna et al. (1993)

Table 3. Scale-up of data from subcellular fraction to organ systems for phase II reactions in the rat liver

Drug	In vitro data					Perfusion data				Predicted E^i			Observed E	References
	Major enzyme[a]	Preparation	K_m[b] (μM)	V_{max}[c] (nmol/min/g)	CL_{int}[d] (ml/min)	Perfusion conditions[e]	$C(0)$ or $CI_{in,ss}$[d] (μM)	f_B[g]	Q[h] (ml/min)	WS	DM	PM		
Procainamide	NAT	S9000 × g SUP*	20300	204	0.1	1% alb, 20% rbc, S	2.6	NA[j]	10	0.010	0.010	0.010	0.823	Schneck et al. (1978), Pang et al. (1984b)
Harmol	AST	Homogenate*	30	300	100									Mulder and Hagedoorn (1974)
	GT	Microsomal*	150	1331	89	1% alb, 15% rbc, S	10	0.60	10	0.919	0.998	1.000	0.850	Koster et al. (1982)
						1% alb, 20% rbc, S	10	0.60	10	0.919	0.998	1.000	0.878	Pang et al. (1981)
7-Hydroxycoumarin	GT	Microsomal*	67	727	109	0% alb, 0% rbc, S	5.0	1.00	35	0.756	0.902	0.955	0.950	Koster and Noordhoek (1982), Conway et al. (1982)
4-Methylumbelliferone	AST	Cytosolic*	1.1	385	3498	1% alb, 20% rbc, S	0.01	0.43	10	0.993	1.000	1.000	0.970	Kauffman et al. (1991), Ratna et al. (1993)
						3% alb, 20% rbc, S	15	0.19	16	0.976	1.000	1.000	1.000	Miyauchi et al. (1989)
p-Nitrophenol	GT	Microsomal[k]	30	15	5.1									Winsnes (1972)
	GT	Microsomal[k,l]	1450	44	0.31									Winsnes (1972)
		Microsomal	360	268	7.4									
		Microsomal	1800	558	3.1									
	GT	Microsomal	240	100	4.2									Lucier et al. (1975)
	GT	Microsomal*	253	180	7.1	2.5% alb, 12.5% rbc, R	500	0.42	15	0.166	0.176	0.180	0.640	Morrison et al. (1986)
	Diabetic: GT	Microsomal*	253	111	4.4	2.5% alb, 12.5% rbc, R	500	0.42	15	0.109	0.114	0.116	0.467	Morrison et al. (1986)
Phenol	AST	Cytosolic*	180	700	39	1% alb, 20% rbc, S	0.53	NA[j]	14	0.741	0.887	0.943	0.980	Belanger et al. (1985), Cassidy and Houston (1984)
Bromosulfophthalein	GST	Cytosolic*	40	9766	2472	0% alb, 0% rbc, S	10	1.00	24	0.990	1.000	1.000	0.500	Folot et al. (1984), Chen et al. (1984)
						1% alb, 20% rbc, S	0.5	0.002	10	0.331	0.371	0.390	0.520	Zhao et al. (1993)
α-Bromoisovalerylurea (R)	GST	Purified enzyme* (2-2)[m]	1400	750	0.5	1% alb, 20% rbc, S	12	0.85	10	0.162	0.172	0.176	0.600	Te Koppele et al. (1988)
		(3-3)[m]	2600	4550	1.8									Te Koppele et al. (1988), Polhuis et al. (1993)
														Te Koppele et al. (1988)
(S)	GST	(1-1)[m]	2000	1110	0.6	1% alb, 20% rbc, S	8	0.83	10	0.235	0.255	0.264	0.350	Te Koppele et al. (1988)
		(2-2)[m]	600	1590	2.7									Te Koppele et al. (1988)
		(3-3)[m]	3100	1510	0.5									Polhuis et al. (1993)

* In vitro data used for the prediction

[a] NAT, N-acetyltransferase; AST, arylsulfotransferase; GT, UDP-glucuronyltransferase; GST, glutathione S-transferase

[b] Corrected for unbound fraction in the reaction mixture, if binding data wwere available

[c] V_{max} value measured in the subcellular fraction of liver (nmol/min/mg protein) was converted to that for liver (nmol/min/g liver) by assuming that there were 51.2 mg microsomal protein/g liver (Lin et al. 1980), 96 mg cytosolic protein/g liver, and/or 127 mg S9 protein/g liver (Pang et al. 1985)

[d] Calculated as V_{max}/K_m where the rat liver weight was assumed to be 10 g   [e] alb, albumin; rbc, blood cells; R, recirculation; S, single pass

[f] Initial or input drug concentration in the perfusate   [g] Unbound fraction in the perfusate

[h] Perfusate flow rate   [i] E, extraction ratio; WS, well-stirred model; DM, dispersion model with $D_N = 0.17$ (St-Pierre et al. 1992); PM, parallel tube model

[j] Not available; f_B was assigned a value of 1.0   [k] Biphasic in vitro kinetics (two sets of K_m's and V_{max}'s) have been reported

[l] Triton X-100 pretreated   [m] Rat GSH isozymes

Table 4. Scale-up of data from isolated hepatocytes to organ systems in the rat

Drug	Major enzymes[a]	K_m[b] (μM)	V_{max}[c] (nmol/min/g)	CL_{int}[d] (ml/min)	Perfusion conditions[e]	$C(0)$ or CIn,ss[f] (μM)	f_B[g]	Q[h] (ml/min)	WS	DM	PM	Observed E	References
Diazepam	Cytochrome P-450*	11	525	500	0% alb, 20% rbc, S	0.35	0.95[j]	10	0.980	1.000	1.000	0.977	Chenery et al. (1987), Rowland et al. (1984)
Imipramine	N-Demethylase*, 2-Hydroxylase*	2.1, 0.7	1024, 66	4875, 932	0% alb, 0% rbc, S	11	1.00	40	0.993	1.000	1.000	0.980	Chiba et al. (1990b), Chiba et al. (1990b), Beaubien and Pakuts (1979)
Acetaminophen	AST*, GT*	30, 2130	136, 163	45, 0.8	1% alb, 20% rbc, S	0.14	1.00	10	0.822	0.958	0.990	0.670	Mizuma et al. (1985a), Mizuma et al. (1985a), Pang and Gillette (1978a), Pang and Terrell (1981b), Fayz et al. (1984), Pang et al. (1988b)
					1% alb, 20% rbc, S	1.5	1.00	10	0.822	0.958	0.990	0.722	
					2% alb, 20% rbc, S	2	1.00	10	0.822	0.958	0.990	0.700	
					1% alb, 20% rbc, S	0.14	1.00	12	0.794	0.936	0.979	0.660	
Harmol	AST*, GT*			716, 225	1% alb, 15% rbc, S	10	0.60	10	0.983	1.000	1.000	0.850	Araya et al. (1984), Araya et al. (1984), Koster et al. (1982), Pang et al. (1981)
					1% alb, 20% rbc, S	10	0.60	10	0.983	1.000	1.000	0.878	
p-Nitrophenol	GT, AST*, GT*	227, 38	896, 125	40, 1200, 33	2.5% alb, 12.5% rbc, R	500	0.42	15	0.972	1.000	1.000	0.390	Eacho et al. (1981), Mizuma et al. (1982), Mizuma et al. (1982), Morrison et al. (1986)
	Diabetic: GT*, Diabetic	295	861	29	2.5% alb, 12.5% rbc, R	500	0.42	15	0.450	0.523	0.558	0.318	Eacho et al. (1981), Morrison et al. (1986)
Salicylamide	AST*, GT*	6, 190	63, 160	104, 8.4	1% alb, 20% rbc, S	30	0.74[k]	10	0.893	0.992	1.000	0.992	Koike et al. (1981), Koike et al. (1981), Xu et al. (1989), Xu et al. (1990)
					1% alb, 20% rbc, S	35	0.74	10	0.893	0.992	1.000	0.998	
4-Methylumbelliferyl sulfate	Sulfatase	750	479	6.4	1% alb, 20% rbc, S	99	0.18[l]	12	0.087	0.090	0.091	0.100	Kauffman et al. (1991), Ratna et al. (1993), Miyauchi et al. (1989)
					3% alb, 20% rbc, S	41	0.18[l]	16	0.067	0.069	0.069	0.054	

* In vitro data used for predictions

[a] GT, UDP-glucuronyltransferase; AST, arylsulfotransferase

[b] Corrected for unbound fraction in the reaction mixture, if binding data were available

[c] V_{max} value obtained with hepatocytes (nmol/min per 10^6 cells or nmol/min/mg cellular protein) was converted to that for the intact liver (nmol/min/g liver) by assuming that there were 125×10^6 cells/g liver (Lin et al. 1980) and 1313 mg cellular protein/g liver (Iwamoto et al. 1984), respectively

[d] Calculated as V_{max}/K_m for a 10-g rat liver   [e] alb, albumin; rbc, blood cells; R, recirculation; S, single pass

[f] Initial or input drug concentration in perfusate   [g] Unbound fraction in perfusate

[h] Perfusate flow rate   [i] E, extraction ratio; WS, well-stirred model; DM, dispersion model $D_N = 0.17$ (St-Pierre et al. 1992); PM, parallel tube model

[j] Predicted based on $C_b/C_p = 1.05$ by St-Pierre and Pang (1992b)   [k] Data of Xu et al. (1990)

[l] Data of Ratna et al. (1993)

Table 5. Scale-up of data from subcellular fraction to whole body for phase I hepatic metabolism

Drug	In vitro data — Major enzyme[a]	Preparation	Species[b]	K_m[c] (μM)	V_{max}[d] (nmol/min/g)	CL_{int}[e] (ml/min)	In vivo data (intravenous) — f_B[f]	Q[g] (ml/min)	Predicted E[h] WS	DM	PM	Observed E	Predicted CL_h[i] WS	DM	PM	Observed CL_{tot} (ml/min)	References
Antipyrine	Cytochrome P-450	Microsomal	Rat	22 000	1760	0.8	1.00	20	0.037	0.038	0.038		0.75	0.76	0.76	2.6	RANE et al. (1977), MCMANUS and ILETT (1979)
		Microsomal*	Rat	3500	272	0.8											
		Microsomal*	Rabbit	5000	325	6.5	1.00	20	0.037	0.038	0.038	0.065	6.26	6.35	6.38	27.0	SINMGH et al. (1991), MCMANUS and ILETT (1979)
							1.00	170	0.037	0.037	0.038						
Benzo[a]pyrene	Cytochrome P-450	Microsomal*	Rat	5.5	41	74	0.14	20	0.342	0.385	0.406		6.9	7.7	8.1	18.4	WIERSMA and ROTH (1983b)
		Microsomal (3MC)*	Rat	0.05	152	28 222	0.14	20	0.995	1.000	1.000		19.9	20.0	20.0	58.0	WIERSMA and ROTH (1983b)
Carbamazepine	Cytochrome P-450	Microsomal	Rat	730	80	1.1	0.22[j]	20	0.049	0.05	0.05		0.97	0.99	1.00	5.0	RANE et al. (1977), WESTENBERG (1980)
		S9000 × g SUP*	Rat	60	28	4.7	0.22[j]	20	0.049	0.05	0.05		0.97	0.99	1.00	4.5	REMMEL et al. (1990)
Diazepam	Cytochrome P-450	Microsomal*	Rat	1.44	22	156	0.14	20	0.522	0.618	0.665						IGARI et al. (1984), IGARI et al. (1983)
			Rat														
			Man									0.650					INABA et al. (1988)
		S9000 × g SUP*	Man			629	0.02	1500	0.007	0.007	0.007		10.4	10.4	10.4	11.5	KLOTZ and REIMANN (1981)
Ethoxybenzamide	Cytochrome P-450	Microsomal*	Rat	378	124	3.3	0.67	20	0.099	0.103	0.104	0.120	1.98	2.05	2.08	2.2	LIN et al. (1980), LIN et al. (1978)
		Microsomal*[k]	Rat	19	88	503											LIN et al. (1982)
			Rabbit	1060	138	14	0.50	170	0.603	0.723	0.782		103	123	133	86.7	LIN et al. (1982), LIN et al. (1982)
Hexobarbital (±)	Cytochrome P-450	S9000 × g SUP	Rat	105	168	16	0.62	20	0.725	0.870	0.929	0.690	14.5	17.4	18.6	12.5	RANE et al. (1977), IGARI et al. (1982)
(±)		Microsomal*	Rat	99	848	86											VERMEULEN (1980)
(±)		Microsomal*	Rat	150	497	33											MIYANO and TOKI (1980)
(+)			Rat				0.55	20	0.477	0.558	0.598	0.940					VAN DER GRAAFF et al. (1983)
(−)		Microsomal*	Rat	300	343	11											MIYANO and TOKI (1983)
(−)			Rat				0.55	20	0.239	0.260	0.270	0.680					VAN DER GRAAFF et al. (1983)

Table 5. *Continued*

Drug	Major enzyme[a]	Preparation	Species[b]	K_m[c] (μM)	V_{max}[d] (nmol/min/g)	CL_{int}[e] (ml/min)	f_B[f]	Q[g] (ml/min)	Pred E[h] WS	DM	PM	Obs E	Pred CL_h[i] (ml/min) WS	DM	PM	Obs CL_{tot} (ml/min)	References
Imipramine	N-Demethylase	Microsomal*	Rat	5.1	411	803											Chiba et al. (1988, 1990b)
	2-Hydroxylase			0.43	63	1476											Chiba et al. (1988, 1990b)
			Rat				0.11	20	0.924	0.998	1.000	0.920					Chiba et al. (1990a)
Lidocaine	Cytochrome P-450	Microsomal	Rat	250	768	31											Nyberg et al. (1977)
	3-Hydroxylase	S9000 × g SUP	Rat	58	476	82											Rane et al. (1977)
	N-Deethylase	Microsomal*	Rat	1.8	15	86											Suzuki et al. (1984)
			Rat	595	502	8.4											Suzuki et al. (1984)
							0.38[l]	20	0.641	0.772	0.833	0.981	12.8	15.4	16.7	17.6	Supradist et al. (1983)
Phenacetin	Cytochrome P-450	Microsomal*	Rat			19											Roberts and Rowland (1985)
				NA[m]	20				0.486	0.570	0.611	0.130	9.72	11.4	12.2	1.86	Klippert et al. (1983)
Phenytoin	Cytochrome P-450	Microsomal (p HPPH)*	Rat	92	16	100											Blake et al. (1978)
		(H2DIOL)*	Rat	84	0.72	1247											Blake et al. (1978)
							0.30	20	0.026	0.027	0.027		0.53	0.53	0.53	1.03	Collins et al. (1978)
	Cytochrome P-450	Microsomal (p HPPH)*	Rat[n]	97	7												Blake et al. (1978)
		(H2DIOL)*	Rat[n]	87	0.91												Blake et al. (1978)
																	Collins et al. (1978)
Propranolol	Cytochrome P-450	Microsomal	Rat	5	50	100	0.28	20	0.012	0.012	0.012	0.012	0.24	0.24	0.24	0.98	Shand and Oates (1971)
		Microsomal MS: (4-hydroxylation)*[k]	Rat	0.16	20	1247											Hori et al. (1985)
			Rat	0.17	20	1156											Ishida et al. (1992)
			Rat	194	29	1.5											Ishida et al. (1992)
		(5-hydroxylation)*[k]	Rat	0.05	2	434											Ishida et al. (1992)
		(7-hydroxylation)*	Rat	68	3	0.43											Ishida et al. (1992)
		(N-desisopropylation)*	Rat	0.18	11	599											Ishida et al. (1992)
			Rat	109	33	3.1											Ishida et al. (1992)
			Rat				0.14		0.939	0.999	1.000	0.959	18.8	20.0	20.0	19.2	Terao and Shen (1983)
			Rat				0.15	20	0.941	0.999	1.000	0.892	18.8	20.0	20.0	17.8	Iwamoto et al. (1985)
			Rat				0.17	20	0.900	0.994	1.000	0.730					Singh et al. (1991)
Quinidine	Cytochrome P-450	Microsomal*	Rat	2.6	46	175											Rakhit and Mico (1985)
			Rat				0.34	20	0.746	0.892	0.947		14.9	17.8	18.9	15.6	Fremstad et al. (1977)
Theophylline	P-450 (3-MX)	Microsomal*	Man	1760	0.11	0.10											Sarkar et al. (1990)
	(1MX)			1680	0.12	0.11											Sarkar et al. (1990)
	(8OH)			4500	1.16	0.39											Sarkar et al. (1990)
			Man				0.44	1500	0.000	0.000	0.000	0.000	0.26	0.26	0.26	45.5	Bieman and Williams (1989)

Drug	Enzyme	In vitro fraction	Species														Reference
Thiopental	Cytochrome P-450	Microsomal*	Rat	103	33	3.2	0.65	20	0.094	0.098	0.099	0.140	1.89	1.95	1.98	2.80	IGARI et al. (1982)
Tolbutamide	Cytochrome P-450	Microsomal*	Rat	960	116	1.2	0.24	20	0.014	0.014	0.014	0.030	0.28	0.28	0.28	0.36	SCHNECK et al. (1978); SUGITA et al. (1981, 1982)
		Microsomal*	Man	120	14	175	0.04	1500	0.005	0.005	0.005		6.96	6.97	6.97	17.0	VERONESE et al. (1989); BALANT (1981)
Warfarin (R)-(+)	Cytochrome P-450	Microsomal*	Man		24		0.01	1500	0.000	0.000	0.000		0.24	0.24	0.24	3.0	RETTIE et al. (1988)
(R)-(+)																	HOLFORD (1987)
(S)-(-)		Microsomal*	Man		121		0.01	1500	0.001	0.001	0.001		1.2	1.2	1.2	4.1	RETTIE et al. (1989)
(S)-(-)																	HOLFORD (1986)
Ethanol	MEOS	Microsomal	Rat	20000	420	0.21											CLEAN and CEDERBAUM (1989)
	ADH	Cytosolic	Rat	26	1344	517											MESSIHA and HUGHES (1979)
	ADH	S4000 × g SUP	Rat	285	1724												CI CERO et al. (1980)
	ADH	Homogenate*	Rat	480	3667												LUMENG and CRABB (1984)
			Rat				1.00	20	0.995	1.000	1.000		20	20	20	1.7	BRAGGINS and CROW (1981)
			Rat				1.00	20	0.995	1.000	1.000		20	20	20	6.4	JULKUNEN et al. (1985)
Meperidine	Esterase	Microsomal	Rat	280	855	31	0.20	20	0.319	0.357	0.357	0.375	6.4	7.1	7.5	43.2	FREEMAN et al. (1977); YEH (1982)
		Microsomal*	Rat	120	563	47	0.20	20	0.319	0.357	0.357	0.375	6.4	7.1	7.5	75.6	KNODELL et al. (1980); DAHLSTROM et al. (1979)

* In vitro data used for predictions

[a] ADH, alcohol dehydrogenase; MEOS, microsomal ethanol oxygenase system; 8OH, 8-hydroxylation; 3MX and 1MX, 3- and 1-methylxanthine formation

[b] Liver and body weight were assumed to be 10 and 300 g for rat: 100 g and 2.75 kg for rabbit; and 1500 g and 70 kg for man, respectively

[c] Corrected by unbound fraction in the reaction mixture if binding data were available

[d] V_{max} value obtained in the subcellular fraction of liver (nmol/min/mg protein) was converted to that for intact liver (nmol/min/g liver) by assuming that there were 51.2 mg microsomal protein/g liver (LIN et al. 1980), 96 mg cytosolic protein/g liver, and 127 mg S9 protein/g liver (PANG et al. 1985)

[e] Calculated as V_{max}/K_m

[f] Unbound fraction in the blood

[g] Hepatic blood flow rate assumed (rat: 20 ml/min; rabbit: 170 ml/min; man: 1500 ml/min)

[h] E, extraction ratio; WS, well-stirred model; DM, dispersion model with $D_N = 0.17$ (ST-PIERRE et al. 1992); PM, parallel tube model

[i] CL_H, hepatic clearance, used to predict in vivo total body clearance (CL_{tot})

[j] Data of REMMEL et al. (1990)

[k] Biphasic in vitro kinetics (two sets of K_m's and V_{max}'s) have been reported

[l] Data of SHIBASAKI et al. (1988)

[m] Not available, assigned as 1.0

[n] 20–21 days pregnant

Table 6. Scale-up of data from subcellular fractions to whole body for hepatic and intestinal phase II metabolism

Drug	Major enzyme[a]	Preparation[b]	Species[c]	K_m[d] (μM)	V_{max}[e] (nmol/min/g)	CL_{int}[f] (ml/min)	f_B[g]	Q^h (ml/min)	Predicted E^i WS	DM	PM	Observed E	Predicted CL_n^j WS	DM	PM	Observed CL_{tot} (ml/min)	References
Liver																	
Procainamide	NAT	S9000 × g SUP*	Rat	20300	205	0.1			0.004	0.004	0.004		0.08	0.08	0.08	31	Schneck et al. (1978)
			Rat				0.84	20	0.004	0.004	0.004		0.08	0.08	0.08	19	Pang et al. (1984b)
			Rat				0.84	20									Schneck et al. (1978)
Buprenorphine	GT	Microsomal*	Rat	36	40	11	0.12	20	0.063	0.065	0.065	0.720					Mistry and Houston (1987)
Morphine	GT	Microsomal	Rat	300	41	1.4											Sanchez and Tephly (1974)
		Microsomal*	Rat	212	33	1.6	0.63	20	0.047	0.048	0.048	0.470					Mistry and Houston (1987)
Naloxone	GT	Microsomal*	Monkey	3.2	311	13264	0.63[k]	200	0.977	1.000	1.000	0.687					Rane et al. (1984)
	GT	Microsomal*	Rat	76	39	5.2	0.58	20	0.131	0.137	0.140	0.800					Mistry and Houston (1987)
Harmol	AST	Homogenate*	Rat	30	300	100										71	Mulder and Hagedoorn (1974)
	GT	Microsomal*	Rat	150	1331	89											Mulder and Hagedoorn (1974)
			Rat														Mulder et al. (1984)
4-Methylumbelliferone	AST	Cytosolic*	Rat	1.1	291	2644	NA[l]	20	0.904	0.995	1.000	0.700	18.1	19.9	20.0		Kauffman et al. (1991)
			Rat				0.10	20	0.930	0.999	0.999	0.970	19	20	20	14	Anundi et al. (1986)
			Rat				0.10[m]	20	0.930	0.999	0.999	0.820	19	20	20	30	Morita et al. (1986)
p-Nitrophenol	GT	MS*	Rat	253	180	7.1											Morrison et al. (1986)
	GT	MS[n]	Rat	30	15.4	5.1											Winsnes (1972)
		MS[n]		1450	44	0.3											
	GT	MS[n,o]	Rat	360	268	7.4											Winsnes (1972)
		MS[n,o]		1800	558	3.1											
	GT	MS		240	100	4.2											
Phenol	AST	Cytosolic*	Rat	180	700	39	0.17	20	0.057	0.058	0.059	0.470	1.14	1.16	1.17	24	Lucier et al. (1975) Mizuma et al. (1982) Machida et al. (1982)
			Rat				0.17[p]	20	0.057	0.058	0.059	0.430					Belanger et al. (1985)
			Rat				NA[l]	20	0.660	0.795	0.857	0.880	13	16	17	24	Cassidy and Houston (1984)

Compound / Enzyme[a]	Preparation[b]	Species	V_{max}[e]	K_m		E[i]	Flow[h]	Predicted CL (WS, DM, PM)[i][j]		Ratio		Reference
α-Bromoisovalerylurea (R) GST	Purified* (2-2)[q] (3-3)[q]	Rat	1400 2600	750 4550	0.5 1.8			0.050 0.051 0.051		1.0 1.0	32	Te Koppele et al. (1988) / Te Koppele et al. (1988) / Polhuijs et al. (1989)
(S) GST	(1-1)[q] (2-2)[q] (3-3)[q]		2000 600 3100	1110 1590 1510	0.6 2.7 0.5	0.46[r]	20	0.078 0.081 0.082		1.6 1.6	1.6 8.4	Te Koppele et al. (1988) / Te Koppele et al. (1988) / Polhuijs et al. (1989)
Intestine						0.46[r]	20					
Buprenorphine GT	Microsomal*	Rat	91 11		0.9	0.12	10	0.011 0.011 0.011	0.480			Mistry and Houston (1987)
Morphine GT	Microsomal	Rat	500 320	6.3 4.0	0.1 0.1	0.63	10	0.006 0.006 0.006	0.330			Villar et al. (1974) / Mistry and Houston (1987)
GT	Microsomal*	Rat				0.63[k]	10	0.006 0.006 0.006	0.660			Iwamoto and Klaassen (1977)
Naloxone GT	Microsomal*	Rat	530 13.5		0.2	0.58	10	0.012 0.012 0.012	0.570			Mistry and Houston (1987)

* In vitro data used for prediction

[a] NAT, N-acetyltransferase; GT, UDP-glucuronyltransferase; AST, arylsulfotransferase; GST, glutathione S-transferase

[b] Purified, purified enzyme

[c] Liver and body weight were assumed to be 10 and 300 g for rat and 135 g and 5 kg for monkey, respectively

[d] Corrected for unbound fraction in the reaction mixture, if binding data were available

[e] V_{max} value obtained in subcellular fraction of liver (nmol/min/mg protein) was converted to that in the intact liver (nmol/min/g liver) by assuming that there were 51.2 mg microsomal protein/g liver (LIN et al. 1980), 96 mg cytosolic protein/g liver, and 127 mg S9 protein/g liver (PANG et al. 1985). Similarly, the V_{max} value obtained for intestinal microsomes (nmol/min/mg protein) was converted to that for the intact intestine by assuming 25 mg intestinal microsomal protein/intestine (MISTRY and HOUSTON 1987)

[f] Calculated as V_{max}/K_m where the rat intestine weights were assumed to be 8 g

[g] Unbound fraction in blood

[h] Hepatic or intestinal blood flow rate assumed (rat hepatic blood flow: 20 ml/min; monkey hepatic blood flow: 200 ml/min; rat intestinal blood flow rate: 10 ml/min)

[i] E, extraction ratio; WS, well-stirred model; DM, dispersion model with $D_N = 0.17$ (ST-PIERRE et al. 1992); PM, parallel tube model

[j] CL_h, or hepatic clearance, was used to predict in vivo total body clearance, CL_{tot}

[k] Data of MISTRY and HOUSTON (1987)

[l] Not available, assumed as 1.0

[m] Data of ANUNDI et al. (1986)

[n] Biphasic in vitro kinetics (two sets of K_m's and V_{max}'s) were reported

[o] Triton X100-treated

[p] Data of MIZUMA et al. (1982)

[q] Rat GST isozymes

[r] Data of TE KOPPELE et al. (1986)

Table 7. Scale-up of data from hepatic and intestinal cells to whole body

Drug	Enzyme[a]	Species[b]	K_m[c] (μM)	V_{max}[d] (mol/min/g)	CL_{int}[e] (ml/min)	f_B[f]	Q[g] (ml/min)	Predicted E[h] WS	DM	PM	Observed E	Predicted CL_h[i] WS	DM	PM	Observed CL_{tot} (ml/min)	References
Liver																
Antipyrine	P-450*	Rat			0.369	1.00	20	0.018	0.018	0.018	0.065					SINGH et al. (1991)
Diazepam	P-450*	Rat			306	0.14	20	0.682	0.821	0.883	0.650	13.6	16.4	17.7	11.5	CHENERY et al. (1987) IGARI et al. (1983)
	P-450*	Rabbit			985	0.13	170	0.426	0.492	0.524		72	84	89	48	CHENERY et al. (1987) TSANG and WILKINSON (1982)
	P-450*	Man			10503	0.02	1500	0.139	0.146	0.149		210	220	224	47	CHENERY et al. (1987) KLOTZ et al. (1976)
		Man				0.02	1500	0.104	0.108	0.110		156	162	165	12	KLOTZ and REIMANN (1981)
	P-450*	Dog			11817	0.07	150	0.854	0.977	0.997		128	147	150	420	CHENERY et al. (1987) KLOTZ et al. (1976)
Ethoxybenzamide	P-450*	Rat	459	86	1.88	0.67	20	0.059	0.061	0.061	0.120	1.19	1.21	1.22	2.2	LIN et al. (1978, 1980)
Imipramine	N-Demethylase*	Rat	2.1	1024	4875	0.11	20	0.969	1.000	1.000	0.920					CHIBA et al. (1990b) CHIBA et al. (1990b) CHIBA et al. (1988, 1990a)
	2-Hydroxylase*	Rat	0.7	66	931											
Nordiazepam	P-450*	Man			2954	0.06	1500	0.107	0.111	0.113		160	166	169	14	CHENERY et al. (1987) KLOTZ et al. (1976)
		Man														
Propranolol	P-450*	Rat			1078	0.17	20	0.900	0.994	1.000	0.730					SINGH et al. (1991)
Acetaminophen	AST*	Rat	30	136	45	1.00	20	0.698	0.839	0.901	0.440	14	17	18	8.4	MIZUMA et al. (1985a)
	GT*	Rat	2130	163	0.8	1.00	20	0.698	0.839	0.901		14	17	18	9.5	MIZUMA et al. (1985a)
		Rat				1.00	20	0.698	0.839	0.901		14	17	18	8.3	PANG and GILLETTE (1978a) LIN and LEVY (1982)
		Rat				1.00	20	0.698	0.839	0.901		14	17	18	16	WATARI et al. (1983) GREGUS et al. (1988)
Harmol	GT*	Rat			225	NA[j]	20	0.979	1.000	1.000	0.700	19.6	20	20	71	ARAYA et al. (1984) ARAYA et al. (1984)
	AST*	Rat			716											MULDER et al. (1984)
p-Nitrophenol	GT	Rat	227	896	40	0.17	20	0.913	0.997	1.000	0.470	18.3	20	20	24.4	EACHO et al. (1981) MIZUMA et al. (1982)
	AST*	Rat			1200											MIZUMA et al. (1982)
	GT*	Rat	38	125	33	0.17[k]	20	0.913	0.997	1.000	0.430		20	20		MIZUMA et al. (1982) MACHIDA et al. (1982)

Substrate	System	Species	(a)	(b)	(c)	f_u	Blood flow	Predicted E	Obs E	Predicted CL	Obs CL	Reference
1-Naphthol	AST*	Rat	30	54	18	0.14[l]	20	0.170 0.181 0.186	0.180	3.4 3.6 3.7	70.8	Schwarz (1980)
	GT*	Rat	57	70	13							Schwarz (1980)
												Mistry and Houston (1985)
Oxazepam	GT*	Dog	4158			0.10	150	0.737 0.882 0.939		111 132 141	380	Chenery et al. (1987)
	GT*	Dog										Alvan et al. (1977)
	GT*	Man	5121			0.04	1500	0.123 0.128 0.131		184 192 196	74	Chenery et al. (1987)
	GT*	Man										Greenblatt et al. (1980)
Salicylamide	AST*	Rat	6.0	63	104	0.33[m]	20	0.647 0.778 0.840		13 16 17	23	Shibasaki et al. (1981)
	GT*	Rat	190	160	8.4							Shibasaki et al. (1981)
												Houston and Levy (1976)
Temazepam	GT*	Man	1641			0.10	1500	0.099 0.102 0.104		148 153 155	89	Chenery et al. (1987)
		Man										Locniskar and Greenblatt (1990)
Intestine												
Phenacetin	P-450*	Rat	57	0.3	0.04	NA[j]	10	0.004 0.004 0.000				Klippert et al. (1982)
	P-450 (3MC)*	Rat	38	2.7	0.58	NA[j]	10	0.054 0.056 0.530				Klippert et al. (1982)
Morphine	GT*	Rat	170	3.8	0.18	0.63	10	0.011 0.011 0.330				Koster et al. (1985a)
	GT*	Rat				0.63[n]	10	0.011 0.011 0.660				Mistry and Houston (1987)
	GT*	Rat										Iwamoto and Klaassen (1977)
1-Naphthol	GT*	Rat	2	25	100	0.14[l]	10	0.576 0.689 0.744	0.460			Koster et al. (1985b)
		Rat										Mistry and Houston (1985)

* In vitro data used for prediction

[a] P-450, cytochrome P-450; GT, UDP-glucuronyltransferase; AST, arylsulfotransferase; 3MC, 3-methylcholanthrene treated

[b] Liver and body weight were assumed to be 10 and 300 g for rat; 100 g and 2.75 kg for rabbit; 500 g and 12 kg for dog; and 1500 g and 70 kg for man, respectively

[c] Corrected by unbound fraction in the reaction mixture, if binding data were available

[d] V_{max} value obtained in hepatocytes (nmol/min/10⁶ cells and nmol/min/cellular protein) was converted to that in the intact liver (nmol/min/g liver) by multiplying by the factor, 125×10^6 cells/g liver (Lin et al. 1980) or 1313 mg cellular protein/g liver (Iwamoto et al. 1984). Similarly, the V_{max} value in the intestinal mucosal cell (nmol/min/10⁶ cells and nmol/min/mucosal cellular protein) was converted to that in the intact intestine by the factor 60×10^6 cells/g intestine (Klippert et al. 1982) or 37.5 mucosal cellular protein/g intestine (Koster et al. 1985a), respectively

[e] Calculated as V_{max}/K_m where rat intestine weight was assumed to be 8 g

[f] Unbound fraction in the blood

[g] Hepatic or intestinal blood flow rate assumed (rat hepatic blood flow: 20 ml/min; rabbit hepatic blood flow: 170 ml/min; dog hepatic blood flow: 1500 ml/min; human hepatic blood flow: 1500 ml/min; rat intestinal blood flow: 10 ml/min)

[h] E, extraction ratio; WS, well-stirred model; DM, dispersion model with $D_N = 0.17$ (St-Pierre et al. 1992); PM, parallel tube model

[i] CL_b, hepatic clearance, used to predicted in vivo total body clearance

[j] Not available, assumed to be 1.0

[k] Data of Mizuma et al. (1982)

[l] Calculated based on the data of Redegeld et al. (1988) and Tremaine et al. (1984)

[m] Predicted based on the binding parameters of Xu et al. (1990)

[n] Data of Mistry and Houston (1985)

kinetics for comparison to in vivo events (Yasuhara et al. 1985; Hirayama et al. 1989).

1. From In Vitro to In Vivo: Compartmental Modeling

The intestine, liver, and lung are three drug-metabolizing organs involved in the first-pass effect of orally administered substrates (Gibaldi et al. 1971; Rowland 1972; Pang and Gillette 1978c; Colburn 1979; Klippert and Noordhoek 1983). Due to the anatomical placement of these organs, the intestine, being anterior, reduces the flux of substrate entering the liver and, in turn, the contribution of hepatic and then lung metabolism. The intestine is often overlooked as a metabolic organ. However, it has been shown that the intestine possesses an abundance of drug-metabolizing activities (Dollery et al. 1971; Iwamoto and Klaassen 1977; Mulder et al. 1984, 1985; Shibasaki et al. 1981; Klippert et al. 1983; Xu et al. 1989; Zimmerman et al. 1991). Studies performed with isolated intestinal fragments and cells have revealed a gradient of enzymatic activities from the duodenal to the ileal end (Hoensch et al. 1976; Koster et al. 1985b; Schwenk and Locher 1985). Higher cytochrome P-450 reductase and cytochrome P-450 contents (Wattenberg et al. 1963; Hoensch et al. 1975, 1976; Dawson and Bridges 1981; Dubey and Singh 1988a) and conjugation enzymes (Dubey and Singh 1988b) were found at the upper villus than in the mucosal crypt on the villi of the rat. Since substrates in lumen are more exposed to the upper villus tip than to crypt cells, this differential gradient of drug-metabolizing activities along the villus can be used to explain the differences in drug metabolism between luminal and intrasuperior mesenteric routes of administration. Additionally, bacterial enzymatic sources in the lumen are another contributing factor which renders discrepant availabilities. For these compounds, the first-pass effect due to intestinal–luminal metabolism could be considered as a preabsorptive event that occurs during drug absorption and will not recur on subsequent passes, due to the inaccessibility of enzymes to systemically delivered substrates. These intestinally formed metabolites may be absorbed as well as serve as substrates for further hepatic metabolism prior to their reaching the general circulation.

Due to the importance of these organs in presystemic drug removal, numerous methods have been developed to investigate their roles in the metabolism of xenobiotics in vivo. The creation of a portal systemic shunt (Gugler et al. 1975) or portacaval transposition (Effeney et al. 1982) in the dog was utilized to bypass liver metabolism, whereas a portacaval shunt was used in the rat (Kravetz et al. 1987) to investigate intestinal first-pass removal with oral administration. Other techniques, including the in vivo perfused intestinal loop (Barr and Riegelman 1970) with sampling across organs, have been exploited to examine the extent and rate of drug removal by the two first-pass organs, the intestine and the liver. Examination of first-pass metabolism in vivo has utilized steady-state infusion with sampling of arterial and venous blood across the organs/tissues to provide organ availabilities and, in turn, organ clearances (MULDER et al. 1985; HIRAYAMA et al. 1990). Another routine method of assessment of organ availability in vivo is by the comparison of area under the curve [AUC or integral of concentration versus time plot, from time $= 0$ to ∞, $\int_0^\infty C(t)dt$] with various modes of administration. The dose, when given intra-arterially, is considered as completely available, excepting the case of blood metabolism. The premise of linearity of the system with respect to dose, which leads to a constancy in clearance (CL $=$ dose/AUC), is usually taken. Under this condition, first-pass metabolism which accompanies oral drug administration may be obtained by a comparison of the dose-corrected area under the curve to yield the systemic availability, F_{sys}:

$$F_{sys} = \frac{[AUC_{po}/dose_{po}]}{[AUC_{ia}/dose_{ia}]} = F_{abs}F_IF_HF_L, \tag{19}$$

which is a product of the fraction absorbed intact into the portal circulation (F_{abs}) and the availabilities of the first-pass organs, the intestine, liver, and lung (F_I, F_H, and F_L). Alternate routes of administration, such as the superior mesenteric artery (SMA), intraportal (pv), and intravenous (iv), reveal the availabilities of individual first-pass organs (CASSIDY and HOUSTON 1980, 1984; MISTRY and HOUSTON 1985):

$$F_L = \frac{[AUC_{iv}/dose_{iv}]}{[AUC_{ia}/dose_{ia}]}, \tag{20}$$

$$F_H = \frac{[AUC_{pv}/dose_{pv}]}{[AUC_{iv}/dose_{iv}]}, \tag{21}$$

$$F_I = \frac{[AUC_{SMA}/dose_{SMA}]}{[AUC_{pv}/dose_{pv}]}, \tag{22}$$

which in turn may be compared to data obtained in vitro. In making in vitro and in vivo correlations, however, it is very commonly assumed that the liver is the only first-pass organ or the sole organ for drug elimination. Hence data obtained in vitro are used to predict the systemic availability or the hepatic clearance (with assumption of complete absorption of the intact drug into the portal circulation).

2. From In Vitro to In Vivo: Physiological Modeling

Another method to relate in vitro data to in vivo is by way of physiological modeling, which has a long history (HIMMELSTEIN and LUTZ 1979). In this approach, organs are interconnected by way of the circulation in accordance with their anatomy (Fig. 4). Physiological volumes and flows are utilized, together with biochemical data obtained from in vitro studies: K_m and V_{max}, partitioning of substrate in that tissue in relation to plasma ($\lambda =$ concentration in tissue/venous plasma concentration), and the extent of protein binding in blood/plasma. The basic premise of the physiological model is

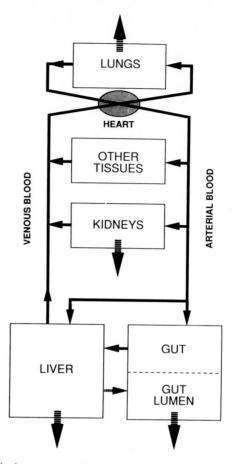

Fig. 4. A physiological representation of the body, with organs and tissues inter-connected by the circulation. Eliminating organs shown are the gut lumen, the liver, the lung, and the kidney

that each organ tissue is to be viewed as a discrete, well-mixed compartment for which venous equilibration exists, such that the concentration emerging from the organ can be related to the concentration within the organ or tissue by the partition ratio, λ, the estimation of which has been fully discussed previously (CHEN and GROSS 1979; KHOR and MAYERSOHN 1991).

For a noneliminating organ, the muscle (subscripted m) for example (Fig. 5A), the rate of change of drug within the organ can be given as:

$$V_m \frac{dC_m}{dt} = Q_m C_A - Q_m C_{m,Out} = Q_m (C_A - C_m/\lambda_m), \tag{23}$$

where C_A and $C_{m,Out}$ are the arterial and venous concentrations, respectively, Q_m is the flow, and V_m, the physiological volume.

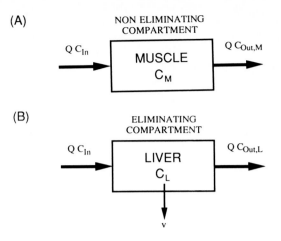

Fig. 5A,B. Rates in and rates out in a noneliminating compartment such as the muscle (**A**) and an eliminating compartment such as the liver (**B**)

For a drug-metabolizing organ such as the liver (subscripted L) (Fig. 5B), which receives flows from the hepatic artery (HA) and portal vein (PV), which receives the venous outflow from the intestine (I),

$$V_L \frac{dC_L}{dt} = Q_{HA}C_A + Q_{PV}C_I/\lambda_L - Q_LC_L/\lambda_L - \frac{V_{max}C_L}{K_m + C_L}. \tag{24}$$

Technically, it is almost impossible to include all organs and tissues, and "lumping" of the organ and tissues with common perfusion rates and partitioning characteristics is often performed. For example, the skin and muscle are poorly perfused tissues, and may be lumped as a "lean tissue" compartment, in contrast to the adipose tissue, or organs that are lumped as "visceral" organs. Bischoff noted that there is no simple way to describe which body regions should be included, and which might be excluded; the initial choice may be to consider the flow, pharmacokinetics, and physicochemical characteristics of the drug as well as the anatomy and physiology of the organs (BISCHOFF 1975). Mass balance equations are then constructed for computer simulation, usually with numerical approaches, to solve for the concentrations within organs and tissues of known partitioning ratios and metabolic constants, and ultimately to yield the time profiles of the drug and its related chemicals.

Physiological modeling has been used to describe nonlinear protein binding and metabolism of thiopental (BISCHOFF and DEDRICK 1968), chlorinated biphenyls (LUTZ et al. 1977), halogenated hydrocarbons (BUNGAY et al. 1979), lidocaine (BENOWITZ et al. 1974), ethoxybenzamide (LIN et al. 1982), methotrexate (BISCHOFF et al. 1971; DEDRICK et al. 1973), actinomycin D (LUTZ et al. 1977), and other compounds. The method has also been described for overdose kinetics (CHEN et al. 1978) and drug–drug interactions between sulfonamides and tolbutamide (Sugita et al. 1982). More detailed events may be described by subdividing individual compartments into blood, interstitial space, and a cellular compartment for the description of transport barriers (Dedrick et al. 1973). Metabolite kinetics are viewed in similar fashion, as exemplified by the bioactivation of trichloroethylene to trichloroacetic acid with various routes of administration in the rat and mouse (Fisher et al. 1991), fetal exposure during pregnancy (Fisher et al. 1989), and the lactating rat and nursing pup (Fisher et al. 1990).

3. From Perfused Organs to In Vivo

a) Organs in Series for First-Pass Effect

The intestine and liver must be viewed as an anatomical series with respect to flow. A drug enters the intestine via the superior mesenteric artery (SMA), then drains into the portal vein for perfusion of the liver, which also receives arterial blood (25% of total liver blood flow) from the hepatic artery. The overall removal by the intestine and liver is represented as the overall loss across the intestine and liver, and an effective extraction ratio (E_{IL}) across these two tissues/organs is given by:

$$E_{IL} = \frac{Q_{PV}C_A + Q_{HA}C_A - Q_{HV}C_{HV}}{Q_{PV}C_A + Q_{HA}C_A} = \frac{C_A - C_{HV}}{C_A} = 1 - F_{IL} \qquad (25)$$

and $C_{HV} = F_{IL}C_A$, where F_{IL} is the overall availability across the intestine and liver; C_A and C_{HV} denote the steady-state drug concentrations in the hepatic artery and hepatic vein, respectively; and Q_{HV}, Q_{PV}, and Q_{HA} represent the hepatic venous, portal venous, and hepatic arterial flows, respectively.

Individually, the steady-state extraction ratios of the intestine, E_I, and liver, E_L, are given by the rate of elimination divided by the rate of presentation at steady state:

$$E_I = \frac{Q_{PV}(C_A - C_{PV})}{Q_{PV}C_A} = \frac{C_A - C_{PV}}{C_A} = 1 - F_I \qquad (26)$$

and $C_{PV} = F_I C_A$, where F_I is the availability across the intestine. The steady-state hepatic extraction ratio, E_H, is given as follows:

$$
\begin{aligned}
E_H &= \frac{Q_{HA}C_A + Q_{PV}C_{PV} - Q_{HV}C_{HV}}{Q_{HA}C_A + Q_{PV}C_{PV}} \\
&= \frac{C_A(Q_{HA} + Q_{PV}F_I) - Q_{HV}C_{HV}}{C_A(Q_{HA} + Q_{PV}F_I)} \\
&= 1 - \frac{Q_{HV}F_{IL}}{Q_{HA} + Q_{PV}F_I}.
\end{aligned}
\qquad (27)
$$

Upon substitution and rearrangement of Eqs. 25–27, the overall availability across the intestine and liver is related to the product of the intestinal and hepatic availabilities:

$$F_{IL} = \frac{F_H(Q_{HA} + Q_{PV}F_I)}{Q_{HV}}. \tag{28}$$

Consideration of the drug metabolism during the first-pass effect for drug absorbed into the intestine only requires a modification of Eqs. 25 and 27, since mass balance concerns only the passage of drug from the intestine to the liver without any contribution from the hepatic artery.

$$E_{H(1st\ pass)} = \frac{Q_{PV}C_{PV} - Q_{HV}C_{HV}}{Q_{PV}C_{PV}} = 1 - \frac{Q_{HV}}{Q_{PV}}\frac{C_{HV}}{C_A F_I} \tag{29}$$

and

$$E_{IL(1st\ pass)} = \frac{Q_{PV}C_A - Q_{HV}C_{HV}}{Q_{PV}C_A} = 1 - \frac{Q_{HV}}{Q_{PV}}\frac{C_{HV}}{C_A} \tag{30}$$

$$F_{IL(1st\ pass)} = \frac{Q_{HV}}{Q_{PV}} \cdot \frac{C_{HV}}{C_A}. \tag{31}$$

Upon substitution of Eq. 31 into Eq. 29, the overall availability across the intestine and liver during the first-pass effect is the product of the corresponding intestinal and hepatic availabilities:

$$F_{IL(1st\ pass)} = F_{I(1st\ pass)}F_{H(1st\ pass)}. \tag{32}$$

The impact of intestinal metabolism on hepatic metabolism and the overall first-pass effect has been examined by Xu et al. (1989). The simplest case of first-pass metabolite formation is the formation of conjugates (mi) (as primary and terminal metabolite) which may be further excreted into bile. The hepatic venous concentration of the conjugate $C_{HV}(mi)$ consists of total metabolite arising from both intestine and liver metabolism, after discounting that which is excreted into bile. Hence, at steady state, hepatic formation rates are obtained as follows:

$$v_H^{mi} = Q_{HV}C_{HV}(mi) + \frac{\Delta A_e(mi)}{\Delta t} - Q_{PV}C_{PV}(mi), \tag{33}$$

where v_H^{mi} is the hepatic formation rate for the conjugate mi; $Q_{PV}\{mi\}$ and $C_{HV}(mi)$ are the portal and hepatic venous concentrations of the conjugate, respectively; and $\Delta A_e(mi)/\Delta t$ is the biliary excretion rate of mi at steady state.

The contribution of the intestine and liver to the overall elimination is given by the ratio of the rate of intestine or liver metabolism to the total rate of elimination across the two organs, at steady state:

$$\frac{v_I}{v_{total}} = \frac{E_I Q_{PV}C_A}{(E_I C_A + E_H C_{PV})Q_{PV}} = \frac{E_I}{E_I + E_H(1 - E_I)}, \tag{34}$$

$$\frac{v_H}{v_{total}} = \frac{E_H Q_{PV}C_{PV}}{(E_I C_A + E_H C_{PV})Q_{PV}} = \frac{E_H(1 - E_I)}{E_I + E_H(1 - E_I)}. \tag{35}$$

Table 8. Comparison of intestinal and liver metabolism in the once-through vascularly perfused rat intestine–liver preparation, in the perfused rat liver preparation, and in the rat in vivo

Compound	Intestine–liver perfusion			Liver perfusion		In vivo			References
	C_{In} (μM)	E_I	E_H	C_{In} (μM)	E_H	Condition	E_I	E_H	
Salicylamide	41	0.262	0.992	35	0.998	i.v. and p.o. bolus, dose = 30 mg/kg; portal vein infusion at 3 mg/kg per min for 10 min	0.35	0.65	Xu et al. (1989) Xu et al. (1990) Iwamoto et al. (1983)
Gentisamide	2.56	0.327	0.837	2.44	0.885	i.v. infusion of tracer at 18.8 nmol/min	0.26	0.37	Hirayama and Pang (1990) Morris et al. (1988b) Hirayama et al. (1990)
4-Methylumbelliferone	0.001 32.3	0.60 0.36	0.92 0.94	0.005 64	0.970 0.970	i.v. infusion at 1.2 mg/kg per min	0.40	0.97	Zimmerman et al. (1991) Zimmerman et al. (1991) Ratna et al. (1993) Ratna et al. (1993) Mulder et al. (1985)

The perfused rat small intestine and liver preparation has been developed and applied to study first-pass metabolism in the rat (HIRAYAMA et al. 1989). In this single-pass preparation, the intestine is perfused with blood containing drug that enters via the superior mesenteric artery, whereas the liver receives blank perfusate into the hepatic artery (25% of total liver blood flow) as well as venous drainage from the intestine. Individual extraction ratios of the intestine and liver as well as the overall intestine–liver extraction ratio are readily determined in the preparation, at steady state, by examination of the drop across the organ/tissue. This preparation has been used to examine the intestinal–liver conjugation of various phenolic substrates, salicylamide (XU et al. 1989), gentisamide (HIRAYAMA et al. 1990), and 4-methylumbelliferone (ZIMMERMAN et al. 1991), which are glucuronidated by the intestine and almost completely removed ($E \approx 1$) via sulfation by the liver at trace input concentrations. The occurrence of intestinal glucuronidation has reduced the flow of substrate to the liver and the contribution of the latter to first-pass metabolism. Moreover, the proportions of metabolites formed will also differ. Higher input concentration will readily saturate intestinal metabolism, allowing residual substrate flow to the liver for subsequent hepatic conjugation. Comparison of trace data for the perfusion series and in vivo shows good promise. After correction of the flow differences employed for perfusion in relation to those in vivo, quite good correlation was found (Table 8).

b) Organs in Parallel

The interorgan metabolic relationships between the liver and kidney have recently been studied with a combined rat liver and kidney preparation, perfused in parallel, with (DE LANNOY and PANG 1993) or without (DAUGAARD et al. 1987) erythrocytes. The correlation between the dual-organ erythrocyte-free perfusion technique and in vivo was sought by YASUHARA et al. (1985), who compared the disposition of phenolsulfophthalein with both control and acute renal failure (ARF, treated with uranyl acetate) rats. Although individual organ clearances were not explored, a lack of change in total body clearance was obtained for both ARF and control rats in vivo, as well as for dual-organ perfusion with control and ARF donors. Total body clearance in vivo was, however, threefold that found for combined organ perfusion, with correspondingly higher in vivo excretion of both unconjugated and conjugated phenosulfophthalein into bile and urine. The differences may be attributed to the higher unbound fraction and higher perfusion flow rate in vivo, as well as reduced organ function for the dual-organ perfusion technique in the absence of red blood cells.

The combined technique was also utilized to examine aldosterone (EGFJORD et al. 1991) and enalapril (DE LANNOY and PANG 1993) metabolism by the rat liver, kidney, and the combined liver–kidney preparations. The use of this dual-organ perfusion technique for metabolite kinetics was illustrated by [^{14}C]enalapril and [^{3}H]enalaprilat (De Lannoy et al. 1989, 1993; De Lannoy and Pang 1993). Although the organ–in vivo relationship was not explored in these studies, the property of additivity of organ clearances for drug was tested. This was found for enalapril (De Lannoy and Pang 1993) but not for aldosterone, which exhibited a lower combined organ clearance, attributed to the production of renal inhibitory factors, in relation to hepatic clearance (Egfjord et al. 1991). Despite the recognition that differences in flow and unbound fractions do exist in the two systems, varied success for correlation of data was obtained. The predictive power of the dual-organ technique remains to be further tested. Good organ viability with adequate flow rates that are comparable to those in vivo may improve the correlation.

C. Poor Correlations Between In Vitro and Perfused Organs

Widely disparate correlations are found between in vitro data and organ perfusion data (Tables 1–4). The probability of success is low and appears random for drugs of low and intermediate E. A good correlation for E and CL was found for compounds with high in vitro CL_{int}. But as discussed below, this is due to the rate limitation of flow and not the closeness between in vitro and in vivo intrinsic clearances. There are many reasons for the poor correlations.

I. Inadequacy of In Vitro Estimates

1. Estimation of Enzymatic Parameters

In order to incorporate metabolic parameters (K_m and V_{max}) into the clearance equations, it is necessary to determine accurately the appropriate initial velocity in vitro. The Michaelis-Menten equation is a steady-state approximation: the rate of change of the enzyme–substrate (ES) complex is time invariant. Some phase I metabolism catalyzed by the cytochrome P-450s for various lipophilic, basic substrates such as propranolol (Ishida et al. 1992), benzo[a]pyrene (Wiersma and Roth 1983a,b), lidocaine (Suzuki et al. 1984), imipramine, and desipramine (Chiba et al. 1988) and phase II sulfation are characterized by high-affinity enzymatic systems ($K_m = 0.5$–$2.0\,\mu M$). Sometimes the high-affinity component is overlooked due to an inadequate concentration range because of limitations in drug assay, and this may lead to an underestimation of the true rate of reaction at the lower concentration range. The general rule of thumb for incubation studies is to employ a substrate concentration such that substrate is not rate limiting, yielding a velocity which is linear with time.

As an illustration, the time courses of the disappearance of substrate were simulated for different ratios (1000 and 100) of initial substrate $[S_0]$ to enzyme concentration $[E_0]$, based on Chance's algorithm (1960). k_2, the rate constant for formation of product, was varied (100 to $10\,min^{-1}$) and was kept much lower than the off binding rate constant of the ES complex (k_{-1} = 10^5 and $10^3\,min^{-1}$), whereas the ratio of the on/off rate constants, k_1/k_{-1} (0.01), and the $K_m[(k_{-1} + k_2)/k_1, 100\,\mu M]$ were both maintained constant;

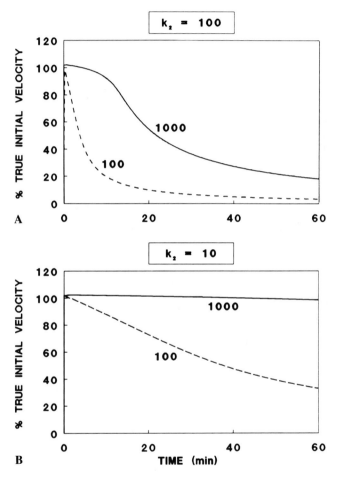

Fig. 6A,B. The initial velocity, expressed as a percentage of the true, theoretical initial velocity, versus incubation time for different initial substrate/enzyme $[S_0]/[E_0]$ ratios (1000 and 100). The rate constant for product formation, k_2, was varied from $100\,min^{-1}$ (**A**) to $10\,min^{-1}$ (**B**); the K_m was kept constant at $100\,\mu M$, whereas the ratio of the on and off binding rate constants, k_1/k_{-1}, was constant at 0.01 (1001/ 100000 or 11/1000), with $k_{-1} \ll k_2$. Note that good estimate of the initial velocity is provided only at $[S_0]/[E_0]$ = 1000 at low k_2 ($10\,min^{-1}$)

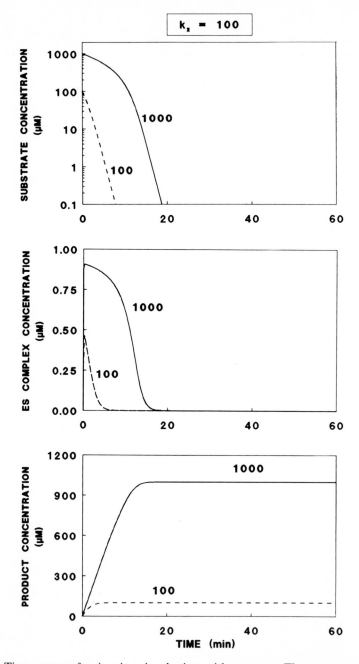

Fig. 7. Time course for in vitro incubation with enzyme. The concentrations of substrate [S] (*upper panel*), the enzyme–substrate complex [ES] (*middle panel*), and product [P] (*lower panel*) were plotted against incubation time. $[S_0]/[E_0]$ ratios were 1000 and 100; $K_m = 100\,\mu M$; k_1/k_{-1}, was constant at 0.01 (1001/100 000 or 11/1000), with $k_{-1} \ll k_2$, and $k_2 = 100\,min^{-1}$ (same as in the upper panel of Fig. 6A)

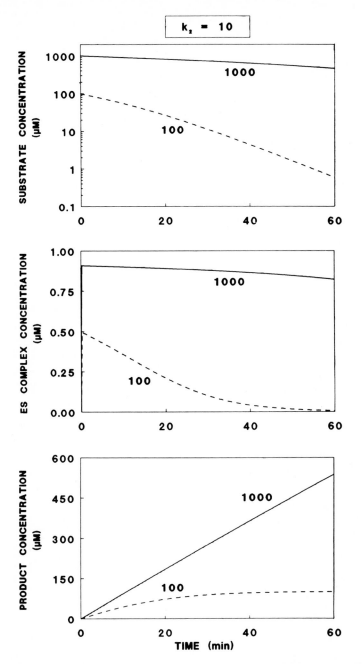

Fig. 8. Time course for in vitro incubation with enzyme. The concentrations of substrate [S] (*upper panel*), the enzyme–substrate complex [ES] (*middle panel*), and product [P] (*lower panel*) were plotted against incubation time. $[S_0]/[E_0]$ ratios were 1000 and 100; $K_m = 100\,\mu M$; k_1/k_{-1} was constant at 0.01 (1001/100 000 or 11/1000), with $k_{-1} \ll k_2$, and $k_2 = 10\,\text{min}^{-1}$ (same as Fig. 6B)

$k_2 \times$ [ES] or the initial velocity, v, and $k_2 \times$ [E_0] or V_{max} also varied. At the higher k_2 (cf. Fig. 6A), v was not adequately estimated for the given [S_0]/[E_0] ratios (1000 or 100) due to substrate depletion (cf. Fig. 7, upper panel), such that the rates of changes of the ES complex were not zero (Fig. 7, middle panel); the same comment applies to the case of the lower k_2 at low [S_0] ($100\,\mu M$) (Fig. 8, middle panel). By contrast, at the low k_2 (cf. Fig. 6B), a lack of appreciable substrate depletion occurred at [S_0] $= 1000\,\mu M$, for which steady state was approached for the ES complex (Fig. 8, upper and middle panels). Hence, estimation of the initial velocity (v) by product formation is accurate only for this case. For other combinations of k_1, k_{-1}, and k_2, the initial velocity, v, was underestimated despite the apparent linear relationship observed in some cases (see Figs. 7 and 8, lower panels). Thus, [S_0]/[E_0] must be maintained sufficiently high for proper estimates of v. This condition will become further complicated when a multiplicity of enzymes of different K_m or k_2 are present.

2. Multiplicity of Enzymes

Experiments conducted with purified enzyme systems will inadvertently yield results which differ from those for subcellular fragments such as the microsomal or cytosolic fractions, for the cell with its full complement of enzymes, and for the organ, where different cell types of different functionalities (NOVIKOFF 1959; DE LEEUE and KNOOK 1984) are present. This is due to the presence of the multiplicity of isoenzymes and different enzymatic systems. Most drug-metabolizing enzymes are a multigene family and display multisubstrate and overlapping substrate specificities. Among these are the well-studied cytochrome P-450s (NEBERT et al. 1987, 1989, 1991), the flavin-containing monooxygenases or Ziegler's enzymes (OZOLS 1989, 1991; YAMADA et al. 1990; ZIEGLER 1990; LAWTON et al. 1991), the sulfotransferases (CAMPBELL et al. 1987; NAKAMURA et al. 1987; DUFFEL and JAKOBY 1981; BINDER and DUFFEL 1988), UDPG-glucuronosyltransferases (BURCHELL 1978; FALANY and TEPHLY 1983; ROY CHOWDHURY et al. 1986; SIEST et al. 1988), the glutathione S-transferases (MEYER et al. 1984; ÅLIN et al. 1985; WANG et al. 1986; TU and REDDY 1985; SOMA et al. 1986; IGARASHI and SATOH 1989), amidases and esterases (ARNDT et al. 1973; ARNDT and KRISCH 1973; HAUGEN and SUTTIE 1974a,b; HEYMANN 1980; ROBBI and BEAUFAY 1983; MENTLEIN et al. 1980, 1984a,b, 1985, 1988; MENTLEIN and HEYMANN 1984), and N-acetylases (HEARSE and WEBER 1973; GRANT et al. 1991; KIRLIN et al. 1989; TRINIDAD et al. 1989). More than 60 cytochrome P-450 isozymes have been isolated and classified into 13 super families based on the sequence homology of amino acids (NEBERT et al. 1987). From the point of view of enzymology, the cytochrome P-450s possess an unusually broad substrate specificity that is partly due to a multiplicity of isozymes. For example, it has been shown that most of the 15 purified isozymes of the cytochrome P-450s from rat liver have the capacity to metabolize both propranolol and lidocaine, although some forms have higher substrate specificity (ODA et al. 1989; FUJITA et al. 1990).

In some cases, formation of the same metabolite may be accomplished by different enzymatic systems; the N-dealkylation of tertiary and secondary amines is mediated by microsomal flavin-containing monooxygenases (MFMOs), better known as Ziegler's enzymes, as well as by the cytochrome P-450s (PROUGH and ZIEGLER 1977; ZIEGLER 1980, 1990). Typical examples include: the N-dealkylation of *p*-chloro-*N*-methylaniline (PROUGH and ZIEGLER 1977) and methamphetamine (YAMADA et al. 1984) and the N-hydroxylation of norcocaine (KLOSS et al. 1982) and 2-aminofluorene (FREDERICK et al. 1982). The stability of these enzymes in NADPH differs in incubation systems (PROUGH and ZIEGLER 1977; ZIEGLER 1980); NADPH stabilizes Ziegler's enzymes, whereas the presence of NADPH during pre-incubation is known to destroy cytochrome P-450 due to formation of peroxidative products. When the reaction in the test tube is initiated by addition of an NADPH generating system to microsomal proteins, the in vitro protocol favors the estimation of cytochrome P-450 metabolic rate and underestimates the contribution of the MFMOs.

When multiple isoforms or enzymatic systems participate in the metabolism of a substrate, the contribution of each isoform or enzymatic system to the reaction product is governed by the amount of the enzyme and its affinity (Michaelis-Menten equation). For isoforms or enzymes of widely varying K_ms, enzymatic parameters may not be pooled to provide an average estimate of the K_m. The overall metabolic rate (v_{tot}) may be calculated by the sum of the Michaelis-Menten equation as follows,

$$v_{tot} = \sum_{i=1}^{n} \frac{V_{max,i}[S]}{K_{m,i} + [S]},$$ (36)

where $V_{max,i}$ and $K_{m,i}$ represent V_{max} and K_m value for the *i*-th isozyme. The contribution of each isoform/enzyme to the overall metabolic rate is highly dependent on the substrate concentration.

The relative abundance of each enzyme in subcellular fractions (microsomal or cytosolic fraction) is controlled by factors such as chemical agents (GUENGERICH et al. 1982; MURRAY and REIDY 1990), sex (KAMATAKI et al. 1983), age (FUJITA et al. 1985, 1989; KAMATAKI et al. 1985), and hormonal control (YAMAZOE et al. 1989). These additional biological variations can affect enzymatic systems differentially.

3. Membrane-Bound Enzymes

The UDP-glucuronosyltransferases (UDGPTs) are a group of membrane-bound enzymes. Substrates for glucuronidation must be nonpolar such that they partition into microsomal milieu and the rate of glucuronidation is independent of substrate concentration in cytosol (Zakim and Vessey 1977; Whitmer et al. 1984). The UDPGTs exhibit poorer activities in vitro than in vivo owing to the fact that the active site of UDPGTs suffers from direct exposure to acceptor substrates (Winsnes 1969). A "latency" (ratio of activities in detergent-treated versue intact microsomes) exists for this group of tightly membrane-bound enzymes (Eleter et al. 1973), which are prone to activation by divalent ions such as Mg^{2+}, Mn^{2+}, and CO^{2+} (Lucier et al. 1971), sonication, freezing, heating, phospholipase C digestion, detergent, and UDP-N-glucosamine treatments (Winsnes 1969, 1972; Graham and Wood 1972). Phospholipids are important in restoring activities from purified enzymes (Graham et al. 1974; Tukey et al. 1979; Tukey and Tephly 1980); those with a phosphorylcholine head, acyl chain length, and unsaturation appear to be most effective in increasing V_{max} and the binding of the enzyme to aglycone and uridine disphosphoglucuronic acid (UDPGA) (Erickson et al. 1978). A topological model for UDPGT has recently been put forward to describe the phenomenon of latency (Jansen et al. 1992). This model proposes that an intraluminal orientation of the active site exists. It is based on the works of Zakim and Vessey (Hochman et al. 1981), who first proposed that the binding of UDPGA to enzyme requires distortion of substrate and/or the enzyme which can be achieved by phospholipid activators. Addition of phospholipids to purified, delipidated enzymes failed to restore their native microsomal activities (Erickson et al. 1978); however, addition of microsomes from Gunn rats which are deficient in UDPGT almost completely restored all of the native activities (Burchell 1982). The conformational changes in UDPGT may vary with membrane fluidity induced by dietary deprivation of fatty acids (Castuma and Brenner 1983). Due to their conformational constraint, the UDPGTs in native microsomes may not be dynamically stable, necessitating stabilization by protein–phospholipid interactions (Tukey et al. 1979; Tukey and Tephly 1980; Dannenberg et al. 1990). Hence native microsomal proteins display reduced activities unless treated with detergents, and variations of enzymatic activity in the presence or absence of detergents have been found (Miners et al. 1988; Rane et al. 1984). The in vivo activities were about 10- to 30-fold higher than those in vitro (Mistry and Houston 1987).

4. Time-Dependent Kinetics

Impairment or induction of enzyme activity occurring only with long-term exposure to substrate and/or metabolities will not be adequately reflected within the time-frame of in vitro incubation systems. The same comment may be made about the interaction between substrate and the formed metabolites, i.e., the accumulation of a metabolite with time may be attained only with perfused organs or in vivo. These conditions constitute time-dependent kinetics for parent drugs as well as metabolites.

a) End Product Inhibition

Some metabolic interactions between parent drug and its metabolites noted in vitro have been found to directly reflect events in vivo. Examples include lidocaine (SUZUKI et al. 1984; KAWAI et al. 1983; PANG and ROWLAND 1977c), ethoxybenzamide (LIN et al. 1984), phenytoin (BORONDY et al. 1972; ASHLEY and LEVY 1972), and imipramine (CHIBA et al. 1988, 1990a), wherein in vivo events are predicted well. For other examples such as diazepam (KLOTZ and REIMANN 1981), in vitro prediction of end product inhibition in vivo is not possible because of lack of accumulation of metabolites due to either a low formation clearance or high metabolite clearance.

b) Enzyme Inactivation

Long-term dosing of the drug could also irreversibly alter the metabolic activity. The metabolic rate catalyzed by the cytochrome P-450s is known to be impaired by chronic exposure to parathion (ORITZ DE MONTELLANO and KUNTZE 1980; ORITZ DE MONTELLANO et al. 1982), chloramphenicol (MURRAY and REIDY 1990), and a series of acetylenes (HOPKINS et al. 1992). This is due to the irreversible binding of reactive intermediate such as S-oxide and the oxamyl derivative to the active site of the cytochrome P-450 protein. Propranolol is also known to be suicide substrate (SCHNECK and PRITCHARD 1981; SHAW et al. 1987) which binds specifically to a cytochrome P-450 isozyme irreversibly after long-term dosing, consequently impairing its own metabolism (MASUBUCHI et al. 1991, 1992). There have been other reports attempting to explain the unusual time course of the N-deethylated metabolite of lidocaine (MEGX) based on time-dependent irreversible inactivation of the MEGX formation rate (GRAY et al. 1987; SAVILLE et al. 1987). In such cases, a time-dependent decrease in the metabolic rate has to be taken into account for proper interpretation of data at the organ or whole-body level.

c) Enzyme Activation

A decrease in the half-life or in the steady-state concentration has been observed clinically after multiple dosing of drugs such as carbamazepine (LEVY et al. 1975; PITLICK and LEVY 1977; BERTILSSON 1978; PATEL et al. 1978; MCNAMARA et al. 1979; BERTILSSON et al. 1980), chlorpromazine (HARASZTI and DAVIS 1978), clonazepam (ROGERS et al. 1977; WINDORFER and SAUER 1977), diazepam (RICHENS 1977), and rifampicin (CURCI et al. 1972; ZILLY et al. 1975). Enzyme activation or induction due to drug or autoinduction has occurred. In vitro studies revealed that autoinduction of rifampicin (JEZEQUEL et al. 1971; HAKIM et al. 1973; PESSAYRE and MAZEL 1976), erythromycin (DANAN et al. 1981), oleandomycin (PESSAYRE et al. 1982), and triacetyloleandomycin (PESSAYRE et al. 1981) had caused increases in total cytochrome P-450 content and liver weight. However, induction is isozyme-specific since not all metabolic activities are induced. Pharmacokinetic approaches which incorporate the time-dependent kinetics into the model have also been reported (Levy and Dumain 1979; Levy et al. 1979a,b; Abramson 1986a,b), and may provide an invaluable framework for the quantitative scale-up of in vitro induction kinetics to in vivo time-dependent disposition. Failure to recognize this, however, will lead to poor correlates.

II. Structural Considerations and Physiological Variables

Two physiological variables – organ blood flow and biological membranes – distinguish between the subcellular and perfused organs. Although biological membranes are present for the cellular system and for the intact liver, the inherent architecture of the liver with respect to flow is absent. A substrate entering an organ via the blood flow must gain access to the inside of the cell through the cell membrane, a first potential barrier, before it can utilize the metabolic/excretory systems within cells; these enzymatic activities and cosubstrates are parceled and localized zonally in discrete regions. In addition, the binding of substrate to proteins in blood and tissues occurs, and each factor can become rate limiting under varying circumstances. The structure of the organ and its attendant heterogeneities need to be considered for the metabolism of drugs (for reviews, see Pang and Xu 1988; Pang et al. 1991b, 1992; Goresky et al. 1992). For the above reasons, observations in vitro often deviate from the results obtained in vivo. In vitro data often provide the metabolic profiling but do not necessarily reveal the rate-controlling factor or yield quantitative information on formation of metabolites within the intact organ.

Theoretical examinations have considered the fates of precursor drug (P) and its primary (M_1), secondary (M_2), and tertiary (M_3) metabolites or preformed metabolites (Pang et al. 1985; St-Pierre et al. 1992). In the absence of membrane limitations, the following kinetic phenomenon will apply. For flow-limited precursor drugs and metabolites (that is, rapid entry of all species across liver cell membranes, no barrier limitation), the apparent extraction ratios of the primary and secondary metabolites, $E\{M_1,P\}$ and $E\{M_2,P\}$, respectively, arising from drug (P) differ from the extraction ratios ($E\{M_1\}$ and $E\{M_2\}$) obtained with the administration of the preformed metabolite species M_1 and M_2, respectively. In both systems, a rank order is found: $E\{M_1\} > E\{M_1,P\}$ and $E\{M_2\} > E\{M_2,M_1\} > E\{M_2,P\}$; that is, the extraction ratio of a generated, lipophilic metabolite (M_1 or M_2) will be less than, or at best equal to, that after its administration into the organ as a preformed species. The discrepancy is further augmented by an increasing number of steps involved in the formation of the metabolite (St-Pierre et al. 1992; St-Pierre and Pang, 1993a,b). The simulated example in Fig. 9 also shows the rank order. The extent of sequential metabolism of a generated metabolite is maximal when associated with precursor compounds having high intrinsic clearances for formation relative to the intrinsic clear-

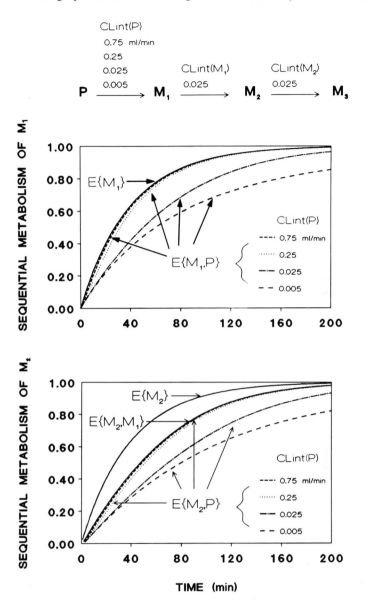

Fig. 9. Simulated sequential metabolism [drug (P) conversion to its primary (M_1), then secondary (M_2) and tertiary (M_3) metabolites] in a well-mixed system (namely, hepatocytes) for a primary metabolite M_1 after administration of P (expressed as $E\{M_1,P\}$) (*upper panel*), and for a secondary metabolite M_2 after administration of P (expressed as $E\{M_2,P\}$) or M_1 (expressed as $E\{M_2,M_1\}$) (*lower panel*). Values of intrinsic clearances (ml/min) for the metabolism of P, M_1, and M_2 are shown. Note the kinetic "lag" in sequential metabolism of the formed metabolites

ance for metabolism of the metabolite, and is least for precursors with very small formation intrinsic clearances. Rapid formation of the primary (or secondary) metabolite furnishes that metabolite for avid metabolism and lessens the "lag" observed when its extent of sequential metabolism is compared to that found for the preformed primary (or secondary) metabolite. When formation of the metabolite is extremely rapid, the extents of metabolism of the preformed and generated primary metabolites become identical, whereas if formation of metabolite is slow, sequential metabolism lags behind that for preformed metabolite, and the rank order hence becomes apparent. This kinetic phenomenon is displayed in the sequential processing of tracer [^{14}C]phenacetin to [^{14}C]acetaminophen and [^{14}C]acetaminophen sulfate conjugate and the metabolism of [^{3}H]acetaminophen to [^{3}H]acetaminophen sulfate conjugate in rat isolated hepatocytes (Pang et al. 1985), which represent a well-mixed system (Pang and Gillette 1978a). In this apparently homogeneous pool of hepatocytes comprising cells from all regions of the liver, preformed acetaminophen (labeled with tritium) and the precursor phenacetin are sufficiently lipophilic for both drug and metabolite to gain ready access into cells; the membrane barrier appears to be absent. [^{14}C]Acetaminophen formed from [^{14}C]phenacetin, however, yields proportionately less labeled sulfate than preformed [^{3}H]acetaminophen under first-order conditions (Fig. 10). The kinetic effect on metabolite formation is observed in the sequential metabolism of diazepam (DZ) and nordiazepam (NZ) to oxazepam (OZ) in the mouse liver preparation: $E\{OZ,DZ\} \approx E\{NZ,DZ\} \approx 0.06 < E\{OZ\}$ or 0.125 (St-Pierre et al. 1990; St-Pierre and Pang 1993a,b).

For the intact organ, the kinetic phenomenon exists for drug and metabolite processing, since uptake is a distributed-in-space phenomenon with repeated processes of influx, removal and excretion, and efflux. A concentration profile in space is created during the steady state, declining from inlet to outlet when the substrate is taken up and irreversibly metabolized (Goresky et al. 1973; Winkler et al. 1974; Pang and Rowland 1977a). This concentration profile of substrate in space (with its corresponding input–output concentration difference) is related to, and must be accounted for by, the underlying hepatic microcirculatory structure and physiological and biochemical processes. The events are dependent on substrate influx for recruitment of metabolic/excretory activities and efflux in a fashion linked to the delivery by flow (Goresky et al. 1973; Pang and Stillwell 1983; Goresky and Groom 1984); the influx, elimination, and efflux characteristics are modulated by substrate binding to red blood cells (Goresky et al. 1975, 1988; Pang et al. 1988a) and plasma proteins (Schary and Rowland 1983; Rowland et al. 1984; Wolkoff et al. 1979; Gärtner et al. 1983; Goresky et al. 1992), the perfusing medium, and tissue (Rubin and Tozer 1986; Fleischner et al. 1975; Goresky et al. 1978; Gärtner et al. 1983). The unbound species is considered that which freely exchanges between plasma and cell and is the species eliminated (Barnhart and

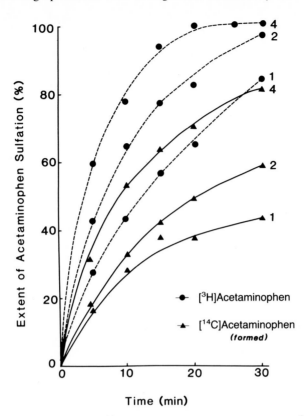

Fig. 10. Reduced sulfation for [^{14}C]acetaminophen generated from [^{14}C]phenacetin compared with preformed [^{3}H]acetaminophen in isolated rat hepatocytes. Incubation was performed in 5 ml, containing 4-, 2-, and 1-ml cell suspensions (*numbers appearing on graph*). (Data from PANG et al. 1985)

CLARENBURG 1973; ØIE and LEVY 1975). A similar consideration is given to metabolites formed within hepatocytes; after its formation, each metabolite is either potentially subjected to immediate additional metabolic and/or excretory events or reenters the sinusoid and then is exposed to the interactions with hepatocytes downstream from its site of formation before it finally leaves the liver (PANG et al. 1983, 1991b; PANG and STILLWELL 1983). For this reason, a metabolite formed within the liver is expected to undergo different degrees of metabolism/excretion, including the formation of various metabolites, in comparison to that found for the preformed, administered metabolite. This disparity is due to different points of metabolite introduction into the organ, even though the same transport and elimination mechanisms are involved in subsequent processing. The distributed-in-space drug and metabolite processing in the intact organ cannot be mimicked by a homogeneous pool of enzymatic activities, although identical amounts of enzymes are present.

1. Flow

A major difference between in vitro and organ systems is the presence of flow in the latter. The precise manner in which hepatic blood flow rate influences the overall rate of substrate disappearance has been described with various models of hepatic drug clearance covered earlier. Although the implications of flow for substrate removal differ among models, similar conclusions are reached. For rapidly equilibrating substances, liver cell entry is controlled only by delivery through blood flow. With high enzymatic activity, drug elimination proceeds at rates limited only by the delivery of substrate via perfusion and the substrate will be almost completely removed; organ clearance becomes rate limited by flow rate with E approaching unity. For this reason, flow, or the limiting value of clearance, will not provide adequate estimates of enzymatic constants in vivo (Pang et al. 1978); the decay rate constant, ordinarily reflecting the intrinsic clearance, will be dictated by the ratio of flow to volume of distribution. Substrates that are metabolized with low intrinsic clearances are poorly cleared substrates, and these will be subjected to the underlying low capacity for overall substrate removal and not to blood flow (Rowland et al. 1973; Wilkinson and Shand 1975; Pang and Rowland 1977a; Wilkinson 1987).

The effect of organ blood flow on hepatic processing has been well studied, especially in perfused organ studies involving drug entry via the portal vein. With a reduction in liver blood flow rate, the extraction ratio of drug is expected to increase, albeit to varying degrees, due to a longer sojourn in the liver. With an elevation in flow rate, the extraction ratio of drug will be diminished due to a more rapid transit of drug through the liver. The inverse relationship between hepatic blood flow rate and drug hepatic extraction ratio for poorly cleared substrates is well known (Pang and Rowland 1977a; Brauer et al. 1956a,b; Whitsett et al. 1971), whereas for highly cleared substrates, drug availability rather than extraction ratio changes proportionally with flow (Pang and Rowland 1977a,b; Ahmad et al. 1983; Keiding and Chiarantini 1978; Roberts and Rowland 1986b). Nonconformity with these predictions (Keiding and Steiness 1984; Miller and Oliver 1986) has been found to be due to a "derecruitment" of hepatocytes (Pang et al. 1988b) and invalidates the basic assumption that the tissue spaces containing enyzmatic activities which are accessible to substrates remain unaltered. The lack of a full opening of the vasculature, as maintained by Brauer (1963) and co-workers (Brauer et al. 1953, 1956a,b), was supported by parallel patterns of oxygen consumption rates (Keiding et al. 1980). This condition of derecruitment of hepatocytes and their associated enyzmatic activities (Pang et al. 1988b) may be another underlying reason for failure of in vitro–in vivo correlations.

The effect of organ blood flow on the formation and appearance of metabolites has been studied only to a limited extent. For MEGX, a metabolite formed from lidocaine, and acetaminophen, a metabolite formed from phenacetin, an increase in flow brings about reduced sequential metabolism of the metabolite, in a fashion similar to that found for drug (PANG and ROWLAND 1977c; DAWSON et al. 1985). The effect of flow on the formation of conjugates via competitive pathways, however, differs for these parallel pathways. This aspect will be covered in Sect. B.II.5.

2. Protein Binding

The influence of drug–protein binding on drug disposition has been well recognized (JUSKO and GRETCH 1976; ROWLAND 1984; ØIE 1986) and intensively studied both theoretically (JANSEN 1981; HUANG and ØIE 1984; XU et al. 1992) and experimentally (GUMUCIO et al. 1981, 1984; WOLKOFF et al. 1979; SCHARY et al. 1983; ROWLAND et al. 1984; JONES et al. 1984; SMALLWOOD et al. 1988b; SORRENTINO et al. 1989). The dogma is that the unbound drug is related to its pharmacological activity and is also the form that is eliminated by drug-metabolizing/excretory organs. Hence changes in the unbound concentrations may elicit toxic or subtherapeutic events. This is especially true for highly bound drugs, e.g., warfarin, bilirubin, dicoumarol, and valproic acid (WOSALAIT and GARTEN 1972; ØIE and LEVY 1975; WIEGARD et al. 1980).

When equilibrative exchange is readily achieved between bound and unbound drug (rapid on and off rates), the dependence of the unbound plasma fraction (f_P) on substrate concentration, the binding constants, the association constant (K_A), and the number of binding sites (N), as well as the classes of identical binding sites is well known (MARTIN 1965; COFFEY et al. 1971). Prediction of the greatest rate of change in the unbound fraction can be achieved at given protein concentrations, K_A, and N (XU et al. 1993). JANSEN (1981) has examined the influence of binding kinetics on drug metabolism or excretion from the sinusoids based on assumptions inherent in the well-stirred and parallel tube models of drug clearances. He commented that when the dissociation rate constant is maintained at the maximal level, no delimiting effect on elimination will be observed. HUANG and ØIE (1984) concluded that concentration-dependent binding is important for drugs of high intrinsic clearances. SMALLWOOD et al. (1988b) also investigated the changes in the total (C_B) and unbound ($C_{B,u}$) steady-state concentrations over a wide intrinsic clearance range. The change in sinusoidal unbound fraction along the length of the sinusoid and its effect on drug removal has recently been explored. When nonlinear drug binding occurs, the unbound fraction can be anticipated to decrease during the steady-state (single-pass) traverse of a drug in a distributed-in-space fashion when rapid drug elimination occurs (XU et al. 1993). Again, drugs which are relatively highly cleared and bound are prone to greater induced changes in f_B at any point x along the length of the sinusoid (or $f_{B,x}$). Large changes in $f_{B,x}$ can occur, resulting in large %f_B (between inlet and outlet) for drugs which undergo extensive removal; the extent is highly dependent on enzymatic parameters,

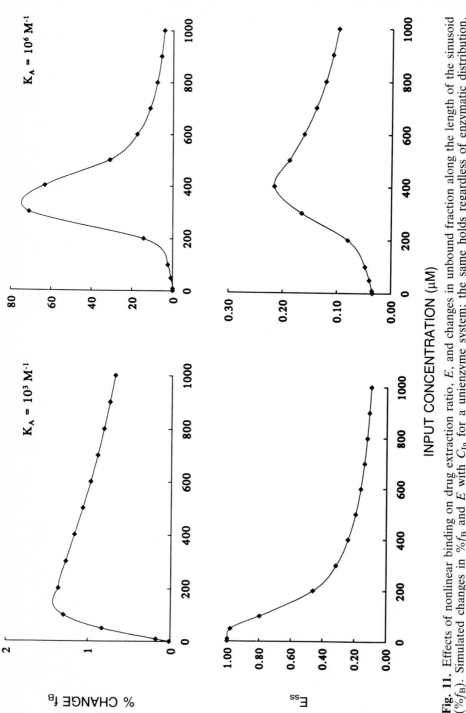

Fig. 11. Effects of nonlinear binding on drug extraction ratio, E, and changes in unbound fraction along the length of the sinusoid ($\%f_B$). Simulated changes in $\%f_B$ and E with C_{In} for a unienzyme system; the same holds regardless of enzymatic distribution. Simulated data were based on $K_m = 10\,\mu M$, $V_{max} = 1000\,$nmol/min, and $K_A = 10^3$ (*left panel*) and 10^6 (*right panel*) M^{-1}

K_m and V_{max}, in addition to the binding constants, K_A and N. Protein binding may become the rate-limiting factor in drug removal for highly cleared and bound compounds (Fig. 11), resulting in an unusual parabolic pattern for the extraction ratio (or clearance) with concentration. This observation can be used to explain the increased total body clearance of prednisolone with increased infusion rates (LEGLER et al. 1982) and the parabolic rise in E with 4-methylumbelliferyl sulfate concentration in the perfused rat liver (Fig. 12) (CHIBA and PANG 1993).

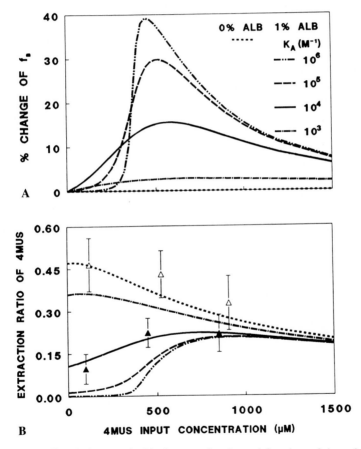

Fig. 12A,B. Predicted changes in % change of unbound fraction of 4-methylumbelliferyl sulfate (*4MUS*) in blood perfusate between the inlet and outlet of the liver (%f_B) (**A**), and the corresponding steady-state extraction ratio of 4MUS (**B**) with different K_A values versus perfusate 4MUS input concentration. Predictions were carried out by varying K_A values, as shown, according to CHIBA and PANG (1993). The observed steady-state extraction ratios, plotted as mean ± SD, for 1% and 0% albumin were taken from RATNA et al. (1993) and CHIBA and PANG (1993) respectively

Given the distributed-in-space nature of drug processing which induces changes in the unbound fraction, parameter estimates for metabolic pathways were reexamined in the presence of constant and nonlinear protein binding. Bass and colleagues had emphasized the use of the logarithmic average concentration ($\bar{C}$) in the Michaelis-Menten equation for parameter estimations, though this applies to galactose removal involving only one enzymatic system and absence of binding (see Winkler et al. 1974). Morris and Pang (1987) further assessed usage of the logarithmic average concentration in parameter estimations of multiple enzymatic systems with concentration-invariant binding and commented that an apparent K_m (which is K_m/f_B) will be obtained: in fact, this is true only for the high-affinity pathways and not for the low-affinity pathways. With nonlinear protein binding, the unbound drug, or the species equilibrating between sinusoids and hepatocytes and acted on by enzymes, should be used for estimation of enzymatic parameters. Use of unbound logarithmic average concentration ($\hat{C}_u$) for estimation of kinetic constants was proposed by Xu et al. (1993), who also found appropriate estimates for the high-affinity pathways but not the low-affinity pathways; however, improved estimations of the K_m for the lower affinity pathways are provided when the high-affinity pathway is suppressed using inhibitors.

It has been widely accepted that only unbound drug passes through the hepatocyte membrane, and uptake rate is predicted on the basis of the unbound fraction measured in plasma or perfusing medium. However, the initial uptake rates of some highly bound compounds (unbound fraction of 0.0001 to 0.1) such as free fatty acids (Weisiger et al. 1981), taurocholate (Forker and Luxon 1981), bilirubin (Weisiger et al. 1980; Wolkoff et al. 1979), rose bengal (Forker et al. 1982; Forker and Luxon 1983), sulfobromophthalein (Weisiger et al. 1980; Mizuma et al. 1985b), iopanoic acid (Barnhart et al. 1985), and warfarin (Tsao et al. 1986, 1988; Horie et al. 1988) were higher than those predicted from unbound uptake kinetics measured in the absence of albumin. This phenomenon was also observed in perfusing medium containing α_1-acid glycoprotein (Øie et al. 1987). An albumin effect has also been demonstrated in mutant analbuminemic rats (Inoue et al. 1983, 1985).

Numerous mechanisms have been proposed to explain the observations. An albumin receptor hypothesis (Weisiger et al. 1981) was rejected since albumin-specific receptors have not been identified on the surface of plasma membranes (Stremmel et al. 1983). Dissociation of the albumin-bound complex was not identified (Weisiger and Ma 1987), and the conventional theory on protein binding was consistent with many data in the literature (Rowland et al. 1984; Sorrentino et al. 1989). Moreover, a protein effect was also found for substrates which do not bind to albumin (Øie et al. 1987). A conformational change of albumin on the surface of the plasma membrane (Horie et al. 1988; Reed and Burrington 1989) or variations in membrane potential (Stremmel 1987) may cause dissociation of the ligand-albumin

Table 9. Effect of transmembrane barrier on the extent of elimination of preformed versus formed metabolites

Metabolite		Preformed metabolite $E(M_1)$[a]	Generated metabolite $E(M_1,P)$	Precursor	References
Enalaprilat		0.053	0.256[b]	Enalapril	Pang et al. (1984a) Pang et al. (1984a)
Acetaminophen sulfate		0.003	0.03[b]	Acetaminophen	Goresky et al. (1992) Pang and Terrell (1981b)
4-Methylumbelliferyl glucuronide		0.073	0.479[b] 0.647[b]	4-Methylumbelliferone 4-Methylumbelliferyl sulfate	Ratna et al. (1993) Ratna et al. (1993) Ratna et al. (1993)
α-Bromoisovalerylurea glutathione conjugate	(R)	0.0003	0.79[c]	(R)-α-Bromoisovalerylurea	Polhuijs et al. (1991) Polhuijs et al. (1992) Polhuijs et al. (1991) Polhuijs et al. (1992)
	(S)	0.0003	1.00[c]	(S)-α-Bromoisovalerylurea	

[a] Extraction ratio of the preformed, administered metabolite

[b] These metabolites primarily undergo biliary excretion; $E(M_1,P)$ was estimated as: $\left(\dfrac{\text{biliary excretion rate of metabolite}}{\text{formation rate of metabolite}} \right)$

[c] This glutathione conjugate undergoes cleavage; $E(M_1,P)$ was estimated as: $\left(1 - \dfrac{\text{Metabolite appearance rate in venous perfusate}}{\text{formation rate of metabolite}} \right)$

bound complex and result in a higher unbound ligand concentration at the surface. Alternatively, disequilibrium at the interstitial space (Weisiger 1985), or a codiffusion of bound and unbound ligands (Pond et al. 1992) across the unstirred water layer adjacent to hepatocyte surfaces, may increase delivery of unbound ligand to the cell surface (Bass and Pond 1988). The exact mechanism of the protein effect in substrate uptake, however, remains unclear (Wolkoff 1987; Berk et al. 1987).

3. Transmembrane Limitation

The major difference between subcellular and cellular/organ studies is the presence of a cellular membrane. The biological membrane imposes a substantial barrier to the entry of substrates. For a major eliminating organ such as the liver, transmembrane transport is a process which can constitute the rate-determining factor in the overall uptake of a substrate. The rate of entry of lipophilic substrates is sustained by passive diffusion, and flux across the membrane is sufficiently high that the membrane is seldom rate limiting. Many organic anions, neutral compounds, cations, and bile acids are known to utilize specific transport carriers to enter the liver cell (for review, see Nathanson and Boyer 1991). Hydrophilic compounds (Pang et al. 1984a; De Lannoy et al. 1989; Miyauchi et al. 1987; Schwab et al. 1990; Goresky et al. 1992) will be barred from entry and their uptake is often retarded. The behaviors of drug and metabolite for the well-stirred model, with barrier, are given by the following equations.

For the parent drug, E is (Gillette and Pang 1977) given as follows:

$$E = \frac{f_B CL_{int} CL^{in}}{QCL^{ef} + f_B CL_{int} CL^{in} + QCL_{int}}, \tag{37}$$

and the extraction ratio of the formed metabolite, $E\{M_1,P\}$ is

$$E\{M_1,P\} = \frac{QCL_{int(M1)} + f_{B(M1)}CL_{int(M1)}CL^{in}_{(M1)}}{QCL^{ef}_{(M1)} + f_{B(M1)}CL_{int(m1)}CL^{in}_{(M1)} + QCL_{int(M1)}}, \tag{38}$$

where CL^{in} and CL^{ef} are the drug influx and efflux clearances (or permeability surface area product PS), and $CL^{in}_{(M1)}$ and $CL^{ef}_{(M1)}$ are the influx and efflux clearances for the metabolite, M_1. Note that $E\{M_1,P\}$ is independent of the intrinsic clearance of formation of the metabolite (fraction of total drug intrinsic clearance) as well as parameters (transmembrane clearances and intrinsic clearance) pertaining to its parent compound.

Modification of Eqs. 12 and 13, with inclusion of membrane barriers for the parallel tube model, yield the following expressions:

For the parent drug,

$$E = 1 - e^{-\left\{\frac{f_B CL_{int} CL^{in}}{Q(CL_{int} + CL^{ef})}\right\}} \tag{39}$$

and for the metabolite,

$$E\{M_1,P\} = 1 -$$

$$\left\{\frac{f_B CL_{int} CL^{in}}{[f_B CL_{int} CL^{in}(CL_{int(M1)} + CL^{ef}{}_{(M1)}) - f_{B(M1)} CL_{int(M1)} CL^{in}{}_{(M1)}(CL_{int} + CL^{ef})]}\right\}$$

$$\times \; \frac{e^{-\frac{f_{B(M1)} CL_{int(M1)} CL^{in}{}_{(M1)}}{Q(CL_{int(M1)} + CL^{ef}{}_{(M1)})}} - e^{-\frac{f_B CL_{int} CL^{in}}{Q(CL_{int} + CL^{ef})}}}{\left(1 - e^{-\frac{f_B CL_{int} CL^{in}}{Q(CL_{int} + CL^{ef})}}\right)}. \tag{40}$$

Note that $E\{M_1,P\}$ is again independent of the intrinsic clearance of formation of metabolite (fraction of total intrinsic clearance of drug), but is dependent on other parameters (binding, transmembrane clearances, and intrinsic clearance) pertaining to the parent compound.

The existence of such a barrier causes drastic differences in the apparent handling between in vitro and organ perfusion studies due to different access to enzymatic sites. In organ perfusion studies, the hepatocyte membrane barrier may give rise to differences in handling between a preformed (administered) product and a product generated within cells or organ (derived from precursor); an apparent enhancement of the removal of the generated, polar product in relation to that of the preformed product results (PANG et al. 1984a; DE LANNOY and PANG 1987; DE LANNOY et al. 1989; GORESKY et al. 1992; RATNA et al. 1993) (Table 9). Such barriers need to be considered for in vitro–in vivo correlations.

4. Cosubstrate

The role of cofactors in phase II reactions is de-emphasized in incubation studies which involve excess amounts of cosubstrates. Conjugation reactions require the presence of cosubstrates, such as 3'-phosphoadenosine-5'-phosphosulfate (PAPS), uridine disphosphoglucuronic acid (UDPGA), and glutathione (GSH) for conjugation reactions. In rats, as much as 77 nmol PAPS/g liver has been reported (BREZNICKA et al. 1987) for ultimate transfer to acceptor substrates in the formation of sulfate conjugates (HERBAI 1970; MULDER and KEULEMANS 1978). The biosynthesis of PAPS from inorganic sulfate is rapid, especially when a high turnover rate of PAPS is required at high substrate supply (MULDER and KEULEMANS 1978; KRIJGSHELD et al. 1981; SCHWARZ and SCHWENK 1984; LIN and LEVY 1982; SWEENY and REINKE 1988). UDPGA levels in liver vary from 0.41 µmol/g wet weight in guinea pig to 0.02 µmol/g in carp (DUTTON 1980). The hepatic synthesis rate of both UDP-glucose (UDPG) and UDPGA in rats has been determined to be 100 nmol/g liver (DILLS and KLAASSEN 1987). Fasting (FELSHER et al. 1979; REINKE et al. 1981; CONWAY et al. 1985; PRICE et al. 1986; PRICE and JOLLOW 1988), diabetes (PRICE and JOLLOW 1982), pretreatment with phenobarbital, 3-methylcholanthrene, and other inducers (WATKINS and KLAASSEN 1983), diethyl ether anesthesia (AUNE et al. 1981; ERIKSSON and STRATH 1981; DILLS and KLAASSEN 1984; SHIPLEY and WEINER 1985), the energy state

(DILLS and KLAASSEN 1984, 1986a, 1987), and oxygen supply (AW and JONES 1982) have been shown to dramatically alter hepatic UDPGA levels in rat hepatocytes and in rat liver in vivo. The liver GSH concentration is higher than the PAPS and UDPGA concentrations. GSH is present at around $4.5-6\,\mu$mol/g rat liver and $2\,\mu$mol/g rat kidney (TORRES et al. 1986; MOHANDAS et al. 1984; LAUTERBURG and MITCHELL 1981) and is found in macrophages and type II and Clara cells in the rabbit lung (HORTON et al. 1987) and many other tissues (KOSOWER and KOSOWER 1978). The synthesis, efflux into sinusoid (KAPLOWITZ et al. 1980; AW et al. 1986; OOHKTENS et al. 1985; SIES and GRAF 1985) and bile (BALLOTORI et al. 1986), and degradation rate (ELING et al. 1986) maintain the intrahepatic GSH pool at a fairly constant level. GSH is synthesized readily from cysteine, glutamine, and glycine, with the rate of incorporation of cysteine being rate limiting (LAUTERBURG et al. 1980). Methionine also serves as an alternative precursor amino acid to cysteine (FINKELSTEIN and MUDD 1967; REED and ORRENIUS 1977; TATEISHI et al. 1981; MEISTER and ANDERSON 1983). The GSH turnover rate is also prone to feedback inhibition (LAUTERBURG and MITCHELL 1981; LAUTERBURG et al. 1982) and is affected by age, fasting, anesthestics (ZUMBIEL et al. 1978), and pretreatment with diethyl maleate (LAUTERBURG et al. 1980) or D,L-buthionine S,R-sulfoximine (GRIFFITH and MEISTER 1979) and other chemicals (PLUMMER et al. 1981).

In the depleted state, however, the supply of cosubstrates may limit the rate of conjugation. The dependency of the rate of reaction on cosubstrate supply becomes apparent when faster rates of conjugation are obtained upon repletion of precursors of cosubstrates, e.g., inorganic sulfate for PAPS (KRIJGSHELD et al. 1979, 1982; GALINSKY and LEVY 1981; LIN and LEVY 1986; HJELLE et al. 1985) and glucose for UDPGA (CONWAY et al. 1985). The limiting role of inorganic sulfate in controlling periportal necrosis due to the highly reactive sulfate conjugate of N-hydroxy-2-acetylamino-fluorene (MEERMAN and MULDER 1981) has revealed indirectly the importance of PAPS precursors. There are also indications that cellular UDPGA may be a determinant of glucuronidation in vivo (SINGH and SCHWARZ 1981; HOWELL et al. 1986; HJELLE et al. 1985). The amount of UDPGA required for glucuronidation of acetaminophen after a therapeutic dose was nearly equal to the total content of UDPGA in the liver; after a toxic dose, the UDPGA demand was more than 100-fold greater than the normal basal level (PRICE and JOLLOW 1984). Like PAPS and UDPGA, GSH is rapidly depleted with loading of acceptor substrates (TATEISHI et al. 1974; ORRENIUS et al. 1983; MEISTER and ANDERSON 1983; KAPLOWITZ et al. 1985) such as acetaminophen (JOLLOW et al. 1974; LAUTERBURG et al. 1980, 1982; LAUTERBURG and MITCHELL 1981), styrene oxide (SMITH et al. 1983), and α-bromoisovaleryl urea (TE KOPPELE et al. 1987). The depletion is associated with reduced rates of glutathione adduct formation. All of these effectively reduce the intrahepatic GSH concentrations or alter intrahepatic energy supply, which influences GSH synthesis (DILLS and KLAASSEN 1986b). The kinetics of phase II conjugation with a second-order reaction have been recently explored by CHEN and GILLETTE (1988) for the conjugation of the reactive metabolite of acetaminophen with glutathione. With incorporation of the synthesis and degradation rates of glutathione, remarkably good agreement was obtained between the predictions and the observed plasma acetaminophen concentrations and time course of intrahepatic GSH depletion described by JOLLOW et al. (1974).

5. Acinar Heterogeneity

The intact liver is an organ of known heterogeneities (NOVIKOFF 1959; DE LEEUE and KNOOK 1984; MILLER et al. 1979; JUNGERMAN and KATZ 1982; GUMUCIO et al. 1978), with well-defined zonation of the microcirculation (RAPPAPORT 1958, 1980), enzymes (THURMAN et al. 1987), biliary excretion (BOYER et al. 1979; GUMUCIO et al. 1978), transport (BURGER et al. 1989), and protein binding (BASS et al. 1989). The metabolic zonation within the liver has been known to influence drug and metabolite processing within the liver. The correlation sought between in vitro data and organ perfusion or in vivo studies fails to account for many of the known functional heterogeneities within the context of the microcirculatory events in the liver.

a) Zonal Localization of Enzymes

In analogy to the microcirculation, which may be classified into three zones according to the intralobular oxygen gradient (RAPPAPORT 1980), zonal enzymatic distribution has been divided into periportal, midzonal, and perivenous (pericentral) regions. Enzymatic heterogeneity is one of the most important determinants of metabolite formation and immediate sequential metabolism of the nascent metabolite within the liver. Direct and indirect techniques have shown an enriched presence of the cytochrome P-450s, epoxide hydrolase, glutathione S-transferases, and carboxylesterases, and both a perivenous abundance and an even distribution of UDP-glucuronosyl-transferases in the perihepatic venous region (zone 3) have been found; sulfation activities are mainly periportal (Table 10). Phagocytosis by Kupffer cells predominates in zone 3 (TE KOPPELE and THURMAN 1990). Elimination of a substrate/metabolite occurs only when it is present along the sinusoid and if it gains access into hepatocytes. Given the marked enzyme heterogeneities noted for phase I and phase II reactions, the nature and proportion of conjugates formed as primary or secondary metabolites arising from parallel or sequential pathways are expected to differ.

The roles of enzyme zonation on competitive and sequential drug metabolism have been illustrated both theoretically and experimentally. Conceptually, and enzymatic distribution describes the density of the enzyme or $V_{max,x}$ along the length of the sinusoid, L, such that $\int_0^\infty V_{max,x} dx/L$ is the average activity of the enzyme. Two such enzymatic systems are depicted schematically in Fig. 13. For these two systems, the relative locations of

Table 10. Enzymatic activities found by immunohistochemical and staining techniques, by microdissection, and by prograde and retrograde perfusions and HAPV and HAHV perfusion of the rat liver

Noted metabolic heterogeneities			Drug examples	References
Anterior	Even	Posterior		
		Mixed-function oxidases		BARON et al. (1982a,b)
		Cytochrome P-450		TAIRA et al. (1981)
		NADPH cytochrome P-450 c reductase		
		UDP-glucuronyltransferase		ULLRICH et al. (1984); KNAPP et al. (1988)
		Epoxide hydrolase		KAWABATA et al. (1981)
		Glutathione S-transferase		REDICK et al. (1982)
		Alcohol dehydrogenase		YAMAUCHI et al. (1988); KATO et al. (1990)
	Arylsulfatase			ANUNDI et al. (1986); EL MOUELHI and KAUFFMAN (1986)
	β-Glucuronidase			ibid
	Ethanol oxidation		Ethanol	KASHIWAGI et al. (1982)
Sulfation			Acetaminophen	PANG and GILLETTE (1978a); PANG and TERRELL (1981a); PANG et al. (1988b)
Sulfation			N-OH-2-acetylaminofluorene	DE BAUN et al. (1971); MEERMAN and MULDER (1981)
		O-Deethylation	Phenacetin	PANG and GILLETTE (1978a); PANG and TERRELL (1981a); PANG et al. (1988b)
		Carboxylester hydrolysis	Enalapril	PANG et al. (1991a)
Sulfation	Glucuronidation		Gentisamide	MORRIS et al. (1988a)
Sulfation	Glucuronidation		Harmol	DAWSON et al. (1985)
Sulfation	Glucuronidation		7-Hydroxycoumarin	CONWAY et al. (1987)
		Glucuronidation	7-Hydroxycoumarin	CONWAY et al. (1982, 1984)
Sulfation	Glucuronidation		Salicylamide	XU and PANG (1989)
Sulfation	Hydroxylation	Hydroxylation N-Deethylation	Lidocaine	PANG et al. (1986)
		Glycine conjugation	Benzoic acid	CHIBA et al. (1994)
		Glutathione conjugation	Bromosulfophthalein	ZHAO et al. (1993)

HAPV, hepatic artery–portal vein; HAHV, hepatic artery–hepatic vein

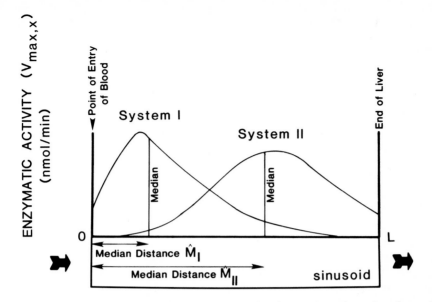

Fig. 13. The distributed-in-space phenomenon in drug processing. A schematic representation of uneven distribution of drug-metabolizing enzymes in the liver, systems I and II, which are involved in parallel, competing, or sequential metabolic pathways. Drug processing occurs along the direction of flow of substrate, from *left* to *right*, in a distributed-in-space fashion. The enzymatic distributions of systems I and II are described by the median distances, the distance from the inlet of the liver to the median (plane which divides the amount of enzyme into equal halves). As shown, system I is anteriorly localized relative to system II along the direction of flow of substrate

each system may be described with respect to its median (or center) of enzymatic distribution, the plane which divides total enzymatic activity into halves, and the median distance is the distance between the inlet of the liver and the median. System I is viewed as an anterior pathway in relation to system II, since its median (or center) of distribution precedes that for system II. These two systems (I and II) may represent competitive pathways or sequential pathways.

Conjugation by sulfation and glucuronidation of most phenolic substrates is the simplest example of parallel, metabolic pathways. Sulfation is often a higher affinity, lower capacity anterior pathway in relation to glucuronidation. A substrate coming into contact with hepatocytes along the direction of flow first accesses the anterior sulfation system; glucuronidation with the posteriorly located competitive system occurs when residual substrate arrives downstream for recruitment of such activities. Hence the concentration of substrate at x is related to its removal at points preceding x and at x, and substrate recruitment of glucuronidation activities occurs only when substrate is able to reach that region. Hence, the sulfation pathway strongly influences the extent of glucuronidation due to substrate depletion; the effect is greatest

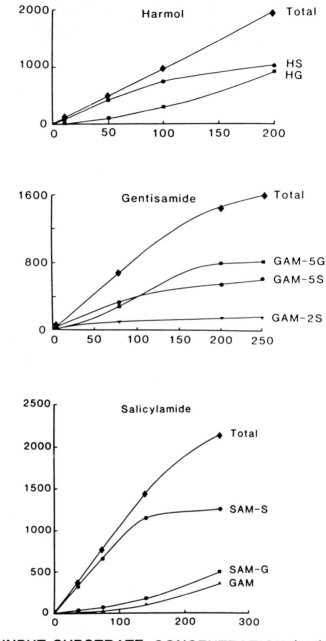

Fig. 14. Observed sulfation (S) and glucuronidation rates (G) of harmol, salicylamide, and gentisamide with input concentration in the single-pass perfused rat liver preparation. Note the disproportionate increase in G upon saturation of S with increasing substrate concentration

at low concentrations, when not all downstream hepatocytes are metabolically recruited because of substrate depletion due to upstream metabolism. At intermediate concentrations that are saturating for the anteriorly located sulfation system, a disproportionally higher substrate flux reaches the downstream region to effect glucuronidation, yielding disproportionately higher glucuronidation rates; at higher concentration ($\gg K_m$'s), all enzymatic systems (anterior and posterior) will be recruited by the substrate, and the role of enzymatic heterogeneity in metabolite formation becomes attenuated and unimportant (PANG et al. 1986; MORRIS and PANG 1987). Salicylamide, gentisamide, and harmol are highly cleared phenolic substrates which exhibit the typical compensatory rise in glucuronidation rate with concentration (Fig. 14). With suppression of sulfation by a specific inhibitor, 2,6-dichloro-4-nitrophenol, the aberrancy observed previously for glucuronidation of harmol and salicylamide disappears; Michaelis-Menten-like kinetics are observed for glucuronidation. This enzymatic pattern also influences sulfate and glucuronide formation with changes in flow: two opposing factors are altered by flow at low substrate supply; these are the transit time of drug and the supply of substrate (PANG and MULDER 1990). With increased flow, harmol sulfation was found to be decreased, as expected, owing to shortened drug transit time; harmol glucuronidation, however, was unchanged (DAWSON et al. 1985) since the effects of substrate sparing from sulfation and a reduced drug transit time with downstream glucuronidation sites counterbalanced each other (PANG and MULDER 1990). Thus, enzyme heterogeneity will cause differential changes in metabolite formation (Fig. 15).

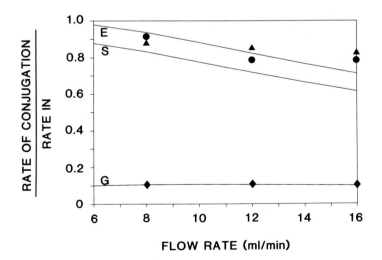

Fig. 15. Influence of organ blood flow on the extraction ratio of harmol ($10\,\mu M$) and the formation of harmol sulfate and harmol glucuronide conjugates. The flow-induced changes of harmol sulfation (▲) paralleled those for harmol extraction ratio (●). No apparent changes were seen for harmol glucuronidation (◆). See text for details. (Data from PANG and MULDER 1990; reproduced from DAWSON et al. 1985)

Sequential pathways are strongly subjected to similar considerations when heterogeneous localization of enzymes occurs. Because metabolite formation must necessarily precede metabolite elimination, events such as drug uptake followed by biotransformation would affect further metabolism/excretion of the immediately formed metabolite. Thus, the "lag" described for subcellular and cellular incubations also exists within the intact organ. The extent of metabolite formation and further metabolism is independent of the presence of competing pathways under first-order conditions (St-Pierre et al. 1992), but is strongly modulated by the heterogeneous distribution of enzymes for the formation and metabolism of the metabolite (Pang and Terrell 1981a). For enzymatic distributions that are unfavorably staggered (enzymes for metabolism of metabolite being placed anterior to enzymes for formation of metabolite), the extent of sequential metabolism of the metabolite will be reduced. When compared to that for a preformed metabolite, which is entering as input to the organ, its removal is independent of the kinetic behavior of drug and is accessible to its full complement of enzymes. The degree to which differences exist between the handling of formed and of preformed metabolite thus becomes dependent on the enzyme stacking and on the intrinsic clearances for the precursors. The behavior of sequential metabolism parallels that found for the parent drug: with increased flow, reduced sequential metabolism ensues (Dawson et al. 1985; Pang and Mulder 1990).

b) Flow

The liver receives a dual supply from the portal vein (PV) and the hepatic artery (HA). Although the artery enters the sinusoids by way of the peribiliary plexus and/or portal vein, it also has direct drainage to the sinusoids (Ohtani and Murakami 1978; Nopanitaya et al. 1978; Nakai et al. 1979; Yamamoto et al. 1985); direct connections of the hepatic artery to the sinusoids are, however, species dependent (Yamamoto et al. 1985). Complete mixing between arterial and portal venous flows is assumed. Arterial flow is regulated in a fashion which conserves the total liver blood flow rate (Lautt et al. 1985; Lautt and Greenway 1987) and may indirectly affect cellular zonation within the hepatic microcirculatory unit, the acinus. Low oxygenation is known to cause zone 2 cells to become zone 3 cells; a high oxygen tension may recruit zone 2 cells to become zone 1 cells (Rappaport 1958, 1980). Apart from this phenomenon, substrates entering via the hepatic artery may affect drug/metabolite processing at two levels: those of biliary excretion and metabolism. Differences in perfusion of the sinusoids by the HA could occur as a result of its intermittent high pressure and propulsion of flow and potentially produce a faster vascular drug transit time within the liver. Preservation of total hepatic blood flow, consisting of both HA and PV, at varying HA/PV flow ratios, could thus result in discrepancies regarding drug and metabolite processing, even though the total rate of delivery of substrate to the liver is preserved.

Reports on the handling of xenobiotics with respect to arterial and portal venous delivery are scarce and confounding. With an increased HA/PV flow ratio, decreased extraction ratios have been observed in the perfused rat liver for lidocaine, meperidine (AHMAD et al. 1984), gentisamide (HIRAYAMA et al. 1990; MORRIS et al. 1988a), acetaminophen, and phenacetin (PANG et al. 1993). The hepatic clearance of krypton-85 following portal venous injection has been found to be both higher (BLUMGART et al. 1977) and unchanged (HOLLENBERG and DOHERTY 1966) compared to that for hepatic arterial injection to the dog. Similarly, the extraction ratios for vitamin D_3 (GASCON-BARRE et al. 1988) and bromosulfophthalein (BRAUER et al. 1959) were unchanged when given into either the HA or the PV.

Reports on the vascular volume for tracers injected into the HA versus that for tracers injected into the PV are also equivocal. Shorter transit times have been found following HA injection (COHN and PINKERTON 1969; RABINOVICI and VARDI 1965). These studies suggest potential bypass of some of the sinusoidal surface for elements entering via the HA as opposed to via the PV, but with evident differences in the large vessel pathways. By contrast, in other studies no difference was found for the accessible vascular spaces for transit time measurements from outflow dilution profiles with HA and PV injections (AHMAD et al. 1984; CONWAY et al. 1985). Yet in more recent studies, slightly enlarged (total or cellular) water and interstitial spaces were found (REICHEN and SAGESSER 1988; PANG et al. 1994) with HA versus PV injection; the excess spaces are associated with the peribiliary capillary plexus. The velocity for HA flow was found, by intravital microscopy, to be faster than PV flow, and the HA streaming was confined to discrete acini (SHERMAN et al. 1991). The concept of arterial streaming, within sinusoids and the presence of a common shared space for HA and PV flow were suggested by FIELD and ANDREWS (1968). The inference is that there is likely a somewhat incomplete mixing of flows at the sinusoidal level. Moreover, a more enriched arterial contribution is known to exist for hepatic capsular flow (GOUMA et al. 1986; ARVIDSSON et al. 1988). With this new evidence on heterogeneous micromixing, it can be concluded that drug metabolism in the intact organ is further modulated by the HA–PV mixing regime. The fate of substrates entering via the HA or PV may thus deviate substantially, depending upon how these traverse the liver. Since most in vitro studies of liver perfusion are conducted with perfusion via the portal vein (ligation of the HA is often performed), the situation differs from that in vivo; this may exacerbate in vitro–in vivo discrepancies.

c) Cosubstrate

A periportal distribution of GSH has been reported (ASGHER et al. 1975; SMITH et al. 1979; MURRAY et al. 1986). The observation stems from studies on labeling of thiol groups that have revealed an enrichment for the periportal region of the rat liver. Recent reports further suggest that GSH in the circulation is removed by the guinea-pig liver, which is enriched with γ-

glutamyltransferases (Speisky et al. 1990). Ectoactivity of the γ-glutamyl-transferases, recently found to be present on the sinusoidal pole (Lança and Israel 1991), will somewhat diminish the heterogeneous distribution of GSH, since as much as 60% GSH can be cleaved to its cysteinyl-glycine dipeptide metabolite, which can be taken up for resynthesis of GSH downstream.

d) Membrane Transport

Acinar transport mechanisms have been recently examined by autoradiography of zonal labeling with antibodies or radiolabeled substrate entering progradely or retrogradely, or uptake by zonally enriched hepatocytes prepared by digitonin/collagenase perfusion (Quistorff 1985; Lindros and Penttilä 1985). These studies have mainly examined influx mechanisms: efflux mechanisms are rarely investigated. Recent observations have suggested uptake of histidine and glutamine by cultured perivenous cells (Burger et al. 1989); histoautoradiography following prograde or retrograde injection of glutamate, aspartate, and α-ketoglutarate confirmed this finding (Stoll et al. 1991). The asialoglycoprotein receptor has been found to be preferentially attached to the periportal liver cells (McFarlane et al. 1990), whereas with prograde and retrograde perfusion, ^{125}I-orosomucoid was found to be taken up by zone 3 cells (Casey et al. 1991) as well as to be more concentrated in the perivenous region (Van Der Sluijs et al. 1988). In interpreting the findings on the tissue distribution of labeled substrates, it needs to be borne in mind that the distribution is highly dependent on plasma and tissue binding properties and intracellular metabolism and efflux, in addition to influx transport mechanisms. The presence of acinar, heterogeneous transport mechanisms is an added complication in the interpretation of in vitro–in vivo correlations.

e) Protein Binding

Little work has been done on the heterogeneity in tissue protein binding. A recent report suggests that the fatty acid binding protein exhibits preferential binding to periportal cells (Bass et al. 1989). The tissue distribution of rhodamine B was found to be time dependent: high levels were initially found in zone 1, and later in zone 3 (Braakman et al. 1987). This phenomenon has been thought to be due to efflux of rhodamine B followed by reuptake and avid binding in zone 3 (Braakman et al. 1989).

D. Reasons for Poor Correlations Between In Vitro, Perfused Organs, and In Vivo

The distributed-in-space behavior of drug and metabolite processing and acinar heterogeneity of the organ are major limitations on in vitro–organ correlations. For the whole body, the same factors prevail among the multiple eliminating organs which exist for drug biotransformation and excretion. These multiple eliminating organs represent additional sites for formation of the same and/or different metabolites, though the enzymatic constants K_m and V_{max} and the rate-controlling factor may differ for each organ in respect of the formation of a common metabolite. The contribution of each organ to metabolism is defined by the size of the organ, perfusion rate, total enzymatic activity, and cosubstrate content in relation to other eliminating organs. Saturability and the dominance of the metabolic pathways within organs vary according to the administered dose and the route of administration (KLIPPERT and NOORDHOEK 1983). Despite all these facts, clearance concepts for drugs are well established with respect to organs in parallel and organs in series. Failure to obtain good in vitro–in vivo correlations may be due to omission of organ-tissue as potential metabolizing organs for in vitro esti-mates or to inadequate estimation of these parameters.

Metabolite clearances, however, are far less well defined. A metabolite formed within an eliminating organ is prone to undergo immediate metab-olism and/or excretion prior to leaving that organ. Metabolite clearances are not additive, even among eliminating organs, as exemplified in a simple scheme where the formed primary metabolite undergoes immediate excretion (DE LANNOY and PANG 1993). The metabolite is likely to enter other elimi-nating organs and be subjected to further metabolism before reaching the site of sampling; a common metabolite formed via multiple organs may endure different fates among the organs. Thus many of these metabolic events will be obscured unless the organs for metabolite formation and elim-ination are identified in vivo (PANG and KWAN 1983; PANG 1985; KLIPPERT and NOORDHOEK 1985). Because of the above, direct correlations of in vitro data with in vivo findings on metabolite disposition are rarely performed.

E. Conclusions

In vitro studies are aimed at providing baseline data for prediction of data in vivo. The common bases for extending in vitro data to the organ and whole body are described. Extrapolation to the organ necessitates consideration of clearance models. Many of the limitations encountered are due to the nature of processing and heterogeneities in the organ. Improved correlations can be achieved only when detailed biochemical data are obtained; for example, in physiological modeling. However, due to the inherent functional hetero-geneity of the organ (as outlined for the liver), the nature and the amount of metabolite(s) formed as well as sequential handling of the metabolite(s) may not be adequately reflected with physiological modeling, which is basically a series of well-stirred compartments representing tissue and organs. Extension of the distributed-in-space models (developed for single-pass systems) for recirculation will undoubtedly represent an improvement over the existing methods.

Acknowledgements. This work was supported by the Medical Research Council of Canada (Faculty Development Award MA-9104, MA-9765) and the National Institutes of Health (GM-38250).

References

Abramson FP (1986a) Kinetic models of induction. I. Persistence of the inducing substance. J Pharm Sci 75:223–228

Abramson FP (1986b) Kinetic models of induction. II. Decreased turnover of a product of its precursor. J Pharm Sci 75:229–232

Ahmad AB, Bennett PN, Rowland M (1983) Models of hepatic drug clearance: discrimination between the "well-stirred" and "parallel-tube" models. J Pharm Pharmacol 35:219–224

Ahmad AB, Bennett PN, Rowland M (1984) Influence of route of hepatic administration on drug availability. J Pharmacol Exp Ther 230:718–725

Ålin P, Jensson H, Guthenberg C, Danielson H, Tahir MK, Mannervik (1985) Purification of major basic glutathione transferase isoenzymes from rat liver by use of affinity chromatography and fast protein liquid chromatofocusing. Anal Biochem 146:313–320

Alvan G, Jonsson M, Sundwall A, Vessman J (1977) First pass conjugation and enterohepatic recycling of oxazepam in dogs: intravenous tolerance of oxazepam in propylene glycol. Acta Pharmacol Toxicol (Copenh) 40:16–27

Anundi RM, Kauffman FC, El-Mouelhi M, Thurman RG (1986) Hydrolysis of organic sulfates in periportal and pericentral regions of the liver lobule: studies with 4-methylumbelliferyl sulfate in the perfused rat liver. J Pharmacol Exp Ther 29:599–605

Araya H, Mizuma T, Horie T, Hayashi M, Awazu S (1984) Heterogeneous distribution of conjugation activities of harmol in isolated rat liver cells. J Pharmacobiodyn 7:624–629

Arndt R, Krisch K (1973) Catalytic properties of an unspecific carboxylesterase. Eur J Biochem 36:129–134

Arndt R, Heymann E, Junge W, Krisch K, Hollandt H (1973) Purification and molecular properties of an unspecific carboxylesterase (E1) from rat-liver microsomes. Eur J Biochem 36:120–128

Arvidsson D, Svensson H, Haglund U (1988) Laser-Doppler flowmetry for estimating liver blood flow. Am J Physiol 254:G471–G476

Asgher K, Reddy BK, Krishna G (1975) Histochemical localization of glutathione in tissues. J Histochem Cytochem 23:774–779

Ashley JJ, Levy G (1972) Inhibition of diphenylhydantoin elimination by its major metabolite. Res Commun Chem Pathol Pharmacol 4:297–306

Aune H, Olsen H, Morland J (1981) Diethyl ether influence on the metabolism of antipyrine, paracetamol and sulphanilamide in isolated rat hepatocytes. Br J Anaesth 53:621–626

Aw TY, Jones DP (1982) Secondary bioenergetic hypoxia: inhibition of sulfation and glururonidation reactions in isolated hepatocytes at low O_2 concentration. J Biol Chem 257:8997–9004

Aw TY, Ookhtens RC, Kaplowitz N (1986) Kinetics of glutathione efflux from isolated rat hepatocytes. Am J Physiol 250:G236–G243

Babiak LM, Cherry WF, Fayz S, Pang KS (1984) Kinetics of meperidine N-demethylation in the perfused rat liver preparation. Drug Metab Dispos 12:698–704

Balant L (1981) Clinical pharmacokinetics of sulphonylurea-hypoglycaemic agents. Clin Pharmacokinet 6:215–241

Ballatori N, Jacob R, Boyer JL (1986) Intrabiliary glutathione hydrolysis: a source of glutamate in bile. J Biol Chem 261:7860–7865

Barnhart JR, Clarenburg R (1973) Factors determining the clearance of bilirubin in perfused rat liver. Am J Physiol 225:497–508

Barnhart JL, Witt BL, Hardison WG, Berk RN (1985) Uptake of iopanoic acid by isolated rat hepatocytes in primary culture. Am J Physiol 244:G630–G636

Baron J, Redick RA, Guengerich FP (1982a) An immunohistochemical study on the localizations and distributions of phenobarbital- and 3-methylcholanthrene-inducible cytochrome P-450 within the livers of untreated rats. J Biol Chem 256:15200–15203

Baron J, Redick RA, Guengerich FP (1982b) Effect of 3-methylcholanthrene, β-naphthoflavone, and phenobarbital on the 3-methylcholanthrene inducible isozyme of cytochrome P-450 within centrilobular, midzonal, and periportal hepatocytes. J Biol Chem 257:953–957

Barr W, Riegelman S (1970) Intestinal drug absorption and metabolism. I. Comparison of methods and models to study physiological factors of in vitro and in vivo intestinal absorption. J Pharm Sci 59:154–163

Bass L, Pond SM (1988) The puzzle of rates of cellular uptake of protein-bound ligands. In: Pecile A, Resigno A (eds) Pharmacokinetics. Plenum, London, pp 245–269

Bass L, Robinson P, Bracken AJ (1978) Hepatic elimination of flowing substrates: the distributed model. J Theor Biol 72:161–184

Bass L, Roberts RS, Robinson PJ (1987) On the relation between extended forms of the sinusoidal perfusion and of the convection-dispersion models of hepatic elimination. J Theor Biol 126:457–482

Bass NM, Barker ME, Manning JA, Jones AL, Ockner RK (1989) Acinar heterogeneity of fatty acid binding protein expression in livers of male, female, and clofibrate-treated rats. Hepatology 9:12–21

Beaubien AR, Pakuts AP (1979) Influence of dose on first-pass kinetics of ^{14}C-imipramine in the isolated perfused rat liver. Drug Metab Dispos 7:34–39

Belanger PM, Lalande G, Labrecque, Dore FM (1985) Diurnal variation in the transferases and hydrolases involved in glucuronide and sulfate conjugation of rat liver. Drug Metab Dispos 13:386–389

Benowitz N, Forsyth RP, Melmon KC, Rowland M (1974) Lidocaine disposition kinetics in monkeys and man. I. Prediction by a perfusion model. Clin Pharmacol Ther 16:87–109

Berk PD, Potter JB, Stremmel W (1987) Role of plasma membrane ligand-binding proteins in the hepatocellular uptake of albumin-bound organic anions. Hepatology 7:165–176

Bertilsson L (1978) Clinical pharmacokinetics of carbamazepine. Clin Pharmacokinet 3:128–143

Bertilsson L, Hojer B, Tybring G, Osterioh EJ, Rane A (1980) Autoinduction of carbamazepine metabolism in children examined by a stable isotope technique. Clin Pharmacol Ther 27:83–88

Bierman CW, Williams PV (1989) Therapeutic monitoring of theophylline: rationale and current status. Clin Pharmacokinet 17:377–384

Binder TP, Duffel MW (1988) Sulfation of benzylic alcohols catalyzed by arylsulfotransferase IV. Mol Pharmacol 33:477–479

Bischoff KB (1975) Some fundamental considerations of the applications of pharmacokinetics to cancer chemotherapy. Cancer Chemother Rep 59:777–793

Bischoff KB, Dedrick RL (1968) Thiopental pharmacokinetics. J Pharm Sci 57:1346–1351

Bischoff KB, Dedrick RL, Zaharko DS, Longstreth LA (1971) Methotrexate pharmacokinetics. J Pharm Sci 60:1128–1133

Blake DA, Collins JM, Miyasaki BC, Cohen F (1978) Influence of pregnancy and folic acid on phenytoin metabolism by rat liver microsomes. Drug Metab Dispos 6:246–250

Blumgart LH, Harper AM, Lieberman DP, Mathie RT (1977) Liver blood flow measurement with [85]krypton clearance from portal venous and hepatic arterial routes of injection (Abstr). Proc Br Pharmacol Soc 60:278P

Börg KO, Eklund B, Skanberg J, Wallborg M (1974) Metabolism of alprenolol in liver microsomes, perfused liver and conscious rat. Acta Pharmacol Toxicol (Copenh) 35:169–179

Borondy P, Chang T, Glazko F (1972) Inhibition of diphenylhydantoin (DPH) hydroxylation by 5-(p-hydroxyphenyl)-5-phenylhydantoin (p-HPPH) (Abstr). Fed Proc 31:582

Boxenbaum H (1980) Interspecies variation in liver weight, hepatic blood flow, and antipyrine intrinsic clearance: extrapolation of data to benzodiazepines and phenytoin. J Pharmacokinet Biopharm 8:165–176

Boxenbaum H, Ronfeld R (1983) Interspecies pharmacokinetic scaling and the Dedrick plots. Am J Physiol 245:R768–R775

Boyer JL, Elias E, Layden TJ (1979) The paracellular pathway and bile formation. Yale J Biol Med 52:61–67

Braakman I, Groothuis GMM, Meijer DKF (1987) Acinar heterogeneity in hepatic transport of the organic cation rhodamine B in rat liver. Hepatology 7:849–855

Braakman I, Groothuis GMM, Meijer DKF (1989) Zonal compartmentation of perfused rat liver: plasma reappearance of rhodamine B explained. J Pharmaol Ther 239:869–873

Braggins TJ, Crow KE (1981) The effects of high ethanol oxidation in rats. A reassessment of factors controlling rates of ethanol oxidation in vivo. Eur J Biochem 119:633–640

Brauer RW (1963) Liver circulation and function. Physiol Rev 43:115–213

Brauer RW, Leong GF, Prescott RL (1953) Vasomotor activity of the isolated perfused rat liver. Am J Physiol 174:304–312

Brauer RW, Leong GF, McElroy RF, Holloway RJ (1956a) Circulatory pathways in the rat liver as revealed by P^{32} chromic phosphate colloid uptake in the perfused rat liver. Am J Physiol 184:593–598

Brauer RW, Leong GF, McElroy RF Jr, Holloway RJ (1956b) Hemodynamics of the vascular tree of the isolated rat liver preparation. Am J Physiol 186:537–542

Brauer RW, Shill OS, Krebs JS (1959) Studies concerning functional differences between liver regions supplied by the hepatic artery and by the portal vein. J Clin Invest 38:2202–2214

Breznicka EA, Hazelton GA, Klaasen CD (1987) Comparison of adenosine 3'-phosphate 5'-phosphosulfate concentrations in tissues from different laboratory animals. Drug Metab Dispos 15:133–135

Bungay PM, Dedrick RL, Matthews HB (1979) Pharmacokinetics of halogenated hydrocarbons. Ann NY Acad Sci 320:257–270

Burchell B (1978) Substrate specificity and properties of uridine diphosphate glucuronyltransferase purified to apparent homogeneity from phenobarbital-treated rat liver. Biochem J 173:749–757

Burchell B (1982) Reconstitution of purified Wistar rat liver bilirubin UDP-glucuronyltransferease into Gunn-rat liver microsomes. Biochem J 201:653–656

Burger HJ, Gebhardt R, Mayer C, Mecke D (1989) Different capacities for amino acid transport in periportal and perivenous hepatocytes isolated by digitonin/collagenase perfusion. Hepatology 9:22–28

Campbell NRC, van Loon JA, Weinshilboum RM (1987) Human liver phenol sulfotransferase: assay conditions, biochemical properties and partial purification of isoenzymes of the thermostable form. Biochem Pharmacol 36:1435–1446

Casey CA, Kragskow SL, Sorrell MF, Tuma DJ (1991) Zonal difference in ethanol-induced impairments in receptor-mediated endocytosis of asialoglycoproteins in isolated rat hepatocytes. Hepatology 13:260–266

Cassidy MK, Houston JB (1980) In vivo assessment of extrahepatic conjugative metabolism in first pass effects using the model compound phenol. J Pharm Pharmacol 32:57–59

Cassidy MK, Houston JB (1984) In vivo capacity and extrahepatic enzymes to conjugate phenol. Drug Metab Dispos 12:619–624

Castuma C, Brenner RR (1983) Effect of fatty acid deficiency on microsomal membrane fluidity and cooperativity of the UDP-glucuronyltransferase. Biochim Biophys Acta 729:9–16

Chance B (1960) Analogue and digital representations of enzyme kinetics. J Biol Chem 235:2440–2443

Chang SL, Levy RH (1985) Inhibition of epoxidation of carbamazepine by valproic acid in the isolated perfused rat liver. J Pharmacokinet Biopharm 13:453–466

Chen CN, Coleman DL, Andrade JD, Temple AR (1978) Pharmacokinetic model for salicylate in cerebrospinal fluid, blood, organs, and tissues. J Pharm Sci 67:38–45

Chen H-S, Gross JF (1979) Estimation of tissue-to-plasma partition coefficients used in physiological pharmacokinetic models. J Pharmacokinet Biopharm 7: 117–125

Chen EH, Gumucio JJ, Ho NH, Gumucio DL (1984) Hepatocytes of zone 1 and zone 3 conjugate sulfobromophthalein with glutathione. Hepatology 4:467–476

Chen R, Gillette JR (1988) Pharmacokinetic procedures for the estimation of organ clearances for the formation of short-lived metabolites. Acetaminophen induced glutathione depletion in hamster. Drug Metab Dispos 16:373–385

Chenery RJ, Ayrton A, Oldeham HG, Standring P, Norman SJ, Seddon T, Kirby R (1987) Diazepam metabolism in cultured hepatocytes from rat, rabbit, dog, guinea pig and man. Drug Metab Dispos 15:312–317

Chiba M, Pang KS (1993) Effects of protein binding on 4-methylumbelliferyl sulfate desulfation kinetics in perfused rat liver. J Pharmacol Exp Ther 266:492–499

Chiba M, Fujita S, Suzuki T (1988) Parallel pathway interactions in imipramine metabolism in rats. J Pharm Sci 77:944–947

Chiba M, Fujita S, Suzuki T (1990a) Pharmacokinetic correlation between in vitro hepatic microsomal enzyme kinetics and in vivo metabolism of imipramine and desipramine in rats. J Pharm Sci 79:281–287

Chiba M, Fujita S, Suzuki T (1990b) Kinetic properties of the metabolism of imipramine and desipramine in isolated rat hepatocytes. Biochem Pharmacol 39:367–372

Chiba M, Poon K, Hollands J, Pang KS (1994) Localization of glycine conjugation activities towards benzoic acid in perfused rat liver: studies with the multiple indicator dilution technique. J Pharmacol Exp Ther 268:1–8

Chindavijak B, Belpaire FM, Bogaert MG (1987) Effect of inflammation and proadifen on the disposition of antipyrine, lignocaine and propranolol in rat isolated perfused liver. J Pharm Pharmacol 39:997–1002

Cicero TJ, Bernard JD, Newman K (1980) Effect of castration and chronic morphine administration on liver alcohol dehydrogenase and the metabolism of ethanol in the male Sprague-Dawley rat. J Pharmacol Exp Ther 215:317–324

Clejan LA, Cederbaum AI (1989) Comparison of the interaction of pyrazole and its metabolite 4-hydroxypyrazole with rat liver microsomes. Drug Metab Dispos 18:393–397

Coffey JJ, Bullock FJ, Schoenemann PT (1971) Numerical solution of nonlinear pharmacokinetic equations: effects of plasma protein binding on drug distribution and elimination. J Pharm Sci 60:1623–1628

Cohn JN, Pinkerton AL (1969) Intrahepatic distribution of hepatic arterial and portal venous flows in the dog. Am J Physiol 216:285–289

Colburn WA (1979) A pharmacokinetic model to differentiate preabsorptive, gut epithelial, and hepatic first-pass metabolism. J Pharmacokinet Biopharm 4:407–415

Colburn WA (1981) Albumin does not mediate removal of taurocholate by the rat liver. J Pharm Sci 71:373–375

Collins JM, Blake DA, Egner PG (1978) Phenytoin metabolism in the rat. Pharmacokinetic correlationship between in vitro hepatic microsomal enzyme activity and in vivo elimination kinetics. Drug Metab Dispos 6:251–257

Conway JG, Kauffman FC, Ji S, Thurman RG (1982) Rates of sulfation and glucuronidation of 7-hydroxycoumarin in periportal and pericentral regions of the liver lobule. Mol Pharmacol 22:509–516

Conway JG, Kauffman FC, Tsukada T, Thurman RG (1984) Glucuronidation of 7-hydroxy-coumarin in periportal and pericentral regions of the liver lobule. Mol Pharmacol 25:487–493

Conway JG, Popp JA, Thurman RG (1985) Microcirculation in periportal and pericentral region of the lobule in perfused rat liver. Am J Physiol 249: G449–G456

Conway JG, Kauffman FC, Tsukuda T, Thurman RG (1987) Glucuronidation of 7-hydroxy-coumarin in periportal and pericentral regions of the lobule in livers from untreated and 3-methylcholanthrene-treated rats. Mol Pharmacol 33: 111–119

Curci G, Bergamini N, Veneri FD, Ninni A, Nitti V (1972) Half-life of rifampicin after repeated administration of different doses in humans. Chemotherapy 17:373–381

Dahlstrom BE, Paalzow LK, Lindberg C, Bogentoft C (1979) Pharmacokinetics and analgesic effect of pethidine (meperidine) and its metabolites in the rat. Drug Metab Dispos 7:108–112

Danan G, Descatorire V, Pessayre D (1981) Self-induction by erythromycin of its own transformation into a metabolite forming an inactive complex with reduced cytochrome P-450. J Pharmacol Exp Ther 218:509–514

Dankwerts PV (1953) Continuous flow systems. Distribution of residence times. Chem Eng Sci 2:1–13

Dannenberg AJ, Kavecansky J, Scarlata S, Zakim D (1990) Organization of microsomal UDP-glucuronosyltransferase. Activation by treatment at high pressure. Biochemistry 29:5961–5967

Daugaard H, Egjford M, Olgaard K (1987) Short communication. Isolated perfused rat kidney and liver combined. A new experimental model. Pflugers Arch 409:220–222

Dawson JR, Bridges JW (1981) Intestinal microsomal drug metabolism. A comparison of rat and guinea-pig enzymes, and of rat crypt and villous tip cell enzymes. Biochem Pharmacol 30:2415–2420

Dawson JR, Weitering JG, Mulder GJ, Stillwell RN, Pang KS (1985) Alteration of transit time and direction of flow to probe the heterogeneous distribution of conjugation activities for harmol in the perfused rat liver preparation. J Pharmacol Exp Ther 234:691–697

De Baun JR, Smith JYR, Miller EC, Miller JA (1971) Reactivity in vivo of the carcinogen N-hydroxy-2-acetylaminofluorene: increase by sulfate ion. Science 167:184–186

Dedrick RL, Bischoff KB, Zaharko DZ (1970) Interspecies correlation of plasma concentration history of methotrexate (NSC-740). Cancer Chemother Rep 54:95–101

Dedrick RL, Zaharko DS, Lutz RJ (1973) Transport and binding of methotrexate in vivo. J Pharm Sci 62:882–890

De Lannoy IAM, Pang KS (1987) Diffusional barriers on drug and metabolite kinetics. Drug Metab Dispos 15:51–58

De Lannoy IAM, Pang KS (1993) Combined recirculation of the rat liver and kidney: studies with enalapril and enalaprilat. J Pharmacokinet Biopharm 21:423–456

De Lannoy IAM, Nespeca R, Pang KS (1989) Renal handling of enalapril and its metabolite, enalaprilat, in the isolated red blood cell-perfused rat kidney. J Pharmacol Exp Ther 251:1211–1222

De Lannoy IAM, Barker F III, Pang KS (1993) Differences in metabolite excretion clearances in formation organs: studies with enalapril and enalaprilat in the single pass and recirculating perfused rat liver. J Pharmacokinet Biopharm 21:395–421

De Leeue AM, Knook DL (1984) The ultrastructure of sinusoidal liver cells in the intact rat at various ages. In: van Bezooijen CFA (ed) Pharmacological, morphological and physiological aspects of aging. Eurage, Rijswik, pp 91–96

Dills RL, Klaassen CD (1984) Decreased glucuronidation of bilirubin by diethyl ether anesthesia. Biochem Pharmacol 33:2813–2814

Dills RL, Klaassen CD (1986a) Effect of reduced hepatic energy state on acetaminophen conjugation in rats. J Pharmacol Exp Ther 238:463–472

Dills RL, Klaassen CD (1986b) The effect of inhibitors of mitochondrial energy production on hepatic glutathione, UDP-glucuronic acid, and adenosine 3'-phosphate-5'-phosphosulfate concentrations. Drug Metab Dispos 14:190–196

Dills RL, Klaassen CD (1987) Hepatic UDP-glucose and UDP-glucuronic acid synthesis rates in rats during a reduced energy state. Drug Metab Dispos 15:281–288

Dollery CT, Davis DS, Connally MB (1971) Differences in the metabolism depend upon their route of administration. Ann NY Acad Sci 79:108–112

Dubey RK, Singh J (1988a) Localization and characterization of drug metabolizing enzymes along the villous-crypt surface of the rat small intestine. I. Monooxygenases. Biochem Pharmacol 37:169–176

Dubey RK, Singh J (1988b) Localization and characterization of drug metabolizing enzymes along the villous-crypt surface of the rat small intestine. II. Conjugases. Biochem Pharmacol 37:177–184

Duffel MW, Jakoby WB (1981) On the mechanism of aryl sulfotransferase. J Biol Chem 256:11123–11127

Dutton GJ (1980) Glucuronidation of drugs and other compounds. CRC, Boca Raton

Eacho PI, Sweeny D, Weiner (1981) Conjugation of p-nitroanisole and p-nitrophenol in hepatocytes isolated from streptozotocin diabetic rats. J Pharmacol Exp Ther 218:34–40

Effeney DJ, Pond SM, Lo M-W, Silber BM, Riegelmans (1982) A technique to study hepatic and intestinal drug metabolism separately in the dog. J Pharmacol Exp Ther 221:507–511

Egfjord M, Daugaard H, Olgaard K (1991) Aldosterone metabolism in combined isolated perfused rat liver and kidney. Am J Physiol 260:F536–F548

El Mouelhi M, Kauffman FC (1986) Sublobular distribution of transferases and hydrolases associated with glucuronide, sulfate, and glutathione conjugation in human liver. Hepatology 6:450–456

Eleter S, Zakim D, Vessey DA (1973) A spin-label study of the role of phospholipids in the regulation of membrane-bound microsomal enzymes. J Mol Biol 78:351–362

Eling TE, Curtis JF, Harman LS, Mason RP (1986) Oxidation of glutathione to its thiyl free radical metabolite by prostaglandin H synthase. J Biol Chem 261:5023–5028

Erickson G, Strath D (1981) Decreased UDP-glucuronic acid in rat liver after ether narcosis. FEBS Lett 124:39–42

Erickson RH, Zakim D, Vessey DA (1978) Preparation and properties of a phospholipid-free form of microsomal UDP-glucuronyltransferase. Biochemistry 17:3706–3711

Falany CN, Tephly TR (1983) Separation, purification and characterization of three isoenzymes of UDP-glucuronyltransferase from rat liver microsomes. Arch Biochem Biophys 227:248–258

Fayz S, Cherry WF, Dawson JR, Mulder GJ, Pang KS (1984) Inhibition of acetaminophen sulfation by 2,6-dichloro-4-nitrophenol in the perfused rat liver preparation. Lack of a compensatory increase of glucuronidation. Drug Metab Dispos 12:323–329

Felsher BF, Carpio NM, VanCouvering K (1979) Effect of fasting and phenobarbital on hepatic UDP-glucuronic acid formation in rat. J Lab Clin Med 93:414–427

Field CD, Andrews WH (1968) Investigation of the hepatic arterial "space" under various conditions of flow in the isolated perfused dog liver. Circ Res 23: 611–622

Finkelstein TD, Mudd SH (1967) Trans-sulfuration in mammals: the methionine-sparing effect of cysteine. J Biol Chem 242:873–880

Fisher JW, Temistocles A, Taylor WDH, Clewell HJ III, Andersen ME (1989) Physiologically based pharmacokinetic modeling of the pregnant rat. A multiroute exposure model for trichloroethylene and its metabolite, trichloroacetic acid. Toxicol Appl Pharmacol 99:395–414

Fisher JW, Temistocles A, Taylor WDH, Clewell HJ III, Andersen ME (1990) Physiologically based pharmacokinetic modeling of the lactating rat and nursing pup: a multiroute exposure model for trichloroethylene and its metabolite, trichloroacetic acid. Toxicol Appl Pharmacol 102:497–513

Fisher JW, Gargas ML, Allen BC, Andersen ME (1991) Physiologically based pharmacokinetic modeling with trichloroethylene and its metabolite, trichloroacetic acid, in the rat and mouse. Toxicol Appl Pharmacol 108:183–195

Fleischner G, Meijer DKF, Levine WG, Gatmaitan Z, Gluck R, Arias IM (1975) Effect of hypolipidemic drugs, nafenopin and clofibrate, on the concentration of ligandin and Z protein in rat liver. Biochem Biophys Res Commun 67:1401–1407

Foliot A, Touchard D, Celier C (1984) Impairment of hepatic glutathione S-transferase activity as a cause of reduced biliary sulfobromophthalein excretion in clofibrate-treated rats. Biochem Pharmacol 33:2829–2834

Forker EL, Luxon BA (1981) Albumin helps mediated removal of taurocholate by rat liver. J Clin Invest 67:1517–1522

Forker EL, Luxon BA (1983) Albumin-mediated transport of rose bengal by perfused rat liver. J Clin Invest 72:1764–1771

Forker EL, Luxon BA, Snell M, Shurmantine WD (1982) Effect of albumin binding on the hepatic transport of rose bengal: surface-mediated dissociation on limited capacity. J Pharmacol Exp Ther 223:342–347

Frederick CB, Mays JB, Ziegler DM, Guengerich FP, Kadlubar FF (1982) Cytochrome P-450- and flavin-containing monooxygenase-catalyzed formation of the carcinogen N-hydroxy-2-aminofluorene and its covalent binding to nuclear DNA. Cancer Res 42:2671–2677

Freeman DS, Gjika HB, Vunakis HV (1977) Radioimmunoassay for normephridine: studies on the N-dealkylation of meperidine and anileridine. J Pharmacol Exp Ther 203:203–212

Fremstad D, Jacobsen S, Lunde PKM (1977) Influence of serum protein binding on the pharmacokinetics of quinidine in normal and anuric rats. Acta Pharmacol Toxicol (Copenh) 41:161–176

Fujita S, Kitagawa H, Chiba M, Suzuki T, Ohta M, Kitani K (1985) Age and sex associated differences in the relative abundance of multiple forms of cytochrome P-450 in rat liver microsomes. A separation by HPLC of hepatic microsomal P-450 species. Biochem Pharmacol 34:1861–1864

Fujita S, Morimoto R, Chiba M, Kitani K, Suzuki T (1989) Evaluation of the involvement of a male specific cytochrome P-450 isozyme in senescence-associated decline of hepatic drug metabolism in male rats. Biochem Pharmacol 38:3925–3931

Fujita S, Ishida R, Kagimoto N, Suzuki K, Masubuchi Y, Chiba M, Funae Y, Suzuki T (1990) Mechanism of alterations of non-linearity in hepatic first-pass metabolism of propranolol: alterations in the relative abundance of cytochrome P-450 isozymes in the liver microsomes in relation to the organ-level metabolic activities. J Pharmacobiodyn 13:s-98

Galinsky RE, Levy G (1981) Dose- and time-dependent elimination of acetaminophen in rats: pharmacokinetic implications of cosubstrate depletion. J Pharmacol Exp Ther 210:14–20

Gärtner U, Stockert RJ, Levine WG, Wolkoff AW (1983) Effect of nafenopin on the uptake of bilirubin and sulfobromophthalein by the isolated perfused rat liver. Gastroenterology 83:1163–1169

Gascon-Barre M, Huet P-M, St-Onge-Brault G, Brault A, Kassissia I (1988) Liver extraction of vitamin D_3 is independent of its hepatic venous or arterial route of delivery. Studies in isolated perfused rat liver preparations. J Pharmacol Exp Ther 245:975–981

Gibaldi M, Boyes RN, Feldman S (1971) Influence of first-pass effect on availability of drugs on oral administration. J Pharm Sci 60:1338–1340

Gillette JR (1971) Factors affecting drug metabolism. Ann NY Acad Sci 179:43–46

Gillette JR, Pang KS (1977) Theoretical aspects of pharmacokinetic drug interactions. Clin Pharmacol Ther 22:623–639

Goresky CA (1963) A linear method for determining liver sinusoidal and extravascular volumes. Am J Physiol 204:626–640

Goresky CA, Groom AC (1984) Microcirculatory events in the liver and spleen. In: Renkin EM, Michel CA (eds) The cardiovascular system: microcirculation. American Physiological Society, Bethesda, pp 689–780 (The handbook of physiology)

Goresky CA, Bach GG, Nadeau BE (1973) On the uptake of materials by the intact liver. The transport and net removal of galactose. J Clin Invest 52:991–1009

Goresky CA, Bach GG, Nadeau BE (1975) Red cell carriage of label. Its limiting effect on the exchange of materials in the liver. Circ Res 36:328–351

Goresky CA, Daly DS, Mishkin S, Arias IM (1978) Uptake of labeled palmitate by the liver: role of intracellular binding sites. Am J Physiol 234:E542–E553

Goresky CA, Schwab AJ, Rose CP (1988) Xenon handling in the liver: red cell capacity effect. Circ Res 63:767–778

Goresky CA, Pang KS, Schwab AJ, Barker F III, Cherry WF, Bach CG (1992) Uptake of a protein bound polar compound, acetaminophen sulfate, by perfused rat liver. Hepatology 16:173–190

Goresky CA, Schwab AJ, Pang KS (1993) Kinetic models of hepatic transport at the organ level. In: Tavoloni N, Berk PD (eds) Hepatic anion transport and bile secretion: physiology and pathophysiology. Raven, New York, pp 11–39

Gouma DJ, Coelho JCU, Schlegel J, Fisher JD, Li YF, Moody FG (1986) Estimation of hepatic blood flow by hydrogen gas clearance. Surgery 99:439–445

Graham AB, Wood GC (1972) Studies on the activation of UDP-glucuronyltransferse. Biochim Biophys Acta 276:392–398

Graham AB, Woodcock BG, Wood GC (1974) The phospholipid-dependence of uridine diphosphate glucuronyltransferase. Biochem J 137:567–574

Grant DM, Blum M, Beer M, Meyer UA (1991) Monomorphic and polymorphic human arylamine N-acetyltransferases: a comparison of liver isozymes and expressed products of two cloned genes. Mol Pharmacol 39:184–191

Gray MR, Tam YK (1986) The series-compartment model for hepatic elimination. Drug Metab Dispos 15:27–31

Gray MR, Saville BA, Tam YK (1987) Mechanism of lidocaine kinetics in the isolated perfused rat liver. III. Evaluation of liver models for time-dependent behavior. Drug Metab Dispos 15:22–26

Greenblatt DJ, Divoll M, Harmat JS, Shacler RJ (1980) Oxazepam kinetics: effect of age and sex. J Pharmacol Exp Ther 215:86–91

Gregus Z, Madhu C, Goon D, Klaassen CD (1988) Effect of galactosamine-induced hepatic UDP-glucuronic acid depletion on acetaminophen elimination in rats. Dispositional differences between hepatically and extrahepatically formed glucuronides of acetaminophen and other chemicals. Drug Metab Dispos 16:527–533

Griffith OW, Meister A (1979) Translocation of intracellular glutathione to membrane-bound gamma-glutamyltranspeptidase as a discrete step in the gamma-glutamyl cycle: glutathionuria after inhibition of transpeptidase. Proc Natl Acad Sci USA 76:268–272

Guengerich FP, Dannan GA, Wright ST, Martin MV, Kaminsky LS (1982) Purification and characterization of liver microsomal cytochrome P-450: electrophoretic, spectral, catalytic, and immunochemical properties and inducibility of eight isozymes isolated from rats treated with phenobarbital or beta-naphthoflavone. Biochemistry 21:6019–6030

Gugler R, Lain P, Azarnoff DL (1975) Effect of portacaval shunt on the disposition of drugs with and without first-pass effect. J Pharmacol Exp Ther 195:416–422

Gumucio JJ, Balabaud C, Miller DL, Demason LF, Appleman HD, Stoecker TJ, Franzblau DR (1978) Bile secretion and liver cell heterogeneity in the rat. J Lab Clin Med 91:350–362

Gumucio JJ, Miller DL, Krauss MD, Zanolli CC (1981) Transport of fluorescent compounds into hepatocytes and the resultant zonal labeling of the hepatic acinus in the rat. Gastroenterology 80:639–646

Gumucio DL, Gumucio JJ, Wilson JAP, Cutter C, Krauss M, Caldwell R, Chen E (1984) Albumin influences sulfobromophthalein transport by hepatocytes of each acinar zone. Am J Physiol 246:G86–G95

Hakim J, Feldmann G, Boivin P, Troube H, Boucherot J, Pnenaud J, Guibout P, Kreis B (1973) Comparative study of hepatic bilirubin and paranitrophenol glucuronyl transferase activities. III. Effect of rifampicin alone or associated with streptomycin and isoniazid in mam. Pathol Biol (Paris) 21:255–263

Haraszti JS, Davis JM (1978) Psychotropic drug interactions. In: Clark G, del Giudice J (eds) Principles of psychopharmacology. Academic, New York, pp 495–510

Haugen DA, Suttie JW (1974a) Purification and properties of rat liver microsomal esterase. J Biol Chem 9:2717–2722

Haugen DA, Suttie JW (1974b) Fluoride inhibition of rat liver microsomal esterase. J Biol Chem 9:2723–2731

Hearse DJ, Weber WW (1973) Multiple N-acetyltransferase and drug metabolism. Tissue distribution, characterization and significance of mammalian N-acetyltransferase. Biochem J 132:519–526

Herbai G (1970) A double isotope method for determination of the miscible inorganic sulfate pool of the mouse applied to in vivo studies of sulfate incorporation into costal cartilage. Acta Physiol Scand 80:470–491

Heymann E (1980) Carboxylesterses and amidases. In: Jakoby WB (ed) Enzymatic basis of detoxication. Academic, New York, pp 291–323

Himmelblau DM, Bischoff KB (1968) Process analysis and simulation. Deterministic systems. Wiley, New York, pp 91–112

Himmelstein KJ, Lutz RL (1979) A review of the application of physiologically based pharmacokinetic modeling. J Pharmacokinet Biopharm 7:125–127

Hirayama H, Pang KS (1990) First-pass metabolism of gentisamide: influence of intestinal metabolism on hepatic formation of conjugates. Studies in the once-through vascularly perfused rat intestine-liver preparation. Drug Metab Dispos 18:588–594

Hirayama H, Xu X, Pang KS (1989) Viability of the recirculating perfused rat intestine and intestine-liver preparations. Am J Physiol 257:G249–G258

Hirayama H, Morgado J, Gasinska I, Pang KS (1990) Estimations of intestinal and liver extraction in the in vivo rat: studies on gentisamide conjugation. Drug Metab Dispos 18:580–587

Hjelle JJ, Hazelton GA, Klaassen CD (1985) Acetaminophen decreases adenosine 3'-phosphate 5'-phosphosulfate and uridine diphosphoglucuronic acid in rat liver. Drug Metab Dispos 13:35–41

Hochman Y, Zakim D, Vessey DA (1981) A kinetic mechanism for modulation of the activity of microsomal UDP-glucuronyltransferase by phospholipids. J Biol Chem 256:4783–4788

Hoensch H, Woo CH, Schmid R (1975) Cytochrome P-450 and drug metabolism in intestinal villous and crypt cells of rats: effect of dietary iron. Biochem Biophys Res Commun 65:399–406

Hoensch H, Woo CH, Raffin SB, Schmid R (1976) Oxidative metabolism of foreign compounds in rat small intestine: cellular localization and dependence on dietary iron. Gastroenterology 70:1063–1070

Holford NHG (1987) Clinical pharmacokinetics and pharmacodynamics of warfarin: understanding the dose-effect relationship. Clin Pharmacokinet 11:483–504

Hollenberg M, Doherty J (1966) Liver blood flow by portal venous and hepatic arterial with Kr^{85}. Am J Physiol 210:926–932

Hopkins NE, Foroozesh MK, Alworth WL (1992) Suicide inhibitors of cytochrome P450 1A1 and P450 2B1. Biochem Pharmacol 44:787–796

Hori R, Okumura K, Yasuhara M, Katayama H (1985) Reduced hepatic uptake of propranolol in rats with acute renal failure. Biochem Pharmacol 34:2679–2683

Horie T, Mizuma T, Kawai S, Awazu S (1988) Conformational change in plasma albumin due to interaction with isolated rat hepatocyte. Am J Physiol 254: G465–G470

Horton JK, Meredith MJ, Bend JR (1987) Glutathione biosynthesis from sulfur-containing amino acids in enriched populations of Clara and type II cells and macrophages freshly isolated from rabbit lung. J Pharmacol Exp Ther 240:376–380

Houston JB, Levy G (1976) Effect of route of administration on competitive drug biotransformation interaction. Salicylamide-ascorbic acid interaction in rats. J Pharmacol Exp Ther 198:284–294

Howell SR, Hazelton GA, Klaassen CD (1986) Depletion of hepatic UDP-glucuronic acid by drugs that are glucuronidated. J Pharmacol Exp Ther 236:610–614

Huang JD, Øie S (1984) Hepatic elimination of drugs with concentration-dependent serum protein binding. J Pharmacokinet Biopharm 12:67–81

Igarashi T, Satoh T (1989) Sex and species differences in glutathione S-transferase activities. Drug Metabol Drug Interact 7:191–212

Igari Y, Sugiyama Y, Awazu S, Hanano M (1982) Comparative physiologically based pharmacokinetics of hexobarbital, phenobarbital and thiopental in the rat. J Pharmacokinet Biopharm 10:53–75

Igari Y, Sugiyama Y, Sawada Y, Iga T, Hanano M (1983) Prediction of diazepam disposition in the rat and man by a physiologically based pharmacokinetic model. J Pharmacokinet Biopharm 11:577–593

Igari Y, Sugiyama Y, Sawada Y, Iga T, Hanano M (1984) In vitro and in vivo assessment of hepatic and extrahepatic metabolism of diazepam in the rats. J Pharm Sci 73:826–828

Inaba T, Tait A, Nakano M, Mahon WA, Kalow W (1988) Metabolism of diazepam in vitro by human liver. Independent variability of N-demethylation and C3-hydroxylation. Drug Metab Dispos 16:605–608

Inoue M, Okajima K, Nagase S, Morino Y (1983) Plasma clearance of sulfobromophthalein and its interaction with hepatic binding proteins in normal and analbuminemic rats: is plasma albumin essential for vectorial transport of organic anions in the liver? Proc Natl Acad Sci USA 80:7654–7659

Inoue M, Hirata E, Morino Y, Nagase S, Roy Chowdhury J, Roy Chowdhury N, Arias IM (1985) The role of albumin in the hepatic transport of bilirubin: studies in mutant analbuminemic rats. J Biochem 97:737–743

Ishida R, Obara S, Masubuchi Y, Narimatsu S, Fujita S, Suzuki T (1992) Induction of propranolol metabolism by the azo dye sudan III in rats. Biochem Pharmacol 43:2489–2492

Iwamoto K, Klaassen CD (1977) First-pass effect of morphine in rats. J Pharmacol Exp Ther 200:236–244

Iwamoto K, Arakawa Y, Watanabe J (1983) Gastrointestinal and hepatic first-pass effects of salicylamide in rats. J Pharm Pharmacol 35:687–689

Iwamoto K, Furune Y, Watanabe J (1984) Difference in hepatic uptake kinetics of aspirin and salicylamide in rats. Biochem Pharmacol 33:3089–3095

Iwamoto K, Watanabe J, Araki K, Satoh M, Deguchi N (1985) Reduced hepatic clearance of propranolol induced by chronic carbon tetrachloride treatment in rats. J Pharmacol Exp Ther 234:470–475

Jansen JA (1981) Influence of plasma protein binding kinetics on hepatic clearance assessed from a "tube" model and a "well-stirred" model. J Pharmacokinet Biopharm 19:15–26

Jansen PLM, Mulder GJ, Burchell B, Bock KW (1992) New developments in glucuronidation research: report of a workshop on "glucuronidation", its role in health and disease. Hepatology 15:532–544

Jezequel AM, Orlandi F, Tenconi LT (1971) Changes of the smooth endoplasmic reticulum induced by rifampicin in human and guineapig hepatocytes. Gut 12:984–987

Jollow DJ, Thorgeirsson SS, Potter WZ, Hashimoto M, Mitchell JR (1974) Acetaminophen-induced hepatic necrosis. VI. Metabolic disposition of toxic and nontoxic doses of acetaminophen. Pharmacology 12:251–271

Jones DB, Morgan DJ, Mihaly GW, Webster LK, Smallwood RA (1984) Discrimination between venous equilibrium and sinusoidal models of hepatic drug elimination in isolated perfused rat liver by perturbation of propranolol protein binding. J Pharmacol Exp Ther 229:522–526

Julkunen RJK, Padova CD, Lieber CS (1985) First-pass metabolism of ethanol – a gastrointestinal barrier against the systemic toxicity of ethanol. Life Sci 37:567–573

Jungerman K, Katz N (1982) Functional hepatocellular heterogeneity. Hepatology 2:385–395

Jusko WJ, Gretch M (1976) Plasma and tissue protein binding of drugs in pharmacokinetics. Drug Metab Rev 5:43–140

Kamataki T, Maeda K, Yamazoe Y, Nagai T, Kato R (1983) Sex difference of cytochrome P-450 in the rat: purification, characterization and quantitation of constitutive forms of cytochrome P-450 from liver microsomes of male and female rats. Arch Biochem Biophys 225:758–770

Kamataki T, Maeka K, Shimada M, Kitani K, Nagai T, Kato R (1985) Age-related alteration in activities of drug-metabolizing enzymes and contents of sex-species forms of cytochrome P-450 in liver microsomes from male and female rats. J Pharmacol Exp Ther 233:222–228

Kaplowitz N, Kuhlenkamp J, Goldstein L, Reeve J (1980) Effect of salicylates and phenobarbital on hepatic glutahione in the rat. J Pharmacol Exp Ther 212:240–245

Kaplowitz N, Aw TK, Ookhtens M (1985) The regulation of hepatic glutathione. Annu Rev Pharmacol Toxicol 25:715–744

Kashiwagi T, Ji S, Lemasters JJ, Thurman RG (1982) Rates of alcohol dehydrogenase-dependent ethanol metabolism in periportal and pericentral regions of the perfused rat liver. Mol Pharmacol 21:438–443

Kato S, Ishii H, Aiso S, Yamashita S, Ito D, Tsuchiya M (1990) Histochemical and immunohistochemical evidence for hepatic zone 3 distribution of alcohol dehydrogenase in rats. Hepatology 12:66–69

Kauffman FC, Whittaker M, Anundi I, Thurman RG (1991) Futile cycling of a sulfate conjugate by isolated hepatocytes. Mol Pharmacol 39:414–420

Kawabata TT, Guengerich FP, Baron J (1981) An immuno-histochemical study on the localization and distribution of epoxide hydrolase within livers of untreated rats. Mol Pharmacol 20:709–714

Kawai R, Tatsuno J, Fujita S, Suzuki T (1983) Lidocaine-lidocaine metabolite interaction in their metabolism. J Pharmacobiodyn 6:s-79

Keiding S, Chiarantini E (1978) Effect of sinusoidal perfusion on galactose elimination in perfused rat liver. J Pharmacol Exp Ther 205:465–478

Keiding S, Prisholm K (1984) Current models of hepatic pharmacokinetics: flow effects on kinetic constants of ethanol elimination in perfused rat liver. Biochem Pharmacol 33:3209–3212

Keiding S, Steiness E (1984) Flow dependence of propranolol elimination in perfused rat liver. J Pharmacol Exp Ther 230:474–477

Keiding S, Johansen S, Midtbøll I, Rabøl A (1979) Ethanol elimination kinetics in human liver and pig liver in vivo. Am J Physiol 237:E316–E324

Keiding S, Vilstrup H, Hansen L (1980) Importance of flow and haematocrit for metabolic function of perfused rat liver. Scand J Clin Lab Invest 40:355–359

Kety SS (1951) Theory and application of the exchange of inert gas at the lungs and tissues. Pharmacol Rev 3:1–41

Khor SP, Mayersohn M (1991) Potential error in the measurement of tissue to blood distribution coefficients in physiological pharmacokinetic modeling. Residual tissue blood. I. Theoretical considerations. Drug Metab Dispos 19:478–485

Kirlin WG, Trinidad AN, Yerokun T, Ogolla F, Ferguson RJ, Andrews AF, Brady PK, Hein DW (1989) Polymorphic expression of acetyl coenzyme A-dependent arylamine N-acetyltransferase and acetyl coenzyme A-dependent O-acetyltransferase mediated activation of N-hydroxyarylamines by human bladder cytosol. Cancer Res 49:2448–2454

Kilppert PJM, Noordhoek J (1983) Influence of administration route and blood sampling site on the area under the curve: assessment of gut wall, liver, and lung metabolism from a physiological model. Drug Metab Dispos 11:62–66

Klippert PJM, Noordhoek J (1985) The area under the curve of metabolites for drugs and metabolites cleared by the liver and extrahepatic organs. Its dependence on the route of precursor drug. Drug Metab Dispos 13:97–101

Klippert PJM, Borm P, Noordhoek J (1982) Prediction of intestinal first-pass effect of phenacetin in the rat from enzyme kinetic data – correlation with in vivo data using mucosal blood flow. Biochem Pharmacol 31:2545–2548

Klippert PJM, Littel JJ, Noordhoek J (1983) In vivo O-deethylation of phenacetin in 3-methylcholanthrene-pretreated rats: gut wall and liver first-pass metabolism. J Pharmacol Exp Ther 225:153–157

Kloss MW, Cavagnaro J, Rosen GM, Rauckman EJ (1982) Involvement of FAD-containing monooxygenase in cocaine-induced hepatotoxicity. Toxicol Appl Pharmacol 64:88–93

Klotz U, Reimann I (1981) Clearance of diazepam can be impaired by its major metabolite desmethyldiazepam. Eur J Clin Pharmacol 21:161–163

Klotz U, Antonin KH, Biek PR (1976) Pharmacokinetics and plasma binding of diazepam in man, dog, rabbit, guinea pig and rat. J Pharmacol Exp Ther 199:67–73

Knapp SA, Green MD, Tephly TR, Baron J (1988) Immuno-histochemical demonstration of isozyme- and strain-specific differences in the intralobular localizations and distributions of UDP-glucuronosyltransferases in livers of untreated rats. Mol Pharmacol 33:14–21

Knodell RG, Brooks DA, Allen RC, Kyner WT (1980) Alterations in pentobarbital and meperidine pharmacokinetics induced by bile duct ligation in the rat. J Pharmacol Exp Ther 215:619–625

Koike M, Sugeno K, Hirata M (1981) Sulfoconjugation and glucuronidation of salicylamide in isolated rat hepatocytes. J Pharm Sci 70:308–311

Koo A, Liang IY, Cheng KK (1975) The terminal hepatic microcirculation in the rat. Q J Exp Physiol 60:261–266

Kosower NS, Kosower EM (1978) The glutathione status of cells. Int Rev Cytol 54:109–160

Koster AS, Noordhoek J (1982) Similarity of rat intestinal and hepatic microsomal 7-hydroxycoumarin-UDP-glucuronyltransferase: in vitro activation by triton X-100, UDP-N-acetylglucosamine and MgCl$_2$. Biochem Pharmacol 31:2701–2704

Koster H, Halsema I, Scholtens E, Pang KS, Mulder GJ (1982) Kinetics of sulfation and glucuronidation of harmol in the perfused rat liver preparation. Disappearance of aberrances in glucuronidation kinetics by inhibition of sulfation. Biochem Pharmacol 31:3023–3028

Koster AS, Frankhuijzen-Sierevogel C, Noordhoek J (1985a) Glucuronidation of morphine and six beta2-sympathomimetics in isolated rat intestinal epithelial cells. Drug Metab Dispos 13:232–237

Koster AS, Frankhuijzen-Sierevogel AC, Noordhoek J (1985b) Distribution of glucuronidation capacity (1-naphthol and morphine) along the rat intestine. Biochem Pharmacol 34:3527–3532

Kravetz D, Arderiu M, Bosch J, Fuster J, Visa J, Casamitjana R, Rodes J (1987) Hyperglucagonemia and hyperkinetic circulation after portacaval shunt in the rat. Am J Physiol 252:G257–G261

Krijgsheld KR, Frankena H, Scholtens E, Zweens J, Mulder GJ (1979) Absorption, serum levels and urinary excretion of inorganic sulfate after oral administration of sodium sulfate in the conscious rat. Biochim Biophys Acta 586:492–500

Krijgsheld KR, Scholtens E, Mulder GJ (1981) An evaluation of methods to decrease the availability of inorganic sulfate for sulfate conjugation in the rat in vivo. Biochem Pharmacol 30:1973–1979

Krijgsheld KR, Scholtens E, Mulder GJ (1982) The dependence of the rate of sulphate conjugation on the plasma concentration of inorganic sulphate in the rat in vivo. Biochem Pharmacol 31:3997–4000

Kutt H, Fouts JR (1971) Diphenylhydantoin metabolism by rat liver microsomes and some of the effects of drug or chemical pretreatment on diphenylhydantoin metabolism by rat liver microsomal preparations. J Pharmacol Exp Ther 176:11–26

Lança AJ, Israel Y (1991) Histochemical demonstration of sinusoidal gamma-glutamyltransferase activity by substrate protection fixation: comparative studies in rat and guinea pig liver. Hepatology 14:857–863

Lauterburg BH, Mitchell JR (1981) Regulation of hepatic glutathione turnover in rats in vivo and evidence for kinetic homogeneity of the hepatic glutathione pool. J Clin Invest 67:1415–1424

Lauterburg BH, Vaishnav Y, Stillwell WG, Mitchell JR (1980) The effect of age and glutathione depletion on hepatic glutathione turnover in vivo determined by acetaminophen probe analysis. J Pharmacol Exp Ther 213:54–58

Lauterburg BH, Smith CV, Hughes H, Mitchell JR (1982) Determinants of hepatic glutathione turnover: toxicological significance. Trends Pharmacol Sci 2:245–248

Lautt WW, Greenway CV (1987) Conceptual review of the hepatic vascular bed. Hepatology 7:952–963

Lautt WW, Legare DJ, d'Almeida MS (1985) Adenosine as putative regulator of hepatic arterial flow (the buffer response). Am J Physiol 248:H331–H338

Lawton MP, Kronbach T, Johnson EF, Philpot RM (1991) Properties of expressed and native flavin-containing monooxygenase: evidence of multiple forms in rabbit liver and lung. Mol Pharmacol 40:692–698

Legler UF, Frey FJ, Benet LZ (1982) Prednisolone clearance at steady-state in humans. J Clin Endocrinol Metab 55:762–767

Levenspiel O (1970) Chemical reaction engineering. Wiley, New York, pp 253–261

Levy RH, Dumain MS (1979) Time-dependent kinetics. VI. Direct relationship between equations for drug levels during induction and those involving constant clearance. J Pharm Sci 68:934–936

Levy RH, Lockard JS, Green JR, Friel P, Martis L (1975) Pharmacokinetics of carbamazepine in monkeys following intravenous and oral administration. J Pharm Sci 64:302–307

Levy RH, Dumain MS, Cook JL (1979a) Time-dependent kinetics. V. Time course of drug levels during enzyme induction (one-compartment model). J Pharmacokinet Biopharm 7:557–578

Levy RH, Lai AA, Dumain MS (1979b) Time-dependent kinetics. IV. Pharma-cokinetic theory of enzyme induction. J Pharm Sci 68:398–399

Lin JH, Levy G (1982) Effect of experimental renal failure on sulfate retention and acetaminophen pharmacokinetics in rats. J Pharmacol Exp Ther 221:80–84

Lin JH, Levy G (1986) Effect of prevention of inorganic sulfate depletion on the pharmacokinetics of acetaminophen in rats. J Pharmacol Exp Ther 239: 94–98

Lin JH, Hayashi M, Awazu S, Hanano M (1978) Correlation between in vitro and in vivo drug metabolism rate: oxidation of ethoxybenzamide in rat. J Pharma-cokinet Biopharm 6:327–337

Lin JH, Sugiyama Y, Awazu S, Hanano M (1980) Kinetic studies on the deethylation of ethoxybenzamide. A comparative study with isolated hepatocytes and liver microsomes of rat. Biochem Pharmacol 29:2825–2830

Lin JH, Sugiyama Y, Awazu S, Hanano M (1982) Physiological pharmacokinetics of ethoxybenzamide based on biochemical data obtained in vitro as well as on physiological data. J Pharmacokinet Biopharm 10:649–661

Lin JH, Sugiyama Y, Awazu S, Hanano M (1984) Effect of product inhibition on elimination kinetics of ethoxybenzamide in rabbits: analysis by physiological pharmacokinetic model. Drug Metab Dispos 12:253–256

Lindros KO, Penttilä KE (1985) Digitonin-collagenase perfusion for efficent separa-tion of periportal and perivenous hepatocytes. Biochem J 228:757–760

Locniskar A, Greenblatt DJ (1990) Oxidative versus conjugative biotransformation of temazepam. Biopharm Drug Dispos 11:499–506

Lucier GW, McDaniel OS, Matthews HB (1971) Microsomal rat liver UDP glucuronyl-transferase: effects of piperonyl butoxide and other factors on en-zymatic activity. Arch Biochem Biophys 145:520–530

Lucier GW, McDaniel OS, Hook GER (1975) Nature of the enhancement of hepatic uridine diphosphate glucuronyltransferase activity by 2,3,7,8-tetrachlorodibenzo-p-dioxin in rats. Biochem Pharmacol 24:325–334

Lumeng L, Crabb DW (1984) Rate-determining factors for ethanol metabolism in fasted and castrated male rats. Biochem Pharmacol 33:2623–2628

Lutz RJ, Dedrick RL, Matthews HB, Eling TE, Anderson MW (1977) A preliminary pharmacokinetic model for several chlorinated biphenyls in the rat. Drug Metab Dispos 5:386–396

Machida M, Morita Y, Hayashi M, Awazu S (1982) Pharmacokinetic evidence for the occurrence of extrahepatic conjugative metabolism of p-nitrophenol. Biochem Pharmacol 31:787–791

Martin BK (1965) Potential effect of the plasma proteins on drug distribution. Nature 207:274–276

Masubuchi Y, Fujita S, Chiba M, Kagimoto N, Umeda S, Suzuki T (1991) Impair-ment of debrisoquine 4-hydroxylase and related monooxygenase activities in the rat following treatment with propranolol. Biochem Pharmacol 41:861–865

Masubuchi Y, Suzuki K, Fujita S, Suzuki T (1992) A possible mechanism of the impairment of hepatic microsomal monooxygenase activities after multiple administration of propranolol in rats. Biochem Pharmacol 43:757–762

McFarlane BM, Spios J, Gove CD, McFarlane IJ, Williams R (1990) Antibodies against the hepatic asialoglycoprotein receptor perfused in situ preferentially attach to periportal liver cells in the rat. Hepatology 11:408–415

McManus ME, Ilett KF (1979) Comparison of rate of hepatic metabolism in vitro and half-life for antipyrine in vivo in three species. Xenobiotica 9:107–118

McNamara PJ, Colburn WA, Gibaldi M (1979) Time course of carbamazepine self-induction. J Pharmacokinet Biopharm 7:63–68

Meerman JHN, Mulder GJ (1981) Prevention of the hepatotoxic action of N-hydroxy-2-acetylaminofluorene in the rat by inhibition of N-O-sulfation by pentachlorophenol. Life Sci 21:2361–2365

Meister A, Anderson ME (1983) Glutathione. Annu Rev Biochem 52:711–760

Mentlein R, Heymann E (1984) Hydrolysis of ester- and amide-type drugs by the purified isoenzymes of nonspecific carboxylesterase from rat liver. Biochem Pharmacol 33:1243–1248

Mentlein R, Desbaillets L, Masters YF, Okabe S (1980) Simultaneous purification and comparative characterization of six serine hydrolases from rat liver microsomes. Arch Biochem Biophys 200:547–559

Mentlein R, Chumann M, Heymann E (1984a) Comparative chemical and immunological characterization of five lipolytic enzymes (carboxylesterases) from rat liver microsomes. Arch Biochem Biophys 234:612–621

Mentlein R, Suttorp M, Heymann E (1984b) Specificity of purified monoacylglycerol lipase, palmitoyl-CoA hydrolase, palmitoyl-carnitine hydrolase, and nonspecific carboxylesterase from rat liver microsomes. Arch Biochem Biophys 228:230–236

Mentlein R, Berge R, Heymann E (1985) Identity of purified monoacylglycerol lipase, palmitoyl-CoA hydrolase and aspirin-metabolizing carboxylesterase from rat liver microsomal fractions. A comparative study with enzymes purified in different laboratorires. Biochem J 232:479–483

Mentlein R, Rix-Matzen H, Heymann E (1988) Subcellular localization of non-specific carboxylesterases, acylcarnitine hydrolase, monoacylglycerol lipase and palmitoyl-CoA hydrolase in rat liver. Biochim Biophys Acta 964:319–328

Messiha FS, Hughes MJ (1979) Liver alcohol and aldehyde dehydrogenase: inhibition and potentiation by histamine agonists and antagonists. Clin Exp Pharmacol Physiol 6:281–292

Meyer DJ, Christodoulides LG, Tan KH, Ketterer B (1984) Isolation, properties and tissue distribution of rat glutathione transferase E. FEBS Lett 173:327–330

Miller DL, Zanolli CS, Gumucio JJ (1979) Quantitative morphology of the sinusoids of the hepatic acinus. Gastroenterology 76:965–969

Miller R, Oliver IF (1986) The influence of oxygen tension on theophylline clearance in the rat isolated perfused liver. J Pharm Pharmacol 38:236–238

Miners JO, Lillywhite KJ, Matthews AP, Jones ME, Birkett DJ (1988) Kinetic and inhibitor studies of 4-methylumbelliferone and 1-naphthol glucuronidation in human liver microsomes. Biochem Pharmacol 37:665–671

Mistry M, Houston JB (1985) Quantitation of extrahepatic metabolism. Pulmonary and intestinal conjugation of naphthol. Drug Metab Dispos 13:740–745

Mistry M, Houston JB (1987) Glucuronidation in vitro and in vivo. Comparison of intestinal and hepatic conjugation of morphine, naloxone, and buprenorphine. Drug Metab Dispos 15:710–717

Miyano K, Toki S (1980) Stereoselective hydroxylation of hexobarbital enantiomers by rat liver microsomes. Drug Metab Dispos 8:104–110

Miyauchi S, Sugiyama Y, Sawada Y, Iga T, Hanano M (1987) Conjugative metabolism of 4-methylumbelliferone in the rat liver: verification of the sequestration process in multiple indicator dilution experiments. Chem Pharm Bull (Tokyo) 35:4241–4248

Miyauchi S, Sugiyama Y, Iga T, Hanano M (1989) The conjugative metabolism of 4-methylumbelliferone and deconjugation to the parent drug examined by isolated perfused liver and in vitro homogenate of rats. Chem Pharm Bull (Tokyo) 37:475–480

Mizuma T, Machida M, Hayashi M, Awazu S (1982) Correlation of drug conjugative metabolism rates between in vivo and in vitro: glucuronidation and sulfation of p-nitrophenol as a model compound in rat. J Pharmacobiodyn 5:811–817

Mizuma T, Hayashi M, Awazu S (1985a) Factors influencing drug sulfate and glucuronic acid conjugation rates in isolated rat hepatocytes: significance of preincubation time. Biochem Pharmacol 34:2573–2575

Mizuma T, Horie T, Awazu S (1985b) The effect of albumin on the uptake of bromosulfophthalein by isolated rat hepatocytes. J Pharmacobiodyn 8:90–94

Mohandas J, Marshall JJ, Duggin GG, Horvath JS, Tiller DJ (1984) Differential distribution of glutathione and glutathione-related enzymes in rabbit kidney. Biochem Phamracol 33:1801–1807

Morita K, Sugiyama Y, Hanano M (1986) Pharmacokinetic study of 4-methylumbel-liferone in rats: influence of dose on its first-pass hepatic elimination. J Pharmacobiodyn 9:117–124

Morris ME, Pang KS (1987) Competition between two enzymes for substrate removal in liver: modulating effects due to substrate recruitment of hepatocyte activity. J Pharmacokinet Biopharm 15:473–496

Morris ME, Yuen V, Pang KS (1988a) Competing pathways in drug metabolism. II. Enzymic systems for 2- and 5-sulfo-conjugation are distributed anterior to 5-glucuronidation in the metabolism of gentisamide by the perfused rat liver. J Pharmacokinet Biopharm 16:633–656

Morris ME, Yuen V, Tang BK, Pang KS (1988b) Competing pathways in drug metabolism. I. Effect of varying input concentrations on gentisamide conjugation in the once-through in situ perfused rat liver preparation. J Pharmacol Exp Ther 245:614–652

Morrison MH, Barber HE, Foschi PG, Hawksworth GM (1986) The kinetics of 4-nitrophenol conjugation by perfused livers and hepatic microsomes from streptozocin-induced diabetic rats. J Pharm Pharmacol 38:188–194

Mulder GJ, Hadgedoorn AH (1974) UDP-glucuronyltransferase and phenolsulfotrans-ferase in vivo and in vitro. Conjugation of harmol and harmalol. Biochem Pharmacol 23:2101–2109

Mulder GJ, Keulemans K (1978) Metabolism of inorganic sulfate in the isolated perfused rat liver. Biochem J 176:959–965

Mulder GJ, Weitering JG, Scholtens E, Dawson JR, Pang KS (1984) Extrahepatic sulfation and glucuronidation in the rat in vivo. Determination of the hepatic extraction ratio of harmol and the extrahepatic contribution to harmol conjugation. Biochem Pharmacol 33:3081–3087

Mulder GJ, Brouwer S, Weitering JG, Scholtens E, Pang KS (1985) Glucuronidation and sulfation in the rat in vivo: the role of the liver and the intestine in the in vivo clearance of 4-methylumbelliferone. Biochem Pharmacol 34:1325–1329

Murray GI, Burke MD, Even SWB (1986) Glutathione lozalization by a novel o-phthaladehyde histofluorescence method. Histochem J 18:434–440

Murray M, Reidy GF (1990) Selectivity in the inhibition of mammalian cytochrome P-450 by chemical agents. Pharmacol Rev 42:85–101

Nakai M, Tamara T, Kamiya A, Togawa T (1979) Control mechanism of intras-inusoidal flow pattern of blood. Jpn J Physiol 29:597–608

Nakamura J, Mizuma T, Horie T, Hayashi M, Awazu S (1987) Arylsulfotransferase in rat liver: multiplicity and substrate specificity. J Pharmacobiodyn 10:736–742

Nathanson MH, Boyer JL (1991) Special article. Mechanisms and regulation of bile secretion. Hepatology 14:551–566

Nebert DW, Adesnik M, Coon MJ, Estbrook RW, Gonzalez FJ, Guengerich FP, Gunsalus IC, Johnson EF, Kemper B, Levin W (1987) The P-450 gene super-family: recommended nomenclature. DNA 6:1–11

Nebert DW, Adesnik M, Coon MJ, Estbrook RW, Gonzalez FJ, Guengerich FP, Gunsalus IC, Johnson EF, Kemper B, Levin W, Phillip IR, Sato R, Waterman MR (1989) The P-450 gene superfamily: updated listing of all genes and recom-mended nomenclature for the chromosomal loci. DNA 8:1–13

Nebert DW, Nelson DR, Coon MJ, Estabrook RW, Feyereisen R, Fujii-Kuriyama Y, Gonzalez FJ, Guengerich FP, Gunsalus IC, Johnson EF, Loper JC, Sato R, Waterman MR, Waxman DJ (1991) The P450 superfamily: update on new sequences, gene mapping, and recommended nomenclature. DNA Cell Biol 10:1–14

Nopanitaya W, Grisham JW, Aghajanian JG, Carson JL (1978) Intrahepatic micro-circulation: SEM study of the terminal distribution of the hepatic artery. In: Johari O, Corvin I (eds) Scanning electron microscopy, vol 2. SEM, O'Hare, IL, pp 837–842

Novikoff AB (1959) Cell heterogeneity within the hepatic lobule of the rat (staining reactions). J Histochem Cytochem 7:240–244

Nyberg G, Karlen B, Hedlund I, Grundin R, von Bahr C (1977) Extraction and metabolism of lidocaine in rat liver. Acta Pharmacol Toxicol (Copenh) 40: 337–346

Oda Y, Imaoka S, Nakahara Y, Asada A, Fujimori M, Fujita S, Funae Y (1989) Metabolism of lidocaine by purified rat liver microsomal cytochrome P-450 isozymes. Biochem Pharmacol 38:4439–4444

Ohtani O, Murakami T (1978) Peribiliary portal system in the rat liver as studied by the injection replica scanning electron microscope method, In: Johari O, Corvin E (eds) Scanning electron microscopy, vol 2. SEM, O'Hare, IL, pp 241–244

Øie S (1986) Drug distribution and binding. J Clin Pharmacol 26:583–586

Øie S, Fiori F (1985) Effects of albumin and alpha-1 acid glycoprotein on elimination of prazosin and antipyrine in the isolated perfused rat liver. J Pharmacol Exp Ther 234:636–640

Øie S, Levy G (1975) Effect of plasma protein binding on elimination of bilirubin. J Pharm Sci 64:1433

Øie S, Fiori F, Chiang J (1987) Decreased elimination of unbound prazosin in the presence of α_1-acid glycoprotein in the rat in vivo. J Pharmacol Exp Ther 241:934–938

Ookhtens M, Hobdy K, Corvasce MC, Aw TY, Kaplowitz N (1985) Sinusoidal efflux of glutathione in the perfused rat liver. Evidence for a carrier-mediated process. J Clin Invest 75:258–265

Orrenius S, Ormstad K, Thor H, Jewell SA (1983) Turnover and functions of glutathione studies with isolated hepatic and renal cells. Fed Proc 42:3177–3188

Ortiz de Montellano PR, Kuntze KL (1980) Self-catalyzed inactivation of hepatic cytochrome P-450 by ethynyl substrates. J Biol Chem 255:5578–5585

Ortiz de Montellano PR, Kuntze KL, Beilan HS, Wheeler C (1982) Destruction of cytochrome P-450 by vinyl fluoride, fluroxene, and acetylene. Evidence for a radical intermediate in olefin oxidation. Biochemistry 21:1331–1339

Ozols J (1989) Liver microsomes contain two distinct NADPH-monooxygenase with NH2-terminal segments homologous to the favin containing NADPH monooxygenase of *Pseudomonas fluorescens*. Biochem Biophys Res Commun 163:49–55

Ozols J (1991) Multiple forms of liver microsomal flavin-containing monooxygenases: complete covalent structure of form 2. Arch Biochem Biophys 290:103–115

Pang KS (1980) Kinetics of conjugation reactions in eliminating organs. In: Mulder GJ (ed) Conjugation reactions in drug metabolism: an integrated approach (GJ Mulder, ed), Taylor and Francis, London, pp 5–39

Pang KS (1983) The effect of intercellular distribution of drug metabolizing enzymes on the kinetics of stable metabolite formation and elimination by liver: first-pass effects. Drug Metab Rev 14:61–76

Pang KS (1985) Metabolite pharmacokinetics: the area under the curve of metabolite and the fractional rate of metabolism of a drug after different routes of administration for renally and hepatically cleared drugs and metabolites. J Pharmacokinet Biopharm 9:477–487

Pang KS, Gillete JR (1978a) Kinetics of metabolite formation and elimination in the perfused rat liver preparation: difference between the elimination of preformed acetaminophen and acetaminophen formed from phenacetine. J Pharmacol Exp Ther 207:178–194

Pang KS, Gillette JR (1978b) Complications in the estimation of hepatic blood flow in vivo by pharmacokinetic parameters: the area under the curve after the con comitant intravenous and intraperitoneal (or intraportal) dose of acetaminophen in rat. Drug Metab Dispos 6:567–576

Pang KS, Gillette JR (1978c) Theoretical relationships between area under the curve and route of administration of drugs and their precursors for evaluating sites and pathways of metabolism. J Pharm Sci 67:703–704

Pang KS, Gillette JR (1979) Sequential first-pass elimination of a metabolite derived from its precursor. J Pharmacokinet Biopharm 7:275–290

Pang KS, Kwan KC (1983) A commentary. Methods and assumptions in the kinetic estimation of metabolite formation. Drug Metab Dispos 11:79–84

Pang KS, Mulder GJ (1990) A commentary: effect of flow on formation of metabolites. Drug Metab Dispos 18:270–275

Pang KS, Rowland M (1977a) Hepatic clearance of drugs. I. Theoretical considerations of a "well-stirred" model and a "parallel-tube" model. Influence of hepatic blood flow, plasma and blood cell binding and hepatocellular enzymatic activity on hepatic clearance. J Pharmacokinet Biopharm 5:625–653

Pang KS, Rowland M (1977b) Hepatic clearance of drugs. II. Experimental evidence for acceptance of the "well-stirred" model over the "parallel tube" model using lidocaine in the perfused rat liver in situ preparation. J Pharmacokinet Biopharm 5:655–680

Pang KS, Rowland M (1977c) Hepatic clearance of drugs. III. Additional experimental evidence supporting the "well-stirred" model, using metabolite (MEGX) generated from lidocaine under varying hepatic blood flow rates and linear conditions in the perfused rat liver in situ preparation. J Pharmacokinet Biopharm 5:681–699

Pang KS, Rowland M, Tozer TN (1978) In vivo evaluation of Michaelis-Menten constants for drug eliminating systems. Drug Metab Dispos 6:197–200

Pang KS, Stillwell RN (1983) An understanding of the role of enzyme localization of the liver on metabolite kinetics: a computer simulation. J Pharmacokinet Biopharm 11:451–468

Pang KS, Terrell JA (1981a) Retrograde perfusion to probe the heterogeneous distribution of hepatic drug metabolizing enzymes in rats. J Pharmacol Exp Ther 216:339–346

Pang KS, Terrell JA (1981b) Conjugation kinetics of acetaminophen by the perfused rat liver preparation. Biochem Pharmacol 30:1959–1965

Pang KS, Xu X (1988) Drug metabolism factors in drug discovery and design. In: Welling PG, Tse FL-S (eds) Pharmacokinetics: regulatory-industrial-academic perspectives. Dekker, New York, pp 383–447

Pang KS, Koster H, Halsema ICM, Scholtens E, Mulder GJ (1981) Aberrant pharmacokinetics of harmol in the perfused rat liver preparation: sulfation and glucuronide conjugations. J Pharmacol Exp Ther 219:134–140

Pang KS, Koster H, Halsema ICM, Scholtens E, Mulder GJ, Stillwell RN (1983) Normal and retrograde perfusion to probe the zonal distribution of sulfation and glucuronidation activities of harmol in the perfused rat liver preparation. J Pharmacol Exp Ther 224:647–653

Pang KS, Cherry WF, Terrell JA, Ulm EH (1984a) Disposition of enalapril and its diacid metabolite, enalaprilat, in a perfused rat liver preparation. Presence of a diffusional barrier into hepatocytes. Drug Metab Dispos 12:309–313

Pang KS, Huang JC, Finkle C, Kong P, Cherry WF, Fayz S (1984b) Kinetics of procainamide N-acetylation in the rat in vivo and in the perfused rat liver preparation. Drug Metab Dispos 12:314–322

Pang KS, Kong P, Terrell JA, Billings RE (1985) Metabolism of acetaminophen and phenacetin by isolated rat hepatocytes. A system in which the spatial organization inherent in the liver is disrupted. Drug Metab Dispos 13:42–50

Pang KS, Terrell JA, Nelson SD, Feuer KF, Clements MJ, Endrenyi L (1986) An enzyme-distributed system for lidocaine metabolism in the perfused rat liver preparation. J Pharmacokinet Biopharm 14:107–130

Pang KS, Barker F III, Schwab AJ, Goresky CA (1988a) Red cell carriage of acetaminophen as studied by the technique of multiple indicator dilution in perfused rat liver (Abstr). Hepatology 8:1384

Pang KS, Lee WF, Cherry WF, Yuen V, Accaputo J, Schwab AJ, Goresky CA (1988b) Effects of perfusate flow rate on measured blood volume, Disse space, intracellular water spaces, and drug extraction in the perfused rat liver preparation: characterization by the technique of multiple indicator dilution. J Pharmacokin Biopharm 16:595–605

Pang KS, Cherry WF, Barker F III, Goresky CA (1991a) Esterases for enalapril hydrolysis is concentrated in the perihepatic venous region of the rat liver. J Pharmacol Exp Ther 257:294–301

Pang KS, Goresky CA, Schwab AJ (1991b) Deterministic factors underlying drug and metabolite clearances in rat liver perfusion studies. In: Ballet F, Thurman RG (eds) Research in perfused liver: clinical and basic applications. INSERM, Paris; Libbey, London, pp 259–302

Pang KS, Xu X, St-Pierre MV (1992) Determinants of metabolite disposition. Annu Rev Pharmacol 32:623–669

Pang KS, Sherman IA, Schwab AJ, Xu N, Barker F III, Dlugosz JA, Cuerrier G, Goresky CA (1994) Role of the hepatic artery in the metabolism of phenacetin and acetaminophen: An intravital microscopic and multiple indicator dilution study in perfused rat liver. Hepatology (accepted)

Patel IH, Levy RH, Trager WF (1978) Pharmacokinetics of carbamazepine-10,11-epoxide before and after autoinduction in rhesus monkeys. J Pharmacol Exp Ther 206:607–613

Perl W, Chinard FP (1968) A convection-diffusion model of indicator transport through an organ. Circ Res 22:273–298

Pessayre D, Mazel P (1976) Induction and inhibition of hepatic drug metabolizing enzymes by rifampin. Biochem Pharmacol 25:943–949

Pessayre D, Descatoire V, Konstantinova-Mitcheva M, Wandscheer JC, Cobert B, Level R, Benhamou JP, Jaouen M, Mansuy D (1981) Self-induction by triacetyloleandomycin of its own transformation into a metabolite forming a stable 456 nm-absorbing complex with cytochrome P-450. Biochem Pharmacol 30:553–558

Pessayre D, Descatoire V, Tinel M, Larrey D (1982) Self-induction by oleandomycin of its own transformation into a metabolite forming an inactive complex with reduced cytochrome P-450. Comparison with troleandomycin. J Pharmacol Exp Ther 221:215–221

Pitlick WH, Levy RH (1977) Time-dependent kinetics. I. Exponential autoinduction of carbamazepine in monkeys. J Pharm Sci 66:647–649

Plummer JL, Smith BR, Sies H, Bend JR (1981) Detoxication and drug metabolism: conjugation and related systems. Methods Enzymol 77:50–59

Polhuijs M, Te Koppele JM, Fockens E, Mulder GJ (1989) Glutathione conjugation of the alpha-bromoisovaleric acid enantiomers in the rat in vivo and its stereo-selectivity. Pharmacokinetics of biliary and urinary excretion of the glutahione conjugation and the mercapturate. Biochem Pharmacol 38:3957–3962

Polhuijs M, Meijer DKF, Mulder GJ (1991) The fate of diastereomeric glutathione conjugates of alpha-bromoisovalerylurea in blood in the rat in vivo and in the perfused liver. Stereoselectivity in biliary and urinary excretion. J Pharmacol Exp Ther 256:458–461

Polhuijs M, Gasinska I, Mulder GJ, Pang KS (1993) Stereoselectivity in glutathione conjugation and amidase-catalyzed hydrolysis of the 2-bromoisovalerylurea enantiomers in the single pass perfused rat liver. J Pharmacol Exp Ther 265: 1402–1412

Pond SM, Davis CKC, Bogoyevitch MA, Gordon RA, Weisiger WA, Bass L (1992) Uptake of palmitate by hepatocyte suspensions – facilitation by albumin. Am J Physiol 262:G883–G894

Price VF, Jollow DJ (1982) Increased resistance of diabetic rats to acetaminophen induced hepatotoxicity. J Pharmacol Exp Ther 220:504–513

Price VF, Jollow DJ (1984) Role of UDPGA flux in acetaminophen clearance and hepatotoxicity. Xenobiotica 7:553–559

Price VF, Jollow DJ (1988) Mechanism of decreased actaminophen glucuronidation in the fasted rat. Biochem Pharmacol 37:1067–1075

Price VF, Schulte JM, Spaethe SM, Jollow DJ (1986) Mechanism of fasting-induced suppression of acetaminophen glucuronidation in the rat. Adv Exp Med Biol 197:697–706

Prough RA, Ziegler DM (1977) The relative participation of liver microsomal amine oxidase and cytochrome P-450 in N-demethylation reactions. Arch Biochem Biophys 180:363–373

Quistorff B (1985) Gluconeogenesis in periportal and perivenous hepatocytes in rat liver, isolated by a new high yield digitonin/collagenase perfusion. Biochem J 229:221–226

Rabinovici N, Vardi J (1965) The intrahepatic portal vein-hepatic artery relationship. Surg Gynecol Obstet 120:38–44

Rakhit A, Mico B (1985) Kinetics of microsomal metabolism of quinidine in rats. Res Commun Chem Pathol Pharmacol 49:109–124

Rane A, Wilkinson GR, Shand DG (1977) Prediction of hepatic extraction ratio form in vitro measurement of intrinsic clearance. J Pharmacol Exp Ther 200: 420–424

Rane A, Lindberg SB, Svensson J-O, Garle M, Erwald R, Jorulf H (1984) Morphine glucuronidation in the rhesus monkey: a comparative in vivo and in vitro study. J Pharmacol Exp Ther 229:51–576

Rappaport AM (1958) The structural and functional unit in the human liver (liver acinus). Anat Rec 130:673–689

Rappaport AM (1980) Hepatic blood flow: morphologic aspects and physiologic regulation. Int Rev Physiol 21:1–63

Ratna S, Chiba M, Bandyophdhyay L, Pang KS (1993) Futile cycling between 4-methylumbelliferone and its conjugates in perfused rat liver. Hepatology 17: 838–853

Redegeld FA, Hofman GA, Noordhoek J (1988) Conjugative clearance of 1-naphthol and disposition of its glucuronide and sulfate conjugates in the isolated perfused rat kidney. J Pharmacol Exp Ther 244:263–267

Redick JA, Jakoby WB, Baron J (1982) Immunohistochemical localization of glutathione-S-transferase in livers of untreated rats. J Biol Chem 257:15200–15203

Reed RG, Burrington CM (1989) The albumin receptor effect may be due to a surface-induced conformational change in albumin. J Biol Chem 264:9867–9872

Reed RG, Orrenius S (1977) The role of methionine in glutathione biosynthesis by isolated hepatocytes. Biochem Biophys Res Commun 77:1257–1264

Reichen J, Sagesser H (1988) Role of the hepatic artery in canalicular bile formation by the perfused rat liver. A multiple indicator dilution study. J Clin Invest 81:1462–1469

Reinke LA, Belinsky SA, Evans RK, Kauffman FC, Thurman RG (1981) Conjugation of p-nitrophenol in the perfused rat liver: the effect of substrate concentration and carbohydrate reserves. J Pharmacol Exp Ther 217:863–870

Remmel RP, Sinz MW, Cloyd JC (1990) Dose-dependent pharmacokinetics of carbamazepine in rats: determination of the formation clearance of carbamazepine-10,11-epoxide. Pharm Res 7:513–517

Rettie AE, Eddy AC, Heimark LD, Gibaldi M, Trager WF (1989) Characteristics of warfarin hydroxylation catalyzed by human liver microsomes. Drug Metab Dispos 17:265–270

Richens A (1977) Interactions with antiepileptic drugs. Drugs 13:266–275

Robbi M, Beaufay H (1983) Purification and characterization of various esterases from rat liver. Eur J Biochem 137:293–301

Roberts MS, Rowland M (1985) Correlation between in vitro microsomal enzyme activity and whole organ hepatic elimination kinetics: analysis with a dispersion model. J Pharm Pharmacol 38:177–181

Roberts MS, Rowland M (1986a) A dispersion model of hepatic elimination. I. Formulation of the model and bolus considerations. J Pharmacokinet Biopharm 14:227–260

Roberts MS, Rowland M (1986b) A dispersion model of hepatic elimination. II. Steady-state considerations – influence of hepatic blood flow, binding within blood, and hepatocellular activity. J Pharmacokinet Biopharm 14:261–288

Roberts MS, Rowland M (1986c) A dispersion model of hepatic elimination. III. Application to metabolite formation and elimination kinetics. J Pharmacokinet Biopharm 14:289–308

Roberts MS, Fraser S, Wagner A, McLeod L (1990) Residence time distributions of solutes in perfused rat liver using a dispersion model of hepatic elimination. II. Effect of pharmacological agents, retrograde perfusions, and enzyme inhibition on Evans blue, sucrose, water, and taurocholate. J Pharmacokinet Biopharm 18:235–258

Rogers HJ, Haslam RA, Longstreth J (1977) Phenytoin intoxication during concurrent diazepam therapy. J Neurol Neurosurg Psychiatry 40:890–895

Rowland M (1972) Influence of route of administration on drug availability. J Pharm Sci 61:70–74

Rowland M (1984) Protein binding and drug clearance. Clin Pharmacokinet 9 Suppl 1:10–17

Rowland M, Benet LZ, Graham GG (1973) Clearance concepts in pharmacokinetics. J Pharmacokinet Biopharm 1:123–136

Rowland M, Leitch D, Fleming G, Smith B (1984) Protein binding and hepatic clearance: discrimination between models of hepatic clearance with diazepam, a drug of high intrinsic clearance, in the isolated perfused rat liver preparation. J Pharmacokinet Biopharm 12:129–147

Roy Chowdhury J, Roy Chowdhury N, Falany CN, Tephly TR, Arias IM (1986) Isolation and characterization o multiple forms of rat liver UDP-glucuronate glucuronosyltransferase. Biochem J 233:827–837

Rubin GM, Tozer TN (1986) Hepatic binding and Michaelis-Menten metabolism of drugs. J Pharm Sci 75:660–663

Sanchez E, Tephly TR (1974) Morphine metabolism. I. Evidence for separate enzymes in the glucuronidation of morphine and p-nitrophenol by rat hepatic microsomes. Drug Metab Dispos 2:247–253

Sarkar M, Polk RE, Guzelian PS, Hunt C, Karnes HT (1990) In vitro effect of fluoroquinolones on theophylline metabolism in human liver microsomes. Antimicrob Agents Chemother 34:594–599

Saville BA, Gray MR, Tam YK (1987) Mechanism of lidocaine kinetics in the isolated perfused rat liver. II. Kinetics of steady-state elimination. Drug Metab Dispos 15:17–21

Sawada Y, Sugiyama Y, Miyamoto Y, Iga T, Hanano M (1985) Hepatic clearance model: comparison among the distributed, parallel-tube and well-stirred models. Chem Pharm Bull (Tokyo) 33:319–326

Schary WL, Rowland M (1983) Protein binding and hepatic clearance: studies with tolbutamide, a drug of low intrinsic clearance, in the isolated perfused rat liver preparation. J Pharmacokinet Biopharm 11:225–243

Schneck DH, Pritchard JF (1981) The inhibitory effect of propranolol pretreatment on its own metabolism in the rat. J Pharmacol Exp Ther 218:575–581

Schneck DW, Sprouse JS, Hayes AH, Shiroff RA (1978) The effect of hydralazine and other drugs on the kinetics of procainamide acetylation by rat liver and kidney N-acetyltransferase. J Pharmacol Exp Ther 204:212–218

Schwab AJ, Barker F III, Goresky CA, Pang KS (1990) Transfer of enalaprilat across rat liver cell membranes is barrier limited. Am J Physiol 258:G461–G475

Schwarz LR (1980) Modulation of sulfation and glucuronidation of 1-naphthol in isolated rat liver cells. Arch Toxicol 44:137–145

Schwarz LR, Schwenk M (1984) Sulfation in isolated enterocytes of guinea-pig: dependence on inorganic sulfate. Biochem Pharmacol 33:3353–3356

Schwenk M, Locher M (1985) 1-Naphthol conjugation in isolated cells from liver, jejunum, colon and kidney of the guinea pig. Biochem Pharmacol 34:697–701

Shand DG, Oates JA (1971) Metabolism of propranolol by rat liver microsomes and its inhibition of phenothiazine and tricyclic antidepressant drugs. Biochem Pharmacol 20:1720–1723

Shand DG, Kornhauser DM, Wilkinson GR (1975) Effect of route of administration and blood flow on hepatic drug elimination. J Pharmacol Exp Ther 195:424–432

Shaw L, Lennard MS, Tucker GT, Bax NDS, Woods HF (1987) Irreversible binding and metabolism of propranolol by human liver microsomes – relationship to polymorphic oxidation. Biochem Pharmacol 36:2283–2288

Sherman IA, Pang KS, Dlugosz JA, Barker F III, Perelman V (1991) Incomplete mixing of hepatic arterial and portal venous flows in the perfused rat liver preparation (Abstr). Hepatology 14:242A

Shibasaki J, Konishi R, Koike M, Imamura A, Sueyasu M (1981) Some quantitative evaluation of first-pass metabolism of salicylamide in rabbit and rat. J Pharmacobiodyn 4:91–100

Shibasaki S, Kawamata Y, Ueno F, Koyama C, Itho H, Nishigaki R, Umemura K (1988) Effects of cimetidine on lidocaine distribution in rats. J Pharmacobiodyn 11:785–793

Shipley LA, Weiner M (1985) Lack of inhibition of glucuronidation in isolated rat hepatocytes by diethyl ether anesthesia. Biochem Pharmacol 34:4179–4180

Sies H, Graf P (1985) Hepatic thiol and glutathione efflux under the influence of vasopressin, phenylephrine and adrenaline. Biochem J 226:545–549

Siest G, Antoine B, Fournel-Gigleux S, Magdalou J, Thomassin J (1988) The glucuronosyltransferase: what progress can pharmacologists expect from molecular biology and cellular enzymology? Biochem Pharmacol 36:983–989

Singh J, Schwarz LR (1981) Dependence of glucuronidation rate on UDP-glucuronic acid levels in isolated hepatocytes. Biochem Pharmacol 30:3252–3254

Singh K, Tripp SL, Dunton AW, Douglas FL, Rakhit A (1991) Determination of in vivo hepatic extraction ratio from in vitro metabolism by rat hepatocytes. Drug Metab Dispos 19:990–996

Smallwood RH, Morgan DJ, Mihaly GW, Jones DB, Smallwood RA (1988a) Effect of plasma protein binding on elimination of taurocholate by isolated perfused rat liver: comparison of venous equilibration, undistributed and distributed sinusoidal, and dispersion models. J Pharmacokinet Biopharm 16:377–396

Smallwood RH, Mihaly GW, Smallwood RA, Morgan DJ (1988b) Effect of a protein binding change on unbound and total plasma concentrations for drugs of intermediate hepatic extraction. J Pharmacokinet Biopharm 16:529–542

Smallwood RH, Mihaly GW, Smallwood RA, Morgan DJ (1988c) Propranolol elimination as described by the venous equilibrium model using flow perturbations in the isolated perfused rat liver. J Pharm Sci 77:330–333

Smith BR, van Anda J, Fouts JR, Bend JR (1983) Estimation of the styrene 7,8-oxide-detoxifying potential of epoxide hydrolase in glutathione-depleted, perfused rat liver. J Pharmacol Exp Ther 227:491–498

Smith MT, Loveridge N, Wills ED, Chayen J (1979) The distribution of glutathione content in the rat liver lobule. Biochem J 182:103–108

Soma Y, Satoh K, Sato K (1986) Purification and subunit-structural and immunological characterization of five glutathione S-transferases in human liver, and the acidic form as a hepatic tumor marker. Biochim Biophys Acta 869:247–258

Sorrentino D, Robinson RB, Kiang C-L, Berk PD (1989) At physiologic albumin/oleate concentrations oleate uptake by isolated hepatocytes, cardiac myocytes, and adipocytes is a saturable function of the unbound oleate concentration. Uptake kinetics are consistent with the conventional theory. J Clin Invest 84:1325–1333

Speisky H, Shackel N, Varghese G, Wade D, Israel Y (1990) Role of hepatic γ-glutamyltransferase in the degradation of circulating glutathione: studies in the intact guinea pig perfused liver. Hepatology 11:843–849

Stoll B, McNelly S, Buscher H-P, Häussinger D (1991) Functional hepatocyte heterogeneity in glutamate, aspartate, and α-ketoglutarate uptake: a histoautoradiographical study. Hepatology 13:247–253

St-Pierre MV, Pang KS (1987) Determination of diazepam and its metabolites by high-performance liquid chromatography and thin-layer chromatography. J Chromatogr 421:291–307

St-Pierre MV, Pang KS (1993a) Kinetics of sequential metabolism of metabolites. I. Formation and metabolism of oxazepam from nordiazepam and temazepam in the perfused murine liver. J Pharmacol Exp Ther 265:1429–1436

St-Pierre MV, Pang KS (1993b) Kinetics of sequential metabolism of metabolites. II. Formation and metabolism of nordiazepam and oxazepam from diazepam in the perfused murine liver. J Pharmacol Exp Ther 265:1437–1445

St-Pierre MV, van den Berg D, Pang KS (1990) Physiological modeling of drug and metabolite: disposition of oxazepam and oxazepam glucuronides in the recirculating, perfused rat liver preparation. J Pharmacokinet Biopharm 18:423–448

St-Pierre MV, Lee PI, Pang KS (1992) A comparative investigation of hepatic clearance models: predictions of metabolite formation and elimination. J Pharmacokinet Biopharm 20:105–145

Stremmel W (1987) Translocation of fatty acid across the basolateral rat plasma membrane is driven by an active potential sensitive sodium-dependent system. Proc Natl Acad Sci USA 83:3584–3588

Stremmel W, Potter BJ, Berk PD (1983) Studies of albumin binding to rat liver plasma membranes. Implications for the albumin receptor hypothesis. Biochim Biophys Acta 756:20–27

Sugita O, Sawada Y, Sugiyama Y, Iga T, Hanano M (1981) Prediction of drug–drug interaction from in vitro plasma protein binding. A study of tolbutamide-sulfonamide interaction in rats. Biochem Pharmacol 30:3347–3354

Sugita O, Sawada Y, Sugiyama Y, Iga T, Hanano M (1982) Physiologically based pharmacokinetics of drug-drug interaction: a study of tolbutamide-sulfonamide interaction in rats. J Pharmacokinet Biopharm 10:297–316

Supradist S, Notarianni LJ, Bennett PN (1983) Lignocaine kinetics in the rat. J Pharm Pharmacol 36:240–243

Suzuki T, Fujita S, Kawai R (1984) Precursor-metabolite interaction in the metabolism of lidocaine. J Pharm Sci 73:136–138

Sweeny DJ, Reinke LA (1988) Sulfation of acetaminophen in isolated rat hepatocytes. Relationship to sulfate ion concentrations and intracellular levels of 3′-phosphoadenosine-5′-phosphosulfate. Drug Metab Dispos 16:712–715

Taira Y, Redick JA, Baron J (1981) An immunohistochemical study on the localization and distribution of NADPH cytochrome c P-450 reductase in rat liver. Mol Pharmacol 17:374–381

Tam YK, Yau M, Berzins R, Montgomery PR, Gray M (1987) Mechanism of lidocaine kinetics in the isolated perfused rat liver. I. Effect of continuous infusion. Drug Metab Dispos 15:12–16

Tateishi N, Higashi T, Shinya S, Naruse A, Sakamoto Y (1974) Studies on the regulation of glutathione level in rat liver. J Biochem 75:93–103

Tateishi N, Higashi T, Naruse A, Hikita K, Sakamoto Y (1981) Relative contributions of sulfur atoms of dietary cysteine and methionine to rat liver glutathione and proteins. J Biochem 90:1603–1610

Te Koppele JM, Thurman RG (1990) Phagocytosis by Kupffer cells predominates in pericentral regions of the liver lobule. Am J Physiol 259:G814–G821

Te Koppele JM, Dogterom P, Vermeulen NPE, Meijer DKF, van der Gen A, Mulder GJ (1986) Alpha-bromoisovalerylurea as model substrate for studies on pharmacokinetics of glutathione conjugation in the rat. II. Pharmacokinetics and stereoselectivity of metabolism and excretion in vivo and in the perfused liver. J Pharmacol Exp Ther 239:905–914

Te Koppele JM, De Lannoy IAM, Pang KS, Mulder GJ (1987) Stereoselective glutathione conjugation and amidase-catalyzed hydrolysis of alpha-bromoisovalerylurea enantiomers in isolated rat hepatocytes. J Pharmacol Exp Ther 243:349–355

Te Koppele JM, Coles B, Ketterer B, Mulder GJ (1988) Stereoselectivity of rat liver glutathione transferase isoenzymes for alpha-bromoisovaleric acid and alpha-bromoisovalerylurea enantiomers. Biochem J 252:137–142

Terao N, Shen DD (1983) Alterations in serum protein binding and pharmacokinetics of l-propranolol in the rat elicited by the presence of an indwelling venous catheter. J Pharmacol Exp Ther 227:369–375

Thurman RG, Kauffman FC, Jungerman K (1987) Regulation of hepatic metabolism. Intra- and intercellular compartmentation. Plenum, New York

Torres AM, Rodriguez JV, Ochoa JE, Elias MM (1986) Rat kidney function related to tissue glutathione levels. Biochem Pharmacol 35:3355–3358

Tremaine LM, Diamond GL, Quebbemann AJ (1984) In vivo quantification of renal glucuronide and sulfate conjugation of 1-naphthol and p-nitrophenol in the rat. Biochem Pharmacol 33:419–427

Trinidad A, Kirlin WG, Ogolla F, Andrews AF, Yerokun T, Ferguson RJ, Brady PK, Hein DW (1989) Kinetic characterization of acetylator genotype-dependent and -independent N-acetyltransferase isozymes in homozygous rapid and slow acetylator inbred hamster liver cytosol. Drug Metab Dispos 17:238–247

Tsang C-F, Wilkinson GR (1982) Diazepam disposition in mature and aged rabbits and rats. Drug Metab Dispos 10:413–416

Tsao SC, Sugiyama Y, Sawada Y, Nagase S, Iga T, Hanano M (1986) Effect of albumin on hepatic uptake of warfarin in normal and analbuminemic mutant rats. Analysis by multiple indicator dilution method. J Pharmacokinet Biopharm 14:51–64

Tsao SC, Sugiyama Y, Sawada Y, Iga T, Hanano M (1988) Kinetic analysis of albumin-mediated uptake of warfarin by perfused rat liver. J Pharmacokinet Biopharm 16:165–181

Tu CPD, Reddy CC (1985) On the multiplicity of rat liver glutathione S-transferases. J Biol Chem 260:9961–9964

Tukey RH, Tephly T (1980) Phospholipid dependency of purified estrone and p-nitrophenol UDP-glucuronyltransferase. Life Sci 27:2471–2476

Tukey RH, Billings RE, Autor AP, Tephly TR (1979) Phospholipid-dependence of oestrone UDP-glucuronyltransferase and p-nitrophenol UDP-glucuronyltransferase. Biochem J 179:59–65

Ullrich D, Fisher G, Katz N, Bock KW (1984) Intralobular distribution of UDP-glucuronosyltransferase in livers from untreated, 3-methylcholanthrene- and phenobarbital-treated rats. Chem Biol Interact 48:181–190

Van der Graaff M, Vermeulen NPE, Joeres RP, Breimer DD (1983) Disposition of hexobarbital enantiomers in the rat. Drug Metab Dispos 11:489–493

Van der Sluijs P, Braakman I, Meijer DKF, Groothuis GMM (1988) Heterogeneous acinar localization of the asialoglycoprotein internalization system in rat hepatocytes. Hepatology 6:1521–1529

Vermeulen NPE (1980) The epoxide-diol pathway in the metabolism of hexobarbital and related barbiturates. PhD thesis, University of Leiden, The Netherlands

Veronese ME, McManus ME, Laupattarakasemm P, Miners JO, Birkett DJ (1989) Tolbutamide hydroxylation by human, rabbit and rat liver microsomes and by purified forms of cytochrome P-450. Drug Metab Dispos 18:356–361

Villar ED, Sanchez E, Tephly TR (1974) Morphine metabolism. II. Studies on morphine glucuronyltransferase activity in intestinal microsomes of rats. Drug Metab Dispos 2:370–374

Wang IY, Tung E, Wang A-C, Argenbright L, Wang R, Pickett, Lu AYH (1986) Multiple Ya subunits of glutathione S-transferase detected by monoclonal antibodies. Arch Biochem Biophys 245:543–547

Watari N, Iwai M, Kaneniwa N (1983) Pharmacokinetic study of the fate of acetaminophen and its conjugates. J Pharmacokinet Biopharm 11:245–272

Watkins JB, Klaassen CD (1983) Chemically-induced alteration of UDP-glucuronic acid concentration in rat liver. Drug Metab Dispos 11:37–40

Wattenberg LW, Leong JL, Strand PJ (1963) Benzyperene hydroxylase activation in the gastrointestinal tract. Cancer Res 22:1120–1125

Weisiger RA (1985) Dissociation from albumin. A potentially rate-limiting step in clearances of substances by the liver. Proc Natl Acad Sci USA 82:1563–1567

Weisiger RA, Ma W-L (1987) Uptake of oleate from albumin solutions by rat liver: failure to detect catalysis of the dissociation of oleate from albumin by an albumin receptor. J Clin Invest 79:1070–1077

Weisiger RA, Gollan J, Ockner R (1980) An albumin receptor on the liver cell may mediate hepatic uptake of sulfobromophthalein and bilirubin: bound ligand, not free, is the major uptake determinant (Abstr). Gastroenterology 79:1065

Weisiger RA, Gollan J, Ockner R (1981) Receptor for albumin on the liver cell surface may mediate uptake of fatty acids and other albumin-bound substances. Science 211:1048–1050

Westenberg HGM (1980) Bioanalysis and pharmacokinetics of carbamazepine. PhD thesis, University of Groningen, The Netherlands

Whitmer DI, Ziurys JC, Gollan JL (1984) Hepatic microsomal glucuronidation of bilirubin in unilamellar liposomal membranes. J Biol Chem 259:11969–11975

Whitsett JL, Dayton PG, McNay TL (1971) The effect of hepatic blood flow on the hepatic removal rate of oxyphenbutazone in the dog. J Pharmacol Exp Ther 177:246–255

Wiegard UW, Hintze KL, Slattery JT, Levy G (1980) Protein binding of several drugs in serum and plasma of healthy subjects. Clin Pharmacol Ther 27:297–300

Wiersma DA, Roth RA (1980) Clearance of 5-hydroxytryptamine by rat lung and liver: the importance of relative perfusion and intrinsic clearance. J Pharmacol Exp Ther 212:97–102

Wiersma DA, Roth RA (1983a) The prediction of benzo(a)pyrene clearance by rat liver and lung from enzyme kinetic data. Mol Pharmacol 24:300–308

Wiersma DA, Roth RA (1983b) Total body clearance of circulating benzo(a)pyrene in conscious rats: effect of pretreatment with 3-methylcholanthrene and the role of liver and lung. J Pharmacol Exp Ther 226:661–667

Wilkinson GR (1987) Clearance approaches in pharmacology. Pharmacol Rev 39: 1–47

Wilkinson GR, Shand DG (1975) Commentary. A physiological approach to hepatic drug clearance. Clin Pharmacol Ther 18:377–390

Windorfer A Jr, Sauer W (1977) Drug interactions during anticonvulsant therapy in childhood: diphenylhydantoin, primidone, phenobarbitone, clonazepam, nitrazepam, carbamazepine and dipropylacetate. Neuropadiatrie 8:29–41

Winkler K, Keiding S, Tygstrup N (1973) Clearance as a quantitative measure of liver function. In: Presig R, Paumgartner P (eds) The liver: quantitative aspects of structure and function. Karger, Basel, pp 144–155

Winkler K, Bass L, Keiding S, Tygstrup N (1974) The effect of hepatic perfusion on the assessment of kinetic constants. In: Lundquist F, Tygstrup N (eds) Regulation of hepatic metabolism. Munksgaard, Copenhagen, pp 797–807

Winsnes A (1969) Studies on the activation in vitro of glucuronyltransferase. Biochim Biophys Acta 191:279–291

Winsnes A (1972) Kinetic properties of different forms of hepatic UDPglucuronyl-transferase. Biochim Biophys Acta 284:394–405

Wolkoff AW (1987) The role of an albumin receptor in hepatic organic anion uptake: the controversy continues. Hepatology 7:777–779

Wolkoff AW, Goresky CA, Sellin J, Gatmaitan Z, Arias IM (1979) Role of ligandin in transfer of bilirubin from plasma into liver. Am J Physiol 236:E638–E648

Wosalait WD, Garten S (1972) Computation of unbound anticoagulant values in plasma. Res Commun Chem Pathol Pharmacol 3:285–291

Xu X, Pang KS (1989) Hepatic modeling of metabolite kinetics in sequential and parallel pathways: salicylamide and gentisamide metabolism in perfused rat liver. J Pharmacokinet Biopharm 17:645–671

Xu X, Hirayama H, Pang KS (1989) First-pass metabolism of salicylamide: studies in the once-through vascularly perfused rat intestine-liver preparation. Drug Metab Dispos 17:556–563

Xu X, Tang K, Pang KS (1990) Sequential metabolism of salicylamide exclusively to gentisamide 5-glucuronide and not gentisamide sulfate conjugates in single-pass in situ perfused rat liver. J Pharmacol Exp Ther 253:965–973

Xu X, Selick P, Pang KS (1993) Nonlinear protein binding and heterogeneity of drug metabolizing enzymes: effect on hepatic drug removal. J Pharmacokinet Biopharm 21:43–74

Yamada H, Baba T, Hirata Y, Oguri K, Yoshimura H (1984) Studies on N-demethylation of methamphetamine by liver microsomes of guinea-pigs and rats: the role of flavin-containing mono-oxygenase and cytochrome P-450 systems. Xenobiotica 14:861–866

Yamada H, Yuno K, Oguri K, Yoshimura H (1990) Multiplicity of liver microsomal flavin-containing monooxygenase in the guinea pig: its purification and characterization. Arch Biochem Biophys 280:305–312

Yamamoto K, Sherman I, Phillips MJ, Fisher MM (1985) Three-dimensional observations of the hepatic arterial terminations in rat, hamster, and human liver by scanning electron microscopy of microvascular casts. Hepatology 5:452–456

Yamauchi M, Potter JJ, Mezey E (1988) Lobular distribution of alcohol dehydrogenase in the rat liver. Hepatology 8:243–247

Yamazoe Y, Shimada M, Murayama N, Nagata K, Kato R (1989) Hormonal regulation of hepatic cytochrome P-450. In: Kato R, Estabrook RW, Cayen MN (eds) Xenobiotic metabolism and disposition. Taylor and Francis, London, pp 37–44

Yasuhara M, Katayama H, Kujiwara J, Okumura K, Hori R (1985) Influence of acute renal failure on pharmacokinetics of phenolsulfonphthalein in rats: a comparative study in vivo and in the simultaneous perfusion system of the liver and kidney. J Pharmacobiodyn 8:377–384

Yeh SY (1982) Localization and characterization of meperidine esterase of rats. Drug Metab Dispos 10:319–325

Zakim D, Vessey DA (1977) Membrane-bound estrone as substrate for microsomal UDP-glucuronyltransferase. J Biol Chem 252:7534–7537

Zhao Y, Snel CAW, Mulder GJ, Pang KS (1992) Glutathione conjugation of bromosulfophthalein in perfused rat liver: studies with the multiple indicator dilution technique. Drug Metab Dispos 21:1070–1078

Ziegler DM (1980) Microsomal flavin-containing monooxygenase: oxygenation of nucleophilic nitrogen and sulfur compounds. In: Jakoby WB (ed) Enzymatic basis of detoxication, vol 1. Academic, New York, pp 201–227

Ziegler DM (1990) Flavin-containing monooxygenase: enzymes adapted for multisubstrate specificity. Trends Pharmacol Sci 11:321–324

Zilly W, Breimaer DD, Richter E (1975) Induction of drug metabolism in man after rifampicin treatment measured by increased hexobarbital and tolbutamide clearance. Eur J Clin Pharmacol 9:219–227

Zimmerman C, Ratna S, LeBoeuf E, Pang KS (1991) A high pressure liquid chromatographic assay for 4-methylumbelliferone and its conjugates. J Chromatogr 563:83–94

Zumbiel MA, Fiserova-Bergerova V, Malinin TI, Holaday DA (1978) Glutathione depletion following inhalation anesthesia. Anesthesiology 49:102–108

CHAPTER 6

Gastrointestinal Transport of Peptide and Protein Drugs and Prodrugs

J.P.F. BAI, B.H. STEWART, and G.L. AMIDON

A. Introduction

The oral absorption of peptide and protein drugs, an important class of therapeutic agents, is generally poor. Significant pharmacological effects of peptide and protein drugs have been observed even though oral bioavailability is in the single digit range (LEE et al. 1991). A trace amount of intact protein molecules is indeed absorbed into the systemic circulation (O'HAGAN et al. 1987; WARSHAW et al. 1971; GONNELLA and WALKER 1987). Cyclosporin is an orally active peptide; furthermore, significant membrane transport of enkephalin and renin inhibitors was observed when peptidase inhibitors were used, and oral efficacy of insulin and vasopressin was improved, though still too low to be useful, using peptidase inhibitors or stable analogs, respectively. These results indicate that oral delivery is feasible if proteolysis is avoided (SAFFRAN et al. 1988; TAKAORI et al. 1986; FRIEDMAN and AMIDON 1991; KIDRON et al. 1982; WOOD et al. 1983). Peptide and protein drugs are transported across the intestinal epithelium by various mechanisms depending on their physicochemical properties.

Di-/tripeptides are absorbed in the mammalian intestine by a common carrier-mediated process with broad substrate specificity (MATTHEWS and PAYNE 1980). Though hydrophilic and ionized at intestinal pH, di-/tripeptide type drugs such as β-lactam antibiotics and angiotensin-converting enzyme (ACE) inhibitors are efficiently absorbed through the peptide transporter (FRIEDMAN and AMIDON 1989a,b; HU et al. 1988; HU and AMIDON 1988; SINKO and AMIDON, 1988 1989; TSUJI et al. 1986, 1987a,b). Targeting the peptide carrier can achieve significant oral availability of di-/tripeptide-type drugs or drugs with low membrane permeability in the form of di-/tripeptide prodrugs (BAI et al. 1992; HU et al. 1989).

By a theoretical analysis of macroscopic mass balance, a correlation is obtained between the permeability from the in situ studies and the fraction dose absorbed in humans for both passively and nonpassively absorbed drugs, and for both peptide-type and nonpeptide drugs (AMIDON et al. 1988). This theoretical analysis is valuable for screening drugs for desired oral availability. This chapter will briefly review the current knowledge of intestinal transport processes, the recent development of structural requirements for the peptide transporter, the transport of small peptide drugs, the correlation between the in situ membrane permeability and the fraction dose absorbed in humans, and the use of peptide prodrug strategies to improve intestinal drug absorption.

B. Mucosal Cell Absorption

The nature of transport processes of polypeptide and protein drugs are ambiguous in mature mammalian gastrointestinal tract. Energy-required, nonactive, and passive transport processes have been reported for quite a few polypeptide and protein drugs (MARCON-GENTY et al. 1989; SCHILLING and MITER 1990; RAO et al. 1990; FRICKER et al. 1991). It is not clear whether these phenomena are due to several distinct transport mechanisms for peptide and protein drugs or simply due to laboratory variations. The general understanding of various transport processes across the intestinal epithelium is discussed below.

I. Paracellular Absorption

Paracellular diffusion is a process whereby molecules diffuse through the intercellular tight junctions of the intestinal epithelium. Morphologically, the tight junction links the brush-border membrane of adjacent enterocytes into a continuum, while functionally it acts as a pore and allows very small molecules to pass through. The paracellular pathway is selective for cations and excludes molecules with hydrodynamic radii greater than 0.4–0.8 nm at the resting state. By activating contraction of epithelial cytoskeletal elements, D-glucose or L-amino acids can open tight junctions to permit transport of nutrients and low-molecular-weight drugs by solvent drag through paracellular channels (LU et al. 1992; PAPPENHEIMER et al. 1987). A recent report indicated that a polypeptide (mol. wt.: 1900) penetrated tight junctions selectively at sites of dilatation which was elicited by D-glucose (ATISOOK and MADARA 1991). However, horseradish peroxidase (mol. wt.: 40 000) was excluded from the open tight junctions.

II. Transcellular Absorption

Transcellular absorption processes across the intestinal epithelial cells include simple diffusion, carrier-mediated transport, and endocytosis.

1. Simple Diffusion

Substances can partition into and diffuse through the membrane by thermodynamic driving forces. The membrane flux, J, is a function of lipophilicity and concentration gradient.

$$J = \frac{DK}{h} \Delta C, \tag{1}$$

where D is the diffusion coefficient of a substance in the biomembrane, K is the membrane versus water partition coefficient, h is the membrane thickness, and ΔC is the concentration gradient across the membrane. Peptide and protein drugs have a high degree of hydrogen bonding with water. The total desolvation enthalpies of peptide drugs are high such that their membrane/water partition coefficients are usually low (Ho et al. 1990).

2. Carrier-Mediated Process

The carrier-mediated transport of substances involves a membrane protein acting as the carrier and an ion gradient as the driving force. The process can operate against a concentration gradient. The transport rate per unit surface area, J, of a carrier-mediated process is determined by carrier permeability, J_{max}/K_m:

$$J = \frac{J_{max}}{K_m}\left(\frac{[S]}{1 + \frac{[S]}{K_m}}\right),$$ (2)

where J_{max} is the maximum flux, K_m is the Michaelis constant, and $[S]$ is the substrate concentration. Certain unique structural features are required to be a substrate of a carrier system. For example, D-glucose, amino acids, and small peptides are transported by distinct and specific intestinal carrier-mediated systems (CRANE 1985; MUNCK 1987; MATTHEWS and PAYNE 1980).

3. Endocytosis

Processes include pinocytosis (fluid phase) and receptor-mediated endocytosis (RME). In mammals, endocytosis usually occurs in the neonatal small intestine (WALKER 1981). Initially macromolecules come into contact with the cell membrane, invagination takes place, and small vesicles are formed. After being endocytosed, vesicles (phagosomes) migrate into the interior of cells and coalesce with the lysosomes. The intravesicular digestion occurs therein, and those molecules that survive enzymatic digestion and digested residues are deposited into the intercellular space (exocytosis). In RME, ligands first bind to membrane receptors and endosomes are formed from invagination (FARQUHAR 1983). Via a membrane-bound proton pump, endosomes undergo progressive acidification which promotes dissociation of the receptor–ligand complex. Ligands may be degraded via the lysosomal pathway or exported from the cell. Transcellular transport of macromolecules has been documented in M cells of Peyer's patches of adult mammalian intestine (HUGHSON and HOPKINS 1990). Small but significant amounts of protein molecules are transported intact across the intestinal epithelium of mature animals (MARCON-GENTY et al. 1989; O'HAGAN et al. 1987; WARSHAW et al. 1971; GONNELLA and WALKER 1987). However, the actual mechanisms are unknown.

C. Mucosal Cell Transport of Peptide Drugs

I. Characteristics of Small Peptide Transport

Di-/tripeptides are absorbed by a carrier-mediated system, which has broad substrate specificity, in various species (Mattews and Payne 1980). Di-/tripeptides share a common transport mechanism, while the absorption of Gly-Gly-Gly-Gly and Gly-Sar-Sar-Sar was concluded to be passive (Addison et al. 1975b; Boyd and Ward 1982). Characterization of the small peptide transporter in the intestinal mucosal cell is complicated by hydrolysis. Moreover, there are more than 480 possible dipeptides and 10^4 possible tripeptides, and the number of existing peptide carriers is unknown. Currently only one protein isolated from the brush-border membrane has been reported as the peptide transporter (Kramer et al. 1990). Di-/tripeptides are cotransported with proton and Na^+ is only indirectly involved in the process (Ganapathy and Leibach 1985). According to Leibach's hyothesis, the Na^+-H^+ exchanger generates and maintains the inward proton gradient, while the Na^+-K^+-ATPase in the basolateral membrane maintains a low intracellular sodium concentration (Fig. 1). Thus the Na^+-H^+ exchanger coupled with the Na^+-K^+-ATPase drives the transport of di-/tripeptides into the intestinal epithelial cells.

1. Substrate Structural Requirements

a) N-terminal α-Amino Group

Imidodipeptides, Pro-X, where X is an amino acid, are compatible with the peptide carrier (Addison et al. 1974; Das and Radhakrishnan 1975). Methylation, acetylation, or other modifications of the N-terminal A-amino

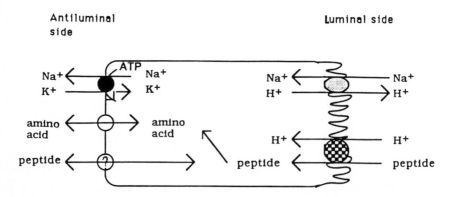

Fig. 1. The transport of di/tripeptides is energized by a proton (H^+) gradient across the brush-border membrane. Adapted from the model proposed by Ganapathy and Leibach (1985)

group reduces or abolishes the capability to inhibit di-/tripeptide transport. Examples include Sar-Gly, *N*-benzyloxycarbonyl-Gly-Leu, and *N*-acetyl-Gly-Gly (ADDISON et al. 1974, 1975a; DAS and RADHAKRISHNAN 1975; RUBINO et al. 1971). A β-amino acid at either side of the dipeptide amide bond is compatible with the peptide transporter. For example, β-alanyl-histidine (carnosine), β-Ala-Gly-Gly, bestatin, and His-β-Ala are transported by this carrier system (ADDISON et al. 1974, 1975a; TOMITA et al. 1990). However, small peptides containing a γ-amino acid are incompatible with the peptide transporter (ADDISON et al. 1975a; DAS and RADHAKRISHNAN 1975).

b) Other Functional groups

Modification of the C-terminal carboxyl group leads to a reduction or an abolition of affinity with the transporter. Examples include Gly-GlyNH$_2$, Gly-Gly-GlyNH$_2$, and Asp-PheOCH$_3$ (ADDISON et al. 1974, 1975a). Gly-Sar, Gly-Sar-Sar, and dipeptides of X-Pro and X-Hyp are absorbed by the peptide transporter (ADDISON et al. 1975a,b; RAJENDRAN et al. 1985), suggesting that di-/tripeptides with imide bond(s) are compatible with the peptide transporter.

c) Stereospecificity

Dipeptides with a D-amino acid on either side of the amide bond are substrates for the peptide transporter (ASATOOR et al. 1973; BURSTON and MATTHEWS 1987; CHEESEMAN and SMYTH 1972). Nevertheless, uptake is stereospecific and dipeptides of L-L forms are transported more readily than their isomers containing a D-amino acid. Dipeptides of L-L form have the highest uptake rates, followed by mixed type of isomers (L-D and D-L) and then D-D isomers.

II. Carrier-Mediated Transport of Peptide Drugs

1. β-Lactam Antibiotics

With free N-terminal α-amino and C-terminal carboxyl groups, amino-β-lactam antibiotics (including cyclacillin, amoxicillin, ampicillin, cefaclor, cefadroxil, cephalexin, cefatrizine, and cephradine) are transported by the peptide transporter (SINKO and AMIDON 1988, 1989, 1989; OH et al. 1989). The Michaelis-Menten parameters describing their transport characteristics are summarized in Table 1. The intestinal absorption of amino-β-lactam antibiotics is inhibited by di-/tripeptides but not by amino acids. Moreover, as shown in Fig. 2, antibiotic absorption shows mutual inhibition. β-Lactam antibiotics without a free N-terminal α-amino group (including cefixime, FK089, and ceftibuten) manifest nonlinear absorption profiles as well and their uptake is competitively inhibited by di-/tripeptides (TSUJI et al. 1987b;

Table 1. Summary of the membrane absorption parameters[a] of β-lactam antibiotics

Compound	J^*_{max} (mM)	K_m (mM)	P^*_c	P^*_m
Cyclacillin[b]	16.30 (3.40)	14.00 (3.30)	1.14 (0.05)	0
Amoxicillin[b]	0.04 (0.02)	0.06 (0.03)	0.56 (0.06)	0.76 (0.09)
Ampicillin[b]	11.78 (1.88)	15.80 (2.92)	0.75 (0.04)	0
Cefaclor[c]	21.30 (4.00)	16.10 (3.60)	1.30 (0.10)	0
Cefadroxil[c]	8.40 (0.80)	5.90 (0.80)	1.40 (0.10)	0
Cephalexin[c]	9.10 (1.20)	7.20 (1.10)	1.30 (0.10)	0
Cefatrizine[c]	0.70 (0.20)	0 60 (0.20)	1.30 (0.10)	0.20 (0.03)
Cephardine[c]	1.60 (0.80)	1.50 (0.80)	1.10 (0.10)	0.30 (0.10)

[a] Reported values are mean ± SD
[b] Adapted from OH et al. (1989)
[c] Adapted from SINKO and AMIDON (1989)

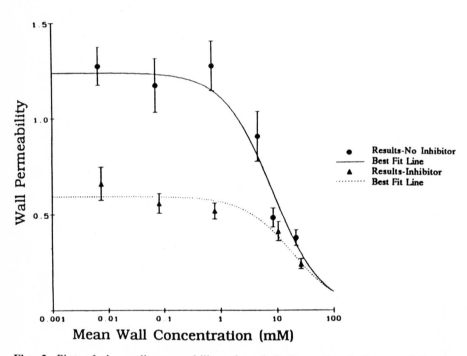

Fig. 2. Plot of the wall permeability of cephalexin perfused alone and in the presence of a competitive inhibitor, cefadroxil (7 mM). The results are reported as the mean wall permeability ±SEM. (Adapted from SINKO and AMIDON 1989)

OH et al. 1990; YOSHIKAWA et al. 1989). Clearly these β-lactam antibiotics without a free N-terminal α-amino group are also transported by the peptide transporter. The transport parameters of cefixime are as follows: J^*_{max}, 0.02 ± 0.01 mM; K_m, 0.03 ± 0.01 mM; P^*_c, 0.52 ± 0.05; P^*_m, 0.18 ± 0.04 (OH et al. 1990). Cefixime absorption is energized by a proton gradient, as is

Table 2. Intestinal transport parameters of ACE inhibitors

Compounds	J_{max}^* (mM)	K_m (mM)	P_c^*	P_m^*
Captopril[a]	12.3 (2.8)	5.91 (1.65)	2.08 (0.19)	0.75
SQ 29852[b]	0.16 (0.04)	0.08 (0.01)	2.00 (0.20)	0.25 (0.07)
Lisinopril[b]	0.18 (0.004)	0.056 (0.003)	0.33 (0.03)	0.06 (0.05)
Enalapril[c]	0.13	0.07	1.9	0.35
Benazepril[d]	0.072	0.075	0.962	0.749
Quinapril[d]	1.703	2.341	0.728	0.621

[a] From Hu and Amidon (1988)
[b] From Friedman et al. (1989b)
[c] From Friedman et al. (1989a)
[d] From Yee and Amidon (1990)

absorption of small peptides (Tsuji et al. 1987b). Uptake of d-cephalexin is saturable and inhibited by its l-isomer, which is absorbed by the peptide transporter (Sinko and Amidon 1988; Tamai et al. 1988).

2. ACE Inhibitors

Recent findings suggest that ACE inhibitors (including captopril, SQ 29852, enalapril, lisinopril, benazepril, and quinapril) are transported by the peptide transporter (Friedman and Amidon 1989a,b; Hu and Amidon 1988; Yee and Amidon 1990; Stewart et al. 1990). Without a free N-terminal α-amino group, these compounds show nonlinear absorption, as summarized in Table 2. Moreover their uptake is significantly inhibited by small peptides and cephradine. The diacid ACE inhibitors (including enalaprilate, quinaprilate, and benazeprilate) are poorly absorbed, while their ester prodrugs (including enalapril, quinapril, and benazepril) are absorbed by the transporter. However, lisinopril, with two free carboxyl groups at similar positions as enalaprilat, is absorbed by the transporter with a low permeability, as is FK089, a β-lactam antibiotic (Friedman and Amidon 1989a,b; Tsuji et al. 1987a; Yee and Amidon 1990). Further investigation of the substrate specificity of the peptide transporter is needed to understand this binding/transport phenomenon.

D. Estimating Extent of Drug Absorption

I. Fraction of Dose Absorbed–Permeability Correlation

Based on a macroscopic mass balance, a theoretical analysis was established by Amidon et al. (1988) to quantitatively predict the fraction dose absorbed in humans from the in situ permeability results in rats. Using the macroscopic mass balance of a drug absorption in the intestine:

$$\frac{-dM}{dt} = Q\,(C_{\mathrm{o}} - C_{\mathrm{m}}) = \int\!\!\int J_{\mathrm{w}}dA, \tag{3}$$

and the steady-state flux, J_{w}, of the film diffusion model across the intestinal wall is estimated as:

$$J_{\mathrm{w}} = P_{\mathrm{e}}C_{\mathrm{w}}. \tag{4}$$

The fraction dose absorbed in humans was estimated from the in situ dimensionless wall permeability:

$$F = 4\mathrm{Gz}P_{\mathrm{e}}^{*} \int_{0}^{1} C_{\mathrm{w}}^{*}dz^{*}. \tag{5}$$

In these equations, M is the total mass in the tube, Q is the fluid flow rate, C_{o} and C_{m} are the inlet and outlet drug concentrations, respectively, P_{e}^{*} is the effective membrane permeability, C_{w} is the wall concentration, and the Graetz number, Gz, is defined as the ratio of the axial convection to radial diffusion time (ELLIOTT et al. 1980):

$$\mathrm{Gz} = \frac{\pi DL}{2Q}.$$

The dimensionless wall permeability and wall concentration are defined as follows:

$$P_{\mathrm{e}}^{*} = \frac{P_{\mathrm{e}}R}{D}$$

and

$$C_{\mathrm{w}}^{*} = \frac{C_{\mathrm{w}}}{C_{\mathrm{o}}}.$$

In these equations, D is diffusivity of a drug and L is length of intestinal tube. A correlation between fraction dose absorbed and permeability was established for several classes of drugs (AMIDON et al. 1988; SINKO et al. 1991).

II. Comparison of Passive and Carrier-Mediated Transport

The membrane permeability of drug transported by both carried-mediated and diffusion processes is:

$$P_{\mathrm{w}}^{*} = \frac{J_{\mathrm{max}}^{*}}{K_{\mathrm{m}}\left(1 + \dfrac{C_{\mathrm{w}}}{K_{\mathrm{m}}}\right)} + P_{\mathrm{m}}^{*} \tag{6}$$

where J_{max}^{*} is defined as $J_{\mathrm{max}}^{*}(R/D)$. Considering compounds that are absorbed by both passive permeability and carrier-mediated processes, a mean permeability is required to determine the permeability–fraction dose absorbed correlation. Based on the first moment of probability theory, the average wall permeability is defined as:

$$\overline{P_w^*} = \frac{\int_{C_o}^{0} P_w^* dC}{\int_{C_o}^{0} dC},$$

(7)

where C_o equals the ratio of dose to luminal volume. After integration, the average membrane permeability becomes:

$$\overline{P_w^*} = P_m^* + P_c^* \frac{K_m}{C_o} \ln\left(1 + \frac{C_o}{K_m}\right),$$

(8)

where P_c^* is J_{max}^*/K_m. When the fraction dose absorbed from the human studies is plotted versus the in situ membrane permeability, a good correlation between the theoretical curve and observed values is obtained for drugs transported by either a carrier-mediated or a passive process, as shown in Fig. 3. The carrier-mediated drugs include β-lactam antibiotics and

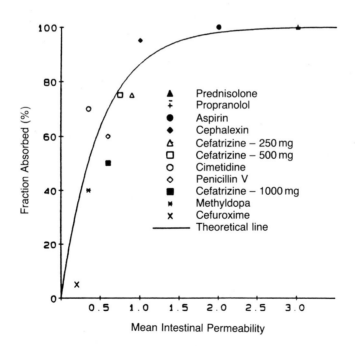

Fig. 3. Plot of the fraction dose absorbed (%) versus the mean dimensionless intestinal wall permeability. Wall permeabilities were calculated from steady-state rat intestinal perfusion experiments. (Adapted from AMIDON et al. 1988)

L-α-methyldopa, which are transported by the peptide and amino acid transporters, respectively. This analysis, based on the in situ permeability and fraction dose absorbed in humans for both carrier-mediated and passive transport drugs, is applicable to peptide as well as nonpeptide-type drugs.

E. Peptide Prodrug Approaches to Improving Intestinal Absorption

As shown above, the key parameter for the fraction dose absorbed is membrane permeability. The intestinal peptide transporter with broad substrate specificity can be utilized to achieve good oral availability of hydrophilic drugs with poor membrane permeability as peptide prodrugs.

I. Peptide Prodrugs of α-Methyldopa

Though sharing an amino acid carrier, L-α-methyldopa, an amino acid analog, has variable and low intestinal absorption (MERFELD et al. 1986; HU et al. 1989). The dipeptidyl derivatives of L-α-methyldopa, Phe-L-α-methyldopa, L-α-methyldopa-Phe, and L-α-methyldopa-Pro, demonstrate more than ten times higher wall permeability than L-α-methyldopa, as illustrated in Table 3 (HU et al. 1989; BAI et al. 1992). Hence the membrane permeability is significantly increased by the peptide prodrug strategy targeting the intestinal peptide transporter (HU et al. 1989; TSUJI et al. 1990). L-α-Methyldopa-Pro is hydrolyzed by prolidase with Michaelis-Menten parameters K_m and V_{max} of $0.09 \pm 0.022 \, \mathrm{m}M$ and $3.98 \pm 0.250 \, \mu\mathrm{mol}/$ min per mg protein, respectively. Clearly L-α-methyldopa-Pro is absorbed via the peptide carrier and hydrolyzed by cytosolic prolidase, whose substrates are usually poorly hydrolyzed by brush-border membrane peptidases (ADIBI and KIM 1981). Therefore, oral availability of poorly absorbed drugs can be improved by targeting prodrugs to the peptide carrier to increase

Table 3. Wall permeabilities ($P_w^* \pm$ SE) of L-α-methyldopa and its dipeptidyl derivatives (from HU et al. 1989)

Compound	Concentration (mM)		
	1.0	0.1	0.01
L-α-Methyldopa (I)	0.41 (0.11)	0.4 (0.22)	0.43 (0.14)
Gly-I		4.34 (0.27)	
Pro-I		1.68 (0.23)	
I-Pro		5.41 (0.55)	
Phe-I		5.29 (1.57)	
I-Phe	4.30 (0.30)	10.22 (0.45)	10.9 (1.8)

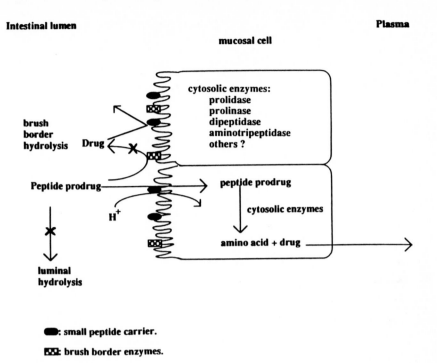

Intestinal lumen **Plasma**

mucosal cell

cytosolic enzymes:
  prolidase
  prolinase
brush   dipeptidase
border   aminotripeptidase
hydrolysis   Drug   others ?

Peptide prodrug   peptide prodrug

cytosolic enzymes

H⁺

amino acid + drug

luminal
hydrolysis

●: small peptide carrier.

▨: brush border enzymes.

Fig. 4. Schematic presentation of a peptide prodrug strategy for improving oral absorption. (Adapted from BAI et al. 1992)

membrane permeability and utilizing cytosolic enzymes to release parent drugs, as illustrated in Fig. 4.

II. Peptide Prodrug Approaches for Acidic Drugs

Small peptide drugs without an N-terminal α-amino group are transported by the peptide transporter, suggesting that peptide prodrugs of acidic drugs can target the peptide transporter to achieve good oral availability. The structures and intestinal permeability of dipeptide prodrugs of small aromatic acids (including phenylpropionic acid, phenylacetic acid, and benzoic acid) are summarized in Table 4. Proline, glycine, and α-methyldopa are used as the C-terminal amino acids (BAI et al. 1991). Absorption of the peptide analog was nonlinear and inhibition by small peptides and/or cephradine but not by amino acids was observed, as shown in Fig. 5. The transport parameters (mean $\pm$ SD) of phenylpropionylproline and N-benzoylproline are as follows: J^*_{max}, 0.037 ± 0.019 mM; K_m, 0.045 ± 0.027 mM; P^*_c, 0.830 ± 0.130; P^*_m, 0.673 ± 0.049 and J^*_{max}, 1.34 ± 0.24 mM; K_m, 1.31 ± 0.30 mM; P^*_c, 1.02 ± 0.11; P^*_m, 0, respectively. The permeability–concentration profile

Table 4. Permeabilities of dipeptide analogs investigated for the need of N-terminal α-amino group (adapted from Bai et al. 1991)

Compound	Chemical structure	P_w^{*a}
Phe-Pro		2.01 ± 0.54
Phenylpropionyl-proline		1.19 ± 0.16
Phenylacetyl-proline		0.84 ± 0.15
N-Benzoylproline		0.90 ± 0.06
Hippuric acid		0.18 ± 0.03
Phenylacetyl-α-methyldopa		0.61 ± 0.07

[a] All compounds were studied at 0.1 mM, except phenylacetyl-α-methyldopa, which was studied at 0.05 mM

of N-benzoylproline is shown in Fig. 6. Consequently, these dipeptide analogs are absorbed by the peptide transporter. The results indicate that peptide analogs are indeed recognized by the peptide carrier. These findings parallel results with β-lactam antibiotics and ACE inhibitors, which also lack an N-terminal α-amino group.

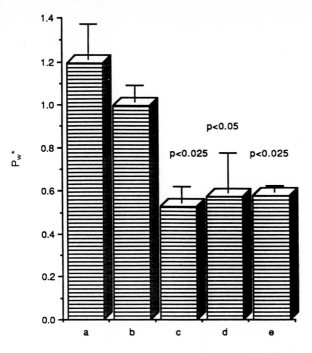

Fig. 5. Inhibition of 0.1 mM phenylpropinylproline permeability: *a*, control; *b*, 27 mM Met; *c*, mixed dipeptides (60 mM Gly-Gly, 2 mM Gly-Phe, 2 mM Pro-Phe); *d*, 1 mM cephradine; *e*, 27 mM Gly-Pro. (Adapted from BAI et al. 1991)

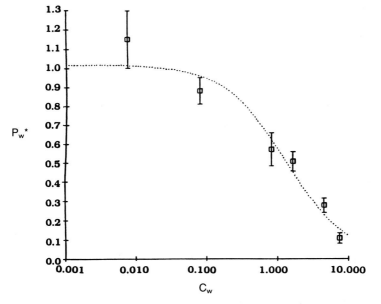

Fig. 6. Transport kinetics of *N*-benzoylproline. The values of P_w^* shown are means $\pm$ SE. (Adapted from BAI et al. 1991)

III. Other Peptide Prodrugs

The oral absorption of lipophilic drugs is often limited by solubility. A small solubility-to-dose ratio will result in poor oral availability, as demonstrated in an extended analysis of the macroscopic mass balance approach (SINKO et al. 1991). By introducing an ionizable group, peptide prodrugs can increase aqueous solubility by the pK_a and solubility relationship (AMIDON 1981). The membrane metabolic reconversion of peptide prodrugs to parent drugs can avoid the solubility/membrane permeability trade-off. Adjacent to the brush-border membrane, the outer membrane glycocalyx, into which the brush-border enzymes (including aminopeptidases, phosphatases, and other proteolytic enzymes) protrude, is an ideal prodrug reconversion site, as shown in Fig. 7 (AMIDON et al. 1985). The lipophilic parent drugs are released by the interfacial enzymes and then permeate through the brush-border membrane readily; thus precipitation of insoluble parent drugs is

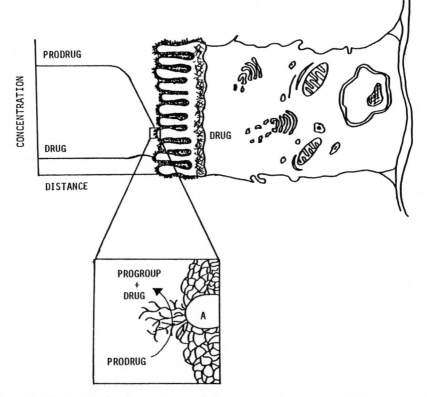

Fig. 7. Mechanism for improving oral absorption of water insoluble compounds. (Adapted from AMIDON et al. 1985)

minimized. At concentrations exceeding aqueous solubility of estrone, a significant increase in absorption rates of estrone is due to a five orders of magnitude increase in solubility by a lysine ester prodrug (AMIDON 1981). The solubility of hydrocortisone phosphate, a substrate of brush-border alkaline phosphatase, is three orders of magnitude greater than that of hydrocortisone (AMIDON et al. 1985; STEWART et al. 1986). It was shown that phosphate esters of hydrocortisone were well absorbed in dogs (FLEISHER et al. 1986).

F. Summary

Large peptide and protein drugs can be transported intact across the intestinal epithelium and pharmacological effects are observed. The actual mechanisms in the mature mammalian intestine remain to be understood. Energized by a H^+ gradient, the intestinal di-/tripeptide transporter has a broad substrate specificity. Small peptide-type drugs with or without an N-terminal α-amino group, such as β-lactam antibiotics and ACE inhibitors, are transported by this carrier system. The macroscopic mass balance analysis of membrane permeability predicts well the fraction dose absorbed in humans from the in situ studies for both peptide or nonpeptide drugs. The use of the peptide transporter and brush-border membrane peptidases to improve oral absorption of di-/tripeptide drugs and/or drugs as peptide prodrugs may be an effective oral delivery strategy in the future.

References

Adibi SA, Kim YS (1981) Peptide absorption and hydrolysis. In: Johnson LR (ed) Physiology of the gastrointestinal tract, 1st edn. Raven, New York, p 1037

Addison JM, Matthews DM, Burston D (1974) Evidence for active transport of the dipeptide carnosine (β-alanyl-L-histidine) by hamster jejunum in vitro. Clin Sci Mol Med 46:707–714

Addison JM, Burston D, Dalrymple JA, Matthews DM, Payne JW, Sleisenger MH, Wilkinson S (1975a) A common mechanism for transport of di- and tri-peptides by hamster jejunum in vitro. Clin Sci Mol Med 49:313–322

Addison JM, Burston D, Payne JW, Wilkison S, Matthews DM (1975b) Evidence for active transport of tripeptides by hamster jejunum in vitro. Clin Sci Mol Med 49:305–312

Amidon GL (1981) Drug derivatization as a means of solubilization: physicochemical and biochemical strategies. In: Yalkowsky SH (ed) Techniques of solubilization of drugs. Dekker, New York, p 183

Amidon GL, Stewart BH, Pogany S (1985) Improving the intestinal mucosal cell uptake of water insoluble compounds. J Control Rel 2:13–26

Amidon GL, Sinko PJ, Fleisher D (1988) Estimating human oral fraction dose absorbed: a correlation using rat intestinal membrane permeability for passive and carrier-mediated compounds. Pharm Res 5:651–654

Asatoor AM, Chadha A, Milne MD, Prosser DI (1973) Intestinal absorption of stereoisomers of dipeptides in the rat. Clin Sci Mol Med 45:199–212

Atisook K, Madara JL (1991) An oligopeptide permeates intestinal tight junctions at glucose-elicited dilations. Gastroenterology 100:719–724

Bai PF, Subramanian P, Mosberg HI, Amidon GL (1991) Structural requirements for the intestinal mucosal cell peptide transporter: the need for N-terminal α-amino group. Pharm Res 8:593–599

Bai PF, Hu M, Subramanian P, Mosberg HI, Amidon GL (1992) Utilization of peptide carrier system to improve the intestinal absorption: targeting prolidase as a prodrug converting enzyme. J Pharm Sci 81:113–116

Boyd CAR, Ward MR (1982) A micro-electrode study of oligopeptide absorption by the small intestinal epithelium of *Necturus maculosus*. J Physiol (Lond) 324:411–428

Burston D, Matthews DM (1987) Effects of sodium replacement on uptake of the dipeptide glycylsarcosine by hamster jejunum in vitro. Clin Sci 73:61–68

Cheeseman CI, Smyth DH (1972) Specific transfer process for intestinal absorption of peptides. Proc Physiol Soc Nov:45p–46p

Crane RK (1985) Comments and experiments on the kinetics of Na^+ gradient-coupled glucose transport as found in rabbit jejunal brush-border membrane vesicles. Ann NY Acad Sci 456:36–46

Das M, Radhakrishnan AN (1975) Studies on a wide-spectrum intestinal dipeptide uptake system in the monkey and in the human. Biochem J 146:133–139

Elliott RL, Amidon GL, Lightfoot EN (1980) A convective mass transfer model for determining intestinal wall permeabilities: laminar flow in a circular tube. J Theor Biol 87:757–771

Farquhar MG (1983) Multiple pathways of exocytosis, endocytosis, and membrane recycling: validation of a Golgi route. Fed Proc 42:2407–2413

Fleisher D, Johnson KC, Stewart BH, Amidon GL (1986) Oral absorption of 21-corticosteroid esters: a function of aqueous stability and intestinal enzyme activity and distribution. J Pharm Sci 75:934–939

Fricker G, Bruns C, Munzer J, Briner U, Albert R, Kissel T, Vonderscher J (1991) Intestinal absorption of the octapeptide SMS 201-995 visualized by fluorescence derivatization. Gastroenterology 100:1544–1552

Friedman DI, Amidon GL (1989a) Intestinal absorption mechanism of two prodrug ACE inhibitors in rats: enalapril maleate and fosinopril sodium. Pharm Res 6:1043–1047

Friedman DI, Amidon GL (1989b) The intestinal absorption mechanism of di-peptide ACE inhibitors of the lysyl-proline type: lisinopril and SQ 29,852. J Pharm Sci 78:995–999

Friedman DI, Amidon GL (1991) Oral absorption of peptides: influence of pH and inhibitors on the intestinal hydrolysis of Leu-enkephalin and analogues. Pharm Res 8(1):93–96

Ganapathy V, Leibach FH (1985) Is intestinal peptide transport energized by a proton gradient? Am J Physiol 249:G153–G160

Gonnella PA, Walker WA (1987) Macromolecular absorption in the gastrointestinal tract. Adv Drug Del Rev 1:235–248

Ho NFH, Day JS, Barsuhn CL, Burton PS, Raub TJ (1990) Biophysical model approaches to mechanistic transepithelial studies of peptides. J Controlled Release 11:3–24

Hu M, Amidon GL (1988) Passive and carrier-mediated intestinal absorption components of captopril. J Pharm Sci 77:1007–1011

Hu M, Sinko PJ, DeMeere ALJ, Johnson DA, Amidon GL (1988) Membrane permeability parameters for some amino acids and β-lactam antibiotics: applica-tion of the boundary layer approach. J Theor Biol 131:107–114

Hu M, Subramanian P, Mosberg HI, Amidon GL (1989) Use of the peptide carrier system to improve the intestinal absorption of L-α-methyldopa: carrier kinetics, intestinal permeabilities, and in vitro hydrolysis of dipeptidyl derivatives of L-α-methyldopa. Pharm Res 6:66–70

Hughson EJ, Hopkins CR (1990) Endocytotic pathways in polarized Caco-2 cells: identification of an endosomal compartment accessible from both apical and basolateral surfaces. J Cell Biol 110:337–348

Kidron M, Bar-On H, Berry EM, Ziv E (1982) The absorption of insulin from various regions of the rat intestine. Life Sci 31:2937–2941

Kramer W, Gutjahr U, Girbig F, Leipe I (1990) Intestinal absorption of dipeptides and β-lactam antibiotics. II. Purification of the binding protein for dipeptides and β-lactam antibiotics from rabbit small intestinal brush border membrane. Biochim Biophys Acta 1030:50–55

Lee VHL, Dodda-Kashi S, Grass GM, Rubas W (1991) Oral route of peptide and protein drug delivery. In: Lee VHL (ed) Peptide and protein drug delivery. Dekker, New York, pp 691–738

Lu HH, Thomas J, Fleisher D (1992) Influence of D-glucose-induced water absorption on rat jejunal uptake of two passively absorbed drugs. J Pharm Sci 81:21–25

Marcon-Genty D, Tome D, Kheroua O, Dumontier AM, Heyman M, Desjeux JF (1989) Transport of β-lactoglobulin across rabbit ileum in vitro. Am J Physiol 256:G943–G948

Matthews DM (1987) Mechanisms of peptide transport. Contrib Infusion Ther Clin Nutr 17:6–53

Matthews DM, Payne JW (1980) Transmembrane transport of small peptides. Curr Top Membr Trans 14:331–425

Merfeld AE, Mlodozeniec AR, Cortese MA, Rhodes JB, Dressman JB, Amidon GL (1986) The effect of pH and concentration on α-methyldopa absorption in man. J Pharm Pharmacol 38:815–822

Munck BG (1987) Intestinal absorption of amino acids. In: Johnson LR (ed) Physiology of the gastrointestinal tract, 2nd edn. Raven, New York, p 1097

Oh DM, Sinko PJ, Amidon GL (1989) Characterization of the oral absorption of some penicillins: determination of intrinsic membrane absorption parameters in the intestine in situ. Pharm Res 5:S-91

Oh DM, Sinko PJ, Amidon GL (1990) Peptide transport of β-lactam antibiotics: structural requirements for an α-amino group. Pharm Res 7:S-119

O'Hagan DT, Palin KJ, Davis SS (1987) Intestinal absorption of proteins and macromolecules and the immunological response. CRC Crit Rev Ther Drug Carrier Syst 4:197–221

Pappenheimer JR, Reiss KZ (1987) Contribution of solvent drag through intracellular junctions to absorption of nutrients by the small intestine of the rat. J Membr Biol 100:123–136

Rao RK, Koldovsky O, Korc M, Pollack PF, Wright S, Davis TP (1990) Processing and transfer of epidermal growth factor in developing rat jejunum and ileum. Peptide 11:1093–1102

Rajendran VM, Ansari SA, Harig JM, Adams MB, Khan AH, Ramaswamy K (1985) Transport of glycyl-L-proline by human intestinal brush border membrane vesicles. Gastroenterology 89:1298–1304

Rubino A, Field M, Shwachman H (1971) Intestinal transport of amino acid residues of dipeptides. I. Influx of the glycine residue of glycyl-L-proline across mucosal border. J Biol Chem 246:3542–3548

Saffran M, Bedra C, Kumar GS, Neckers DC (1988) Vasopressin: a model for the study of effects of additives on the oral and rectal administration of peptide drugs. J Pharm Sci 77:33–38

Schilling RJ, Mitra AK (1990) Intestinal mucosal transport of insulin. Int J Pharm 62:53–64

Sinko PJ, Amidon GL (1988) Characterization of the oral absorption of β-lactam antibiotics: I. Cephalosporins. Determination of intrinsic membrane absorption parameters in the rat intestine in situ. Pharm Res 5:645–650

Sinko PJ, Amidon GL (1989) Characterization of the oral absorption of β-lactam antibiotics. II. Competitive absorption and peptide carrier specificity. J Pharm Sci 78:723–726

Sinko PJ, Leesman GD, Amidon GL (1991) Predicting fraction dose absorbed in human using a macroscopic mass balance approach. Pharm Res 8:979–988

Stewart BH, Amidon GL, Brabec RK (1986) Uptake of prodrugs by rat intestinal mucosal cells: mechanism and pharmaceutical implications. J Pharm Sci 75:940–945

Stewart BH, Dando SA, Morrison RA (1990) In vitro uptake of SQ 29,852 by everted rat intestinal rings. Pharm Res 7:S516

Takaori K, Burton J, Donawitz M (1986) The transport of an intact oligopeptide across adult mammalian jejunum. Biochem Biophys Res Commun 137:682–687

Tamai I, Ling HY, Timbul SM, Nishikido J, Tsuji A (1988) Stereospecific absorption and degradation of cephalexin. J Pharm Pharmacol 40:320–324

Tomita Y, Katsura T, Okano T, Inui KI, Hori R (1990) Transport mechanisms of bestatin in rabbit intestinal brush-border membrane: role of H^+/dipeptide cotransport system. J Pharmacol Exp Ther 252:859–862

Tsuji A, Nakashima E, Kagami I, Asano T, Nakashima R, Yamana T (1978) Kinetics of Michaelis Menten absorption of amino-penicillins in rats. J Pharm Pharmacol 30:508–509

Tsuji A, Hirooka H, Tamai I, Terasaki T (1986) Evidence for a carrier-mediated transport system in the small intestine available for FK089, a new cephalosporin antibiotic without an amino group. J Antibiot (Tokyo) 39:1592–1597

Tsuji A, Tamai I, Hirooka H, Terasaki T (1987a) β-Lactam antibiotics and transport via the dipeptide carrier system across the intestinal brush-border membrane. Biochem Pharmacol 36:565–567

Tsuji A, Terasaki T, Tamai I, Hirooka H (1987b) H^+-gradient-dependent and carrier-mediated transport of cefixime, a new cephalosporin antibiotic, across brush-border membrane vesicles from rat small intestine. J Pharmacol Exp Ther 241:594–601

Tsuji A, Tamai I, Nakanishi M, Amidon GL (1990) Mechanism of absorption of the dipeptide α-methyldopa-Phe in intestinal brush-border membrane vesicles. 7:308–309

Walker WA (1981) Intestinal transport of macromolecules. In: Johnson LR (ed) Physiology of the gastroointestinal tract, 1st edn. Raven, New York, pp 1271–1289

Warshaw AL, Walker WA, Cornell R, Isselbacher KJ (1971) Small intestinal permeability to macromolecules. Lab Invest 25:675–684

Wood AJ, Maurer G, Niederberger W, Beveridge T (1983) Cyclosporine: pharmacokinetics, metabolism, and drug interactions. Transplant Proc 15:2409–2410

Yee S, Amidon GL (1990) Intestinal absorption mechanism of three angiotensin-converting enzyme inhibitors: quinapril, benazepril and CGS16617. Pharm Sci 7:S-155

Yoshikawa T, Muranushi N, Yoshida M, Yamada H, Oguma T, Hirano K (1989) Transport characteristics of ceftibuten, a new oral cephem, in rat intestinal brush-border membrane-vesicles – relationship to oligopeptide and amino beta-lactam transport. Pharm Res 6:308–312

D. Classical Problems

CHAPTER 7

Stereoselectivity in Metabolic Reactions of Toxication and Detoxication

J.M. MAYER and B. TESTA

A. Introduction

The present chapter does not aim to review the whole field of stereoselective xenobiotic metabolism and disposition (which many general reviews have already covered), but rather to focus on its significance in *molecular toxicology*. By the latter term, we mean the study of metabolic reactions of toxication and detoxication which affect drugs and all other classes of xenobiotics.

Drugs and other xenobiotics can elicit wanted effects (e.g., therapeutic response, parasite destruction) or unwanted effects (e.g., exaggerated pharmacological response, acute or chronic toxicity), both of which can be due to the parent compound and/or its metabolite(s). Considering only unwanted effects, i.e., toxicity, three situations can be schematized which emphasize the role of biotransformation in molecular toxicology and give an operational definition of toxication and detoxication.

A first possibility (Fig. 1A) is for the xenobiotic to be nontoxic but to give rise to a toxic metabolite (M_1). Very often, this reaction of toxication is competitive with other biotransformation reaction(s) which lead to inactive metabolite(s) (M_2), and as a rule, the toxic metabolite M_1 is itself transformed into an inactive metabolite (M_3) in a typical reaction of detoxication.

A second possibility (Fig. 1B) is for the xenobiotic and its metabolite M_1 to be toxic, in which case both metabolites M_2 and M_3 are products of detoxication reactions. A third possibility, by far the least frequent when chronic toxicity is concerned, is for only the xenobiotic to be toxic and all its metabolites to be inactive – a situation involving only reactions of detoxication.

How does stereoselectivity enter this scene and what is its role? These questions will be answered in Sects. C and D using selected and representative examples, but not before some general principles of stereoselective xenobiotic metabolism are briefly presented.

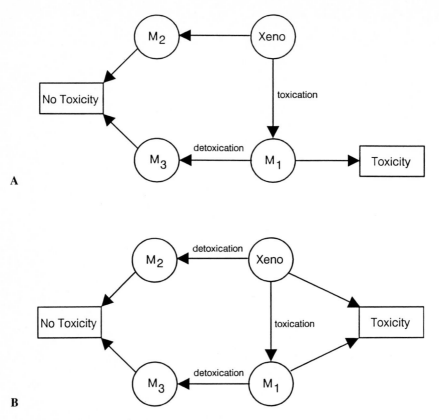

Fig. 1 A,B. Schematic cases of toxication and detoxication encountered in xenobiotic metabolism. In **A**, Xeno is nontoxic; in **B**, Xeno is toxic

B. Principles of Stereoselective Xenobiotic Metabolism

I. Chiral Recognition and Stereoselective Processes in Xenobiotic Metabolism and Disposition

One of the fundamental principles of pharmacodynamics, as formulated by Paul Ehrlich, is that compounds do not act unless bound. However, this rule is of such significance and scope that, far from being restricted to pharmacodynamic events, it also applies to pharmacokinetic and toxicokinetic events. Indeed, many processes in xenobiotic metabolism and disposition involve binding to biological macromolecules or macromolecular assemblies, covering a continuum of energies ranging from weak reversible bonds to covalent bonds. The only pharmacokinetic events not involving biological binding *stricto sensu* are reactions of non-enzymatic biotransformation (Testa 1982) and processes of passive diffusion (transport, excretion), although the passive partitioning into membranes is based on the same weak interactions as reversible binding and is thus conceptually comparable.

These molecular processes are necessary for a proper understanding of the fact that the enantiomers of a chiral drug display differences in their metabolism, protein binding, storage, distribution, and excretion, as abundantly documented in the literature (CAMPBELL 1990; TESTA and MAYER 1988). Indeed, their binding to a chiral biomolecule such as a macromolecule or an enzyme results in diastereomeric complexes and, at least in principle, in *chiral recognition* (TESTA 1979). The latter phenomenon is of fundamental significance in biology and accounts for enantioselective xenobiotic disposition in the organism. In contrast to enantiomers, diastereomers differ in their physicochemical properties and can be discriminated without a chiral tool; but because the tools of the biosphere (enzymes, macromolecules, membranes, etc.) are always chiral, such a theoretical distinction between enantiomers and diastereomers is of little pharmacokinetic relevance in practice.

As far as stereoselectivity is concerned, pharmacokinetic and toxico-kinetic events must be classified into two groups:

1. Only one type of stereoselectivity, namely the differential disposition displayed by stereoisomers, corresponds to the processes of absorption, distribution, binding, and excretion. This situation is comparable to that found in pharmacodynamic events. Thus, a large number of examples document differences, usually modest ones, in the binding of enantiomers to plasma proteins or in their tissue distribution (e.g., IGWEMEZIE et al. 1991; MEHVAR 1991; MÜLLER 1988).

2. Biotransformation reactions (i.e., metabolism in a narrow sense) are more complex than other processes of xenobiotic disposition and can display two basic types of stereoselectivity, namely substrate stereoselectivity and product stereoselectivity (JENNER and TESTA 1973; TESTA and MAYER 1988). The broad applicability of these concepts has been proven, as has their power in extracting valuable additional information from experimental studies (TESTA 1986; TRAGER and TESTA 1985; VERMEULEN and BREIMER 1983; WEERAWARNA et al. 1991); they are discussed further below.

II. Substrate Stereoselectivity and Product Stereoselectivity

Substrate stereoselectivity is seen when stereoisomers are metabolized (a) differentially (in quantitative and/or qualitative terms), and (b) by the "same" biological system under identical conditions. Substrate stereoselectivity, and principally enantioselectivity, is a well-known and abundantly documented phenomenon, be it under in vivo (WALLE and WALLE 1986) or in vitro conditions. Apparent and not absolute substrate stereoselectivity is usually observed. Biological factors, inhibition, competition between several metabolic routes, and concentration effects can all influence the observed selectivity.

Product stereoselectivity occurs when stereoisomeric metabolites are generated (a) differentially (in quantitative or qualitative terms) and (b) from a single chiral, prochiral, or proachiral substrate. Note that only apparent product stereoselectivity can be observed under a given set of experimental conditions.

All documented cases of product enantioselectivity, and most cases of product diastereoselectivity, result from the metabolic generation of a center of chirality from a suitable prochiral center or face. The most representative reactions are ketone reduction, methylene hydroxylation, oxidation of enantiotopic substituents, N-oxygenation, and sulfoxidation.

III. Substrate–Product Stereoselectivity

The question may be asked as to the influence of an existing center of chirality on the metabolic generation of a second such center in a given molecule. This phenomenon is known in synthetic chemistry as *asymmetric induction* and implies the preferential formation of one diastereomeric product from a chiral reactant. In asymmetric induction there is only one chiral tool, namely the preexisting chiral center. This contrasts with xenobiotic metabolism, where an enzyme is most frequently operative as a second chiral tool, implying that the concept of asymmetric induction must take a special meaning when applied to enzymatic reactions. Yet it is a common observation that product stereoselectivity can be different for two enantiomeric substrates, in other words that product stereoselectivity is itself substrate-enantioselective. The term "substrate–product stereoselectivity" was proposed a number of years ago to designate such cases (JENNER and TESTA 1973).

IV. Relevance to Molecular Toxicology

The concepts of substrate, product, and substrate–product stereoselectivity are indeed useful in ordering and clarifying many observations, for example within the perspective of molecular toxicology underlying the present chapter. Thus, substrate stereoselectivity in a reaction of toxication implies that one stereoisomer is preferentially transformed to a toxic metabolite or a reactive intermediate (e.g., Fig. 1A with Xeno being chiral, one enantiomer being metabolized selectively to M_1, and the other to M_2). Product stereoselectivity in reactions of toxication implies a different phenomenon, namely that the two stereoisomeric metabolites or metabolic intermediates formed from a single substrate have different toxicities (e.g., Fig. 1A with M_1 and M_2 being stereoisomers). The latter case, while of obvious toxicological significance, appears less well documented in the literature.

C. Toxicologically Relevant Examples of Stereoselective Metabolism

I. Introduction

As mentioned above, innumerable examples of stereoselective xenobiotic metabolism have been published, and results continue to accumulate at an impressive rate. As an illustration, a few selected and recent examples of stereoselective xenobiotic metabolism have been compiled in Table 1.

Less numerous but not rare are cases for which stereoselective metabolism is of documented or strongly suspected toxicological relevance. This is illustrated in Table 2, in which the examples pertain to drugs and other xenobiotics and reactions of functionalization and conjugation, as well as substrate stereoselectivity and product stereoselectivity. Some of the examples listed in Table 2 are discussed below.

II. Substrate Stereoselectivity in Drug Oxidation: Disopyramide and Mianserin

Disopyramide (Fig. 2A) is a chiral antiarrhythmic agent marketed as the racemic mixture of its $(-)$-(R)- and $(+)$-(S)-enantiomers. In vitro studies using rat hepatocytes revealed a considerably higher cytotoxicity of the (S)-enantiomer, particularly at lower concentrations, as assessed by leakage of lactate dehydrogenase and morphological changes. Metabolic studies conducted under similar conditions revealed an interesting case of substrate stereoselectivity in that N-dealkylation affected mainly the (R)-enantiomer while the (S)-enantiomer appeared to be transformed almost entirely by aromatic oxidation. The low cytotoxicity of the mono-N-dealkylated metabolite and the observed concentration effects were all consistent with the hypothesis that disopyramide elicits its toxicity via aromatic oxidation (LE CORRE et al. 1988).

The antidepressant mianserin (Fig. 2B) revealed analogies and differences with disopyramide. Indeed, aromatic oxidation in human liver microsomes occurred more readily with the (S)-enantiomer, while N-demethylation was the major route for the (R)-enantiomer. At low drug concentrations, cytotoxicity toward human mononuclear leukocytes was due to (R)-mianserin more than to (S)-mianserin, and showed a significant correlation with N-demethylation (RILEY et al. 1989). Thus for mianserin toxicity was associated with N-demethylation rather than aromatic oxidation, while the reverse appeared true for disopyramide. The chemical nature of the actual toxic intermediates was not established, but a comparison between disopyramide and mianserin emphasizes how each drug must be studied for itself.

Table 1. Some recent examples of stereoselective xenobiotic metabolism

Metabolic reaction	Xenobiotic	Enantioselectivity (biological model)	References
Hydroxylation	Propafenone	Stereoselectivity in 5-hydroxylation following incubation of individual isomers: V_{max} of (S)-isomer is twice that of (R)-isomer No stereoselectivity upon incubation of racemate, indicating interaction between enantiomers (Human liver microsomes)	KROEMER et al. (1991)
	Sparteine	(−)-Isomer forms (2S)-hydroxysparteine (+)-Isomer (pachycarpine) forms (4S)-hydroxypachycarpine (Rats)	EBNER et al. (1991)
N-Demethylation	Nicotine	Affects only (+)-(R)-isomer (Guinea pigs)	NWOSU et al. (1988)
O-Demethylation	Gallopamil	More extensive for (S)- than (R)-isomer (Rat, human liver microsomes)	MUTLIB and NELSON (1989)
N-Oxidation	Verapamil	Faster for (S)- than (R)-isomer (Rat, hog liver microsomes and purified FMO)	CASHMAN (1989)
	Nicotine	No selectivity in the formation of cis-(1′R,2′S)- and trans-(1′R,2′S)-N-oxide from (S)-nicotine (R)-nicotine produces only trans-(1′R,2′R)-N-oxide (Pig liver FMO)	DAMANI et al. (1988)

Reaction	Compound	Description	Reference
S-Oxygenation	2-Aryl-1,3-dithiolanes	Cytochrome P450 oxygenates exclusively the *pro-S* sulfur atom FMO oxygenates the *pro-R* sulfur atom (Rabbit lung enzyme preparations)	CASHMAN and WILLIAMS (1989)
Ketone reduction	Fenofibrate	Substrate enantioselectivity for (−)-isomer (Rats, guinea pigs, and dogs, not humans)	WEIL et al. (1989)
	Warfarin	(+)-(R)-isomer preferred substrate, mainly reduced to (RS)-alcohol (Liver cytosol, most species) Species-dependent substrate stereoselectivity (Liver microsomes)	HERMANS and THIJSSEN (1989)
O-Glucuronidation	Ofloxacin	(S)-Isomer better substrate (Rats)	OKAZAKI et al. (1990)
N-Glucuronidation	Verapamil Gallopamil	Stereoselective for (S)-isomer of demethylated metabolites (Rats)	MUTLIB and NELSON (1990)
Sulfation	Terbutaline	K_m identical for both isomers, V_{max} 8 times greater for (+)-isomer (Rat liver cytosol)	WALLE and WALLE (1990)
	4-Hydroxypropranolol	High stereoselectivity toward (+)-isomer (Human platelets)	WALLE and WALLE (1991)
Glutathione conjugation	Bromoisovalerylurea	Faster for (R)-isomer (Rat liver cytosol and microsomes, isolated hepatocytes, perfused liver)	TE KOPPELA et al. (1988)

Table 2. Some recent examples of toxicologically relevant enantioselective biotransformations

Xenobiotic	Enantioselective metabolism (biological model)	Toxicity or potential toxicity	References
Benzo[a]pyrene	Epoxidation to (7R,8S)-oxide followed by stereoselective hydrolysis, then second epoxidation to (7R,8S)-diol-(9S,10R)-epoxide; this isomer is the preferred substrate for glutathione conjugation (Rat liver cytosol and microsomes, purified enzymes)	(7R,8S)-Diol-(9S,10R)-epoxide is the more carcinogenic isomer, but is also efficiently detoxified by glutathione conjugation	Thakker et al. (1988), Yang (1988) Te Koppele and Mulder (1991)
Methylchrysene	Stereoselectively transformed to (1R,2R)-dihydrodiol (Rat, mouse liver and epidermis)	(R,R)-Enantiomer more tumorigenic in mouse skin	Amin et al. (1987)
Primaquine	Oxidative deamination stereoselective for (−)-isomer (Mice)	(−)-Isomer less toxic in mice due to its faster detoxication to carboxyprimaquine	Baker and McChesney (1988)
Disopyramide	N-Dealkylation $R > S$ Aromatic hydroxylation $R < S$ (Rat hepatocytes)	(S)-Enantiomer more cytotoxic due to phenolic metabolites	Le Corre et al. (1988)
Prilocaine	Faster hydrolysis of (−)-(R)-isomer (Mice)	Methemoglobinemia due to product of hydrolysis (o-toluidine)	Akerman and Ross (1970)
Mianserin	(S)-Isomer mainly hydroxylated (R)-isomer mainly N-demethylated (Human liver microsomes)	Cytotoxicity toward mononuclear leukocytes ($R > S$) correlated with N-demethylation	Riley et al. (1989)

Profens	Unidirectional chiral inversion from (R)- to (S)-isomer via stereoselective formation of an acyl-CoA conjugate (Species differences)	(R)-Isomer responsible for: – Long-lasting residues in adipose tissues – Stereospecific inhibition of triacylglycerol synthesis – Inhibition of mitochondrial β-oxidation producing microvesicular steatosis	WILLIAMS et al. (1986) SALLUSTIO et al. (1990) GENEVE et al. (1987)
Nabilone	Ketone reduction stereoselectively produces (SSS)-carbinol (Dog)	Accumulation of (SSS)/(RRR)-carbinol in brain: causative factor for CNS toxicity in chronically treated dogs	SULLIVAN et al. (1987)
Fenvalerate	Reduction minor pathway in monkeys Formation of cholesteryl ester only with (2R,αS)-isomer (Mammals)	Explains low toxicity in monkeys Granulomatous changes in liver, spleen, lymph nodes, and adrenals	KANEKO et al. (1988), MIYAMOTO (1990)
EM12 (an analogue of thalidomide)	Hydrolysis of piperidinedione ring; slower plasma elimination of the (S)-isomer; rapid racemization! (Callithrix jacchus, marmoset monkey)	Glutamic acid metabolites derived from (S)-enantiomer are clearly more embryotoxic and teratogenic	HEGER et al. (1988) SCHMAHL et al. (1988) SCHMAHL et al. (1988)
Phenytoin	Stereoselective p-hydroxylation of pro-S phenyl ring (Humans, animals except dog)	Gingival overgrowth caused by phenyl oxidation	RAO (1983)

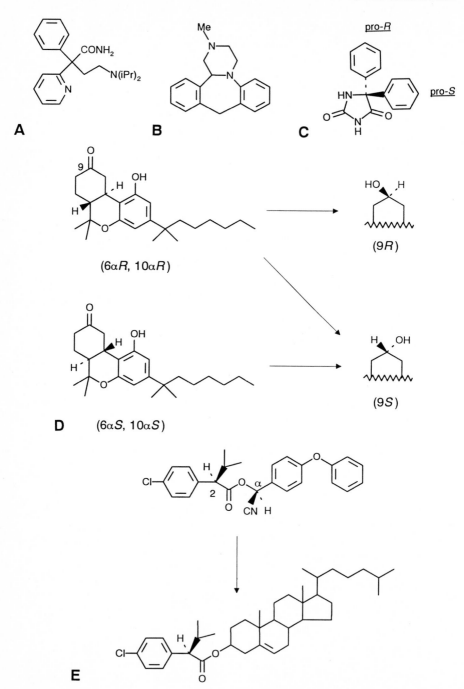

Fig. 2A–E. Chemical structure of disopyramide (**A**), mianserin (**B**), phenytoin (**C**), nabilone enantiomers and their 9-hydroxylated metabolites (**D**), and (2R,αS)-fenvalerate and its cholesterol-containing metabolite (**E**)

III. Product Stereoselectivity in Drug Oxidation and Reduction: Phenytoin and Nabilone

The widely used antiepileptic drug phenytoin (Fig. 2C) is known to induce gingival overgrowth in chronically treated patients. In the absence of surgical removal (gingivectomy), this overgrowth can reach severe stages. Significant levels of phenytoin and its *p*-hydroxylated metabolite were found in the gingivae of patients chronically treated with phenytoin, while in experimental animals both the drug and its metabolite were found to induce gingival overgrowth at concentrations comparable to those achieved in patients. Gingival toxicity is postulated to result from covalent binding of a reactive metabolite formed during phenyl oxidation (RAO 1983).

An inspection of the chemical structure of phenytoin (Fig. 2C) reveals it to be a prochiral compound by virtue of a center of prochirality featuring two enantiotopic phenyl rings. In humans and most experimental animals (an exception being the dog), the 4'-hydroxylated metabolite is predominantly the $(-)$-(S)-enantiomer (the S/R ratio in humans is approximately 10:1) (BUTLER et al. 1976; POUPAERT et al. 1975). This implies an enzymatic discrimination of the two enantiotopic groups with a marked recognition of the *pro-S* ring. Assuming the same product stereoselectivity for gingival cytochrome P450, it would be interesting to establish whether oxidation of the *pro-R* ring (as occurring in the dog) is a reaction of toxication of similar efficacy.

The synthetic 9-ketocannabinoid nabilone is an orally effective antiemetic agent used as the racemic mixture of the $(6aR,10aR)$- and $(6aS,10aS)$-enantiomer (Fig. 2D). The drug undergoes product stereoselective reduction of its prochiral 9-keto group to the corresponding carbinol. In the rat, dog, and monkey, the reaction is substrate stereoselective in that the (S,S)-enantiomer is reduced two- to three times faster than the (R,R)-enantiomer. In addition, reduction of the (S,S)-ketone yields almost exclusively the (S,S,S)-carbinol and is thus essentially product stereospecific, while the (R,R)-ketone yields a species-dependent mixture of the (R,R,R)- and (R,R,S)-carbinol (SULLIVAN et al. 1987).

The toxic consequences of this reaction are partly understood. The carbinol possesses a longer half-life than nabilone and shows a tendency to accumulate in the plasma of chronically treated animals. In addition, long-term studies in dogs revealed drug-related toxicity in the form of convulsions which have been ascribed to brain accumulation of the carbinol metabolite. Interestingly, the carbinol present in brain consisted only of a (nonracemic) mixture of the (S,S,S)- and (R,R,R)-stereoisomer, no (R,R,S)- and (S,S,R)-stereoisomers being found (SULLIVAN et al. 1987). Since the brain concentrations of the carbinol metabolite were five times those observed in plasma, it is conceivable that the $(S,S,S)/(R,R,R)$-carbinol has a better cerebral penetration and hence greater CNS toxicity than the $(S,S,R)/(R,R,S)$-carbinol.

IV. Substrate Stereoselectivity in Xenobiotic
Conjugation: Fenvalerate

The xenobiotic discussed here is not a drug but fenvalerate, a pyrethroid insecticide, while the metabolic reaction is one of conjugation. The compound (Fig. 2E) contains two centers of chirality and is used technically as a mixture of four stereoisomers, the most active (in insects) of which has the $(2S,\alpha S)$ configuration. The compound exhibits a highly complex metabolic behavior and undergoes a wealth of metabolic routes, each of which displays its own stereoselectivity and species differences (MIYAMOTO 1990).

In the course of extensive toxicological studies in mammals, granulomatous changes were observed in liver, spleen, lymph nodes, and adrenals. These changes result from the proliferation and tissue accumulation of mononuclear cells, a tissue response to injury caused by poorly soluble substances. Detailed investigations revealed granuloma formation to be due to a lipophilic conjugate, namely the cholesterol ester of (R)-2-(4-chlorophenyl)isovaleric acid. In addition, this metabolic route was substrate stereospecific since $(2R,\alpha S)$-fenvalerate was the only one of the four isomers to yield the cholesterol conjugate (MIYAMOTO 1990). This is thus a very clear example of substrate stereoselective formation of a toxic metabolite (Fig. 1A).

D. The Case of Profens

I. Metabolic Chiral Inversion: In Vivo and In Vitro Studies

2-Arylpropionic acids (profens) are a major group of nonsteroidal anti-inflammatory drugs (NSAIDs). These compounds exist in two enantiomeric forms due to the presence of an asymmetric carbon atom alpha to the carbonyl function (Fig. 3). In vitro tests have shown that the antiprostaglandin synthase activity of profens resides almost exclusively in the $(+)$-(S)-enantiomers (SHEN 1981), yet all profens except naproxen (Fig. 3A) are marketed as racemates. The profens exhibit enantioselective pharmacokinetics, the most intriguing aspect of which is their unidirectional chiral inversion from the $(-)$-(R)- to the $(+)$-(S)-enantiomer (Fig. 4).

The first evidence of the occurrence of metabolic chiral inversion was produced by MILLS et al. (1973), who observed that urinary metabolites of ibuprofen (Fig. 3B) in humans were dextrorotatory regardless of whether the (R)- or the (S)-enantiomer was administered. Investigation of the plasma levels of both enantiomers in healthy volunteers revealed the unidirectional nature of the inversion process (LEE et al. 1985). Indeed, substantial amounts of (S)-ibuprofen were detectable following administration of (R)-ibuprofen, whereas no (R)-ibuprofen was found after the administration of (S)-ibuprofen.

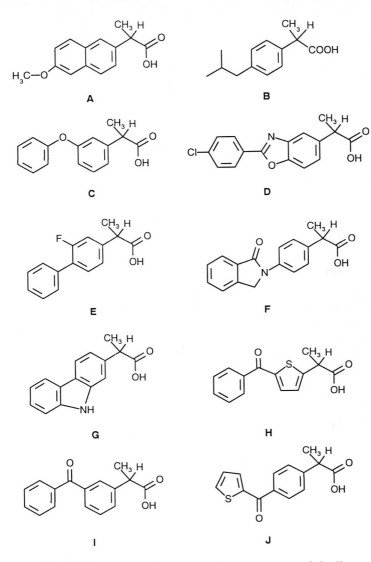

Fig. 3A–J. Chemical structure of some profens: naproxen (**A**), ibuprofen (**B**), fenoprofen (**C**), benoxaprofen (**D**), flurbiprofen (**E**), indoprofen (**F**), carprofen (**G**), tiaprofenic acid (**H**), ketoprofen (**I**), and suprofen (**J**)

However, not all profens undergo metabolic chiral inversion. Only two other profens, fenoprofen (Fig. 3C) (RUBIN et al. 1985) and benoxaprofen (Fig. 3D) (BOPP et al. 1979), have revealed significant inversion in humans. The stereoselective disposition of profens in laboratory animals does not always correspond to that observed in humans. Thus, the inversion half-life of (R)- to (S)-benoxaprofen in rat is about 2.6 h whereas the conversion in

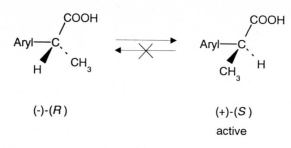

Fig. 4. The unidirectional chiral inversion of profens

humans is much slower (about 108 h) (SIMMONDS et al. 1980). Flurbiprofen (Fig. 3E) (JAMALI et al. 1988), indoprofen (Fig. 3F) (BUTTINONI et al. 1983), and carprofen (Fig. 3G) (KEMMERER et al. 1979) are not inverted in rats and humans. However, profens such as flunoxaprofen, tiaprofenic acid (Fig. 3H), and ketoprofen (Fig. 3I) undergo significant inversion in rats but are not inverted in man (FOSTER and JAMALI 1987; JAMALI 1988; PEDRAZZINI et al. 1988). There are other examples of important interspecies differences. Thus, ketoprofen, which is extensively inverted in the rat, shows less than 10% inversion in the rabbit (ABAS and MEFFIN 1987). No inversion occurs for 2-phenylpropionic acid in the mouse, in contrast to the rat and rabbit

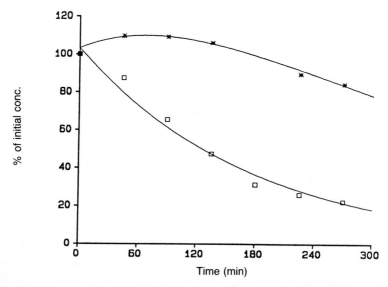

Fig. 5A–C. Time course of metabolic elimination of (−)-(R)-ibuprofen (*empty squares*) and (+)-(S)-ibuprofen (*asterisks*) from rat hepatocytes (5 × 10⁵ cells per ml) suspended in Hanks' buffer containing 0.5% bovine serum albumin (MÜLLER et al. 1990). **A** Incubation of the racemate; **B** incubation of (R)-ibuprofen; **C** incubation of (S)-ibuprofen

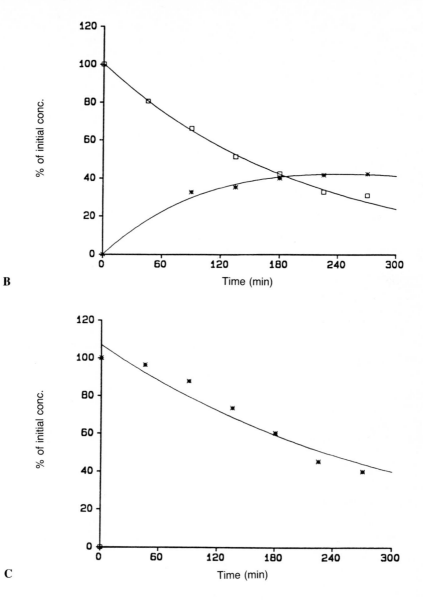

B

C

(Fournel and Caldwell 1986). It appears from this brief compilation that the rate of configurational inversion depends on both animal species and the nature of substrate, but no clear generalization can be made on the basis of the available data.

Early investigations of the chiral inversion of profens using hepatic subcellular fractions were not successful (Mayer et al. 1988), perhaps due to the lack of certain cofactors and/or to the destruction of cellular integrity during homogenization. The latter possibility has been confirmed by the efficiency of isolated hepatocytes and isolated perfused liver preparations in catalyzing the inversion of profens. Indeed, we have demonstrated that isolated rat hepatocytes are a suitable in vitro model for investigation of the metabolic chiral inversion of profens (MÜLLER et al. 1990). Figure 5 shows the concentration–time profiles of ibuprofen enantiomers during incubation. The isolated perfused rat liver preparation was the first biological model which allowed in vitro demonstration of the metabolic chiral inversion of ibuprofen (Cox et al. 1985). No inversion of flurbiprofen, suprofen (Fig. 3J), and naproxen was observed in the perfused liver, in agreement with in vivo results (MAYER 1990).

Oxidation and glucuronidation are major pathways in the biotransformation of profens. Both reactions can be substrate enantioselective and compete for the same substrate, and can therefore influence the rate and extent of chiral inversion. Such an influence has been reported for glucuronidation. In human subjects the coadministration of benoxaprofen and probenecid, an inhibitor of glucuronide formation and tubular secretion, not only reduced the amount of drug excreted as glucuronide but also changed significantly the enantiomeric ratio of the conjugates in favor of the (S)-isomer (SPAHN et al. 1987). Rabbits with renal dysfunction induced by uranyl nitrate showed a similar increase in the fraction of inverted (R)-2-phenylpropionic acid along with reduced clearance by processes other than inversion (MEFFIN et al. 1986). Based on these results it can be concluded that reduced glucuronidation increases the chiral inversion of profens.

Induction of oxidation does not seem to influence the metabolic inversion of profens. Thus, the clearance of (R)-fenoprofen by chiral inversion to (S)-fenoprofen was not affected by phenobarbital pretreatement (HAYBALL and MEFFI 1987). The clearance of (S)-fenoprofen by processes other than glucuronidation and elimination of unchanged drug in urine was induced by phenobarbital whereas that of (R)-fenoprofen remained unchanged. The absence of interaction between oxidative pathways and chiral inversion is also exemplified by the fact that preincubation with the cytochrome P450 inhibitor metyrapone did not detectably affect the chiral inversion of (R)-ibuprofen in isolated rat hepatocytes (SANINS et al. 1990).

II. Mechanism of Inversion

Despite the fact that the first observation of chiral inversion dates back to the early 1970s, the molecular mechanism of this transformation has yet to be fully elucidated. HUTT and CALDWELL (1983) have critically reviewed the various mechanisms postulated. The most likely mechanism involves activation of the 2-arylpropionic acid by formation of the acyl-coenzyme A thioester (NAKAMURA et al. 1981; WECHTER et al. 1974). The unidirectional inversion of configuration is explained in terms of the acyl-CoA formation

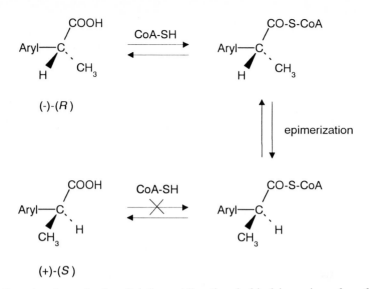

Fig. 6. Postulated mechanism for the unidirectional chiral inversion of profens via epimerization of 2-arylpropanoyl-coenzyme A thioesters (NAKAMURA et al. 1981)

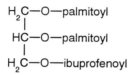

Fig. 7. Hybrid triglyceride: one fatty acid is replaced by a xenobiotic acid

being substrate enantiospecific for the $(-)$-(R)-enantiomer, while the $(+)$-(S)-enantiomer is not a substrate for the acyl-CoA synthetase(s) catalyzing the reaction. The (R)-thioester may then epimerize to the (S)-thioester, since coenzyme A is itself chiral, and the sequence is completed with the hydrolysis of the thioester (Fig. 6).

The first, albeit indirect, evidence of the participation of coenzyme A in the biotransformation of profens came from the demonstration that ibuprofen, ketoprofen, and fenoprofen incubated in rat liver slices are incorporated into "hybrid" triglycerides (Fig. 7) (FEARS et al. 1978). Indeed, this reaction necessarily implies the activation of the xenobiotic acid by formation of its coenzyme A conjugate. It is interesting to note that flurbiprofen (which does not undergo chiral inversion) is not incorporated into lipids (FEARS and RICHARDS 1981). Of particular relevance is the stereoselectivity of profen incorporation into lipids. Following chronic treatment of rats with (S)-ibuprofen, only a negligible amount of drug was incorporated into adipose tissues whereas after the administration of (R)-ibuprofen both

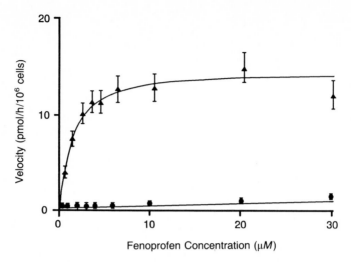

Fig. 8. Synthesis of fenoprofen-containing triacylglycerol by isolated adipocytes incubated in the presence of [³H]glycerol and (*R*)- (*triangles*) or (*S*)-fenoprofen (*circles*). (From Sallustio et al. 1988)

enantiomers were detected at significant levels in the lipids (Williams et al. 1986).

The first direct proof for the formation of hybrid triacylglycerols was obtained in isolated hepatocytes and adipocytes, where the synthesis of hybrid triglycerides from (*R*)-fenoprofen followed Michaelis-Menten kinetics and (*S*)-fenoprofen was a very poor substrate (Fig. 8) (Sallustio et al. 1988). The enzyme catalyzing stereoselectively the formation of (*R*)-fenoprofenoyl-CoA has been identified as the microsomal long-chain fatty acyl-CoA synthetase (EC 6.2.1.3) (Knights et al. 1988).

Studies carried out with regiospecifically deuteriated substrates showed that inversion of the (*R*)-enantiomer results in the loss of its α-methine deuterium (Baillie et al. 1989; Tanaka and Hayashi 1980). It has been proposed that the lability of the methine proton, as induced by the strong acidity-enhancing effect of the thioester bridge (Hilal and El-Aaeser 1985), favors configurational inversion by deprotonation at C(2).

III. Toxicological Consequences of Chiral Inversion

Gastrointestinal ulceration, the most common adverse effect of nonsteroidal anti-inflammatory drugs, is related to the ability of such drugs to inhibit the synthesis of prostaglandins. In this respect (*S*)-profens are more toxic than their (*R*)-antipodes. The observed intersubject variability in the response to profens appears to be influenced by the degree of inversion, which for (*R*)-ibuprofen may vary between 49% and 71% of the dose (Williams and Day 1985).

Unwanted effects may also be due to the formation of acyl-CoA conjugates capable of following the metabolic routes of fatty acids (CALDWELL 1984; CALDWELL and MARSH 1983). Thus, (R)-fenoprofen stereoselectively inhibits lipid biosynthesis (SALLUSTIO et al. 1990). The inhibition of the synthesis of cholesterol observed with racemic mixtures of various profens also appears to be correlated with their capacity to form acyl-CoA conjugates (FEARS and RICHARDS 1981). Pirprofen has been found to exhibit a concentration-dependent inhibition of mitochondrial β-oxidation of fatty acids, a finding postulated to account for the microvesicular steatosis produced by this drug (GENEVE et al. 1987). Ibuprofen and tiaprofenic acid similarly inhibited β-oxidation, but (S)-naproxen was inactive (GENEVE et al. 1987). The formation of long-lasting residues in adipose tissues is another cause of concern (WILLIAMS et al. 1986). And finally, it has been speculated that hybrid triglycerides may be incorporated into membranes and alter their function (CALDWELL and MARSH 1983). These observations suggest that the acyl-CoA conjugates of (R)-profens represent a pivotal point not only in their pharmacological activation but also in toxication pathways.

E. Conclusion

Chirality is an important issue in current drug research and development, and a lively debate is being conducted in industrial, governmental, and academic circles on the relative merits of racemic and optically pure forms of chiral drugs (TESTA and TRAGER 1990). As shown in this review, we have at best a fragmentary knowledge of the influence of stereochemical factors on reactions of toxication and detoxication in xenobiotic metabolism. While a number of examples have been investigated to a fair depth, general rules, if such exist, have failed to appear. We are therefore unable at present to venture generalizations of predictive value and have to continue case-by-case studies on the comparative metabolism of stereoisomers of drugs and other interesting xenobiotics.

But even studies of this type may prove unsatisfactory if they neglect one frequently overlooked phenomenon, namely metabolic interactions between stereoisomers. Indeed, evidence is beginning to accumulate that stereoisomers and particularly enantiomers may influence each other's metabolism, for example by acting as inhibitors (TESTA and TRAGER 1990). In such situations, the metabolic behavior of a racemate will not be the mere sum of the metabolism of its individual enantiomers, presumably leading to a shift in the relative importance of toxication and detoxication reactions. Metabolic interactions between stereoisomers thus add a new level of complexity to the issue under discussion, a level whose toxicological implications cannot be left unexplored.

References

Abas A, Meffin PJ (1987) Disposition of 2-arylpropionic acid nonsteroidal anti-inflammatory drugs. IV. Ketoprofen disposition. J Pharmacol Exp Ther 240: 637–641

Akerman B, Ross S (1970) Stereospecificity of the enzymatic biotransformation of the enantiomers of prilocaine (Citanest^R). Acta Pharmacol Toxicol (Copenh) 28:445–453

Amin S, Huie K, Balanikas G, Hecht SS, Pataki J, Harvey RG (1987) High stereoselectivity in mouse skin metabolic activation of methylchrysenes to tumorigenic dihydrodiols. Cancer Res 47:3613–3617

Baillie TA, Wade J, Adams WJ, Kaiser DG, Olanoff LS, Halstead GW, Harpootlian H, van Giessen GJ (1989) Mechanistic studies of the metabolic chiral inversion of (R)-ibuprofen in humans. J Pharmacol Exp Ther 249:517–523

Baker JK, McChesney JD (1988) Differential metabolism of the enantiomers of primaquine. J Pharm Sci 77:380–382

Bopp RJ, Nash JF, Ridolfo AS, Shepard ER (1979) Stereoselective inversion of (R)-(−)-benoxaprofen to the (S)-(+)-enantiomer in humans. Drug Metab Dispos 7:356–359

Butler TC, Dudley KH, Johnson D, Roberts SB (1976) Studies of the metabolism of 5,5-diphenylhydantoin relating principally to the stereoselectivity of the hydroxylation reactions in man and the dog. J Pharmacol Exp Ther 199:82–92

Buttinoni A, Ferrari M, Colombo M, Cesarini R (1983) Biological activity of indoprofen and its optical isomers. J Pharm Pharmacol 35:603–604

Caldwell J (1984) Xenobiotic acyl-coenzyme A: critical intermediates in the biochemical pharmacology and toxicology of carboxylic acids. Biochem Soc Trans 12:9–11

Caldwell J, Marsh MV (1983) Interrelationships between xenobiotic metabolism and lipid biosynthesis. Biochem Pharmacol 32:1667–1672

Campbell B (1990) Stereoselectivity in clinical pharmacokinetics and drug development. Eur J Drug Metab Pharmacokinet 15:109–125

Cashman JR (1989) Enantioselective N-oxygenation of verapamil by the hepatic flavin-containing monooxygenase. Mol Pharmacol 36:497–503

Cashman JR, Williams DE (1989) Enantioselective S-oxygenation of 2-aryl-1,3-dithiolanes by rabbit lung preparations. Mol Pharmacol 37:333–339

Cox JW, Cox SR, van Giessen G, Ruwart MJ (1985) Ibuprofen stereoisomer hepatic clearance and distribution in normal and fatty in situ perfused rat liver. J Pharmacol Exp Ther 232:636–643

Damani LA, Pool WF, Crooks PA, Kaderlik RK, Ziegler DM (1988) Stereoselectivity in the N′-oxidation of nicotine isomers by flavin-containing monooxygenase. Mol Pharmacol 33:702–705

Ebner T, Meese CO, Eichelbaum M (1991) Regioselectivity and stereoselectivity of the metabolism of the chiral quinolizidine alkaloids sparteine and pachycarpine in the rat. Xenobiotica 21:847–857

Fears R, Richards DH (1981) Association between lipid-lowering activity of aryl-substituted carboxylic acids and formation of substituted glycerolipids in rats. Biochem Soc Trans 9:572–573

Fears R, Baggaley KH, Alexander R, Morgan B, Hindles RM (1978) The participation of ethyl 4-benzoyloxybenzoate (BRL 10894) and other aryl-substituted acids in glycerolipid metabolism. J Lipid Res 19:3–11

Foster RT, Jamali F (1987) Stereoselective pharmacokinetics of ketoprofen in rat: influence of route of administration. Pharm Res 4:S-117

Fournel S, Caldwell J (1986) The metabolic chiral inversion of 2-phenylpropionic acid in rat, mouse and rabbit. Biochem Pharmacol 35:4153–4159

Geneve J, Hayat-Bonan B, Labbe G, Degott C, Letteron P, Freneaux E, Le Dinh T, Larry D, Pessayre D (1987) Inhibition of mitochondrial β-oxidation of fatty acids by pirprofen. Role in microvesicular steatosis due to this nonsteroidal anti-inflammatory drug. J Pharmacol Exp Ther 242:1133–1137

Hayball PJ, Meffin PJ (1987) Enantioselective disposition of 2-arylpropionic acid nonsteroidal anti-inflammatory drugs. III. Fenoprofen disposition. J Pharmacol Exp Ther 240:631–636

Heger W, Klug S, Schmahl HJ, Nau H, Merker HJ, Neubert D (1988) Embryotoxic effects of thalidomide derivatives on the non-human primate *Callithrix jacchus*. III. Teratogenic potency of the EM 12 enantiomers. Arch Toxicol 62:2–3

Hermans JJR, Thijssen HHW (1989) The in vitro ketone reduction of warfarin and analogues. Substrate stereoselectivity, product stereoselectivity and species differences. Biochem Pharmacol 38:3365–3370

Hilal R, El-Aaeser AM (1985) A comparative quantum chemical study of methyl acetate and S-methylthioacetate. Toward an understanding of biochemical reactivity of esters of coenzyme A. Biophys Chem 22:145–150

Hutt AJ, Caldwell J (1983) The metabolic chiral inversion of 2-arylpropionic acids – a novel route with pharmacological consequences. J Pharm Pharmacol 35:693–704

Igwemezie L, Beatch GN, Walker MJA, McErlane KM (1991) Tissue distribution of mexiletine enantiomers in rats. Xenobiotica 21:1153–1158

Jamali F (1988) Pharmacokinetics of enantiomers of chiral non-steroidal anti-inflammatory drugs. Eur J Drug Metab Pharmacol 13:1–9

Jamali F, Berry BW, Tehrani MR, Russell AS (1988) Stereoselective pharmacokinetics of flurbiprofen in humans and rats. J Pharm Sci 77:666–669

Jenner P, Testa B (1973) The influence of stereochemical factors on drug disposition. Drug Metab Rev 2:117–184

Kaneko H, Takamatsu Y, Okuno Y, Abiko J, Yoshitake A, Miyamoto J (1988) Substrate specificity for formation of cholesterol conjugate from fenvalerate analogs and for granuloma formation. Xenobiotica 18:11–19

Kemmerer JM, Rubio FA, McClain RM, Koechlin BA (1979) Stereospecific assay and stereospecific disposition of racemic carprofen in rats. J Pharm Sci 68:1274–1280

Knights KM, Drew R, Meffin PJ (1988) Enantiospecific formation of fenoprofen coenzyme A thioester in vitro. Biochem Pharmacol 37:3539–3542

Kroemer HK, Fischer C, Meese CO, Eichelbaum M (1991) Enantiomer/enantiomer interaction of (S)- and (R)-propafenone for cytochrome P450IID6-catalyzed 5-hydroxylation: in vitro evaluation of the mechanism. Mol Pharmacol 40:135–142

Le Corre P, Ratanasavanh D, Gibassier D, Barthel AM, Sado P, Le Verge R, Guillouzo A (1988) Rat hepatocyte cultures and stereoselective biotransformation of disopyramide enantiomers. Colloq Inserm 164:321–324

Lee EJD, Williams K, Day R, Graham G, Champion D (1985) Stereoselective disposition of ibuprofen enantiomers in man. Br J Clin Pharmacol 19:669–674

Mayer JM (1990) Stereoselective metabolism of anti-inflammatory 2-aryl-propionates. Acta Pharm Nord 2:197–216

Mayer JM, Bartolucci C, Maître JM, Testa B (1988) Metabolic chiral inversion of anti-inflammatory 2-arylpropionates: lack of reaction in liver homogenates, and study of methine proton acidity. Xenobiotica 18:533–543

Meffin PJ, Sallustio BC, Purdie YJ, Jones ME (1986) Enantioselective disposition of 2-arylpropionic acid non-steroidal anti-inflammatory drugs. II. 2-Phenylpropionic acid disposition. J Pharmacol Exp Ther 238:280–287

Mehvar R (1991) Apparent stereoselectivity in propafenone uptake by human and rat erythrocytes. Biopharm Drug Dispos 12:299–310

Mills RFN, Adams SS, Cliffe EE, Dickinson A, Nicholson JS (1973) The metabolism of ibuprofen. Xenobiotica 3:589–598

Miyamoto J (1990) Stereoselective metabolism and toxicology of pyrethroid. In: Holmstedt B, Frank H, Testa B (eds) Chirality and biological activity. Liss, New York, pp 153–168

Müller S, Mayer JM, Etter JC, Testa B (1990) Metabolic chiral inversion of ibuprofen in isolated rat hepatocytes. Chirality 2:74–78

Müller WE (1988) Stereoselective plasma protein binding of drugs. In: Wainer IW, Drayer DE (eds) Drug stereochemistry, analytical methods and pharmacology. Dekker, New York, pp 227–244

Mutlib AE, Nelson WL (1989) Pathways of gallopamil metabolism. Regioselectivity and enantioselectivity of the O-demethylation processes. Drug Metab Dispos 18:309–314

Mutlib AE, Nelson WL (1990) Synthesis and identification of the N-glucuronides of norgallopamil and norverapamil, unusual metabolites of gallopamil and verapamil. J Pharmacol Exp Ther 252:593–599

Nakamura Y, Yamaguchi T, Takahashi S, Hashimoto S, Iwatani K, Nakagawa Y (1981) Optical isomersation mechanism of $R(-)$-hydratropic acid derivatives. J Pharmacobiodyn 4:S-1

Nwosu CG, Godin CS, Houdi AA, Damani LA, Crooks PA (1988) Enantio-selective metabolism during continuous administration of S-$(-)$- and R-$(+)$-nicotine isomers to guinea pigs. J Pharm Pharmacol 40:862–869

Okazaki O, Kurata T, Tachizawa H (1990) Stereoselective metabolic disposition of enantiomers of ofloxacin in rats. Xenobiotica 19:419–429

Pedrazzini S, De Angelis M, Zanoboni MW, Furgione A (1988) Stereochemical pharmacokinetics of the 2-arylpropionic acid non-steroidal antiinflammatory drug flunoxaprofen in rats and in man. Arzneimittelforschung 38:1170–1175

Poupaert JH, Cavalier R, Claessen MH, Dumont PA (1975) Absolute configuration of the major metabolite of 5,5-diphenylhydantoin, 5-(4'-hydrophenyl)-5-phenyl-hydantoin. J Med Chem 18:1268–1271

Rao GS (1983) Drug metabolism in oral soft tissues. Pharm Int 4:103–106

Riley RJ, Lambert C, Kitteringham NR, Park BK (1989) A stereochemical investigation of the cytotoxicity of mianserin in vitro. Br J Clin Pharmacol 27:823–830

Rubin A, Knadler MP, Ho PPK, Bechtol LD, Wolen RL (1985) Stereoselective inversion of R-fenoprofen to S-fenoprofen in humans. J Pharm Sci 74:82–84

Sallustio BC, Meffin PJ, Knights KM (1988) The stereospecific incorporation of fenoprofen into rat hepatocyte and adipocyte triacylglycerols. Biochem Pharmacol 37:1919–1923

Sallustio BC, Knights KM, Meffin PJ (1990) The stereoselective inhibition of endogenous triacylglycerol synthesis by fenoprofen in rat isolated adipocytes and hepatocytes. Biochem Pharmacol 40:1414–1417

Sanins SM, Adams WJ, Kaiser DG, Halstead GW, Baillie TA (1990) Studies on the metabolism and chiral inversion of ibuprofen in isolated rat hepatocytes. Drug Metab Dispos 18:527–533

Schmahl HJ, Nau H, Neubert D (1988) The enantiomers of the teratogenic thalidomide analogue EM 12. I. Chiral inversion and plasma pharmacokinetics in the marmoset monkey. Arch Toxicol 62:200–204

Schmahl HJ, Heger W, Nau H (1989) The enantiomers of the teratogenic thalidomide analogue EM 12. II. Chemical stability, stereoselectivity of metabolism and renal excretion in the marmoset monkey. Toxicol Lett 45:23–33

Shen TY (1981) Nonsteroidal anti-inflammatory agents. In: Wolff ME (ed) Burger's medical chemistry, part 3, 4th edn. Wiley, New York, pp 1205–1261

Simmonds RG, Woodage TJ, Duff SM, Green JN (1980) Stereospecific inversion of (R)-$(-)$-benoxaprofen in rat and man. Eur J Drug Metab Pharmacokinet pp 5:169–172

Spahn H, Iwakawas S, Benet LZ, Lin ET (1987) Influence of probenecid on the urinary excretion rates of diastereoisomeric benoxaprofen glucuronides. Eur J Drug Metab Pharmacokinet 12:233–237

Sullivan HR, Hanasono GK, Miller WM, Wood PG (1987) Species specificity in the metabolism of nabilone. Relationship between toxicity and metabolic routes. Xenobiotica 17:459–468

Tanaka Y, Hayashi R (1980) Stereospecific inversion of configuration of 2-(2-isopropylindan-5yl)-propionic acid in rats. Chem Pharm Bull (Tokyo) 28:2542–2545

Te Koppele J, Mulder GJ (1991) Stereoselective glutathione conjugation by subcellular fractions and purified glutathione S-transferases. Drug Metab Rev 23:331–354

Te Koppele JM, Esajas SW, Brussee J, Van der Gen A, Mulder GJ (1988) Stereoselective glutathione conjugation of the separate alpha-bromo-isovalerylurea and alpha-bromoisovaleric acid enantiomers in the rat in vivo and in rat liver subcellular fractions. Biochem Pharmacol 37:29–35

Testa B (1979) Principles of organic stereochemistry. Dekker, New York

Testa B (1982) Nonenzymatic contributions to xenobiotic metabolism. Drug Metab Rev 13:25–50

Testa B (1986) Chiral aspects of drug metabolism. Trends Pharmacol Sci 7:60–64

Testa B, Mayer JM (1988) Stereoselective drug metabolism and its significance in drug research. Prog Drug Res 32:249–303

Testa B, Trager WF (1990) Racemates versus enantiomers in drug development: dogmatism or pragmatism? Chirality 2:129–133

Thakker DR, Levin W, Wood AW, Conney AH, Yagi H, Jerina DM (1988) Stereoselective biotransformation of polycyclic aromatic hydrocarbons to ultimate cancerinogens. In: Wainer IW, Drayer DE (eds) Drug stereochemistry. Analytical methods and pharmacology. Dekker, New York, pp 271–296

Trager WF, Testa B (1985) Stereoselective drug disposition. In: Wilkinson GR, Rawlins MD (eds) Drug metabolism and disposition: considerations in clinical pharmacology. MTP Press, Lancaster, pp 35–61

Vermeulen NPE, Breimer DD (1983) Stereoselectivity in drug and xenobiotic metabolism. In: Ariëns EJ, Soudijn W, Timmermans PBMWM (eds) Stereochemistry and biological activity of drugs. Blackwell, Oxford, pp 33–53

Walle T, Walle UK (1986) Pharmacokinetic parameters obtained with racemates. Trends Pharmacol Sci 7:155–158

Walle UK, Walle T (1990) Stereoselective sulfatation of terbutaline by rat liver cytosol: evaluation of experimental approaches. Chirality 1:121–126

Walle UK, Walle T (1991) Stereoselective sulfate conjugation of 4-hydroxypropanolol in humans: comparison of platelet and hepatic activity. Drug Metab Dispos 19:838–840

Wechter WJ, Loughhead DG, Reischer RJ, van Giessen GJ, Kaiser DG (1974) Enzymatic inversion at saturated carbon: nature and mechanism of the inversion of $R(-)$ p-iso-butylhydratropic acid. Biochem Biophys Res Commun 61:833–837

Weerawarna SA, Geissühsler SM, Murthy SS, Nelson WL (1991) Enantioselective and diastereoselective hydroxylation of bufuralol. J Med Chem 34:3091–3097

Weil A, Caldwell J, Guichard JP, Picot G (1989) Species differences in the chirality of the carbonyl reduction of [^{14}C]fenofibrate in laboratory animals and humans. Chirality 1:197–201

Williams KM, Day RO (1985) Stereoselective disposition – basis for variability in response to NSAIDs. Agents Actions 17 Suppl:119–126

Williams KM, Day R, Knihinicki R, Duffield A (1986) The stereoselective uptake of ibuprofen enantiomers into adipose tissue. Biochem Pharmacol 35:3403–3405

Yang SK (1988) Stereoselectivity of cytochrome P-450 isoenzymes and epoxide hydrolase in the metabolism of polycyclic aromatic hydrocarbons. Biochem Pharmacol 37:85–92

Interethnic Differences in Drug Disposition and Response: Relevance for Drug Development, Licensing, and Registration

L.P. Balant and P.G. Welling

A. Introduction

In 1982, Kalow introduced his review on "Ethnic differences in drug metabolism" by stating that: "the literature contains a number of examples of differences between populations in drug metabolizing capacity. Although this topic has been discussed previously as part of pharmacogenetics review, it deserves a new effort with different emphasis on a recently expanded data base. The topic should help improve understanding of human biology, and is of practical significance in pharmacology and toxicology." Ten years later the same statement is still true and considerable knowledge has been acquired at the molecular biology level. As a matter of fact, a recently published book on pharmacogenetics (Kalow 1992) contains important and extensive information on interethnic differences in drug metabolism. Accordingly, the authors of the present review decided to concentrate their presentation on aspects related essentially to drug development, licensing, and registration in the context of the new "4 W" environment (i.e., What and Why to present for World Wide drug registration). In this framework, pharmacokinetic/pharmacodynamic (PK/PD) relationships are also becoming of importance, as exemplified by a recent conference (Peck et al. 1992), and the authors felt that their presentation should deal also with some aspects of interethnic differences in drug tolerance and response. However, the wide-ranging subject of interethnic differences in drug response and tolerance will not be discussed in detail in the present review and interested readers are referred to treatises of internal medicine such as the *Harrison's* (Braunwald et al. 1988). Nevertheless, PK/PD relationships will serve as a reference framework for this chapter on interethnic differences in drug metabolism.

In order to concentrate on issues related to drug development, licensing, and registration, the chapter will dwell more on conceptual issues than on scientific bases of interethnic differences in drug metabolism, which are discussed in review articles as indicated in the bibliography. The Appendix to this chapter lists a selected number of publications dealing with the investigation of xenobiotics in different racial groups. They are, however, not discussed in detail in this review. As a consequence, most of the statements will represent personal opinions of the authors rather than established regulatory guidelines, which are essentially nonexistent in the context of interethnic differences or similarities in drug behavior and effects.

B. Case Reports

I. Unexpected Behavior

A parenteral cephalosporin developed in Japan was acquired by a US multinational pharmaceutical company for development and marketing in other countries (including the United States and Western Europe). The new drug had an adequate microbiological profile and an elimination half-life of more than 3h, permitting twice-a-day administration. This property was considered important since most drugs of the same class have a shorter half-life. In addition, elimination in Japanese healthy volunteers was about 50% by renal (CL_R = 20 ml/min) and 50% by nonrenal (CL_{NR} = 20 ml/min) processes.

On the first administration to Caucasian healthy volunteers (ALLAZ et al. 1979), it was surprising to observe that the elimination half-life measured only about 1.7h. Pharmacokinetic analysis showed that renal clearance was identical in Japanese and Caucasian subjects, but that nonrenal clearance in Caucasians was 60 ml/min, reducing renal excretion to 25% of the dose. Careful examination of the microbiological and kinetic data showed that, despite this difference, the drug was still a good candidate for twice-a-day administration in Caucasians, although the difference with similar drugs was not as striking as in Japanese patients.

Another interesting observation was made: some hours after completing the study, two out of eight volunteers showed a probable antabuse reaction when they had a "good" lunch with the money received for their participation in the study (ALLAZ et al. 1979). This reaction, which was confirmed in later studies, had not been detected in Japan. This is probably due to the fact that 50% of the Japanese population is defective in acetaldehyde dehydrogenase and, alcohol-induced flushing being a commonly observed reaction, this interaction had not been detected during phase I-III studies in the country of origin. In contrast, in Switzerland, where "flushes" are extremely rare, the reaction was immediately evident.

This case demonstrates why interethnic differences in behavior and effect must be evaluated early in the transfer of a drug from one racial group to another.

II. A Biopharmaceutical Dilemma

A substance used for the treatment of liver diseases was developed in Japan. Preclinical development was performed in different animal species and led to the conclusion that, from pharmacological and toxicological data, a dose of 600 mg per day (i.e., 10 mg/kg) was adequate for clinical trials in Japan. Systemic concentrations were not available for comparison between animal species and humans (L.P.B., personal observation).

When the drug was acquired by a European multinational company, one of the first steps was to compare the ADME profile between Japanese and Caucasian healthy volunteers. The behavior was indeed identical in the two groups (L.P.B., personal observation). However, Caucasians weighing generally closer to 75 kg than to 60 kg, the question was raised as to the dosage regimen. Since the elimination half-life was relatively short, one could think that steady-state concentrations (i.e., systemic clearance) may not be the most important factor for drug response at the hepatic level and, accordingly, a dose of 750 mg/day was chosen for clinical trials in Europe in order to be consistent with the Japanese hypothesis.

As a consequence, the Japanese formulation could not be used and a formulation had to be developed in Europe, tested for stability, and a bioequivalence trial performed before clinical trials could be started. The consequence was an important delay (as foreseen when the decision for 750 mg was taken) in the development program.

This case is interesting in the sense that it was not a difference in metabolic clearance which was a cause of concern, but body weight.

III. The Drug Which Did Not Become a Case

Early in the development of bufuralol, a β-blocking agent, it was suspected that its metabolism was under the control of a polymorphic enzyme (BALANT et al. 1976). During a phase 1 pharmacokinetic study, a volunteer suffered from marked orthostatic hypotension with simultaneous very high blood concentrations of parent drug and very low concentrations of the hydroxylated metabolite. Further work by the same group confirmed this hypothesis (DAYER et al. 1982, 1983). In Great Britain, investigators of the behavior of debrisoquine, an antihypertensive drug, found that a marked hypotensive response in one volunteer was due to impaired 4-hydroxylation of the drug (MAHGOUB et al. 1977). At about the same time, a group of physicians in Bonn observed increased side-effects associated with decreased oxidative metabolism of sparteine, an antiarrhythmic and oxytocic drug (EICHELBAUM et al. 1979). Since these early observations, numerous investigations have followed, indicating that the proportion of "poor" metabolizers is about 7% in Caucasian populations (see Chap. 9 by KROEMER et al. in the present volume).

Later, the development of bufuralol was stopped because there were already a number of β-blocking agents available. The relatively narrow therapeutic margin combined with the sensitivity of its metabolism to the debrisoquine/sparteine-type polymorphism was an additional reason for this decision.

This case is interesting since today we know the reason for the strange behavior of the volunteer in the early pharmacokinetic experiment. It must, however, be remembered that in 1974, when this early study was performed, polymorphic metabolism was not recognized. Let us imagine that bufuralol could have been synthesized and tested in China or Japan, before being licensed out for clinical testing in the United States and/or Europe. As mentioned above, among Caucasians, between 5% and 10% of subjects are classified as poor metabolizers (PM) (ALVAN et al. 1990). This proportion drops to less than 1% in native Chinese of both Han and Mongolian origin (LOU et al. 1987). Similar results were obtained with mainland Chinese from Hunan (HORAI et al. 1989). Three studies in native Japanese (NAKAMURA et al. 1985; ISHIZAKI et al. 1987; HORAI et al. 1989) have also shown that there is a low proportion of PM in this population (from 0% to 2.5%). It is thus highly probable that in China or Japan, bufuralol would not have shown the adverse properties which led to the interruption of its developmental program. This could have had important consequences in the case of its transfer to North America or Europe. It must also be remembered that bufuralol was a special case among the β-blocking agents, having a relatively narrow therapeutic margin.

The knowledge we have today must also caution those who would be tempted to oversimplify the subject. In further studies of the debrisoquine/ sparteine polymorphism, using genomic leukocyte DNA from some Chinese and analysis of restriction fragment length polymorphisms (RFLPs), a number of Chinese with low metabolic ratios (i.e., EM phenotype) were shown to be genotypically PM (YUE et al. 1989). This study indicates that the antimode for a probe drug determined in one population might not be appropriate for another and that, in the Chinese, the antimode for the debrisoquine-metabolic ratio is probably lower than in Caucasians. The mechanism behind the dissociation between debrisoquine hydroxylation phenotype and genotype is not known. It is possible that the Chinese, in addition to debrisoquine hydroxylase (CYPIID6), have another enzyme able to hydroxylate debrisoquine. Another possibility is that the gene which is inoperative in the Caucasian PM is operational in the Chinese, producing debrisoquine hydroxylase (BERTILSSON 1990).

This case, together with its long history, also helps to distinguish two basically different situations:

1. A drug is developed and it is rapidly detected (using human microsomes or any other appropriate technique) that its metabolism is under the control of a known polymorphism. The situation is well documented in different racial groups and adequate strategies may be devised to overcome potential and foreseeable problems.
2. A drug is developed and its metabolism is under the control of an unknown polymorphism. The facts provided above, and the hypothesis of the discovery of an "oriental bufuralol," demonstrate the complexity

of the potential problems that may be encountered by partners of a licensing agreement.

Finally, it is most probable that genetic polymorphism in drug metabolism does not explain all differences in drug response found between different ethnic groups since environmental factors certainly also play an important role. In addition, it is possible, as discussed below, that pharmacodynamic differences in response exist in different groups. As an example, despite the fact that propranolol is metabolized faster in Chinese subjects than in Caucasians, the Chinese are more sensitive to the β-blocking effect. Stereoselective metabolism of the drug does not explain these differences, suggesting a pharmacodynamic cause for the increased sensitivity (ZHOU and WOOD 1990).

IV. The Drug Which Is Not a Case

Studies in the Chinese and Japanese (NAKAMURA et al. 1985; HORAI et al. 1989) have shown that 15%–22% of these individuals are PM of S-mephenytoin, whereas the proportion is less than 5% among Caucasians (KÜPFER and PREISIG 1984). Although this polymorphism has been found to be of little clinical relevance up to now, the situation might change. For example, the finding that the metabolism of diazepam (mainly N-demethylation) and desmethyl-diazepam (mainly C-hydroxylation to oxazepam) is related to S-mephenytoin hydroxylation, but not to debrisoquine hydroxylation (BERTILSSON et al. 1989), together with the fact that there are more PM of S-mephenytoin among Orientals than among Caucasians, could be of great interest (SANZ et al. 1989). GHONEIM et al. (1981) had indeed shown that Orientals had a lower metabolic clearance than Caucasians. Interestingly, in another study it was noted that "many Hong-Kong physicians routinely prescribe smaller diazepam doses for Chinese than for white Caucasians" (KUMANA et al. 1987).

In the case of diazepam, the therapeutic margin is wide. Accordingly, even if a genetic polymorphism in drug metabolism should be confirmed as a major determinant in interindividual variability, its clinical relevance would be relatively difficult to assess and it might thus well escape detection, even during drug development in different ethnic groups.

C. Basic Concepts and Definitions

Before discussing the pharmacokinetic and pharmacodynamic implications of "interethnic" differences for new drug development, it is important to define some concepts which may have different meanings outside of the scientific field.

Species, *racial*, or *ethnic classifications* have different significance depending on their context of use. The definitions given below are those from *Churchill's Medical Dictionary* (1989).

- *Species* [L (from *specere* to see, observe) a sight, aspect, appearance, form, type, particular kind]. A taxonomic collection of interbreeding populations that are reproductively isolated from other such collections. A group of closely related species forms a genus.
- *Race* [Middle French, from Italian *razza* race, kind]. A subspecies or other division or subdivision of a species. Human races are generally defined in terms of original geographic range and common hereditary traits which may be morphological, serological, hematological, immunological, or biochemical. The traditional division of mankind into several well-recognized racial types such as Caucasoid (white), Negroid (black), and Mongoloid (yellow) leaves a residue of populations that are of problematical classification, and its focus on a limited range of visible characteristics tends to oversimplify and distort the picture of human variation.
- *Ethnic* [Gk *ethnikos* (from *ethnos* a nation, people) national, of a people]. Designating the physical and cultural traits that distinguish members of one society or larger human group from members of other such groups.

Since the scope of this review is to address issues related to drug development and use in large groups of people, without regard for divisions which are merely of a tribal, linguistic, or political nature, the terms "racial" and "ethnic" will be considered as virtually interchangeable in the majority of cases. However, in some cases the term "racial" will be used to focus on genetic traits, whereas "ethnic" will be used to encompass environmental factors as well. As an example, a difference in drug metabolism observed in second-generation Asians living in North America with the same life habits as Caucasians will be termed "racial," whereas the same observation made in Japan or China will be termed "ethnic" as long as the underlying causes (i.e., genetic and/or environmental) have not been elucidated.

Basically, the behavior of all drugs is determined, at least to some extent, by genetic factors. It is thus possible to state that "pharmacogenetics" is a basic component of the interindividual variability of all drugs. It is however, customary to restrict the term *"pharmacogenetics"* to the situation where one or more distinct subpopulations can be identified as far as their metabolic capacities towards drugs or groups of drugs are concerned.

Genetic factors influencing drug metabolism can be mono- or polygenic. If they are of monogenic type, they present either as polymorphisms or as rare phenotypes. A *genetic polymorphism* is a monogenic trait that exists in the population in at least two phenotypes and at least two genotypes, neither of which is rare, i.e., less frequent than 1% (MEYER et al. 1990).

Genetic polymorphisms of drug metabolism usually segregate the population into two groups differing in their ability to metabolize certain drugs.

Individuals with a deficient metabolism are termed "poor metabolizers" (PM), as compared to "extensive metabolizers" (EM).

For more information on genetic polymorphisms, consult Chap. 9 by Kroemer et al. in the present volume.

Drugs may mean different entities depending on the context. The nomenclature adopted here is that of the European Community (COUNCIL DIRECTIVE 1965), according to which:

– A *substance* is a "chemical", e.g., element, naturally occurring chemical material, or chemical product obtained by structural change or synthesis. Insofar as a substance shows pharmacological activity it may be termed an "active substance" or, if intended for use as a medicinal product, a "drug" or the "active drug."

– A *medicinal product* is any substance or combination of substances presented for treating or preventing disease in human beings or animals. The term *drug product* will be used as a synonym.

In this review, the word "drug" will be used as a generic term rather than "medication."

In the context of this review, *clinical trials* imply (a) systematic studies in humans designed to discover or verify the pharmacodynamics, the therapeutic effects, and/or the adverse reactions of medicinal products, and (b) human pharmacokinetic studies as defined by the European Communities. The acceptance of this definition has important consequences, since it implies adherence to some formal rules, including those of good clinical practice.

– *Phase 1 trials* of a new active substance in man are conducted in healthy volunteers, with a few exceptions such as cytostatic agents and immunomodulators. Phase 1 makes reference not only to timing in drug development but also to a basic methodological aspect, in the sense that fate and effects of drugs are investigated in healthy volunteers. Accordingly, phase 1-type studies can be performed at any time in the life cycle of a drug, for example, as bioequivalence studies after the medicinal product has been in clinical use for many years.

– *Phase 2 trials* are pilot therapeutic studies in patients. They are usually explorative (controlled or not) during phase 2a and controlled in phase 2b. One important objective is to provide information on dose–response relationships, or better, on dose–concentration–response relationships. The pharmacodynamic parameters thus obtained are often short-term response parameters, the so-called surrogate endpoints.

– *Phase 3 trials* are the classical clinical trials. Here, drug response is frequently assessed by monitoring short-term parameters.

– *Phase 4 trials* are performed after marketing of the final medicinal product. At this stage, clinical trials exploring new indications, new pharmaceutical formulations, new methods of administration, new dosage regimens, or new target subpopulations are considered as trials of new medicinal products having similar objectives as premarketing trials. Such studies may consequently require trial conditions as defined for phase 1, 2, or 3. This is particularly true for pharmacokinetic and bioavailability studies.

The concepts underlying *pharmacokinetics* in the present review are well known and suitably described in textbooks. The terms "pharmacokinetics" and "drug disposition" are often used interchangeably, whereas "toxicokinetics" and "drug metabolism" have more restricted meanings. These words are applicable to endogenous and exogenous substances alike, while the term "xenokinetics" generally covers the study of any exogenous compound (i.e., xenobiotic), be it a drug, a potential drug, or neither. In order to avoid confusion, the term "pharmacokinetics" will be used in this review as a generic term qualifying the study of the kinetics of absorption, distribution, metabolism, and excretion (ADME) of substances or medicinal products active in preventing or treating human diseases.

The term *metabolite(s)* will be used to define biotransformation products considered pharmacokinetically and/or pharmacodynamically relevant. In some cases, such substances represent an important part of the pharmacokinetic profile in blood or excreta. As a rule of thumb, one may consider that pharmacokinetically relevant metabolites are characterized by blood concentrations similar to or higher than those of the parent compound and/or which individually represent more than 30% of the measurable excreted substances. In other cases, metabolites, even when present in low concentrations, may contribute significantly to the therapeutic or toxic effects of the drug and can be of pharmacodynamic relevance.

D. Integration of Pharmacokinetic, Pharmacodynamic, and Toxicokinetic Principles in Drug Development

I. The Conceptual Framework

The overall benefit that the integration of pharmacokinetics and pharmacodynamics in preclinical and clinical studies can produce is an early identification of optimal dosing regimens, thus shortening the overall time of drug development (PECK et al. 1992). Of equal importance, the increased understanding of drug action derived from PK/PD integration leads to a more informative drug development program, especially with regard to identification of dosage regimens that result in optimal therapeutic outcome through strategies for *individualization of dosage.*

A critical step in the complex process of drug development is to decide whether animal and early human studies of drug response suggest useful clinical activity (HOLFORD 1992). Useful clinical activity is supported initially by demonstrating a potential therapeutic effect. A therapeutic effect may be shown by demonstrating that a significant difference exists in comparison with a placebo or a reference drug. While this kind of binary decision making is presently the normal case in drug development, it does not describe the complexities of using a drug which are usually recognized when it is subsequently widely used. Accordingly, it has been advocated (PECK et al. 1992) to use the PK/PD approach to link dosage with knowledge of drug disposition, and coupling that with observable clinical outcomes. This paradigm is particularly useful for dose finding during phase 1 and phase 2 studies. Since discovery of optimal dosing regimens early in drug development may contribute to efficient drug development programs by mitigating failed clinical trials, it is obvious that this information should be acquired early in the development process. This is even more important if registration is intended in different ethnic groups for which differences in pharmacokinetic and/or pharmacodynamic parameters may be observed.

II. Preclinical Studies

During preclinical studies, determination of systemic drug concentration ranges that are associated with pharmacological action and toxicological effects of a drug [or its metabolite(s)] may aid in development of human dosing regimens and may indicate the likely steepness of the dose–concentration–response curve in humans. In addition, concentration monitoring used to determine extent of exposure during safety evaluation studies (toxicokinetics) is essential to substantiate safety assessments and to assist in interpretation of unanticipated toxicity.

III. Phase 1 Studies

The well-accepted objectives of phase 1 studies are to define the initial parameters of tolerance and effect (if measurable in healthy volunteers) and their relation to dosage and relevant pharmacokinetics of the drug. These studies are also intended to optimize the drug delivery system and to probe potential drug–drug interactions that might be expected to perturb the PK/PD relationship. Accordingly, whenever possible, parallel measurements of systemic concentrations and acute effects should be performed in order to provide data for PK/PD modeling. In this context, it must be stressed that the importance of the dosage form is often unappreciated, leading to premature commitment to suboptimal formulations. Such a premature decision, prior to full characterization of PK/PD relationships, may have severe consequences in future steps in drug development. Clearly, feedback is needed between the results obtained in patients during phase 1 and phase 2 bioavailability studies.

PK/PD modeling during phase 1 studies is restricted to those drugs for which acute effects can be measured in healthy volunteers. Quantitative data analysis too often deals with calculation of pharmacokinetic parameters only and neglects simultaneous consideration of pharmacodynamic aspects. This is a result of the lack of appropriate pharmacological endpoints or because of the difficulty in their quantitative assessment. In addition, in many instances, such an approach is not attempted because it is felt that the measurable effects are without clinical relevance. However, in many cases it is probable that linking measured systemic drug concentrations with observations of acute toxic effects or intolerance (pharmacodynamic) may lead to preliminary definition of maximum safe drug concentrations and doses (PECK 1992). Such an approach is certainly closer to the "pharmacokinetic screen" discussed below than to traditional PK/PD modeling using integrated models. Similar considerations apply for early phase 2 clinical trials during which only a small and selected number of patients are studied.

IV. Phase 2 Studies

The principal goal of phase 2 studies is to provide unequivocal evidence of the desired therapeutic effect. A second major goal is to gain information that will guide phase 3 clinical trials. Often, however, phase 2 is shortened and hence the extra time needed to explore the full dose range and various dose intervals to obtain good dose- and concentration–response information may not be committed. Undoubtedly, this approach can be successful and it can be rapid, but on too many occasions failure to define dose–concentration–response relationships leads to unacceptable toxicity or adverse effects, marginal evidence of effectiveness, and lack of information on how to individualize dosing. This is especially true when phase 3 is designed with a series of concurrent studies that allow no opportunity for the results of one trial to influence the design of subsequent studies. It is in this context that the concept of *randomized concentration-controlled clinical trials* has been proposed (PECK 1992). In these types of studies, subjects are randomized into separate ranges of average plasma drug concentrations achieved by PK-controlled dosage. As discussed below, this concept can certainly be adapted to the particular problems raised by new drug development in different ethnic groups.

V. Phase 3 Clinical Studies

In phase 3 clinical trials, systemic drug concentration data, apart from those related to concentration–response trials (as performed during phase 2), should be routinely obtained on a survey basis to help explain unusual responses, to suggest the possibility of either the presence of or lack of drug–drug and drug–disease interactions, and to identify other unanticipated variability such as metabolic heterogeneity (BALANT et al. 1989). Even a well-developed and carefully planned program cannot anticipate all possibilities. Moreover, specific studies of all possible subsets and interactions are costly, time consuming, and probably unnecessary. The *pharmacokinetic screen* (a small number of blood level measurements taken in some or all patients), coupled with integrated analyses of effectiveness and safety data, or using more *formal population models*, can be used to identify and quantify important demographic and other subset differences.

Large-scale phase 3 clinical trials are usually designed to have maximum efficiency for rejecting the null hypothesis of no treatment effect. The usual design is the *randomized controlled clinical trial*. As such, they are usually one-factor (drug), two-level (zero dose and maximum safe dose) designs which measure a single univariate endpoint per patient (e.g., time to a clinical event), and are generally applied to a homogeneous patient population. When overall efficacy of standard treatments is the central question, such designs serve well. However, the central issue of ultimate efficacy for modern drugs is maximization of the benefit–risk ratio for individual patients (SHEINER 1992). These individuals may come from apparently homogeneous populations, or from populations where racial and/or environmental factors may play a decisive role in drug efficacy and toxicity. In this context, a series of questions must be answered: What is the relationship between input profile and dose magnitude on the one hand, and beneficial or harmful pharmacological effects on the other? How does this relationship vary with individual patient characteristics? Studies designed to answer these questions must be factorial (i.e., study several treatments simultaneously) and multilevel (e.g., study multiple dose magnitudes). They must also measure multiple (overtime), possibly multivariate responses in a deliberately heterogeneous patient population (SHEINER 1992). Heterogeneity may be introduced by age, gender, comedications, concurrent diseases, etc. or racial and life habit diversities. In order to improve the discriminatory power of data analysis, it is probably valuable to obtain some type of information on dose–concentration relationships and, accordingly, it may be of interest to systematically take some blood samples from the patients enrolled in phase 3 clinical trials.

Data interpretation may be based on data collected according to the pharmacokinetic screen concept. In this situation, collection of trough levels during clinical studies is recommended in order to detect patient groups at risk of an altered dose–concentration–effect relationship. A more complex approach termed "population pharmacokinetics," is based on a more intensive data collection scheme, more complex PK/PD models, and a higher level of sophistication of the statistical methodology (VOZEH 1992; EBELIN et al. 1992; see also Chap. 15 by STEIMER et al. in the present volume). These concepts have recently been discussed, and controversial positions have been expressed. It is not the intention of the authors to discuss the advantages or disadvantages of this approach in the development of a new drug under normal conditions. They do, however, feel that these concepts should be considered and possibly adapted to the requirements of drug development in different ethnic groups.

VI. Regulatory Considerations

In the European Communities, similar views have been expressed as in the United States (GUNDERT-REMY 1992). It can be anticipated that in the future, the concept will prevail that a full understanding of the pharmacokinetics and pharmacodynamics of a new drug in preclinical animal species and humans provides a scientific framework for efficient and rational development. There is presently a general consensus on the content of pharmacokinetic documentation needed to support the choice of a dosage regimen with respect to efficacy and safety. The required information will of course depend largely upon the kinetic properties of the active principle(s), the therapeutic margin, the indication(s) for the new drug, and the potential subpopulations such as aged persons or patients with renal insufficiency. It must, however, be stressed that pharmacokinetic programs are based largely on the assumption that the target populations will be of a homogeneous type as far as potential interethnic differences in drug behavior and action are concerned. This will not necessarily be the case in the future because there is growing concern that, with the increased trend for people to migrate to other countries, "minorities" may acquire the status of "subpopulations" which may require special attention during drug development, even if the new medication is not a priori intended for use in parts of the world other than the country of origin.

VII. Interethnic Differences in Drug Behavior and Action and PK/PD Integration

It is clear, as indicated in the previous section, that the potential of an integrated PK/PD approach depends on the interplay between pharmacokinetic and metabolic profiles, pharmacological activity, therapeutic margin, clinical endpoints, indications, and patient populations. Similar considerations certainly apply for the transfer of a medication from one racial group to another. It seems, as illustrated in the "typical cases" (Sect. B), that an understanding of the behavior of the drug in different ethnic groups is of crucial importance. At this stage, it may be of interest, as underlined by KALOW (1982), to discuss briefly some methodological issues. There is a need for systematic distinction between clinical pharmacological studies designed to elucidate the fate and effects of a drug using a few subjects, and studies intended to assess the distribution of drug-metabolizing characteristics in populations: the first type of study emphasizes the drug, the second the people.

In the context of new drug development the pharmaceutical industry can be expected to devote time and resources to investigate the potential impact of interethnic differences in drug metabolism for an active substance for which it can be assumed from preclinical or clinical data that such differences might be clinically relevant. It is, however, not practical to ask industry to perform, systematically, the second type of studies for all new chemical entities intended for human use. Costs and timing would become prohibitive if strategies used for the investigation of the acetylation or debrisoquine/sparteine polymorphisms were adopted as standard procedures for all new chemical entities. Despite these limitations there might nevertheless be a case for utilizing ad hoc population approaches during phase 1–3 clinical trials in order to gain some insight into potential interethnic differences in drug fate and effects. This subject will be addressed in more detail in following sections of this chapter.

E. Preclinical Studies

It is important, in the framework of interethnic differences in drug behavior and response, to briefly discuss some of the problems encountered in interspecies differences in kinetics. A discussion of differences in drug response is too far-reaching for the present review but information can be found in the pharmacological and toxicological literature.

There are two main reasons for conducting animal pharmacokinetic studies during drug development (BALANT et al. 1990). The first is to gain insight into the behavior of the new medication and the second is to consolidate the safety evaluation in animals. The first type of study may be conducted with some degree of freedom in experimental protocols, whereas the second type is much more regulated and must be performed in accordance with good laboratory practice.

Main objectives of formal animal pharmacokinetic studies are:

– Assessment of drug and metabolite concentrations and kinetics in blood, body fluids, and organs; simultaneously metabolite structures can be elucidated and their potential activities investigated
– Gathering of information on the relationship between target organ toxicity and blood or body fluids or organ concentrations
– Assessment of possible enzyme induction and drug accumulation on repeated administration

It is now well recognized that volume of distribution and renal clearance are consistent across species in the sense of the allometric concept, provided plasma protein binding is similar. This is due to the fact that tissue diffusion and renal handling are essentially passive processes, with the exception of tubular secretion. These passive processes are determined in part by the physicochemical properties of the substance (molecular weight, lipophilicity, pK_a, etc.) and by its binding to plasma proteins. In contrast to these passive processes, metabolic reactions are less predictable and very large differences may exist between species. These differences may manifest themselves at both the quantitative and the qualitative level. Accordingly, the metabolism of a new drug must be investigated in all species used in safety evaluation.

This is particularly important if the structure of "endpoint metabolites" suggests that formation of "reactive metabolites" may vary in rate and extent in different mammalian species. The qualitative–quantitative aspects of drug metabolism are important in selecting the animal species best suited for long-term toxicity studies. If no good relationship can be found between a rodent species, a nonrodent species, and humans, it is better to choose an animal species in which all human metabolites are formed, even if quantitative differences exist, than to choose an animal species quantitatively similar for some metabolites, but with qualitative differences as far as potentially active or toxic metabolites are concerned.

In toxicological and toxicokinetic studies, emphasis is placed on the fact that pharmacokinetics should serve as a basis for selection of appropriate species for toxicity testing, and for reliable prediction of human drug safety. Comparative semiquantitative information on blood levels and metabolic patterns in animals and humans represents a minimal requirement. However, it must be realized that the goal of animal species selection based on comparative pharmacokinetic data is seldom achieved in full. Toxicologists argue that it is still preferable to conduct studies in well-known animal species such as the Wistar rat or the Beagle dog (for which there is a considerable amount of information) than in exotic, less well-known species on the ground that their metabolic pattern is closer to the one observed in healthy young human males. Clearly, this is a controversial issue, but the role of the pharmacokineticist remains that of providing the most reliable and relevant information for a rational choice of animal species used for safety assessment. This is particularly difficult if different metabolic patterns are observed in different human racial groups.

F. Phase 1 Studies and Interethnic Differences

I. Investigational Pharmacokinetics

It is now well accepted that, if in vitro data obtained with human microsomes or human hepatocytes indicate that the metabolism of a new compound might be under the control of a known genetic polymorphism, the first studies in healthy volunteers should ideally be performed in panel consisting of both extensive and poor metabolizers (BALANT et al. 1989). If the difference between the two groups shows potential clinical significance, special care must be taken in the development of the new compound. If the contrary is true, drug development may generally proceed without this requirement. Until recently, it was customary to extend this type of targeted pharmacokinetic investigation to ethnic groups other than the main ethnic component of the country of origin of the compound only if it was evident that licensing out to countries with other ethnic majorities was a prime goal in the development of the new medication (see Sect. I). However, today it is becoming increasingly evident that, with the important migrations that characterize the later part of this century, other strategies must be examined if the new drug product is to be marketed in multiethnic countries or different geographical areas.

In this context, as well as for licensing purposes, two situations may be distinguished: (a) the metabolism of the drug is under the control of a known polymorphism, and (b) no defined polymorphism has been detected. In the first case, specific study designs may be used combining ethnic groups and metabolizer status. In the second case no specific recommendations may be given at this stage of drug development and it is probably necessary to wait for phase 3 studies using the pharmacokinetic screen approach (or others) in order to detect eventual ethnic differences in drug metabolism and response (see Sect. H).

One point which needs special attention is the potential difference in *stereoselective metabolism* which might occur in different ethnic groups when specific metabolism pathways are under the control of genetic polymorphisms. This may be exemplified with metoprolol, a β-blocking agent administered as a racemic mixture of its enantiomers. In preliminary reports, stereoselectivity in its disposition (HERMANSSON and VON BAHR 1982) was reported before it was known that metabolism is under the control of the debrisoquine/sparteine polymorphism. Later, the pharmacokinetics of its enantiomers have been investigated in panels of extensive and poor metabolizers following oral racemic administration (LENNARD et al. 1983). Significantly higher plasma concentrations of the active $(S)(-)$-enantiomer as compared to the inactive $(R)(+)$-enantiomer were observed in extensive metabolizers, whereas in poor metabolizers this stereoselectivity was decreased. Maximum plasma concentrations of both enantiomers were higher and the elimination half-life was longer in poor metabolizers. The results of a study in which extensive metabolizers were given an oral dose of pseudoracemic metoprolol indicate that preferential O-demethylation of the inactive $(R)(+)$-enantiomer contributes to its more rapid clearance [relative to the $(S)(-)$-enantiomer] in this phenotypic group. This difference in metabolic rates is probably absent in poor metabolizers. Thus, not only is the overall clearance of metoprolol lower in poor metabolizers, but the ratio of the active and inactive enantiomers is also different in the two groups of subjects. This is an excellent example of pharmacokinetically important differences in drug metabolism. The main question, however, relates to the clinical relevance of this finding when one tries to deduce guidelines for the potential impact of such drug behavior in two hypothetical ethnic groups, one comprising only extensive metabolizers and the other poor metabolizers.

As discussed by LENNARD (1992), the "total plasma" metoprolol concentration β-blockade profile is shifted to the left in extensive metabolizers compared to poor metabolizers, a finding compatible with the higher plasma concentrations of the active isomer in the extensive metabolizer phenotype. Since a greater pharmacological effect would be expected in extensive metabolizers than in poor metabolizers at a given total $[(R) + (S)]$ plasma drug concentration, the magnitude of the difference of drug effect between phenotypes would tend to be less than that indicated by the pharmacokinetics of the sum of the enantiomers. The confounding fact is that there is a large absolute difference in β-blocking action between the two phenotypes, as well as in total drug concentration. Lennard (1992) concludes that these differences cannot be explained by stereoselectivity in the pharmacokinetics of metoprolol. At this stage of this rather complicated story, it would probably be clinically more relevant to conduct a phase 2 trial in hypertensive patients from the two hypothetical ethnic groups, combined with pharmacokinetic analysis in order to gain insight into drug behavior in the target populations.

II. Investigational Pharmacodynamics

There are some well-documented cases of drugs or drug families for which interethnic differences exist in terms of efficacy or tolerance. Thus, among the congenital defects, by far the most common is glucose-6-phosphate dehydrogenase (G6PD) deficiency. Individuals with the Mediterranean-type G6PD have a more unstable enzyme than other genotypes and therefore a much lower overall enzyme activity than, for example, blacks with the A-variant. Such patients are at risk of suffering from a fulminant hemolytic crisis following exposure to oxidants such as sulfa-drugs or some fava beans. Clearly the impact of this defect on the tolerance of a new drug cannot be tested in healthy volunteers and in vitro methods using red blood cells from sensitive subjects must be used. Such a procedure is mandatory, for example, if a new drug with a physicochemical profile close to sulfa-drugs is to be marketed in Sardinia where the Mediterranean type of G6PD is particularly important. This is a situation in which intolerance to a drug is independent of the pharmacokinetic profile. This example emphasizes, as already discussed, that pharmacodynamic aspects should not be neglected in the context of new drug development in different racial or ethnic groups, even if these aspects are only superficially discussed in this chapter.

In other situations, kinetics and dynamics are more closely related. As an example, response to hydralazine therapy is dependent upon the acetylation phenotype. The hypotensive effect of hydralazine is greater in patients who acetylate the drug slowly, and the lupus erythematosus-like syndrome produced by hydralazine occurs almost exclusively in those with slow acetylation. Similarly, early studies in healthy volunteers suggested that side-effects of bufuralol (see Sect. B.III) were to be associated with slow metabolizers (Balant et al. 1976). This finding was later confirmed in a larger panel of healthy subjects (Dayer et al. 1982) and related to the debrisoquine/sparteine phenotype. However, here again, one must distinguish between cases for which a polymorphism in drug metabolism is known and cases for which such knowledge is not available. In the case of bufuralol, the discovery of the polymorphism was accidental, one volunteer out of six in an exploratory pharmacokinetic study being a poor hydroxylator of the drug. It then took years of work to elucidate the mechanism of the observed effects and to define the clinical relevance of this finding. As mentioned before, bufuralol did not finally reach the market place.

Psychopharmacology represents an interesting field in the context of drug behavior and effects in the sense that some scientists have been aware for more than 25 years that there are important "transcultural" differences in response to psychotropic drugs. As shown in the Appendix, and as discussed in Sect. B.IV for diazepam, some of these differences may result from pharmacokinetic factors, but other reasons must also be investigated. In 1979, KATZ et al., discussing methodological problems involved in the "transcultural" development and use of psychotropic medications and focusing on East (i.e., Asia) versus West (i.e., Europe and North America) differences, asked the following questions: "Can a drug which is found to be effective in one country be used equally well but in a significantly smaller dosage in another country? Must clinicians be sensitive to expected differences when applying the result of a clinical trial in one country to other national settings, particularly when the other settings are culturally quite different?" KATZ et al. then concluded that "Despite increasing concern over the past 20 years with these practical problems, there has been little scientific action directed toward solving them." The impetus given to pharmacogenetics and interethnic studies by the discovery of the debrisoquine/sparteine and mephenytoin polymorphisms seems to have changed this attitude. As an example, two review papers addressing such issues for Hispanic and native Americans (MENDOZA et al. 1991), as well as black Americans (STRICKLAND et al. 1991), have been published recently. It is also interesting to note in Sect. III of the Appendix that among the pharmacokinetic studies performed in Asians and Caucasians, a majority concern substances with psychotropic activity.

III. Bioavailability Investigations

Interracial differences have limited potential impact on the outcome of investigations on *relative bioavailability*. Indeed, from the present literature there is no evidence that a drug formulation intended for oral administration will behave differently in the gastrointestinal system of healthy subjects from different racial groups, at least in the fasting state. The situation becomes more complicated if nutritional parameters are included. It can be debated whether such factors should be considered as purely environmental or as part of the "ethnic package." As an example, a drug product used in Japan may show (in its country of origin) different systemic availability than in Japanese subjects living in the United States and having a different lifestyle. From these considerations it appears that in planning relative bioavailability studies, the racial and ethnic components of potential interest should always be considered. However, no formal recommendations may be given in this respect.

The situation is different for *absolute bioavailability* studies, in which hepatic first-pass metabolism may be of importance. In this case differences may occur in different racial groups. Similar considerations to those presented in Sect. F.I apply for study design and interpretation. Experience gained with drugs that are under the control of the debrisoquine/sparteine polymorphism shows that important differences and high interindividual variability may be observed (KUBLI et al. 1982). As an example, in one study of bufuralol, systemic clearance was found to be about 37 l/h in extensive metabolizers and only about 15 l/h in poor metabolizers (DAYER et al. 1985). It was shown that polymorphic metabolism had a major influence on the extent of hepatic first-pass elimination, as judged by the large variability in systemic availability. Since, for safety reasons, the intravenous dose used in the study was smaller than the oral doses, the calculated apparent absolute availability exceeded 100% in a healthy volunteer phenotyped as a "very poor" metabolizer, reflecting the fact that nonlinear kinetics probably occurred at the higher oral doses used.

Finally, it must be stressed that if a substance is prone to produce side-effects in some ethnic groups for pharmacogenetic reasons, care should be taken to select subjects in order to avoid safety problems.

IV. Bioequivalence Studies

Since bioequivalence studies are designed primarily to compare pharmaceutical formulations and not to study the behavior of active principles, it is highly probable that the results of such studies performed with the same formulations in different racial groups under *fasting conditions* would have similar outcomes. However, if the metabolic control by a genetic polymorphism is present at different frequencies in the two racial groups this might alter the results of such investigations. In this case, it may be appropriate to phenotype the volunteers before testing.

The situation is probably not as simple if *food effects* are studied and one might, for example, question the relevance of testing a drug product in China in combination with the typical Anglo-Saxon "high-fat standard" breakfast. There is, however, too little published experience to enable recommendations to be made on this subject.

G. Phase 2 Studies

As stated previously, the results of phase 2 investigations should provide information on dose–concentration–response relationships. In the context of interethnic differences, it is particularly important to obtain kinetic information in order to distinguish between *pharmacodynamic* and *pharmaco-*

kinetic factors. However, as illustrated by a study with angiotensin I in healthy black and white volunteers (JOUBERT and BRANDT 1990), *environmental factors* should also be considered. The study was conducted in order to explore the well-documented fact that black hypertensives tend to respond poorly to some antihypertensive medications. In this study, blacks exhibited a significantly greater angiotensin I sensitivity than whites. Plasma renin activities were similar in the two groups and could thus not explain the observed differences. In contrast, blacks had significantly higher urinary sodium values and it was thus concluded that the differences in the two groups could be due largely to differences in dietary sodium intake.

Although this study is not strictly speaking a phase 2 study since it was performed in healthy volunteers, it underlines the necessity to record all information potentially useful for data interpretation. It also indirectly shows that pharmacokinetic data must be obtained. As a matter of fact, had no sodium effect been detected, the absence of data on plasma concentrations of the angiotensin I would have made data interpretation very difficult. This example underlines, as discussed in earlier sections of this chapter, the potential advantage of including pharmacokinetic data in pharmacodynamic investigations. In the present case, kinetics of the active substance were apparently not involved; this is, however, not always the case, as previously discussed for some psychotropic medications.

The influence of environmental factors on the pharmacokinetics of drugs is very complex, and detailed information on this subject is presented in Chap. 10 by PELKONEN and BREIMER in this volume.

H. Phase 3 Studies

As discussed in Sect. D.V, there is a general tendency to use strict inclusion and exclusion criteria for phase 3 studies in order to maximize the chances of reaching statistically significant results in favor of the drug under development. This leads, however, to "information-poor" data as far as different covariables such as age, race, or concomitant diseases are concerned. It is thus necessary to reconsider this attitude if a new chemical entity is intended to be used in different ethnic settings and, as discussed above, implementation of population approaches such as the pharmacokinetic screen or the more complex population kinetic models might be cost-effective means of detecting interethnic differences in drug effects.

I. Phase 4 Studies in the Context of Drug Product Licensing

If a drug product is developed involving essentially healthy subjects and patients of a single racial group, and if the product is to be commercialized in a geographical area where another racial group is predominant, some precautions must be taken as far as safety and efficacy are concerned. The same measures should be taken if a drug product is licensed from a parent company to its subsidiary or if an agreement is reached between two independent corporations. As an example, Darmansjah and Muchtar (1992) have listed a number of drugs which display a specific action pattern in Indonesia as compared to Europe or North America: a formulation of lesser strength had to be introduced for prochlorperazine used as an antiemetic, lower doses of chlorpromazine are used for the treatment of schizophrenia, and similar measures had to be taken with sympathomimetic and β-adrenergic blocking drugs. The same authors also reported pharmacokinetic differences for rifampicin and diazepam and concluded that "Clinicians and those who conduct trials in Asia should be aware of these differences in drug response, and the industry should be encouraged to look at the problem more thoroughly."

I. Pharmacoanthropological Considerations

As stated by Kalow (1992), "that there are interethnic differences in drug-metabolizing capacity is now a well established fact. . . . Nevertheless, it is not clear how frequent or how widespread genetic differences are, nor is it clear how many differences are dependent on culture, lifestyle, or choice of foods. . . . ." Accordingly, questions are raised as "to what extent these differences are of medical and toxicological consequences? . . . Whether, or under what circumstances, some of the recognized, genetically controlled differences in metabolic capacity can be ignored, and when they need to be considered in order to protect important segments of a population from harmful effects of drugs . . . ?" As already mentioned in Sect. F.II, differences in drug response are also of crucial importance, even if they are only briefly addressed in this review.

In the context of worldwide drug development the interethnic differences in behavior and action of drugs which have not yet been discovered are probably as important as those which have already been discovered. However, literature on this subject is naturally limited and one must rely for the most part on anecdotal reports. In this context it is usual to guess rather than to plan what action should be undertaken in order to provide drugs with maximum efficiency and minimum side-effects in various continents and regions.

Kalow (1984) has proposed that pharmacoanthropology be defined as the branch of pharmacology (or clinical pharmacology?) that deals with interethnic differences in *response to* or *metabolism of* drugs and toxicants. The reference to anthropology is meant to indicate that the inquiry is of scientific rather than political nature, and is not biased by considering only genetic or only cultural factors; it thereby differs from pharmacogenetics, which deals specifically with hereditary variations in drug metabolism.

As discussed in Sect. C, in classical genetics three main human races are recognized: the Caucasoids, the Negroids, and the Mongoloids. In addition, two other races comprising less individuals are distinguished: the Bushmen and the Australian aborigines. However, as far as drug development is concerned, each of the large races consists of subgroups (e.g., characterized by well-defined genetic polymorphisms in drug metabolism) and any group tested will be somewhat different from the "average" Caucasoid, "average" Mongoloid, or "average" Negroid (KALOW 1992). The question then arises to what extent races should be considered when testing new drugs in the context of a world-wide development. As already briefly discussed in Sect. D.VII, it is not possible to test drugs under all possible situations and ad hoc strategies must be developed.

In this context it is appropriate to mention the European Concerned Action COST B1, which resulted in 1989 in the European Consensus Conference on Pharmacogenetics, a conference attended by scientists from academia, the pharmaceutical industry, and regulatory agencies. The conference aimed at reaching a consensus on optimal approaches to deal with polymorphic drug metabolism, particularly with regard to drug development.

II. Studies in Healthy Volunteers

It may be advantageous to perform, at an early stage, comparative pharmacokinetic trials in target populations. There are no specific guidelines for such studies. It is, however, probably wise to use the same pharmaceutical formulation as administered in key pharmacokinetic trials in the country of origin. The protocol should be as close as possible to some reference protocol used to determine the "fingerprint" in the population of origin. Blood concentration curves and urinary excretion and metabolic patterns should be determined under identical conditions.

It could be argued that it would be preferable to conduct the study in parallel in one single setting in order to minimize variables. As an example, one could study Caucasian Americans and Americans of Japanese origin in the United States. Such a study design has the advantage of homogeneity, but it does not take into account nongenetic factors such as food or environmental effects. The alternative is to compare two groups of subjects studied simultaneously in two locations or to use a "historical" control cohort.

III. Studies in Patients

The same considerations as are expressed in Sects. D.IV, D.V, G, and H on phase 2 and 3 studies apply in the context of licensing a drug product from one ethnic setting for use in another. One may once again emphasize the importance of some form of pharmacokinetic information being obtained in such studies. Such data are important not only in order to understand possible interethnic differences but also to provide a rational basis for potential dosage regimen modification or dosage strength changes.

J. Conclusions

Pharmacogenetic differences in drug behavior and effects can be studied in two totally different situations: (a) the drug is under the control of a known polymorphism, and (b) nothing is known about polymorphism regulating enzymes or receptors. In both cases, it must be recognized that differences in the proportion of subjects of one or another phenotype in different racial groups will induce differences in drug response. Interethnicity provides the additional dimension of environmental or life-style factors. A number of combinations of these factors is possible and it is not possible to give guidelines that would be valid on all occasions.

An interesting point in the context of worldwide drug development is the analysis of the impact on research efforts of the knowledge, or not, of the existence of a polymorphism. As seen in the Appendix, the literature on N-acetyltransferase or debrisoquine/sparteine oxidation contains a number of papers related to interethnic differences or ethnic characteristics. If one were to add studies for which an ethnic group is not specifically mentioned in the title of the paper, but which are based essentially on racially homogeneous subjects, then the Appendix would more than double in size. As an example, many recent studies of N-acetyltransferase have examined possible links with diseases so numerous that it is impossible to list them here (EVANS 1992). Another example is the explosive and exponential appearance of papers relating debrisoquine/sparteine polymorphism to possible ethnic groups which could be studied. The fundamental question that must be raised in the context of new drug development is whether the published material is a good indicator of the relevance of the subject. The answer is probably no. This answer is in part substantiated by the fact that there are probably numerous unpublished studies within the archives of pharmaceutical companies showing that their drug products behaved identically in a number of ethnic groups. Accepting this fact allows the problem of interethnic differences during drug development to be tackled in a (hopefully) pragmatic matter.

Despite the numerous potential combinations of genetic and environmental factors, it would appear that for new drug development two basic situations may be envisaged. The consequences for developmental strategies are then clearly different. The simple situation arises when a drug is under the control of a known polymorphism in drug metabolism. The development strategy is then relatively easy in that study design can be deduced from available knowledge, and answers can be obtained in a relatively straightforward manner, allowing eventual dosage regimen adaptations to be envisaged and ad hoc pharmaceutical formulations to be developed.

More complicated is the situation when there is no a priori indication of a polymorphism in drug metabolism, a difference in pharmacodynamic susceptibility, or the impact of environmental or nutritional factors. In such situations a pragmatic attitude from academia, regulatory bodies, and the pharmaceutical industry is of crucial importance if one desires to avoid "nonsense" science. It is indeed interesting and impressive to analyze retrospectively the contribution of chance and the time and effort needed to discover, confirm, and elucidate, for example, the debrisoquine/sparteine polymorphism. Such enormous efforts cannot be provided for each new chemical entity or drug class under development, but it is hoped that some of the ideas presented in this chapter may serve as a basis for a rational approach to investigate potential interethnic differences in drug behavior and effects during drug development, licensing, and registration in the context of a worldwide market for pharmaceuticals.

References

Allaz AF, Dayer P, Fabre J, Rudhardt M, Balant L (1979) Pharmacocinétique d'une nouvelle céphalosporine, la céfopérazone. Schweiz Med Wochenschr 109:1999–2005

Alván G, Bechtel P, Iselius L, Gundert-Remy U (1990) Hydroxylation polymorphisms of debrisoquine and mephenytoin in European populations. Eur J Clin Pharmacol 39:533–537

Balant LP, Gorgia A, Tschopp JM, Revillard C, Fabre J (1976) Pharmacocinétique de deux médicaments bêta-bloquants: détection d'une anomalie pharmacogénétique? Schweiz Med Wochenschr 106:1403–1407

Balant LP, Gundert-Remy U, Boobis AR, von Bahr C (1989) Relevance of genetic polymorphism in drug metabolism in the development of new drugs. Eur J Clin Pharmacol 36:551–554

Balant LP, Roseboom H, Gundert-Remy U (1990) Pharmacokinetic criteria for drug research and development. Adv Drug Res 19:1–139

Bertilsson L (1990) Interethnic differences in drug oxidation polymorphism. In: Alvan G, Balant LP, Bechtel PR, Boobis AR, Gram LF, Pithan K (eds) European consensus conference on pharmacogenetics. Commission of the European Communities, Luxembourg, pp 171–178 (Coordinated action COST B1)

Bertilsson L, Henthorn TK, Sanz E, Tybring G, Säwe J, Villén T (1989) Importance of genetic factors in the regulation of diazepam metabolism: relationship to S-mephenytoin, but not debrisoquine, hydroxylation phenotype. Clin Pharmacol Ther 45:348–355

Braunwald E et al. (eds) (1988) Harrison's principles of internal medicine, 11th edn. McGraw-Hill, New York

Darmansjah I, Muchtar A (1992) Dose-response variation among different populations. Clin Pharmacol Ther 52:449–452

Dayer P, Balant LP, Courvoisier F, Küpfer A, Kubli A, Gorgia A, Fabre J (1982) The genetic control of bufuralol metabolism in man. Eur J Drug Metab Pharmacokinet 7:73–77

Dayer P, Balant LP, Küpfer, A, Courvoisier F, Fabre J (1983) Contribution of the genetic status of oxidative metabolism to variability in the plasma concentrations of beta-adrenoceptor blocking agents. Eur J Clin Pharmacol 24:797–799

Dayer P, Balant LP, Küpfer A, Striberni R, Leemann T (1985) Effect of oxidative polymorphism (debrisoquine/sparteine type) on hepatic first-pass metabolism of bufuralol. Eur J Clin Pharmacol 28:317–320

Ebelin ME, Steimer JL, Laplanche R, Niederberger W (1992) An evaluation
    of population pharmacokinetics during drug development: experiences with
    graphical exploratory analysis for isradipine and tropisetron. In: Rowland M,
    Aarons L (eds) New strategies in drug development and clinical evaluation: the
    population approach. Commission of the European Communities, Luxembourg,
    pp 131–141 (Coordinated action COST B1)
Eichelbaum M, Spannbrucker N, Steincke B, Dengler HJ (1979) Defective N-
    oxidation of sparteine in man: a new pharmacogenetic defect. Eur J Clin
    Pharmacol 16:183–187
Evans DAP (1992) N-acetyltransferase. In: Kalow W (ed) Pharmacogenetics of drug
    metabolism. Pergamon, New York, pp 95–178
Ghoneim MM, Korttila K, Chiang CK, Jacobs L, Schoenwald RD, Mewaldt SP,
    Kabaya KO (1981) Diazepam effects and kinetics in Caucasians and Orientals.
    Clin Pharmacol Ther 29:749–756
Gundert-Remy U (1992) Population approach in pharmacokinetic and pharmaco-
    dynamics – views within regulatory agencies: Europe. In: Rowland M, Aarons L
    (eds) New strategies in drug development and clinical evaluation: the population
    approach. Commission of the European Communities, Luxembourg, pp 153–156
    (Coordinated action COST B1)
Hermansson J, von Bahr C (1982) Determination of (R)- and (S)-alprenolol and (R)-
    and (S)-metoprolol diastereoisomeric derivatives in human plasma by reversed-
    phase liquid chromatography. J Chromatogr 227:113–127
Holford NHG (1992) Parametric models for the time course of drug action: the
    population approach. In: Rowland M, Aarons L (eds) New strategies in drug
    development and clinical evaluation: the population approach. Commission of
    the European Communities, Luxembourg, pp 193–206 (Coordinated action
    COST B1)
Horai Y, Nakano M, Ishizaki T, Ishikawa K, Zhou HH, Zhou BJ, Lia CL, Zhang
    LM (1989) Metoprolol and mephenytoin oxidation polymorphisms in Far Eastern
    Oriental subjects: Japanese versus mainland Chinese. Clin Pharmacol Ther
    46:198–207
Ishizaki T, Eichelbaum M, Horai Y, Hashimoto K, Chiba K, Dengler HJ (1987)
    Evidence for polymorphic oxidation of sparteine in Japanese subjects. Br J Clin
    Pharmacol 23:482–485
Joubert PH, Brandt HD (1990) Apparent racial difference in response to angiotensin
    I infusion. Eur J Clin Pharmacol 39:183–185
Kalow W (1982) Ethnic differences in drug metabolism. Clin Pharmacokinet 7:
    373–400
Kalow W (1984) Pharmacoanthropology: outline, problems, and the nature of case
    histories. Fed Proc 43:2314–2318
Kalow W (1992) Pharmacoanthropology and the genetics of drug metabolism. In:
    Kalow W (ed) Pharmacogenetics of drug metabolism. Pergamon, New York, pp
    865–877
Katz MM, Katz MM, Kato M, Yamamoto J et al. (1979) Transcultural psycho-
    pharmacology in depression: East and West. Psychopharmacol Bull 15:24–31
Kubli A, Balant LP, Dayer P, Balant-Gorgia A, Fabre J (1982) Influence du
    polymorphisme génétique de l'oxydation sur les études de biodisponibilité: à
    propos du bufuralol. J Pharmacol Clin 1:301–315
Kumana CR, Lauder IJ, Chan M, Ko W, Lin HJ (1987) Differences in diazepam
    pharmacokinetics in Chinese and white Caucasians – relation to body lipid
    stores. Eur J Clin Pharmacol 32:211–215
Küpfer A, Preisig R (1984) Pharmacogenetics of mephenytoin: a new drug hydroxy-
    lation polymorphism in man. Eur J Clin Pharmacol 26:753–759
Lennard MS (1992) The polymorphic oxidation of beta-adrenoceptor antagonists. In:
    Kalow W (ed) Pharmacogenetics of drug metabolism. Pergamon, New York, pp
    701–720

Lennard MS, Tucker GT, Silas JH, Freestone S, Ramsay LW, Woods HF (1983) Differential stereoselective metabolism of metoprolol in extensive and poor debrisoquine metabolisers. Clin Pharmacol Ther 34:732–737

Lou YC, Ying L, Bertilsson L, Sjöqvist F (1987) Low frequency of slow debrisoquine hydroxylation in a native Chinese population. Lancet 2:852–853

Mahgoub A, Idle JR, Dring LG, Lancester R, Smith RL (1977) Polymorphic hydroxylation of debrisoquine in man. Lancet 2:584–586

Mendoza R, Smith MW, Poland RE, Lin KM, Strickland TL (1991) Ethnic psychopharmacology: the Hispanic and native American perspective. Psychopharmacol Bull 27:449–461

Meyer UA, Zanger UM, Grant D, Blum M (1990) Genetic polymorphisms of drug metabolism. Adv Drug Res 19:197–241

Nakamura K, Goto F, Ray WA, McAllister CB, Jacqz E, Wilkinson GR, Branch RA (1985) Interethnic differences in genetic polymorphism of debrisoquin and mephenytoin hydroxylation between Japanese and Caucasian populations. Clin Pharmacol Ther 38:402–408

Peck CC (1992) Population approach in pharmacokinetics and pharmacodynamics: FDA view. In: Rowland M, Aarons L (eds) New strategies in drug development and clinical evaluation: the population approach. Commission of the European Communities, Luxembourg, pp 157–168 (Coordinated action COST B1)

Peck CC, Barr WH, Benet LZ, et al. (1992) Opportunities for integration of pharmacokinetics, pharmacodynamics, and toxicokinetics in rational drug development. Clin Pharmacol Ther 51:465–473

Sanz EJ, Villén T, Alm C, Bertilsson L (1989) S-mephenytoin hydroxylation phenotypes in a Swedish population determined after coadministration with debrisoquin. Clin Pharmacol Ther 45:495–499

Sheiner LB (1992) Population approach in drug development: rationale and basic concepts. In: Rowland M, Aarons L (eds) New strategies in drug development and clinical evaluation: the population approach. Commission of the European Communities, Luxembourg, pp 13–27 (Coordinated action COST B1)

Strickland TL, Ranganath V, Lin KM, Poland RE, Mendoza R, Smith MW (1991) Psychopharmacologic considerations in the treatment of black American populations. Psychopharmacol Bull 27:441–448

Vozeh S (1992) Applications of population approach to clinical pharmacokinetics and validation of results. In: Rowland M, Aarons L (eds) New strategies in drug development and clinical evaluation: the population approach. Commission of the European Communities, Luxembourg, pp 107–120 (Coordinated action COST B1)

Yue QY, Bertilsson L, Dahl-Puustinen ML, Säwe J, Sjöqvist F, Johansson I, Ingelman-Sundberg M (1989) Dissociation between debrisoquine hydroxylation phenotype and genotype among Chinese. Lancet 2:870

Zhou HH, Wood AJJ (1990) Differences in stereoselective disposition of propranolol do not explain sensitivity differences between white and Chinese subjects: correlation between the clearance of (−)- and (+)-propranolol. Clin Pharmacol Ther 47:719–723

Appendix
Selected References on Interethnic Differences in Drug Kinetics

The selection of papers presented in this Appendix is centered around racial or ethnic differences in xenobiotic pharmacokinetics. The survey covers essentially the 1980s with some "overflowing" in the late 1970s and early

1990s. Although most of the studies involve pharmacogenetic investigations, this list is not at all representative for this aspect of drug behavior in humans. The absence of references to interethnic differences in alcohol and acetaldehyde is deliberate. Review articles and books are referenced in the bibliography directly related to the text of the chapter.

I. Phenotypes of N-acetylation

Afonia AO, Arharwarien ED, Okotore RO, Femi-Pearse D (1979) Isoniazid acetylator phenotypes of Nigerians. Nigerian Med J 9:86–88

Airaksinen E, Mattila MJ, Olilla O (1969) Inactivation of isoniazid and sulpha-dimidine in Mongoloid subjects. Ann Med Exp Biol Fenn 47:303–307

Armstrong AR, Peart HE (1960) A comparison between the behaviour of Eskimos and non-Eskimos to the administration of isoniazid. Am Rev Respir Dis 81:588–594

Bouayad Z, Chevalier B, Maurin R, Bartal M (1982) Phénotype d'acétylation de l'isoniazide au Maroc. Etude préliminaire sur 100 cas. Rev Maroc Med Sante 4:13–18

Bozkurt A, Basci NE, Tuncer M, Kayaalp SO (1990) N-acetylation phenotyping with sulphadimidine in a Turkish population. Eur J Clin Pharmacol 38:53–56

Bressolette L, Berthou F, Riche C, Mottier D, Floch HH (1990) Polymorphisme génétique d'acétylation et d'hydroxylation dans la population bretonne. Thérapie 45:99–103

Desai M, Jariwala G, Khokhani B, Desai NK, Sheth UK (1973) Isoniazid inactivation in Indian children. Indian Pediatr 10:373–376

Eidus L, Hodgkin MM, Schaeffer O, Jessamine AG (1974) Distribution of isoniazid inactivators determined in Eskimos and Canadian college students by a urine test. Rev Can Biol 33:117–123

Eidus L, Glatthaar E, Hodgkin MM, Nel EE, Kleeberg HH (1979) Comparison of isoniazid phenotyping of black and white patients with emphasis on South African blacks. Int J Clin Pharmac Biopharm 17:311–316

El-Yazigi A, Chaleby K, Martin CR (1989) Acetylator phenotypes of Saudi Arabians by a simplified caffeine metabolite test. J Clin Pharmacol 29:246–250

Evans DAP, Paterson S, Francisco P, Alvarez G (1985) The acetylator phenotype of Saudi Arabian diabetics. J Med Genet 22:479–483

Evans DAP, Wicks J, Higgins J, Assisto M (1991) The acetylator phenotypes of Saudi Arabians with coronary arterial atheroma. J Med Genet 28:192–193

Eze LC (1987) High incidence of the slow nitrazepam acetylator phenotype in a Nigerian population. Biochem Genet 25:225–229

Eze LC, Obidoa O (1978) The acetylation of sulphamethazine in a Nigerian popu-lation. Biochem Genet 16:1073–1077

Fawcett IW, Gammon PT (1975) Determination of the acetylator phenotype in a Northern Nigerian population. Tubercle 56:119–201

Goedde HW, Benkmann HG, Agarwal DP, Kroeger A (1977a) Genetic studies in Ecuador; acetylator phenotypes, red cell enzyme and serum protein poly-morphisms of Shuara indians. Am J Phys Anthropol 47:419–425

Goedde HW, Flatz G, Rahimi AG, Kaifie S, Benkmann HG, Kreise G, Delbrück H (1977b) The acetylator polymorphism in four populations of Afghanistan. Hum Hered 27:383–388

Gupta RC, Nair CR, Jindal SK, Malik SK (1984) Incidence of isoniazid acetylation phenotypes in North Indians. Int Clin Pharmacol Ther Toxicol 22:259–264

Gurumurthy P, Krisnamurthy MS, Nazareth O, Parthasarathy R, Raghupati Sarma G, Somasundaram PR, Tripathy SP, Ellard GA (1984) Lack of relationship between hepatic toxicity and acetylator phenotype in three thousand South

Indian patients during treatment with isoniazid for tuberculosis. Am Rev Respir Dis 129:58–61

Hayward GA (1975) Human acetylation polymorphism in Polynesians. Proc Univ Otago Med Sch 53:67–68

Hilderbrand M, Seifert W (1989) Determination of acetylator phenotype in Caucasians with caffeine. Eur J Clin Pharmacol 37:525–526

Homeida M, Abboud OI, Dawi O, Rahama AM, Awad EH, Ahmed OM (1986) The acetylator phenotype of Sudanese subjects. Arab J Med 5:30–31

Horai Y, Ishizaki T (1988) N-acetylation polymorphism of dapsone in a Japanese population. Br J Clin Pharmacol 25:487–494

Horai Y, Ishizaki T, Sasaki T, Koya G, Matsuyama K, Iguelin S (1982) Isoniazid disposition, comparison of isoniazid phenotyping methods in and acetylator distribution of Japanese patients with idiopathic lupus erythematosus and control subjects. Br J Clin Pharmacol 13:361–374

Horai Y, Zhou HH, Zhang LM, Ishizaki T (1988) Acetylation phenotyping with dapsone in a mainland Chinese population. Br J Clin Pharmacol 25:81–87

Horai Y, Fujita K, Ishizaki T (1989) Genetically determined N-acetylation and oxidation capacities in Japanese patients with non-occupational urinary bladder cancer. Eur J Clin Pharmacol 37:581–587

Inaba T, Arias TD (1987) On phenotyping with isoniazid. The use of urinary acetylation/ratios and the uniqueness of antimodes found in two Amerindian populations. Clin Pharmacol Ther 42:493–497

Irshaid YM, Al-Halidi HF, Abuirjeie MA, Rawasheh NM (1991) N-acetylation phenotyping using dapsone in a Jordanian population. Br J Clin Pharmacol 32:1039–1057

Irshaid YM, Al-Hadidi HF, Abuirjeie MA, Latif A, Sartawi O, Rawashed NM (1992) Acelylator phenotype of Jordanian diabetics. Eur J Clin Pharmacol 43:621–623

Islam SI (1982) Polymorphic acetylation of sulphamethyzine in rural Bedouin and urban-dwellers in Saudi Arabia. Xenobiotica 12:323–328

Jenkins T, Lehmann H, Nurse GP (1974) Public health and genetic constitution of the Sab ("Bushmen"): carbohydrate metabolism and acetylator status of the Kung of Tsumkwe in the North-Western Kalahari. Br Med J 2:23–26

Karim AKMB, Elfellah MS, Evans DAP (1981) Human acetylator polymorphism: estimate of allele frequency in Libya and details of global distribution. J Med Genet 18:325–330

Lee EJD, Lim JME, Feng P-H (1985) Acetylator phenotype in Chinese patients with spontaneous systemic lupus erythematosus. Syngapore Med J 26:295–299

Lilyin ET, Korunskaya MP, Meksin VA, Taelicheva LV, Shapiro EF (1983) The distribution of acetylator phenotypes in Moscow population. Genetika 19:1378–1380

Lilyin ET, Korunskaya MP, Meksin VA, Drozdov ES, Nasarov VV, Monastyrskaya AR (1984) The distribution of acetylator phenotypes in normal individuals and the patients suffering from alcoholism among Moscow urban population. Genetika 20:1557–1559

Lower GM Jr, Nilsson T, Nelson CE, Wolf H, Gamsky TE, Bryan GT (1979) N-acetyltransferase phenotype and risk in urinary bladder cancer: approaches in molecular epidemiology. Preliminary results in Sweden and Denmark. Environ Health Perspect 29:71–79

Nhachi CFB (1988) Polymorphic acetylation of sulphamethazine in a Zimbabwe population. J Med Genet 25:29–31

Odeigah PGC, Okunowo MA (1989) High frequency of the rapid isoniazid acetylator phenotype in Lagos (Nigeria). Hum Hered 39:26–31

Paik YK, Cho YH, Kim IK, Benkmann HG, Goedde HW (1988) Pharmacogenetic studies in South Korea: serum cholinesterase and N-acetyltransferase polymorphisms. Korean J Genet 10:272–278

Parthasarathy R, Raghupati Sarma G, Janardhanam B, Ramachandran P, Santha T, Sivasubramaian S, Somasundaram PR, Tripathy SP (1986) Hepatic toxicity in South Indian patients during treatment of tuberculosis with short-course regimens containing isoniazid, rifampicin and pyrazinamide. Tubercle 67:99–108

Paulsen O, Nilsson LG (1985) Distribution of acetylator phenotype in relation to age and sex in Swedish patients. Eur J Clin Pharmacol 28:311–315

Penketh RJA, Gibreig SFA, Nurse GT, Hopkinson DA (1983) Acetylator phenotypes in Papua New Guinea. J Med Genet 20:39–40

Peters JH, Gordon GT, Karat ABA (1975) Polymorphic acetylation of the antibacterials, sulfamethazine and dapsone, in South Indian subjects. Am J Trop Med Hyg 24:641–648

Sardas S, Karakaya AE, Cok I (1986a) Determination of the acetylator phenotype in a Turkish population. Clin Genet 29:185–186

Tang BK, Kadar D, Qian L, Iriah J, Yip J, Kalow W (1991) Caffeine as a metabolic probe: validation of its use for acetylator phenotyping (Various ethnic groups). Clin Pharmacol Ther 49:648–657

Viznerova A, Slavikova Z, Ellard GA (1973) The determination of the acetylator phenotype of tuberculosis patients in Czechoslovakia using sulphadimidine. Tubercle 54:67–76

II. Phenotypes of Hydroxylation

Alvan G, Bechtel P, Iselius L, Gundert-Remy U (1990) Hydroxylation polymorphisms of debrisoquine and mephenytoin in European populations. Eur J Clin Pharmacol 39:533–537

Arias TD, Jorge LF, Inaba T (1986) No evidence for the presence of poor metabolizers of sparteine in an Amerindian group: the Cunas of Panama. Br J Clin Pharmacol 21:547–548

Arias TD, Jorge LF, Lee D, Barrantes R, Inaba T (1988a) The oxidative metabolism of sparteine in the Cuna Amerindians of Panama: absence of evidence for deficient metabolizers. Clin Pharmacol Ther 43:456–465

Arias TD, Inaba T, Cooke RG, Jorge LF (1988b) A preliminary note on the transient polymorphic oxidation of sparteine in the Ngawbé Guaymí Amerindians: a case of genetic divergence with tentative phylogenetic time frame for the pathway. Clin Pharmacol Ther 44:343–352

Arvela P, Kirjarinta M, Kirjarinta M, Kärki N, Pelkonen O (1988) Polymorphism of debrisoquine hydroxylation among Finns and Lapps. Br J Clin Pharmacol 26:601–603

Benitez J, Llerena A, Cobaleda (1988) Debrisoquin oxidation polymorphism in a Spanish population. Clin Pharmacol Ther 44:74–77

Bressolette L, Berthou F, Riche C, Mottier D, Floch HH (1990) Polymorphisme génétique d'acétylation et d'hydroxylation dans la population bretonne. Therapie 45:99–103

Brøsen K (1986) Sparteine oxidation polymorphism in Greenlanders living in Denmark. Br J Clin Pharmacol 22:415–419

Brøsen K, Otton SV, Gram LF (1985) Sparteine oxidation polymorphism in Denmark. Acta Pharmacol Toxicol (Copenh) 57:357–360

Clasen K, Madsen L, Brøsen K, Albøge K, Misfeldt S, Gram LF (1991) Sparteine and mephenytoin oxidation: genetic polymorphisms in East and West Greenland. Clin Pharmacol Ther 49:624–631

Dayer P, Balant LP, Courvoisier F, Küpfer A, Kubli A, Gorgia A, Fabre J (1982) The genetic control of bufuralol metabolism in man (Switzerland). Eur J Drug Metab Pharmacokinet 7:73–77

Dayer P, Balant L, Küpfer A, Courvoisier F, Fabre J (1983) Contribution of the genetic status of oxidative metabolism to variability in the plasma concentrations of beta-adrenoceptor blocking agents (bufuralol in Switzerland). Eur J Clin Pharmacol 24:797–799

Dick B, Küpfer A, Molnàr J, Braunschweig S, Preisig R (1982) Hydroxylierungsdefekt für Medikamente (Typus Debrisoquin) in einer Stichprobe der Schweizerischen Bevölkerung. Schweiz Med Wochenschr 112:1061–1067

Drøhse A, Bathum L, Brøsen K, Gram LF (1989) Mephenytoin and sparteine oxidation: genetic polymorphism in Denmark. Br J Clin Pharmacol 27:620–625

Eichelbaum M, Woolhouse NM (1985) Inter-ethnic difference in sparteine oxidation among Ghanaians and Germans. Eur J Clin Pharmacol 28:79–83

Evans DAP, Mahgoub A, Sloan TP, Idle JR, Smith RL (1980) A family and population study of the genetic polymorphism of debrisoquine oxidative in a white British population. Br J Med Genet 17:102–105

Horai Y, Ishizaki T, Ishikawa K (1988) Metoprolol oxidation in a Japanese population: evidence for only one poor metabolizer among 262 subjects. Br J Clin Pharmacol 26:807–808

Horai Y, Nakano M, Ishizaki T, Ishikawa K, Zhou HH, Zhou BJ, Lia CL, Zhang LM (1989) Metoprolol and mephenytoin oxidation polymorphisms in Far Eastern Oriental subjects: Japanese versus mainland Chinese. Clin Pharmacol Ther 46:198–207

Inaba T, Jurima M, Nakano M, Kalow W (1984) Mephenytoin and sparteine pharmacogenetics in Canadian Caucasians. Clin Pharmacol Ther 36:670–676

Inaba T, Jorge LF, Arias TD (1988) Mephenytoin hydroxylation in the Cuna Amerindians of Panama. Br J Clin Pharmacol 25:75–79

Ishizaki T, Eichelbaum M, Horai Y, Hashimoto K, Chiba K, Dengler HJ (1987) Evidence for polymorphic oxidation of sparteine in Japanese subjects. Br J Clin Pharmacol 23:482–485

Islam SI, Idle JR, Smith RL (1980) The polymorphic 4-hydroxylation of debrisoquin in a Saudi Arab population. Xenobiotica 10:819–825

Iyun AO, Lennard MS, Tucker GT, Woods HF (1986) Metoprolol and debrisoquin metabolism in Nigerians: lack of evidence for polymorphic oxidation. Clin Pharmacol Ther 40:387–394

Jacqz E, Dulac H, Mathieu H (1988) Phenotyping polymorphic drug metabolism in the French Caucasian population. Eur J Clin Pharmacol 35:167–171

Jurima M, Inaba T, Kadar D, Kalow W (1985) Genetic polymorphism of mephenytoin $p(4^1)$-hydroxylation: difference between Orientals and Caucasians. Br J Clin Pharmacol 19:483–487

Kallio J, Lindberg R, Huuponen R, lisalo E (1988) Debrisoquine oxidation in a Finnish population: the effect of oral contraceptives on the metabolic ratio. Br J Clin Pharmacol 26:791–795

Kalow W, Otton SV, Kadar D, Endrenyi L, Inaba T (1980) Ethnic differences in drug metabolism: debrisoquine 4-hydroxylation in Caucasians and Orientals. Can J Physiol Pharmacol 58:1142–1144

Küpfer A, Preisig R (1984) Pharmacogenetics of mephenytoin: a new drug hydroxylation polymorphism in man (Switzerland). Eur J Clin Pharmacol 26:753–759

Larrey D, Amouyal G, Tinel M, Letteron P, Berson A, Labbe G, Pessayre D (1987) Polymorphism of dextromethorphan oxidation in a French population. Br J Clin Pharmacol 24:676–679

Leclercq V, Desager JP, van Nieuwenhuyze Y, Harvengt C (1987) Prevalence of drug hydroxylator phenotype in Belgium. Eur J Clin Pharmacol 33:439–440

Lennard MS, Tucker GT, Woods HF, Silas JH, Iyun AO (1989) Stereoselective metabolism of metoprolol in Caucasians and Nigerians – relationship to debrisoquin oxidation phenotype. Br J Clin Pharmacol 27:613–616

Lou YC, Ying L, Bertilsson L, Sjöqvist F (1987) Low frequency of slow debrisoquine hydroxylation in a native Chinese population. Lancet 2:852–853

Mahgoub A, Idle JR, Smith RL (1979) A population and familial study of the defective alicyclic hydroxylation of debrisoquine among Egyptians. Xenobiotica 9:51–56

Mbanefo C, Bababunmi EA, Mahgoub A, Sloan TP, Idle JR, Smith RL (1980) A study of the debrisoquine hydroxylation polymorphism in a Nigerian population. Xenobiotica 10:811–818

Nakamura K, Goto F, Ray WA, McAllister CB, Jacqz E, Wilkinson GR, Branch RA (1985) Interethnic differences in genetic polymorphism of debrisoquin and mephenytoin hydroxylation between Japanese and Caucasian populations. Clin Pharmacol Ther 38:402–408

Peart GF, Boutagy J, Shenfield GM (1986) Debrisoquine oxidation in an Australian population. Br J Clin Pharmacol 21:465–471

Relling MV, Cherries J, Schell MJ, Petros WP, Meyer WH, Evans WE (1991) Lower prevalence of the debrisoquin oxidative poor metabolizer phenotype in American black versus white subjects. Clin Pharmacol Ther 50:308–313

Sanz EJ, Villén T, Alm C, Bertilsson L (1989) S-Mephenytoin hydroxylation phenotypes in a Swedish population determined after coadministration with debrisoquin. Clin Pharmacol Ther 45:495–499

Schellens JHM, Danhof M, Breimer DD (1986) The poor metabolizer incidence of sparteine, mephenytoin and nifedipine in a Dutch population. Acta Pharmacol Toxicol (Copenh) Suppl 5:252

Steiner E, Bertilsson L, Säwe J, Bertling I, Sjöqvist F (1988) Polymorphic debrisoquine hydroxylation in 757 Swedish subjects. Clin Pharmacol Ther 44:431–435

Sommers DK, Moncrieff J, Avenant J (1989) Metoprolol α-hydroxylation polymorphism in the San Bushmen of Southern Africa. Hum Toxicol 8:39–43

Sommers DK, Moncrieff J, Avenant J (1989) Non-correlation between debrisoquine and metoprolol polymorphisms in the Venda. Hum Toxicol 8:365–368

Szórády I, Sánta A (1987) Drug hydroxylator phenotype in Hungary. Eur J Clin Pharmacol 32:325

Veronese ME, McLean S (1991) Debrisoquine oxidation polymorphism in a Tasmanian population. Eur J Clin Pharmacol 40:529–532

Vinks A, Inaba T, Otton SV, Kalow W (1982) Sparteine metabolism in Canadian Caucasians. Clin Pharmacol Ther 31:23–29

Ward SA, Goto F, Nakamura K, Jacqz E, Wilkinson GR Branch RA (1987) S-Mephenytoin 4-hydroxylase is inherited as an autosomal-recessive trait in Japanese families. Clin Pharmacol Ther 42:96–99

Wedlund PJ, Aslanian WS, McAllister CB, Wilkinson GR, Branch RA (1984) Mephenytoin hydroxylation deficiency in Caucasians: frequency of a new oxidative drug metabolism polymorphism. Clin Pharmacol Ther 36:773–780

Woolhouse NM, Andoh B, Mahgoub A, Sloan TP, Idle JR, Smith RL (1979) Debrisoquin hydroxylation polymorphism among Ghanaians and Caucasians. Clin Pharmacol Ther 26:584–591

Woolhouse NM, Eichelbaum, Oates NS, Idle JR, Smith RL (1985) Dissociation of co-regulatory control of debrisoquin/phenformin and sparteine oxidation in Ghanaians. Clin Pharmacol Ther 37:512–521

Yue QY, Bertilsson L, Dahl-Puustinen ML, Säwe J, Sjöqvist F, Johansson I, Ingelman-Sundberg M (1989) Dissociation between debrisoquine hydroxylation phenotype and genotype among Chinese. Lancet 2:870

III. Pharmacokinetics

Branch RA, Salih SY, Homeida M (1978) Racial differences in drug metabolizing ability: a study with antipyrine in the Sudan. Clin Pharmacol Ther 24:283–286

Buchanan N, Bill P, Moodley G, Eyberg C (1977) The metabolism of phenobarbitone in black patients. S Afr Med J 52:394–395

Desai NK, Sheth UK, Mucklow JC, Fraser HS, Bulpitt CJ, Jones SW, Dollery CT (1980) Antipyrine clearance in Indian villagers. Br J Clin Pharmacol 9:387–394

Chan E, Ti TY, Lee HS (1990) Population pharmacokinetics of phenytoin in Singapore Chinese. Eur J Clin Pharmacol 39:177–181

De Sommers K, Van Staden DA, Moncrieff J, Schoenman HS (1985) Paracetamol metabolism in African villagers. Hum Toxicol 4:385–389

De Sommers K, Moncrieff J, Avenant JC (1987) Paracetamol conjugation: an interethnic and dietary study. Hum Toxicol 6:407–409

Ghoneim MM, Korttila K, Chiang CK, Jacobs L, Schoenwald RD, Mewaldt SP, Kabaya KO (1981) Diazepam effects and kinetics in Caucasians and Orientals. Clin Pharmacol Ther 29:749–756

Kalow W, Tang BK, Kadar D, Endrenyi L, Chan FY (1979) A method for studying drug metabolism in populations: racial differences in amobarbital metabolism. Clin Pharmacol Ther 26:766–776

Kromann N, Christiansen J, Flachs H, Dam M, Hvidberg EF (1981) Differences in single dose phenytoin kinetics between Greenland Eskimos and Danes. Ther Drug Monit 3:239–245

Kumana CR, Lauder IJ, Chan M, Ko W, Lin HJ (1987) Differences in diazepam pharmacokinetics in Chinese and white Caucasians – relation to body lipid stores. Eur J Clin Pharmacol 32:211–215

Pi EH, Tran-Johnson TK, Walker NR, Cooper TB, Suckow RF, Gray GE (1989) Pharmacokinetics of desipramine in Asian and Caucasian volunteers. Psychopharmacol Bull 25:483–487

Rudorfer MV, Lane EA, Chang WH, Zhang M, Potter WZ (1984) Desipramine pharmacokinetics in Chinese and Caucasian volunteers. Br J Clin Pharmacol 17:433–440

Spector R, Choudhury AK, Chiang CK, Goldberg MJ, Ghoneim MM (1980) Diphenhydramine in Orientals and Caucasians. Clin Pharmacol Ther 28:229–234

Zhou HH, Wood AJJ (1990) Differences in stereoselective disposition of propranolol do not explain sensitivity differences between white and Chinese subjects: correlation between the clearance of (−)-and (+)-propranolol. Clin Pharmacol Ther 47:719–723

Zhou HH, Adedoyin A, Wilkinson GR (1990) Differences in plasma binding of drugs between Caucasians and Chinese subjects. Clin Pharmacol Ther 48:10–17

CHAPTER 9

Clinical Relevance of Pharmacogenetics

H.K. KROEMER, G. MIKUS, and M. EICHELBAUM

A. Introduction

One of the central problems in pharmacotherapy is the interindividual variability in response to drugs. While in vitro experiments show a close relationship between dose and resulting effects, large differences are observed once the same dose is administered to a population of patients.

The variability in response to drugs was already recognized about 500 years ago by Paracelsus, who stated "Every substance is a poison. It is just the dose which determines whether a substance is toxic." This phrase of Paracelsus holds true when a single individual is observed: an increase in the dose of any substance administered to one individual will eventually lead to adverse side-effects.

It was soon observed, however, that in any one population there is pronounced interindividual variability in response to xenobiotics after administration of the same dose. In his pioneering work, Garrod applied the fundamental observations of Gregor Mendel to man and postulated the existence of "inborn errors of metabolism." He observed that patients with alkaptonuria either excrete homogentisic acid in normal amounts or none at all: "its appearance in traces or in gradually increasing or diminishing quantities has never yet been observed" (GARROD 1902). This first description of a multimodal distribution of metabolic patterns based on factors of inheritance represented a watershed in pharmacogenetics. Other work by Garrod suggested the individual response to drugs and constituents of diet to be determined by the individual genetic constitution of a patient (GARROD 1931). In the late 1950s the combined work of Vogel and Motulski led to the contemporary definition of pharmacogenetics: while the term itself was coined by VOGEL (1959), MOTULSKI had suggested in 1957 that exaggerated (unusual) responses to drugs may be a result of genetically determined enzyme deficiencies.

The relevance of such inherited deficiencies had been suggested by clinical observations, and a striking example of the time course of events and discoveries is that of genetically determined deficiencies in butyrylcholinesterase. The depolarizing muscle relaxant succinylcholine was introduced into therapy in 1951 (LOCKRIDGE 1992). The drug gained widespread application due to its rapid onset and short duration of action. Complete paralysis is observed 2 min after intravenous administration of 1 mg/kg body weight. The half-life of 2–6 min leads to total recovery from relaxation within a very short time. Soon after the introduction of succinylcholine it was noted that some patients showed increased susceptibility to the effects of this drug: complete paralysis persisted for several hours and such patients had to be maintained on mechanical ventilators.

The work of Kalow (1956), who is widely recognized as a pioneer of modern pharmacogenetics, provided unequivocal evidence that the prolonged effects of succinylcholine resulted from a defect in its metabolism: in the vast majority of patients succinylcholine is rapidly cleaved by the enzyme butyrylcholinesterase (acylcholine acylhydrolase; EC 3.1.1.8), leading to the inactive succinylmonocholine and choline. Kalow reported an altered function of this enzyme in patients with an unusual response to succinylcholine. The affinity of the drug to the enzyme was very low in these patients, resulting in high concentrations of parent compound which in turn led to prolonged depolarization. Later work by Kalow and Staron (1957) showed the defect to be inherited as an autosomal recessive trait. Kalow and Genest (1957) introduced a very simple test that allowed identification of patients at risk: normal butyrylcholinesterase activity is inhibited to a large degree by dibucaine whereas the deficient variant is less susceptible to inhibition by dibucaine. The degree of inhibition was expressed as the dibucaine number and allowed the identification of patients homozygous for the normal variant and heterozygous or homozygous for the atypical form.

Lately, progress in molecular biology techniques has permitted the genetic defect in patients with deficient butyrylcholinesterase to be examined at the molecular level. The gene located on chromosome 3 which encodes for butyrylcholinesterase shows from nucleotide 208 to 210 the sequence GAT, which encodes for aspartic acid at position 70 of the enzyme. Substitution of a single nucleotide at position 209 leads to GGT, which replaces aspartic acid 70 by glycine (McGuire et al. 1989). Replacing the monoamine dicarbonic aspartic acid by the monoamine monocarbonic acid glycine results in loss of a free carboxylic group which is necessary for binding of the quarternary amine structure of succinylcholine. Therefore, affinity of the drug to the enzyme is reduced, which results in a higher K_m while maximal turnover rate (V_{max}) remains unchanged. Since intrinsic clearance is V_{max}/K_m an increased K_m leads to decreased clearance and hence plasma concentrations of succinylcholine associated with paralysis are sustained for a longer period.

To date a total of seven variants of butyrylcholinesterase which lead to decreased catalytic activity of the enzyme have been described. The most frequent K-variant, named in honor of W. Kalow, has a frequency of 1%. A recent excellent review by Lockridge (1992) summarizes the current knowledge concerning butyrylcholinesterase. This genetically determined enzyme deficiency serves as an example of a closed chain of evidence from a patient's genetic disposition to an abnormal drug effect.

Table 1. Drug-metabolizing enzymes, the activity of which is genetically determined. The references refer to recent reviews

Type of enzyme	Enzyme affected	Clinical consequences of enzyme deficiency	Reference
Esterase	Butyrylcholinesterase	Prolonged action of succinylcholine	LOCKRIDGE (1992)
Transferase	N-Acetyltransferase	See text	EVANS et al. (1992)
	Methyltransferase	Enhanced toxicity of mercaptopurine	WEINSHILBAUM (1992)
	UDP-glucuronosyltransferase	Crigler-Najjar or Gilbert's syndrome	BURCHELL and COUGHTRIE (1992)
Dehydrogenase	Aldehyde dehydrogenase	Flush after ethanol intake	GOEDDE and AGARWAL (1992)
Oxidoreductase	Flavin-containing monooxygenase	Fish odor syndrome	AYESH and SMITH (1992)
P-450-dependent monooxygenase	Sparteine/debrisoquine polymorphism	See text	EICHELBAUM and GROSS (1992)
	Mephenytoin polymorphism	See text	WILKINSON et al. (1992)

Besides the genetically determined variability in butyrylcholine esterase activity, a variety of genetically determined enzyme deficiencies which lead to abnormal drug reactions in man have been described (Table 1). While the deficiency in butyrylcholinesterase shows a low frequency and is therefore defined as a rare genetic variant, other metabolic pathways (N-acetyltransferase, CYP2D6) fulfill the criteria for genetic polymorphism: genetic polymorphism is defined as a monogenic trait which occurs in the population in at least two geno- and phenotypes, neither of which has a frequency of less than 1% (Vogel and Motulski 1979). A phenotype is defined as the visual expression of a genotype.

In this review we focus on the clinical relevance of three genetic polymorphisms in drug metabolism, namely the sparteine/debrisoquine polymorphism, the mephenytoin polymorphism, and the polymorphic N-acetylation. In each case the sequence of discoveries was analogous to that outlined for butyrylcholinesterase. The initial observation of abnormal response to drugs was made by physicians during pharmacotherapy. The next step was evaluation of the biochemical nature of the deficiency, followed by application of methods for assignment of phenotype in order to identify patients at risk. Eventually, the molecular basis of the respective defect was evaluated by means of molecular biology. After reviewing the three polymorphisms, we will outline the relevance of genetic polymorphisms for two other clinically relevant topics, namely development of new drugs the metabolism of which may be genetically determined and drug interactions mediated by polymorphically expressed enzymes. In general, genetic factors in drug metabolism are a source of interindividual variability in the relationship between a given dose and the resulting concentrations and hence drug actions. Knowledge of these factors may allow adaptation of the dosage regimen to the individual metabolic capacity of patients.

The therapeutic consequences arising from such polymorphic drug metabolism are complex and preclude generalizations. The hypothesis that patients with genetic defects in drug-metabolizing enzymes have a high risk of side-effects after administration of a polymorphically oxidized drug is an oversimplification. One problem arises from the fact that only a minor pathway may be mediated by the polymorphically expressed enzyme, the major portion of the drug being biotransformed by other routes. In this case the disposition of parent compound may be independent of phenotype. However, phenotype-dependent drug interactions for the polymorphic enzyme may be observed. Moreover, polymorphic oxidation may be relevant only in certain disease states: If a drug is eliminated by two routes, e.g., renal excretion of parent compound and hepatic metabolism, then the genetically determined defects in drug metabolism may have only a minor impact since they can be compensated by the intact renal function. If, however, a patient suffers from renal failure and has in addition a genetically determined lack of metabolism, both routes of elimination are severely impaired and serious consequences may arise.

If the major metabolic pathway of a drug is catalyzed by a polymorphically expressed enzyme then the clinical consequences depend on whether the drug is activated or inactivated during the course of biotransformation. If the metabolic step leads to inactive metabolites, the active parent compound will accumulate in patients deficient of this pathway and hence toxicity may occur. In contrast, formation of active metabolites via a polymorphic enzyme can lead to lack of drug effects in the subset of patients devoid of metabolic activity.

B. The Genetic Polymorphism of the Sparteine/Debrisoquine Oxidation

As with many observations, the discovery of polymorphic sparteine oxidation was not a result of a planned strategy but rather an incidental observation. During a routine pharmacokinetic study with the antiarrhythmic sparteine, one of the volunteers experienced serious side-effects such as nausea and diplopia characteristic of intoxication with class 1 antiarrhythmics. Analysis of the plasma concentrations revealed the total clearance of sparteine in this volunteer to be 1/5th of that in other volunteers (EICHELBAUM 1975; EICHELBAUM et al. 1979). Urinary excretion of sparteine metabolites was literally absent in this volunteer, and nearly 100% of the drug was excreted unchanged in urine. Subsequent studies revealed that defective sparteine oxidation is inherited as an autosomal recessive trait in about 7%–10% of Caucasians; the persons concerned are referred to as being of poor metabolizer (PM) phenotype, while the extensive metabolizer (EM) phenotype can be assigned to the remainder of the population (EICHELBAUM and GROSS 1992).

A similar "accidental" observation led to the discovery of the debrisoquine polymorphism (MAHGOUB et al. 1977). Again, severe side-effects such as orthostatic hypotension were noted in a volunteer and family studies uncovered the mode of inheritance (EVANS et al. 1980). Later studies established that the two independently discovered polymorphisms of sparteine and debrisoquine cosegregate in Caucasians. Thus, PMs for sparteine have an impaired debrisoquine metabolism and vice versa.

These findings would have been of rather theoretical interest if the defect in oxidation were to be restricted to sparteine or debrisoquine since neither of these drugs can be regarded as essential for therapy. Further investigations, however, have shown that the metabolism of a variety of frequently used drugs cosegregates with polymorphic oxidation of sparteine and debrisoquine (a list is provided in Table 2).

The fact that many drugs are catalyzed by this polymorphically expressed enzyme has sparked considerable research efforts in order to uncover the molecular mechanisms of this defect and the clinical consequences. While the molecular mechanisms have been described in great detail, the clinical

Table 2. Compounds whose metabolism cosegregates with that of sparteine/debriso-quine and the metabolic pathways affected

Compound	Pathway	Reference
Alprenolol	Aromatic hydroxylation	ALVAN et al. (1982)
Amiflamine	N-Demethylation	ALVAN et al. (1984)
Amitriptyline	Benzylic hydroxylation	MELLSTRÖM et al. (1983)
Aprindine	Aromatic hydroxylation	EBNER and EICHELBAUM (1993)
Bufuralol	Aliphatic and aromatic hydroxylation	DAYER et al. (1986)
CGP 15210G	Aromatic hydroxylation	GLEITER et al. (1985)
Clomipramine	Aromatic hydroxylation	BALANT-GORGIA et al. (1986)
Clozapine	–	FISCHER et al. (1992)
Codeine	O-Demethylation	DAYER et al. (1988)
Despiramine	Aromatic hydroxylation	BROSEN et al. (1986)
Dextromethorphan	O-Demethylation	KÜPFER et al. (1984)
Encainide	O-Demethylation	WANG et al. (1984)
Ethylmorphine	O-Deethylation	RANE et al. (1992)
Flecainide	O-Dealkylation	BECKMANN et al. (1988)
Guanoxan	Aromatic hydroxylation	SLOAN et al. (1978)
Haloperidol	–	LLERENA et al. (1992)
Indoramin	Aromatic hydroxylation	PIERCE et al. (1987)
Imipramine	Aromatic hydroxylation	BROSEN et al. (1986)
Methoxyamphetamine	O-Dealkylation	KITCHEN et al. (1979)
Methoxyphenamine	Aromatic hydroxylation and N-demethylation	ROY et al. (1985)
Metoprolol	Aliphatic hydroxylation and O-dealkylation	McGOURTY et al. (1985)
Nortriptyline	Benzylic hydroxylation	NORDIN et al. (1985)
N-Propylajmaline	Aromatic hydroxylation (?)	ZEKORN et al. (1985)
Perhexiline	Aliphatic hydroxylation	COOPER et al. (1984)
Perphenazine	Not identified	DAHL-PUUSTINEN et al. (1989)
Phenformin	Aromatic hydroxylation	OATES et al. (1982)
Propafenone	Aromatic hydroxylation	SIDDOWAY et al. (1987)
Propranolol	Aromatic hydroxylation	RAGHURAM et al. (1984)
Timolol	O-Dealkylation (?)	LEWIS et al. (1985)
Thioridazine	Side chain sulfoxidation	VON BAHR et al. (1991)
Tropisetron	Aromatic hydroxylation	FISCHER (1992)
Tomoxetine	Not identified	FEHER et al. (1988)

implications are not fully established and often illustrated only by case reports.

I. Molecular Mechanisms of the Sparteine/Debrisoquine Polymorphism

It soon became apparent that both sparteine and debrisoquine oxidation are mediated by an enzyme of the cytochrome P-450 family termed CYP2D6. The CYP2D gene cluster consists of CYP2D8, CYP2D7, and CYP2D6 and is located on the long arm of the human chromosome 22 (MEYER et al. 1992; EICHELBAUM et al. 1987). While CYP2D8 and CYP2D7 are most likely pseudogenes, the functional protein is encoded by CYP2D6. Several mutations of CYP2D6 have been described which in most cases lead to the absence of functional protein. The most frequent mechanism is aberrant splicing which is due to replacement of a single nucleotide in the consensus region of a splice site (BROLY et al. 1991; KAGIMOTO et al. 1990; GONZALEZ et al. 1988). Other molecular mechanisms underlying the PM phenotype consist in complete deletion of the CYP2D6 gene (GAEDIGK et al. 1991). Most recently, HEIM and MEYER (1992) reported the observed 44-kb fragment after digestion with the endonuclease Xba_1 to be associated with four CYP2D genes instead of three.

II. Clinical Consequences of the Sparteine/Debrisoquine Polymorphism and Assignment of Genotype or Phenotype

In contrast to the detailed knowledge concerning the molecular nature of the CYP2D6 polymorphism, clinical data on its relevance are largely restricted to anecdotal reports. Although a variety of frequently used drugs are metabolized by CYP2D6 (see Table 2), no prospective clinical trials have been carried out on the therapeutic relevance of this polymorphism. A number of studies, however, indicate that the genetically related variability in plasma concentrations translates into variable responses which, depending on whether bioinactivation or bioactivation results from CYP2D6-mediated metabolism, may lead to side-effects or therapeutic failure.

One of the first described substrates for this enzyme was sparteine, and this drug has been used as a potent oxytocic. However, during clinical trials to assess its efficacy for induction of labor at term a substantial number of tetanic uterine contractions occurred, leading to adverse fetal outcome (NEWTON et al. 1966). The patients affected were in all probability PMs of sparteine who attained very high plasma concentrations associated with an exaggerated pharmacological effect and the observed adverse outcomes. While the individual phenotype was not established in the study of NEWTON et al. (1966), another retrospective investigation addressed the incidence of polyneuropathy after administration of the calcium channel blocker perhexiline. SHAH et al. (1982, 1983) reported that 50% of patients developing peripheral neuropathy were PMs of debrisoquine.

The class 1C antiarrhythmic propafenone is extensively metabolized to 5-hydroxypropafenone and N-desalkylpropafenone. Extreme interindividual variability in plasma concentrations has been described and was associated with the CYP2D6-mediated 5-hydroxylation of the drug (SIDDOWAY et al. 1987; KROEMER et al. 1989). Siddoway and co-workers showed the PM phenotype to be associated with a higher incidence of CNS side-effects (67%) when compared to patients with the EM phenotype. Besides class 1 antiarrhythmic activity, propafenone exerts β-blockade which resides in the parent compound. Hence, this (side)-effect of propafenone is more pronounced in PMs (Lee et al. 1990). In fact, Lee et al. (1990) reported dose-dependent side-effects in PMs receiving 300 mg propafenone q 8 h, leading to termination of their study in two out of five volunteers. The implications of polymorphic oxidation of propafenone for treatment of arrhythmias, however, are in part masked by the activity of 5-hydroxypropafenone: this metabolite has a similar electrophysiological profile to the parent compound and therefore the lack of active metabolite in a PM may be compensated by accumulation of parent compound.

The class 1C antiarrhythmic N-propylajmaline is polymorphically metabolized to inactive compounds cosegregating with sparteine oxidation. Mörike et al. (1990) were able to show that both clearance of N-propylajmaline and the therapeutic response in terms of arrhythmia suppression depend on the individual CYP2D6 activity. Therefore, the dose of this drug should be adjusted according to the phenotype, thereby avoiding intoxication or insufficient plasma concentrations. Again, these assumptions are based on case reports of clinical observations and no prospective study has been carried out which would prove improvement of safety and efficacy once CYP2D6 activity is used for individualization of dose.

The metabolism of some β-adrenoceptor antagonists cosegregates with sparteine/debrisoquine oxidation (propranolol, metoprolol, timolol, and alprenolol; Lennard 1992). While the CYP2D6-mediated hydroxylation constitutes a minor route of propranolol metabolism and hence no significant differences in clearance are observed between EMs and PMs, other drugs such as metoprolol show phenotype-dependent pharmacokinetics (Lennard 1992). PMs attain much higher concentrations of the β-blockers that are polymorphically metabolized than do EMs when comparable doses are administered. If side-effects are concentration related, then PMs are at greater risk of adverse effects than EMs. Nevertheless, a number of literature reports do not substantiate either this postulated higher incidence of PMs amongst patients who experience side-effects when administered β-adrenoceptor antagonists (Clark et al. 1984) or a higher incidence of side-effects for β-blockers which are eliminated by polymorphic oxidation rather than renal elimination (Regardh and Johnson 1984). Again, prospective studies are lacking.

Some neuroleptics and antidepressants are metabolized by CYP2D6. The latter class of drugs has a narrow therapeutic index and carries a problem similar to that of antiarrhythmic agents: the symptoms of excessive drug concentrations are similar to those of the original syndrome requiring treatment (Bertilsson et al. 1981). Although the list of drugs cosegregating with oxidation of sparteine and debrisoquine is steadily growing (with haloperidol being a recently identified member; Gram et al. 1989; Llerena et al. 1992), the clinical relevance of this variable metabolism is still uncertain.

While in general the PM phenotype is expected to be at higher risk for eliciting concentration-related side-effects, this assumption is reversed once drug action requires metabolic activation and the enzyme responsible for this step is polymorphically expressed. An example of this scenario is the CYP2D6 catalyzed O-demethylation of codeine to morphine (CHEN et al. 1988), with the latter carrying the analgesic effect. Therefore, PMs are expected to have a smaller analgesic effect than EMs. A placebo-controlled study by SINDRUP et al. (1990) confirmed these contentions: the pain threshhold determined by copper vapor laser stimuli was significantly increased in EM but not in PM volunteers after administration of codeine.

While prospective data concerning the clinical relevance are rare, methods for rapid assignment of phenotype or genotype are available. "Phenotypization" requires intake of a probe drug such as sparteine (EICHELBAUM 1975), debrisoquine (MAGHOUB et al. 1977), or dextromethorphan (SCHMID et al. 1985). The excretion of parent compound and/or metabolites in urine allows calculation of a metabolic ratio which assigns CYP2D6 activity to the individual patient. A disadvantage is that application of a probe drug is required and that phenotyping may be hampered in patients who receive other CYP2D6 substrates concomitantly, which block metabolism of the probe drug. Such apparent transformation of an EM phenotype to a PM phenotype is termed "phenocopying" (BROSEN et al. 1987; LEEMANN et al. 1986). Finally, dextromethorphan represents the only probe drug which is readily available in most countries (KÜPFER and PREISIG 1984). Unfortunately, dextromethorphan metabolism proceeds simultaneously via non-CYP2D6 enzymes (MORTIMER et al. 1989), thereby reducing specificity of this probe drug.

Assignment of genotype is independent of concomitant administration of other drugs. Isolation of DNA from peripheral lymphocytes is followed by restriction fragment length polymorphism (RFLP; SKODA et al. 1988) and polymerase chain reaction. The combination of both techniques allows unequivocal assignment of genotype in more than 90% of PMs (HEIM and MEYER 1990). The disadvantage of genotyping is the limited information concerning the individual CYP2D6 activity within the EM phenotype. A wide variability may occur within one phenotype and this variability cannot be assessed once "genotypization" is used.

In summary, a general problem in evaluating the therapeutic relevance of polymorphic expression of CYP2D6 is the lack of prospective clinical studies. While the original observation was made by clinicians, rapid progress in molecular biology, and therefore knowledge of the molecular mechanisms of this defect, has preceded studies of therapeutic implications.

C. The Genetic Polymorphism of Mephenytoin Oxidation

Mephenytoin (3-methyl-5-phenyl-5-ethylhydantoin) has been used as an anticonvulsant ever since it was developed in the 1940s. The major metabolic pathways consist of 4'-hydroxylation (4'-hydroxymephenytoin; 4'-

OH-M) and N-demethylation (5-phenyl-5-ethylthydantoin; PEH; Nirvanol). Nirvanol contributes to the anticonvulsive activity after administration of mephenytoin. During pharmakokinetic studies with mephenytoin the urinary metabolic profile of one subject showed a marked impairment in the ability to form 4'-hydroxymephenytoin (KÜPFER et al. 1984). Moreover, stereo-selectivity of mephenytoin disposition, which is due to preferential 4'-hydroxylation of S-mephenytoin and which leads to the predominance of the R-enantiomer plasma, was absent in this volunteer. Further studies revealed that this defect was familial, which was the basis for further detailed research.

I. Molecular Mechanisms of the Mephenytoin Polymorphism

Studies using conventional biochemistry techniques indicated that mepheny-toin 4'-hydroxylation and N-demethylation were mediated by cytochrome P-450 isozymes (JURIMA et al. 1985; MEIER et al. 1985; HALL et al. 1987). P-450MP is a member of the IIC subfamily which is characterized by inducibility by phenobarbital and constitutive expression. The gene for P-450MP is located on the long arm of chromosome 10 (OKINO et al. 1987). At least two enzymes designated as P-450MP1 and P-450MP2 have been isolated which have the capability to 4'-hydroxylate mephenytoin (SHIMADA et al. 1986). Despite intensive work, no detailed insight into the mechanism of the mephenytoin polymorphism has been obtained so far. P-450MP appears to be present in PMs of mephenytoin and the mechanism of the mephenytoin 4'-hydroxylation deficiency may be a minor structural change causing altered function of the cytochrome P-450 isozyme. This hypothesis was supported by using antibodies prepared from sera of patients suffering from tienilic acid-induced hepatitis (MEIER and MEYER 1987). These antibodies are designated anti-LKM2 and are strong inhibitors of P-450MP. Isolation of P-450MP from EM and PM liver microsomes by means of anti-LKM2 immunoaffinity columns revealed similar proteins from both phenotypes. Catalytic activity, however, was impaired in the protein isolated from PM livers. If a minor structural change is indeed responsible for an altered P-450 leading to deficiency in mephenytoin 4'-hydroxylation, molecular biology techniques are likely to detect this alteration. Consequently, expression libraries have been screened and several clones for P-450MP have been isolated. Two of them, called MP-8 and MP-4 (CYP2C9 and CYP2C10; NEBERT et al. 1991), differ by only two bases in the coding region, and both are present in human liver samples, thereby indicating the existence of a multigene family. Heterologous expression studies have revealed the complex situation in the CYP2C family: although yeast microsomes reacted with polyclonal anti-CYP$_{MP-1}$, they had less than 6% of the S-mephenytoin 4'-hydroxylase activity of human liver microsomes but a high activity in hydroxylation of the tolylmethyl moiety of tolbutamide (BRIAN et al. 1989). In summary, the CYP2C family consists of several closely related enzymes with oxidation of mephenytoin and tolbutamide being catalyzed by different enzymes. Mephenytoin 4'-hydroxylation may be catalyzed by CYPs different from CYP2C8-10 (SRIVASTAVA et al. 1991).

II. Clinical Consequences of Polymorphic Mephenytoin Oxidation and Assignment of Genotype or Phenotype

The in vivo metabolism of a number of drugs appears to be coregulated by the same genetic factor(s) involved in the 4'-hydroxylation of mephenytoin (Table 3). KÜPFER and BRANCH (1985) reported that mephobarbital 4'-hydroxylation was essentially absent in PMs of mephenytoin. A similar effect has been described for hexobarbital (KNODELL et al. 1988). These substrates are structurally closely related to mephenytoin and HALL et al. (1987) studied the relationship between structural changes and affinity to P-450MP. He described the minimal requirement for binding to P-450MP to be an aryl or cyclohexenyl ring positioned alpha to the carbonyl carbon of an N-alkyllactam in a five- or six-membered ring. Propranolol 4'-hydroxylation is coregulated with debrisoquine metabolic activity. WARD et al. (1989) reported the formation of another metabolic pathway of propranolol – formation of naphthoxylactic acid – to cosegregate with mephenytoin 4'-hydroxylation. Thus, propranolol appears to be the first substrate described whose metabolism requires both CYP2D6 and P-450MP and is therefore catalyzed by two enzymes which exhibit a genetic polymorphism. More recently, a similar phenomenon has been reported by SKJELBO et al. (1991) for imipramine. N-Demethylation of imipramine was significantly reduced in PMs of mephenytoin. BERTILSSON et al. (1989) reported the plasma clearance of both diazepam and desmethyldiazepam to be reduced in PMs of mephenytoin. By virtue of the fact that benzodiazepines are among the most commonly used drugs, these findings, if confirmed, would yield progress in the understanding of interindividual differences in drug response to benzodiazepines.

The proton pump inhibitor omeprazole exhibits a reduced clearance in PMs of mephenytoin (ANDERSSON et al. 1990). In parallel the drug was shown to induce CYP1A1 and CYP1A2; the latter results, however, were

Table 3. Compounds whose metabolism cosegregate with that of mephenytoin and the metabolic pathways affected

Diazepam	N-Demethylation	BERTILSSON et al. (1989)
Hexobarbital	Hydroxylation	KNODELL et al. (1988)
Imipramine	N-Demethylation	SKJELBO et al. (1991)
Mephobarbital	4-Hydroxylation	KÜPFER and BRANCH (1985)
Omeprazole		ANDERSSON et al. (1990)
Proguanil	Formation of cycloguanil	WARD et al. (1991)
Propranolol	Side chain oxidation	WARD et al. (1989)

inconsistent and variable. Recently, ROST et al. (1992) showed that induction of CYP1A2 activity is restricted to PMs of mephenytoin. The possible consequences of this observation with respect to CYP1A2-dependent bioactivation of carcinogens remain to be elucidated.

The antimalarial agent proguanil is bioactivated to cycloguanil. This metabolic step cosegregates with the mephenytoin oxidation polymorphism, leading to a significantly higher urinary ratio of parent compound to active metabolite (WARD et al. 1991).

Finally, there are some nongenetic factors contributing to mephenytoin disposition characteristics. ARNS et al. (1988) described the S/R ratio in urine to be close to unity in patients with reduced hepatic function or portasystemic shunting. Thus, hepatic dysfunction affects mainly the disposition of S-mephenytoin. Moreover, 4'-hydroxylation of mephenytoin appears to be inducible by rifampin.

To determine the exact frequency of impaired mephenytoin metabolism in a population a robust method of obtaining an index indicative of the individual phenotype is required. However, only traces of unchanged mephenytoin after a single oral dose are excreted in urine in the EM phenotype, which does not allow exact quantification on a routine basis. Thus it has been suggested that the so-called hydroxylation index be used, which represents the molar ratio of the dose of S-mephenytoin and the amount of 4'-hydroxymephenytoin in the urine from 0 to 8h (KÜPFER and PREISIG 1984). A second trait measurement approach takes advantage of the different pharmacokinetic profiles of the mephenytoin enantiomers (WEDLUND et al. 1984). S-Mephenytoin is characterized by a high hepatic extraction ratio and high first-pass metabolism to form 4'-OH-M. In contrast R-mephenytoin is poorly extracted by the liver and mainly N-demethylated to form nirvanol. Consequently AUC and therefore apparent oral clearance exhibit a 200-fold difference. The half-lives for S- and R-mephenytoin average 2.13 ± 0.9h and 76 ± 38h, respectively. In subjects with impaired 4'-hydroxylation of mephenytoin these differences in extraction ratio are absent and the pharmacokinetic profiles of both mephenytoin enantiomers are more similar. Thus it has been suggested that the 0–8h urinary R/S ratio be used as a phenotyping index, with low values representing slow metabolizers and high values representing EMs (JACQZ et al. 1986).

Using both the hydroxylation index and the 8-h urinary enantiomeric ratio to phenotype 156 unrelated Tennessians of Caucasian origin, a complete concordance between the two methods was found and the incidence of slow metabolizers was found to be 2.7% (WEDLUND et al. 1984). Overall, studies performed to date have identified 33 PMs of mephenytoin among 834 Caucasians, which represents a prevalence of 3.7% (WILKINSON et al. 1992). No correlation was found to the debrisoquine metabolizer phenotype (KÜPFER and PREISIG 1984). Family studies revealed that the impaired mephenytoin 4'-hydroxylation is inherited as an autosomal recessive trait which involves at least two alleles at a single gene locus (INABA et al. 1986).

Attempts have been made to establish an RFLP using MP-8 as a probe to test human genomic DNA after digestion with different restriction enzymes (GED et al. 1988). However, RFLP patterns did not match in vivo phenotypes. Therefore, this technique appears to be unsuitable for phenotyping individuals. The exact mechanism of polymorphic mephenytoin 4'-hydroxylation on a genetic level, however, is still unclear and remains to be elucidated.

In summary, mephenytoin 4'-hydroxylation has been the subject of extensive research over the past decade. A genetically determined polymorphism with a frequency of 4% in the Caucasian population has been described and a variety of drugs cosegregate with that polymorphism. As outlined above for the sparteine/debrisoquine polymorphism, data concerning therapeutic implications are lacking.

D. The Genetic Polymorphism of N-Acetylation

Isoniazid was introduced for the treatment of tuberculosis in 1952 (ROBITZEK et al. 1952) and quickly attained widespread popularity. One year later it was reported that a population of 86 patients could be subdivided into two subgroups (BÖNIKE and REIF 1953), with about 50% excreting the drug in N-acetylated form. These findings were expanded upon by MITCHELL and BELL (1957), who described a clear-cut bimodality in parameters describing isoniazid disposition. The major metabolites excreted in urine were identified to be acetylisoniazid and nicotinic acid (HUGHES et al. 1955). The patients who excreted most of the drug as parent compound were referred to as "slow acetylators" as compared to the remaining patients who excreted the drug as N-acetyl conjugate and were termed "rapid acetylators" (EVANS et al. 1960).

In Caucasians the incidence of the rapid acetylator phenotype is approximately 50% (McQUEEN 1980). Family studies have revealed that variability in acetylation is genetically determined by at least two alleles at a single gene locus (ISELIUS and EVANS 1983). Moreover, acetylation capacity is influenced by factors such as age, sex, and weight.

I. Molecular Mechanisms of Polymorphic N-Acetylation

Until recently, the cause of the deficiency in acetylation observed in slow acetylators was unknown. Most information has been obtained using animal models. Liver samples obtained from New Zealand rabbits which could be phenotyped as slow or rapid acetylators contained equal quantities of N-acetyltransferases (ANDERS and WEBER 1986). In contrast, human liver samples from slow and rapid acetylators exhibited differences in kinetic experiments which suggested that the variation in acetylation capacity could be attributed to different quantities of N-acetyltransferases (JENNE 1965).

More recently, GRANT et al. (1990) compared the in vivo acetylation capacity in patients who donated liver wedge biopsy specimens with the in vitro activity of N-acetyltransferase observed in these specimens (GRANT et al. 1990). A significant correlation between in vivo and in vitro activity was noted. Moreover, Western blots from liver samples of slow acetylators showed a decrease in or absence of immunoreactive protein. These data suggest that defective drug acetylation in the slow acetylator phenotype is due to a decrease in the amount of the enzyme present. Isolation of a human gene encoding arylamine N-acetyltransferases has recently been reported (GRANT et al. 1989). Several mutant alleles have been identified (DEGUCHI et al. 1990; BLUM et al. 1991; VATSIS et al. 1991). A radiolabeled cDNA from rabbits was used to screen a human genomic library (BLUM et al. 1990). Three nonoverlapping clusters were identified and termed NAT1, NAT2, and NATP. NAT1 and NAT2 are located on chromosome 8. Expression in COS-1 cells resulted in N-acetyltransferase activity for the substrate sulfamethazine. Moreover, recombinant NAT2 was highly specific in metabolizing polymorphically acetylated substrates. Using RFLP analysis of genomic DNA with restriction endonuclease Kpn1 revealed several mutant alleles of NAT2. The most frequent ones were termed M1 and M2.

II. Clinical Consequences of Polymorphic Acetylation and Assignment of Genotype or Phenotype

The metabolism of a variety of drugs is dependent on acetylator phenotype (Table 4). The relationship between acetylator phenotype and development of certain diseases has been investigated and reviewed by EVANS (1992). A high incidence of slow acetylators has been reported among patients with chemically induced bladder cancer (EVANS et al. 1983). More recently, HORAI et al. (1989) reported no association between acetylator phenotype and the development of spontaneous bladder cancer in a population of 51 Japanese patients who were not exposed to occupational risk factors. Drug-induced lupus erythematosus has been reported to be more frequent in slow acetylators. This subgroup of patients developed antinuclear antibodies at lower doses of procainamide than fast acetylators (WOOSLEY et al. 1978). The data presently available on the possible association between diabetes mellitus and acetylator phenotype are also reviewed by EVANS (1992). In

Table 4. Drugs which are polymorphically acetylated (EVANS 1992)

Aminoglutethimide	Dapsone	Prizidilol
7-Amino nitrazepam	Dipyrone	Procainamide
Amrinone	Endralazine	Sulfamerazine
Caffeine	Hydralazine/hydrazine	Sulfamethazine
Clonazepam metabolites	Isoniazid	Sulfapyridine

European patients the incidence of diabetes is higher among rapid acetylators. Therefore, some diseases appear to be associated with acetylator phenotype. In the case of chemically induced bladder cancer such an association may be anticipated since xenobiotic aromatic amines which have been held responsible for the development of the disease are polymorphically acetylated. The association of acetylator phenotype with Gilbert's syndrome, diabetes, and other disorders is based on the higher incidence of slow acetylators in the populations studied and the underlying causes are not yet understood.

In addition to isoniazid a variety of probe drugs including sulfadimidine (RAO et al. 1970), dapsone (DRAYER and REIDENBERG 1977), and caffeine (GRANT et al. 1984) have been used to establish the acetylator phenotype.

Recent work by BLUM et al. (1991) identified an additional rare mutant allele (M3) and described a genotyping procedure which identifies more than 95% of slow and rapid acetylator alleles. Another genotyping procedure has been developed identifying new allotypic variants of slow acetylators (HICKMAN et al. 1992).

E. Genetic Polymorphisms and Drug Development

While the clinical consequences of genetically determined polymorphisms in drug metabolism are subject to discussion, there is no doubt that these phenomena introduce interindividual variability into the dose–concentration relationship. Thus, administration of the same dose may lead to large differences in the plasma concentrations achieved. This phenomenon is important for development of new drugs. So far volunteers in phase I studies have been selected on the basis of "normal" health status as assessed by certain biochemical parameters. The individual drug-metabolizing capacity was often not taken into account and the use of model compounds for testing drug metabolism (e.g., antipyrine) is of limited value as long as the enzymes involved in metabolism of these compounds are not identified. In order to identify cosegregation of a new compound's metabolism with a polymorphism, volunteers should be phenotyped and/or genotyped for sparteine/debrisoquine hydroxylation, mephenytoin oxidation, and N-acetylation capacity. Metabolic profiles of the new compound in different phenotypes can be compared in a so-called panel approach. One of the rare published examples of this procedure is that of CGP 15210 G by GLEITER et al. (1985), in which significant differences in clearance of CGP 15210 G were observed between EMs and PMs for CYP2D6-mediated sparteine hydroxylation. A disadvantage of this approach is that recognition of genetically determined variability in metabolism of a new compound in the setting of a phase 1 study occurs at a late stage of drug development. Therefore, it would be desirable to develop strategies for prediction of metabolic profiles at early stages of drug development.

Several in vitro approaches have been developed which allow prediction of whether metabolism of a new compound is subject to genetic polymorphism during preclinical testing. In the case of sparteine/debrisoquine polymorphism, attempts were made to use molecular modeling based on common structural features for assignment of metabolic pathways (Islam et al. 1991; Meyer et al. 1986; Guengerich et al. 1986). At present this technique is not sufficient for reliable prediction of affinity to CYP2D6 and extent of CYP2D6-mediated metabolism from structural data.

Stable expression of drug-metabolizing enzymes allows unequivocal assignment of a certain metabolic pathway to an enzyme. Either formation of metabolites of the new compound by stable expressed enzymes or inhibition of the metabolism of known substrates for this enzyme by the new drug can be investigated. Recent work by Fischer et al. (1992) applied this technique to the neuroleptic clozapine. A disadvantage of this appoach is that only one enzyme is stably expressed while – after administration to humans – the new drug may be metabolized by several enzymes via different routes and at different rates.

A complementary technique, therefore, is the use of human liver tissues which host a variety of drug-metabolizing enzymes. The microsomal fraction of human liver allows characterization of phase I pathways involved in the biotransformation of a new compound and estimation of which pathways are controlled by polymorphically expressed enzymes. Such identification and quantitation of metabolic profiles based on in vitro experiments correlating rate of formation of the new drug with that of known substrates, inhibition of metabolic pathways by specific antibodies, and formation via stable expressed enzymes has been successfully applied to metabolism of the antiarrhythmic propafenone (Kroemer et al. 1989; Botsch et al. 1993). Therapeutic implications of CYP2D6-mediated formation of 5-hydroxypropafenone (genetically determined) and CYP3A4-catalyzed formation of N-desalkylpropafenone (environmentally determined) could be predicted on the basis of in vitro experiments.

F. Genetic Polymorphisms and Drug Interactions

If a drug-metabolizing enzyme is subject to a genetic polymorphism then concomitant administration of two drugs which are both metabolized by this enzyme can lead to genetically determined drug interactions. Such interactions will be restricted to the EM phenotype.

This phenomenon has been investigated in detail for CYP2D6 because this enzyme is not only absent in PMs but has a limited metabolizing capacity for many drugs in EMs. Consequently, patients of EM-phenotype show nonlinear pharmacokinetics due to saturation of CYP2D6-catalyzed first-pass metabolism (e.g., propafenone: Siddoway et al. 1987; imipramine: Brosen and Gram 1988). As a result of this finite metabolizing capacity the enzyme is the site of a number of drug interactions the consequences of which depend on the relative affinity of the compounds to CYP2D6. The antiarrhythmic propafenone binds with high affinity to the enzyme and metabolism of other drugs such as metoprolol (WAGNER et al. 1987) may be inhibited.

The interaction of two substrates for CYP2D6 can result in a number of clinical responses. Higher plasma concentrations of parent compound may lead to enhanced pharmacodynamic responses. This has been demonstrated for the combination of ajmaline and quinidine. The latter drug inhibits the first-pass metabolism of ajmaline to such a degree that the area under the plasma concentration vs time curve is increased up to 30-fold (HORI et al. 1984). Combining neuroleptics and antidepressants may result in clinically significant interactions (GRAM and OVERO 1972; GRAM 1975; NELSON and JATLOW 1980).

Such interactions, however, may lead to lack of therapeutic response when pharmacological activity is mediated by an active metabolite. Combination of quinidine and encainide resulted in less pronounced QRS widening than did administration of encainide alone in volunteers with the EM phenotype (FUNCK-BRENTANO et al. 1989). This interaction is explained by inhibition of formation of the active metabolite O-desmethyl-encainide by quinidine.

G. Conclusions

Discovery of genetic polymorphism in drug metabolism has contributed a great deal to understanding the variability in dose–concentration relationships introduced by genetic factors, thereby elucidating the mechanism responsible for certain unexpected drug reactions. This knowledge should find its way into clinical practice in order to make therapy more efficient and safe. Moreover, genetic factors in drug metabolism should be taken into account during drug development. Therefore, in vitro methods for identifying the metabolic pattern of new compounds during early stages of drug development should be improved. The field of pharmacogenetics in general may be broadened in the future and, beside drug metabolism, focus on genetic mechanisms of expression of transporters and receptors for foreign compounds (GONZALEZ 1992).

References

Alvan G, von Bahr C, Seideman P, Sjöqvist F (1982) High plasma concentrations of β-receptor blocking drugs and deficient debrisoquine hydroxylation. Lancet 1:333

Alvan G, Grind M, Graffner C, Sjöqvist F (1984) Relationship of N-demethylation of amiflamine and its metabolite to debrisoquine hydroxylation polymorphism. Clin Pharmacol Ther 36:515–519

Anders HH, Weber WW (1986) N-acetylation pharmacogenetics: Michealis-Menten constants for aryamine drugs as predictors of their N-acetylation rates in vivo. Drug Metab Dispos 14:382–385

Andersson T, Regardh CG, Dahl-Puustinen ML, Bertilsson L (1990) Slow omeprazole metabolizers are also poor S-mephenytoin hydroxylators. Ther Drug Monit 12:415–416

Arns PA, Wilkinson GR, Branch RA (1988) The stereoselective disposition of mephenytoin provides a probe of hepatic function and development of portasystemic shunts in liver disease. Hepatology 8:1277

Ayesh R, Smith RL (1992) Genetic polymorphism of trimethylamine N-oxidation. In: Kalow W (ed) Pharmacogenetics of drug metabolism. Pergamon, New York, pp 315–333

Balant-Gorgia AE, Balant LP, Genet C, Dayer P, Aeschlimann JM, Garrone G (1986) Importance of oxidative polymorphism and levomepromazine treatment on the steady-state blood concentrations of clomipramine and its major metabolites. Eur J Clin Pharmacol 31:449–455

Beckmann J, Hertrampf R, Gundert-Remy U, Mikus G, Gross AS, Eichelbaum M (1988) Is there a genetic factor in flecainide toxicity? Br Med J 297:1326

Bertilsson L, Mellström B, Sjöqvist F, Martensson B, Asberg M (1981) Slow hydroxylation of nortriptyline and concomitant poor debrisoquine hydroxylation: clinical implications. Lancet 1:560–561

Bertilsson L, Henthorn TK, Sanze E, Tybring G, Säwe J, Villen T (1989) Importance of genetic factors in the regulation of diazepam metabolism: relationship to S-mephenytoin, but not debrisoquine hydroxylation phenotype. Clin Pharmacol Ther 45:348–355

Blum M, Grant DM, McBride W, Heim M, Meyer UA (1990) Human arylamine N-acetyltransferase genes: isolation, chromosomal localisation and functional expression. DNA Cell Biol 9:193–203

Blum M, Demierre A, Grant DM, Heim M, Meyer UA (1991) Molecular mechanism of slow acetylation of drugs and carcinogens in humans. Proc Natl Acad Sci USA 88:5237–5241

Bönike R, Reif W (1953) Enzymatische Inaktivierung von Isonicotinsäurehydrazid im menschlichen und tierischen Organismus. Arch Exp Pathol Pharmakol 220:321–333

Botsch S, Gautier JC, Beaune P, Eichelbaum M, Kroemer HK (1993) Identification and characterization of the cytochrome P450 enzymes involved in N-dealkylation of propafenone: molecular base for interaction potential and variable disposition of active metabolites. Mol Pharmacol 43:120–126

Brian WR, Srivastava PK, Umbenhauer DR, Lloyd RS, Guengerich FP (1989) Expression of a human liver cytochrome P-450 protein with tolbutamide hydroxylase activity in Saccharomyces cerevisiae. Biochemistry 28:4993–4999

Broly F, Gaedigk A, Heim M, Eichelbaum M, Mörike K, Meyer UA (1991) Debrisoquine/sparteine hydroxylation genotype and phenotype: analysis of common mutations and alleles of CYP2D6 in a European population. DNA Cell Biol 10:545–558

Brosen K, Gram LF (1988) First-pass metabolism of imipramine and desipramine: impact of the sparteine oxidation phenotype. Clin Pharmacol Ther 43:400–406

Brosen K, Gram LF, Klysner R, Bech P (1986) Steady-state levels of imipramine and its metabolites: significance of dose-dependent kinetics. Eur J Clin Pharmacol 30:43–49

Brosen K, Gram LF, Haghfelt T, Bertilsson L (1987) Extensive metabolizers of debrisoquine become poor metabolizers during quinidine treatment: Pharmacol Toxicol 60:312–314

Burchell B, Coughtrie MWH (1992) UDP-glucuronosyltransferases. In: Kalow W (ed) Pharmacogenetics of drug metabolism. Pergamon, New York, pp 95–165

Chen ZR, Somogyi AA, Bochner F (1988) Polymorphic O-demethylation of codeine. Lancet 2:914–915

Clark DWJ, Morgan AKW, Waal-Manning H (1984) Adverse effects from meto-prolol are not generally associated with oxidation status. Br J Clin Pharmacol 18:965–966

Cooper RG, Evans DAP, Whibley EJ (1984) Polymorphic hydroxylation of perhexi-line maleate in man. J Med Genet 21:27–33

Dahl-Puustinen ML, Liden A, Alm C, Nordin C, Bertilsson L (1989) Disposition of perphenazine is related to the polymorphic debrisoquine hydroxylation in human beings. Clin Pharmacol Ther 46:78–81

Dayer P, Leemann T, Küpfer A, Kronbach T, Meyer UA (1986) Stereo- and re-gioselectivity of hepatic oxidation in man – effect of the debrisoquine/sparteine phenotype on bufuralol hydroxylation. Eur J Clin Pharmacol 31:313–318

Dayer P, Desmeules J, Leemann T, Striberni R (1988) Bioactivation of the narcotic drug codeine in human liver is mediated by the polymorphic monooxygenase catalyzing debrisoquine 4-hydroxylation (cytochrome P-450 db1/buf1). Biochem Biophys Res Commun 152:4161–4165

Deguchi T, Mashimo M, Suzuki T (1990) Correlation between acetylator phenotype and genotypes of polymorphic arylamine N-acetyltransferase in human liver. J Biol Chem 265:12757–12760

Drayer DE, Reidenberg DM (1977) Clinical consequences of polymorphic acetylation of basic drugs. Clin Pharmacol Ther 22:251–258

Ebner T, Eichelbaum M (1993) The metabolism of aprindine in relation to the sparteine/debrisoquine polymorphism. Br J Clin Pharmacol 35:426–430

Eichelbaum M (1975) Ein neuentdeckter Defekt im Arzneimittelstoffwechsel des Menschen: Die fehlende N-Oxidation des Spartein. Habilitationsschrift, Fried-rich-Wilhelms-University, Bonn

Eichelbaum M, Gross AS (1992) The genetic polymorphism of debrisoquine sparteine metabolism – clinical aspects. In: Kalow W (ed) Pharmacogenetics of drug metabolism. Pergamon, New York, pp 625–643

Eichelbaum M, Spannbrucker N, Steincke B, Dengler HJ (1979) Defective N-oxidation of sparteine in man: a new pharmacogenetic defect. Eur J Clin Pharmacol 16:183–187

Eichelbaum M, Baur MP, Dengler HJ, Osikowska-Evers BO, Tieves G, Zekorn C, Rittner C (1987) Chromosomal assignment of human cytochrome P450 (debriso-quine/sparteine type) to chromosome 22. Br J Clin Pharmacol 23:455–458

Evans DAP (1992) N-acetyltransferase. In: Kalow W (ed) Pharmacogenetics of drug metabolism. Pergamon, New York, pp 95–165

Evans DAP, Manley KA, McKusick VA (1960) Genetic control of isoniazid metabo-lism in man. Br Med J 2:485–461

Evans DAP, Mahgoub A, Sloan TP, Idle JR, Smith RL (1980) A family and population study of the genetic polymorphism of debrisoquine oxidation in a white British population. J Med Genet 17:102–105

Evans DAP, Eze LZ, Whibley EJ (1983) The association of the slow acetylator phenotype with bladder cancer. J Med Genet 20:321–329

Feher MD, Lucas RA, Farid NA, Idle JR, Bergstrom RF, Lemberger L, Sever PS (1988) Single dose pharmacokinetics of tomoxetine in poor and extensive meta-bolisers of debrisoquine. Br J Clin Pharmacol 26:231P

Fischer V (1992) Polymorphic drug metabolism and its consequences for drug devel-opment (Abstr). 13th European Workshop on Drug Metabolism, Bergamo

Fischer V, Vogels B, Maurer G, Tynes RE (1992) The antipsychotic clozapine is metabolized by the polymorphic human microsomal and recombinant cyto-chrome P450 2D6. J Pharmacol Exp Ther 260:1355–1360

Funck-Brentano C, Turgeon J, Woosley RL, Roden DM (1989) Effects of low dose quinidine on encainide pharmacokinetics and pharmacodynamics. Influence of genetic polymorphism. J Pharmacol Ther 249:134–142

Gaedigk A, Blum M, Gaedigk R, Eichelbaum M, Meyer UA (1991) Deletion of the entire cytochrome P450 CYP2D6 gene as a cause of impaired drug metabolism in poor metabolizers of the debrisoquine/sparteine polymorphism. Am J Hum Genet 48:943–950

Garrod AE (1902) The incidence of alcaptonuria: a study in chemical individuality. Lancet 2:1616–1620

Garrod AE (1931) The inborn factors of disease. Oxford University Press, London

Ged C, Umbenhauer DR, Bellew TM, Bork RW, Srivastava PK, Shinriki N, Lloyd RS, Guengerich FP (1988) Characterization of cDNAs, mRNAs and proteins related to human liver microsomal cytochrome P450 *S*-mephenytoin 4-hydroxylase. Biochemistry 27:6929–6940

Gleiter CH, Aichele G, Nilsson E, Hengen N, Antonin KH, Bieck PR (1985) Discovery of altered pharmacokinetics of CGP 15210G in poor hydroxylators of debrisoquine during early drug development. Br J Clin Pharmacol 20:81–84

Goedde HW, Agarwal DP (1992) Pharmacogenetics of aldehyde dehydrogenase. In: Kalow W (ed) Pharmacogenetics of drug metabolism. Pergamon, New York, pp 281–314

Gonzalez FJ (1992) Pharmacogenetics redefined. Trends Pharmacol Sci 13:348

Gonzalez FJ, Skoda RC, Kimura S, Umeno M, Zanger UM, Nebert DW, Gelboin HV, Hardwick JP, Meyer UA (1988) Characterization of the common genetic defect in humans deficient in debrisoquine metabolism. Nature 331:442–446

Gram LF (1975) Effects of perphenazine on imipramine metabolism in man. Psychopharmacol Commun 1:165–175

Gram LF, Overo KF (1972) Drug interaction: inhibitory effect of neuroleptics on metabolism of tricyclic antidepressants in man. Br Med J 163:463–465

Gram LF, Debruyne D, Caillard V, Boulenger JP, Lacotte J, Moulin M, Zarifian E (1989) Substantial rise in sparteine metabolic ratio during haloperidol treatment. Br J Clin Pharmacol 27:272–275

Grant DM, Blum M, Demierre A, Meyer UA (1989) Nucleotide sequence for an intronless gene for a human arylamine *N*-acetyltransferase related to polymorphic drug acetylation. Nucleic Acids Res 17:3978

Grant DM, Mörike K, Eichelbaum M, Meyer UA (1990) Acetylation pharmacogenetics. The slow acetylator phenotype is caused by decreased or absent arylamine *N*-acetyltransferase in human liver. J Clin Invest 85:968–972

Grant DM, Tang BK, Kalow W (1984) Polymorphic N-acetylation of a caffeine metabolite. Clin Pharmacol Ther 33:355–359

Guengerich FP, Distlerath LM, Reilly PEB, Wolff T, Shimada T, Umbenhauer DR, Martin MV (1986) Human-liver cytochromes P-450 involved in polymorphisms of drug oxidation. Xenobiotica 16:367–378

Hall SD, Guengerich FP, Branch RA, Wilkinson GR (1987) Characterization and inhibition of mephenytoin 4-hydroxylase activity in human liver microsomes. J Pharmacol Exp Ther 240:216–222

Heim M, Meyer UA (1990) Genotyping of poor metabolizers of debrisoquine by allele specific PCR-amplification. Lancet 336:529–532

Heim M, Meyer UA (1992) Evolution of a highly polymorphic human cytochrome P450 gene cluster: CYP2D6. Genomics 14:49–58

Hickman D, Risch A, Camilleri JP, Sim E (1992) Genotyping human arylamine *N*-acetyltransferase: identification of new allotypic variants. Pharmacogenetics 2:217–226

Horai Y, Fujita K, Ishizaki T (1989) Genetically determined N-acetylation and oxidation capacities in Japanese patients with non occupational urinary bladder cancer. Eur J Clin Pharmacol 37:581–587

Hori R, Okumura K, Inui KI, Yasuhara M, Yamada K, Sakurai T, Kawai C (1984) Quinidine-induced rise in ajmaline plasma concentration. J Pharm Pharmacol 36:202–204

Hughes HB, Schmidt LH, Biehl JP (1955) The metabolism of isoniazide, its implications in therapeutic use. 14th Conference on Chemotherapy in Tuberculosis, Washington DC, US Veterans Adm Army Navy, pp 217–222

Inaba T, Jurima M, Kalow W (1986) Family studies of mephenytoin hydroxylation deficiency. Am J Hum Genet 38:768–772

Iselius L, Evans DAP (1983) Formal genetics of isoniazid metabolism in man. Clin Pharmacol Ther Clin Pharmacokinet 8:541–544

Islam SA, Wolf CR, Lennard MS, Sternberg MJE (1991) A three-dimensional molecular template for substrates of human cytochrome P450 involved in debrisoquine 4-hydroxylation. Carcinogenesis 12:2211–2219

Jacqz E, Hall SD, Branch RA, Wilkinson GR (1986) Polymorphic metabolism of mephenytoin in man: pharmacokinetic interaction with a coregulated substrate, mephobarbital. Clin Pharmacol Ther 39:646–653

Jenne JW (1965) Partial purification and properties of the isoniazide transacetylase in human liver: its relationship to the acetylation of *para*-amino salicylic acid. J Clin Invest 44:1992–2002

Jurima M, Inaba T, Kalow W (1985) Mephenytoin metabolism in vitro by human liver. Drug Metab Dispos 13:151–155

Kagimoto M, Heim M, Kagimoto K, Zeugin T, Meyer UA (1990) Multiple mutations of the human cytochrome P450IID6 gene (CYP2D6) in poor metabolizers of debrisoquine. J Biol Chem 265:17209–17214

Kalow W (1956) Familial incidence of low pseudocholinesterase level. Lancet 2: 576–577

Kalow W, Genest K (1957) A method for the detection of atypical forms of the human serum cholinesterase. Determination of dibucaine numbers. Can J Biochem Physiol 35:339–346

Kalow W, Staron N (1957) On distribution and inheritance of atypical forms of human serum cholinesterase as indicated by dibucaine numbers. Can J Biochem Physiol 35:1305–1320

Kitchen I, Tremblay J, Andre J, Dring LG, Idle JR, Smith RL, Williams RT (1979) Inter-individual and inter-species variation in the metabolism of the hallucinogen 4-methoxyamphetamine. Xenobiotica 9:397–404

Knodell RG, Dubey RK, Wilkinson GR, Guengerich FP (1988) Oxidative metabolism of hexobarbital in human liver: relationship to polymorphic *S*-mephenytoin 4-hydroxylation. J Pharmacol Exp Ther 245:845–849

Kroemer HK, Mikus G, Kronbach T, Meyer UA, Eichelbaum M (1989) In vitro characterization of the human cytochrome P-450 involved in polymorphic oxidation of propafenone. Clin Pharmacol Ther 45:28–33

Küpfer A, Branch RA (1985) Stereoselective mephobarbital hydroxylation cosegregates with mephenytoin hydroxylation. Clin Pharmacol Ther 38:414–418

Küpfer A, Preisig R (1984) Pharmacogenetics of mephenytoin: a new drug hydroxylation polymorphism in man. Eur J Clin Pharmacol 26:753–759

Küpfer A, Schmid B, Preisig R, Pfaff G (1984) Dextromethorphan as a safe probe for debrisoquine hydroxylation polymorphism. Lancet 1:517–518

Lee JT, Kroemer HK, Silberstein DJ, Funck-Brentano C, Lineberry MD, Wood AJJ, Roden DM, Woosley RL (1990) The role of genetically determined polymorphic drug metabolism in the beta-blockade produced by propafenone. N Engl J Med 322:1764–1768

Leemann T, Dayer P, Meyer UA (1986) Single-dose quinidine treatment inhibits metoprolol oxidation in extensive metabolizers. Eur J Clin Pharmacol 29: 739–741

Lennard MS (1992) The polymorphic oxidation of β-adrenoceptor antagonists. In: Kalow W (ed) Pharmacogenetics of drug metabolism. Pergamon, New York, pp 701–720

Lewis RV, Lennard MS, Jackson PR, Tucker GT, Ramsay LE, Woods HF (1985) Timolol and atenolol: relationships between oxidation phenotype, pharmacokinetics and pharmacodynamics. Br J Clin Pharmacol 19:329–333

Llerena A, Dahl MJ, Ekqvist B, Bertilsson L (1992) Haloperidol disposition is dependent on the debrisoquine hydroxylation phenotype: increased plasma levels of the reduced metabolite in poor metabolizers. Ther Drug Monit 14:261–264

Lockridge O (1992) Genetic variants of human serum butyrylcholinesterase influence the metabolism of the muscle relaxant succinylcholine. In: Kalow W (ed) Pharmacogenetics of drug metabolism. Pergamon, New York, pp 15–50

Mahgoub A, Idle JR, Dring LG, Lancaster R, Smith RL (1977) Polymorphic hydroxylation of debrisoquine in man. Lancet 2:584–586

McGourty JC, Silas JH, Fleming JJ, McBurney A, Ward JW (1985) Pharmacokinetics and beta-blocking effects of timolol in poor and extensive metabolisers of debrisoquin. Clin Pharmacol Ther 38:409–413

McGuire MC, Nogueira CP, Bartels CF, Lightstone H, Hajra A, van der Spek AFL, Lockridge O, La Du BN (1989) Identification of the structural mutation responsible for the dibucaine resistant (atypical) variant form of human serum cholinesterase. Proc Natl Acad Sci USA 86:953–957

McQueen EG (1980) Pharmacological bases of adverse drug reactions. In: Avery GS (ed) Drug treatment. Adis, Auckland, pp 202–235

Meier UT, Meyer UA (1987) Genetic polymorphism of cytochrome P450 (S)-mephenytoin 4-hydroxylase. Studies with human autoantibodies suggest a functionally altered P450 enzyme as cause of genetic deficiency. Biochemistry 26: 8466–8474

Meier UT, Dayer P, Male PJ, Kronbach T, Meyer UA (1985) Mephenytoin hydroxylation polymorphism: characterization of the enzymatic deficiency in liver microsomes of poor metabolizers phenotyped in vivo. Clin Pharmacol Ther 38:488–494

Mellström B, Bertilsson L, Lou Y-C, Säwe J, Sjöqvist F (1983) Amitryptiline metabolism: relationship to polymorphic debrisoquine hydroxylation. Clin Pharmacol Ther 34:516–520

Meyer UA, Gut J, Kronbach T, Skoda C, Meier UT, Catin T, Dayer P (1986) The molecular mechanisms of two common polymorphisms of drug oxidation – evidence for functional changes in cytochrome P-450 isozymes catalysing bufuralol and mephenytoin oxidation. Xenobiotica 16:449–464

Meyer UA, Skoda RC, Zanger UM, Heim M, Broly F (1992) The genetic polymorphism of debrisoquine/sparteine polymorphism – molecular mechanisms. In: Kalow W (ed) Pharmacogenetics of drug metabolism. Pergamon, New York, pp 609–624

Mitchell RS, Bell JC (1957) Clinical implications of isoniazide, PAS and streptomycin blood levels in pulmonary tuberculosis. Trans Am Clin Chem Assoc 69:98–105

Mörike K, Hardtmann E, Heimburg P (1990) Interindividual variation of N-propylajmaline dose requirement in patients with ventricular arrhythmia in relation to metabolic capacity of sparteine (Abstr). Naunyn Schmiedebergs Arch Pharmacol 341:110

Mortimer Ö, Lindström B, Laurell H, Bergman U, Rane A (1989) Dextromethorphan: polymorphic serum pattern of the O-demethylated and didemethylated metabolites in man. Br J Clin Pharmacol 27:223–227

Motulsky AG (1957) Drug reactions, enzymes and biochemical genetics. JAMA 165:835–837

Nebert DW, Nelson DR, Feyereisen R, Fuji-Kuriyama Y, Coon MJ, Estabrook RW, Gonzolez FJ, Guengerich FP, Gunsalus IC, Johnson EF, Loper JC, Sato R, Waterman MR, Waxman DJ (1991) The P450 superfamily: update on new sequences, gene mapping and recommended nomenclature. DNA Cell Biol 10:1–14

Nelson JC, Jatlow PI (1980) Neuroleptic effect on desipramine steady-state plasma concentrations. Am J Psychiatry 137:1232–1234

Newton BW, Benson RC, McCarriston CC (1966) Sparteine sulphate: a potent capricious oxytocic. Am J Obstet Cynecol 94:234–241

Nordin C, Siwers B, Benitez J, Bertilsson L (1985) Plasma concentrations of nortriptyline and its 10-hydroxy metabolite in depressed patients – relationship to the debrisoquine hydroxylation ratio. Br J Clin Pharmacol 19:832–835

Oates NS, Shah RR, Idle JR, Smith RL (1982) Genetic polymorphism of phenformin 4-hydroxylation. Clin Pharmacol Ther 32:81–89

Okino ST, Quattrochi LC, Pendurthi UR, McBride OW, Tukey RH (1987) Characterization of multiple human cytochrome P4501 cDNAs: the chromosomal localization of the gene and evidence for alternate RNA splicing. J Biol Chem 262:16072–16079

Pierce DM, Smith SE, Franklin RA (1987) The pharmacokinetics of indoramin and 6-hydroxyindoramin in poor and extensive hydroxylators of debrisoquine. Eur J Clin Pharmacol 33:59–65

Raghuram TC, Koshakji RP, Wilkinson GR, Wood AJJ (1984) Polymorphic ability to metabolize propranolol alters 4-hydroxypropranolol levels but not beta blockade. Clin Pharmacol Ther 36:51–56

Rane A, Modiri AR, Gerdin E (1992) Ethylmorphine O-deethylation cosegregates with the debrisoquin genetic metabolic polymorphism. Clin Pharmacol Ther 52:257–264

Rao KVN, Mitchison DA, Nair NGK, Prema K, Tripathy SP (1970) Sulfadimidine acetylation test for classification of patients as slow or rapid inactivators of isoniazide. Br Med J 3:495–497

Regardh CG, Johnson G (1984) Interindividual variations in metoprolol metabolism – some clinical and other observations. Br J Clin Pharmacol 17:495–496

Robitzek EH, Selikoff IJ, Ornstein GG (1952) Chemotherapy of human tuberculosis with hydrazine derivatives of isonicotinic acid. Q Bull Sea View Hosp NY 13:27–51

Rost KL, Brösicke H, Brockmöller J, Scheffler M, Helge H, Roots I (1992) Increase of cytochrome P4501A2 activity by omeprazole: evidence by the ^{13}C-[N-3-methyl]-caffeine breath test in poor and extensive metabolizers of S-mephenytoin. Clin Pharmacol Ther 52:170–180

Roy SS, Hawes EM, McKay G, Korchinski ED, Midha KK (1985) Metabolism of methoxyphenamine in extensive and poor metabolisers of debrisoquin. Clin Pharmacol Ther 38:128–133

Schmid B, Bircher J, Preisig R, Küpfer A (1985) Polymorphic dextromethorphan metabolism: co-segregation of oxidative O-demethylation with debrisoquin hydroxylation. Clin Pharmacol Ther 38:618–624

Shah RR, Oates NS, Idle JR, Smith RL, Lockhart JDF (1982) Impaired oxidation of debrisoquine in patients with perhexiline neuropathy. Br Med J 284:295–299

Shah RR, Oates NS, Idle JR, Smith RL, Lockhart DF (1983) Prediction of subclinical perhexiline neuropathy in a patient with inborn error of debrisoquine hydroxylation. Am Heart J 105:159–161

Shimada T, Misono KS, Guengerich FP (1986) Human liver microsomal cytochrome P450 mephenytoin hydroxylase, a prototype of genetic polymorphism in oxidative drug metabolism: purification and characterization of two similar forms involved in the reaction. J Biol Chem 261:909–921

Siddoway LA, Thompson KA, McAllister B, Wang T, Wilkinson GR, Roden DM, Woosley RL (1987) Polymorphism of propafenone metabolism and disposition in man: clinical and pharmacokinetic consequences. Circulation 75:785–791

Sindrup SH, Brosen K, Bjerring P, Arendt-Nielsen L, Larsen U, Angelo HR, Gram LF (1990) Codeine increases pain thresholds to copper vapor laser stimuli in extensive but not in poor metabolizers of sparteine. Clin Pharmacol Ther 48:686–693

Skjelbo E, Brosen K, Hallas J, Gram LF (1991) The mephenytoin oxidation polymorphism is partially responsible for the N-demethylation of imipramine. Clin Pharmacol Ther 49:18–23

Skoda R, Gonzalez FJ, Demierre A, Meyer UA (1988) Two mutant alleles of the human cytochrome P450 db1 gene (P450 IID1) associated with genetically deficient metabolism of debrisoquine and other drugs. Proc Natl Acad Sci USA 85:5240–5243

Sloan TP, Mahgoub A, Lancaster R, Idle JR, Smith RL (1978) Polymorphism of carbon oxidation of drugs and clinical implications. Br Med J 2:655–657

Srivastava PK, Yun CH, Beaune P, Ged C, Guengerich FP (1991) Separation of human liver microsomal tolbutamide hydroxylase and S-mephenytoin 4'-hydroxylase cytochrome P450 enzymes. Mol Pharmacol 40:69–79

Vatsis KP, Martell KJ, Weber WW (1991) Diverse point mutations in the human gene for polymorphic N-acetyltransferase. Proc Natl Acad Sci USA 88:6333–6337

Vogel F (1959) Moderne Probleme der Humangenetik. Ergeb Inn Med Kinderheilkol 12:52–125

Vogel F, Motulsky AG (1979) Human genetics. Springer, Berlin Heidelberg New York

Von Bahr C, Movin G, Nordin C, Liden A, Hammarlund-Udenaes M, Hedberg A, Ring H, Sjöqvist F (1991) Plasma levels of thioridazine and metabolites are influenced by the debrisoquine hydroxylation phenotype. Clin Pharmacol Ther 49:234–240

Wagner F, Kalusche D, Trenk D, Jähnchen E, Roskamm H (1987) Drug interaction between propafenone and metoprolol. Br J Clin Pharmacol 24:213–220

Wang T, Roden DM, Wolfenden HT, Woosley RL, Wood AJJ, Wilkinson GR (1984) Influence of genetic polymorphism on the metabolism and disposition of encainide in man. J Pharmacol Exp Ther 228:605–611

Ward SA, Walle T, Walle K, Wilkinson GR, Branch RA (1989) Propranolol's metabolism is determined by both mephenytoin and debrisoquine hydroxylase activities. Clin Pharmacol Ther 45:72–79

Ward SA, Helsby NA, Skjelbo E, Brosen K, Gram LF, Breckenridge AM (1991) The activation of the biguanide antimalarial proguanil cosegregates with the mephenytoin oxidation polymorphism – a panel study. Br J Clin Pharmacol 31:689–692

Wedlund PJ, Aslani WS, McAllister CB, Wilkinson GR, Branch RA (1984) Mephenytoin hydroxylation deficiency in Caucasians: frequency of a new oxidative drug metabolism polymorphism. Clin Pharmacol Ther 36:773–780

Weinshilbaum R (1992) Methyltransferase pharmacogenetics. In: Kalow W (ed) Pharmacogenetics of drug metabolism. Pergamon, New York, pp 179–194

Wilkinson GR, Guengerich FP, Branch RA (1992) Genetic polymorphism of S-mephenytoin hydroxylation. In: Kalow W (ed) Pharmacogenetics of drug metabolism. Pergamon, New York, pp 657–680

Woosley RL, Drayer DE, Reidenberg MM, Nies AS, Carr K, Oates JA (1978) Effect of acetylator phenotype on the rate at which procainamide induces antinuclear antibodies and the lupus syndrome. N Engl J Med 298:1157–1159

Zekorn C, Achtert G, Hausleiter HJ, Moon CH, Eichelbaum M (1985) Pharmacokinetics of N-propylajmaline in relation to polymorphic sparteine oxidation. Klin Wochenschr 63:1180–1186

CHAPTER 10

Role of Environmental Factors in the Pharmacokinetics of Drugs: Considerations with Respect to Animal Models, P-450 Enzymes, and Probe Drugs

O. Pelkonen and D.D. Breimer

No probe drug can as yet replace measurement of the actual drug with which a patient is treated.

D.D. Breimer

A. Introduction

Human beings live in changing environments in which some factors change very rapidly and others more slowly. Organisms must adapt themselves to these changes if they are to survive and reproduce. A specific aspect of the adaptation is the mechanism by which organisms try to maintain homeostasis in respect to the chemical environment. Organisms are endowed with the enzyme machinery which disposes of chemicals that have entered the body. These enzymes are called drug- or xenobiotic-metabolizing enzymes and they have been dealt with in numerous monographs, review articles, and symposia during the past 30 years or so (see, e.g., JENNER and TESTA 1980; ORTIZ DE MONTELLANO 1986; BENFORD et al. 1987; ALVARES and PRATT 1990; TUKEY and JOHNSON 1990).

It became clear very early during the pioneering studies of drug biotransformation that a large number of different environmental and nongenetic host factors can influence the activity of different enzymes participating in the metabolism of foreign-body substances. Even brief perusal of the enormous amount of published literature reveals that almost any exogenous influence has been shown to affect at least a certain aspect of drug metabolism in experimental animals. In human beings, perhaps only practical difficulties in experimentation have prevented a similar conclusion from being reached. However, an effect as such does not mean that it is of importance in terms of physiological, pharmacological, or toxicological outcomes. Similarly, a demonstrated effect on a certain enzyme involved in drug metabolism does not mean that such an effect is discernible in other enzyme systems. Thus, specificity and extent of environmental influences are among the most important considerations of any study, be it experimental or clinical. Even more important, from the practical point of view, is the assessment of "relevance" of the observed effect, regardless of its origin, i.e., genetic or environmental (Breimer 1990).

Consequently, this review on the effects of environmental factors on pharmacokinetics has several objectives. Specific enzymes and isoforms, both in experimental animals and in man, are dealt with in some detail, with special reference to cytochrome P-450 isoforms. Furthermore, an important part of the review will comprise an assessment of probe drugs which are particularly suitable for revealing environmental influences on the activity of oxidative drug-metabolizing enzyme activity in man. The use of a panel or "cocktail" of polymorphic probes is also considered. The clinical pharmacological objectives of using probe drugs to detect environmental influences on drug metabolism are twofold. The first and perhaps the more important objective is the quantitative assessment of differential changes in enzyme activity in vivo due to specific environmental and other factors. This includes the measurement of the activities of specific P-450 isoforms, e.g., for defining the characteristics of a volunteer and/or patient, in analogy to the use of polymorphic probes (see Balant et al. 1989). Alternatively this approach can be used to set up a population study with large interindividual variation as regards a desired metabolic characteristic. Secondly, one might wish to obtain an overall impression of liver function with respect to xenobiotic-metabolizing enzyme activity, as determined by physiological, pathological, and toxicological processes. Naturally, there may be other objectives, and these are also identified during the discussions. Some of the above-mentioned topics have recently been discussed by Alvan et al. (1990a).

B. Relevant Environmental Factors

I. What Are "Relevant" Environmental Factors?

It has been customary to start with the famous circle of Vesell (1982) and list those factors that are definitely environmental (the circle contains quite a number of factors which could rather be described as host factors or physiological determinants) (Fig. 1). All the familiar factors, e.g., cigarette smoking and alcohol drinking, are included, but so too are not so familiar ones such as hyperbaric oxygen. So, which are really relevant and in what context? If we look at the problem from the clinical point of view we can list those factors that are most commonly encountered, and which may compromise drug therapy. These include cigarette smoking, alcohol drinking, and exposure to other recreational chemicals as well as occupational exposure to chemicals. Of particular concern in clinical practice are drug–drug interactions caused by either enzyme induction or inhibition. An interesting question of relevance to drug development or drug therapy is that of specificity of a certain factor. It has been quite amply demonstrated that most environmental influences cause only a few tens of percent change in

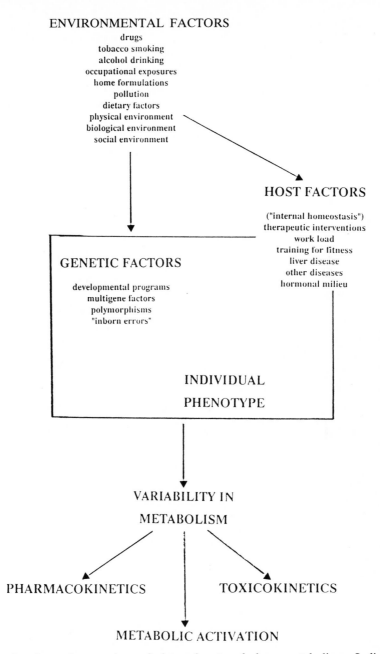

Fig. 1. A schematic overview of determinants of drug metabolism. Individual phenotype is determined by (a) genetic factors, which are preprogrammed potentialities of each individual, (b) host factors, which are more or less "acquired" characteristics of an individual ("life history"), and (c) environmental factors, which are strictly "outside" influences, but which work through, and are influenced by, the genetic and host makeup of an individual

the rate of metabolism or elimination of a given probe drug, with probably minor therapeutic and/or clinical consequences (POULSEN and LOFT 1988). It should be considered most important to detect those environmental factors and those drugs that – if taken together – are likely to cause therapeutic failures or adverse reactions. This issue leads to the question of the relevance of probe drugs in terms of predictive value in respect of other drugs and is directly related to the issue of the specificity of probe drugs. A theoretical example may be used to illustrate this.

An environmental factor α causes a tenfold increase in the amount of a specific enzyme isoform A which is mainly responsible for the metabolism and inactivation of an important experimental drug X. However, α causes barely a 50% increase in the elimination of a commonly used probe drug PD, because PD is also metabolized by other enzymes which are not affected by α. So, while from the point of view of scientific inquiry PD does provide information on the enzyme-inducing capability of α, it is not of practical and predictive relevance to patients to be treated with drug X. We would like to have a probe drug as specific as possible for isoform A, because this probe should predict the patient's kinetic response to α and its consequences for the use of X. As long as this is not the case, "no probe drug can as yet replace measurement of the actual drug with which a patient is being treated" (see introductory quote).

Obviously an important question is whether environmental influences are very specific indeed. We know that phenobarbital is a rather wide-ranging inducing substance, causing increases in a number of P-450 isoforms and other drug-metabolizing enzymes (see WAXMAN and AZAROFF 1992). On the basis of this knowledge we would predict that patients receiving or exposed to phenobarbital-type inducers, be they drugs, industrial chemicals, or pollutants, will eliminate a large and varied number of chemicals more rapidly. However, as we have come to know more about inducing substances, so we have come to appreciate the very variable patterns of seemingly similar inducers. A case in point is the differing patterns of induction caused by a group of substances, all of which increase a P-450 isoform active in coumarin 7-hydroxylation in mouse liver. Phenobarbital, 1,4-bis[2-(3,5-dichloropyridyloxy)]benzene (TCPOBOP), pyrazole, cobalt, and cerium all increase this activity severalfold in mouse liver (see PELKONEN et al. 1993), whereas their effects on other isoforms are highly variable. A P-450 isoform active in pentoxyresorufin O-depentylation is strongly increased by phenobarbital and TCPOBOP, but is either unchanged or decreased by pyrazole, cobalt, and cerium (RAUNIO et al. 1988; ARVELA et al. 1991; HAHNEMANN et al. 1992). One can even demonstrate isoform-dependent differences between phenobarbital and TCPOBOP, both regarded as prototypes of phenobarbital-class inducers (HONKAKOSKI et al. 1992). It is also well established that TCPOBOP is active in mice, but not in rats, for unknown reasons (POLAND et al. 1981).

The above considerations lead us to conclude that it would be desirable to characterize the impact of the most common environmental influences encountered in clinical drug trials and actual drug therapy on drug-metabolizing enzyme activity. Such characterization should preferably address the specificity issue in detail. The environmental factors concerned include commonly used inducing and inhibiting drugs, cigarette smoking, alcohol drinking, and nutrition. With respect to environmental exposures to chemicals there are obvious difficulties, i.e., there is a multitude of chemicals to which people are exposed at work. Because of this immense variation, it is not possible to identify any single measure or index to assess any metabolizing enzyme activity. If it is known beforehand to which chemicals people are exposed, it should in principle be possible to select an appropriate probe drug or a combination of probe drugs. In reality, this approach is certainly not widely practised.

II. Examples

In order to illustrate what is meant by "relevant" environmental factors, representative examples are discussed below (see also PELKONEN and SOTANIEMI 1987; BREIMER 1990). It is important to devote attention to the quantification of the impact of an environmental factor, because such impacts are "dose" dependent. In principle, quantification can be differentiated into two component parts: (a) *quantitation of exposure*, and (b) *quantitation of impact*, which in the context of this review is the change in the enzyme activity, i.e., the change in vivo in drug kinetics and/or dynamics. Together, these two parts provide a dose–response relationship, which is a principal objective of this type of investigation. In addition, the specificity issue is very relevant, as has been discussed in the previous section.

1. Cigarette Smoking

In the Western world, the prevalence of cigarette smoking is variable, but in many societies around 30%–40% of the adult population smoke cigarettes (IARC 1986). Because it has been exhaustively demonstrated that smoking affects many aspects of drug metabolism (JUSKO 1979; DAWSON and VESTAL 1982; PELKONEN and SOTANIEMI 1987; HARRIS 1987), it would be useful to find an objective marker to measure the extent of smoking ("exposure") and a probe drug or drugs that would give an indication of those isoforms which are affected by smoking ("impact"). As to markers, it suffices to say that several markers ranging from carbon monoxide–hemoglobin to specific nicotine metabolites, such as cotinine or 3-hydroxycotinine, are available (IARC 1986; see also IDLE 1990). How these markers reflect the exposure to specific smoke components (more than 4000 are listed!) remains largely unexplored, but this problem is really at the heart of dose–response considerations with regard to cigarette smoking.

2. Alcohol Drinking

In populations of the Western world less than 10% of people do not consume alcohol, and the rate of alcoholism and heavy drinking has been estimated to be anywhere between 5% and 10% in such populations (IARC 1988). Alcohol drinking has profound acute and chronic effects on the liver (LIEBER 1988), which have both direct (inhibition, induction) and indirect long-term (liver injury) consequences for drug metabolism and kinetics, as amply demonstrated in both experimental animals and man (PELKONEN and SOTANIEMI 1982; LIEBER 1991). Although markers for alcohol consumption have been searched for extensively, there is really no consensus on this topic among researchers (IARC 1988). Nevertheless, it would be extremely useful to find a probe or a marker which would indicate the amount and duration of alcohol drinking. It is worth emphasizing that alcohol–drug interactions are certainly among the most common in drug therapy (LANE et al. 1985).

3. Drugs

Drug–drug interactions at the level of metabolism are drug-specific and dose dependent. Much of our basic knowledge on environmental effects on drug metabolism comes from experiments and experience with drugs as inducers and inhibitors of enzyme activity. There are numerous reviews on drug–drug and drug–chemical interactions at the metabolic level and the reader is referred to those for detailed information (see, e.g., PLAA et al. 1987). We will therefore constantly refer to them in this review, but not discuss them in any detail. For drugs to be suitable probe drugs that can be made easily available and widely used, it is preferable for them to be therapeutic substances, as there are then fewer ethical and practical constraints on their application. Some such compounds will be discussed in later sections.

4. Occupational Chemicals

Occupational chemicals are numerous and variable, but there are classes which may be more common and more important than others, e.g., polycyclic aromatic hydrocarbons in certain occupational settings (e.g., coke ovens) and organic solvents in a large number of industries (extensive reviews on various occupational chemicals can be found in the IARC monographs series). It has become routine practice in occupational hygiene to measure environmental levels of these classes of chemicals, and markers and probes for internal exposure have been or are under development. This area cannot be dealt with in detail here, but the reader can find further information in recent reviews and congress monographs (see, e.g., AITIO et al. 1984; IARC 1986, 1988).

5. Other Factors

To the layman one of the most important and threatening environmental factors seems to be environmental pollution, including urban pollution. While there is no doubt about the general significance of this phenomenon, its effects on drug-metabolizing enzymes are somewhat controversial. Estimating environmental pollution in general is certainly a daunting task and linking the exposure with impact as reflected in changes in enzyme activity is even more difficult. However, it must be kept in mind that people are exposed to haloalkanes through chlorinated drinking water, to polycyclic aromatic hydrocarbons and heterocyclic compounds through air and food (e.g., smoke, charcoal-broiled meat), and to all sorts of aliphatic and aromatic solvents and compounds through household items such as paints and glues (see PLAA et al. 1987).

SITAR (1989) has discussed some "environmental" factors implicated in residual variation of drug metabolism in man. Intraindividual (and possibly also interindividual) variation may confound clinical pharmacological studies even if more obvious factors have been taken into consideration (see, e.g., UPTON et al. 1982). As probable contributing factors, Sitar lists cruciferous vegetables, fluid and electrolyte balance, high protein diet, and time of day. Some possible contributing factors include caffeine, high fat diet, composition of intestinal microorganisms, macrobiotic diet, and moderate alcohol ingestion.

As examples of more specific influences which may be very relevant in certain situations one might also mention treatment-induced host reactions such as changes in liver function in connection with transplantation as measured with the metabolite of lidocaine, monoethylglycinexylidide (MEXG) (OELLERICH et al. 1989), and some factors belonging to the physical and biological environment, e.g., the effect of infections and interferons on drug metabolism and kinetics (RENTON and KNICKLE 1990). We shall not discuss these factors in detail, nor shall we discuss disease factors, including liver disease.

C. Animal Models

Most of our knowledge on the effects of environmental factors (meaning chemicals in most cases) on drug metabolism stems from studies in experimental animals, mainly rodents. It is useful in the context of this review (a) to discuss briefly what is known about the environmentally affected P-450 enzymes, and consequent changes in drug kinetics, using the rat as an experimental model species, and (b) to look at similarities and differences between species, with a view to trying to extrapolate from one species to another.

Table 1. Rat hepatic P-450 isoforms, some substrates/reactions and inducers[a]

Isoform	Preferred substrates[b] (sites)	Inducing substances										
		MC	TCDD	BNF	ISF	PCB	PB	EtOH	AC	PCN	Dex	Other inducers
1A1	7-Ethoxycoumarin (O)	+	+	+	+	+	-	-	-	-	-	
	Benzo [a] pyrene (3/9)											
	Zoxazolamine (6)											
	p-Nitroanisole (N)											
1A2	Estradiol (2)	+	+	+	+	+	(+)	-	-	-	-	
	Phenacetin (O)											
	Zoxazolamine (6)											
2A1	Testosterone (7α)	Constitutive										
2A2	Testosterone (15α)			+	+	+	+			+	-	
2B1	Benzphetamine (N)	-	-	-	+	+	+	+	+	+		
	Hexobarbital (3)											
2B2	Benzphetamine (N)	-	-	-	+	+	+	-	-	+	+	
	Hexobarbital (3)											
2C6	Benzphetamine (N)						++	+				
2C7	?											

Isozyme	Substrate[b]					Inducers
2C11	Benzphetamine (N)					Constitutive
	Hexobarbital (3)					
	Testosterone (16α)					
2C12	Androgen-disulfate (15β)					Constitutive
2C13	Benzphetamine (N)					
2D1	Benzphetamine	+				
2E1	Dimethylnitrosamine	+	+			Pyrazole
	Aniline (p)	+	+	+		Isoniazide
						Solvents
3A1	Steroids (6β)	+		+	+	
	Ethylmorphine (N)					
	Nifedipine (oxidation)					
3A2	Steroids (2β, 6β)	+				TAO
4A1–3	Fatty acids (ω and ω-1)	–	–	–		Clofibrate

AC, acetone; BNF, β-naphthoflavone; Dex, dexamethasone; EtOH, ethanol; ISF, isosafrole; MC, 3-methylcholanthrene; PB, phenobarbital; PCB, polychlorinated biphenyl; PCN, pregnenolone-16α-carbonitrile; TAO, triacetyloleandomycin; TCDD, tetrachlorodibenzo-p-dioxin

[a] Data in this table are compiled from review articles by GUENGERICH (1987b), LEVIN (1990), MURRAY and REIDY (1990), OKEY (1990), WOLF et al. (1990), and SOUCEK and GUT (1992)

[b] Substrate preferences have to be understood in relative terms, because more often than not a substrate is metabolized by more than one isozyme (see, e.g., benzphetamine)

I. Environmental Regulation of P-450 Isoforms in the Rat

In Table 1 we have tried to summarize in a relatively concise manner what is known about rat hepatic P-450 isoforms and their regulation by environmental factors. These include predominantly chemicals or classes of chemicals affecting specific P-450 isoforms. In the rat, a rather clear and detailed picture of the phenomenology of induction by various chemical agents can be obtained, because inducers can be administered one at a time and specific effects recorded directly in the target tissue. Unfortunately, it is quite difficult to translate this extensive body of knowledge into the consequences for pharmacokinetics in vivo for the following reasons: (a) In practice, these isoforms have been and still are being identified by their typical metabolic reactions, and the substrates used are primarily selected on the basis of analytical ease rather than their wide use or clinical importance or in vivo suitability. (b) Because those substances are more often than not metabolized by several isoforms, their isozyme specificity is only relative.

II. Similarities and Differences Between Species

How safe is the extrapolation from one species to another? Several studies and review articles have been published on this subject (see SMITH 1987, 1991). If we consider the question at the level of some specific substances and P-450 isoforms metabolizing these substances (Table 2), both close similarities and profound differences have been shown to exist between different species, giving rise to overall confusion. In terms of substrate

Table 2. Metabolism of some model substances by P-450 isoforms in different species[a]

Substrate/reaction	Principal isoform			
	Rat	Mouse	Rabbit	Man
Ethoxyresorufin O-dealkylation	1A	1A	1A	1A
Phenacetin O-dealkylation	1A	1A	1A	1A
Coumarin 7-hydroxylation	NK[b]	2A	2A	2A
Benzphetamine N-demethylation	2B	2B	2B	3A?
S-Mephenytoin 4-hydroxylation	3A	2C	2C	2C
Hexobarbital 1'-hydroxylation	2C	2C	2C	2C
Tolbutamide hydroxylation	2B	NK	3A	2C
Debrisoquine 4-hydroxylation	2D	NK	2D	2D
Aniline p-hydroxylation	2E	2E	2E	2E
Nifedipine oxidation	2C	–	3A	3A
Lidocaine N-deethylation	2C	–	3A	3A

[a] For the original references see the text and SMITH (1987, 1991), GONZALEZ (1990), and NEBERT et al. (1989, 1991)
[b] NK, not known; i.e., the isozyme responsible has not been identified, but it is not the isoform catalyzing the reaction in other species

specificities of various isoforms, for certain gene families, such as CYP1A and CYP2E, substrate specificity is quite highly conserved, whereas for other families there are numerous and important differences in substrate specificities between species. The reasons for conservation of the properties of some members and not of others are poorly understood. Furthermore, some authors believe that "safe" extrapolation is not possible even within those gene families which are best conserved (see, e.g., JUCHAU 1990).

A good example of differences in substrate specificity of orthologous enzymes is the CYP2D family. Human and rat enzymes hydroxylate debrisoquine, but the corresponding mouse enzyme is not able to catalyze this reaction (WONG et al. 1987). Human and rat enzymes are noted for their polymorphisms (GONZALEZ and MEYER 1991; KAHN et al. 1985). The mouse enzyme exhibits testosterone 16α-hydroxylase activity, whereas human or rat enzymes do not display this activity (WONG et al. 1987). The mouse enzyme is also male-specific, but neither human nor rat enzymes display any sex dependence.

Another interesting example is tolbutamide, which appears to be hydroxylated by CYP2B1/2 in rats, partially by CYP3A6 in rabbits, and by CYP2C8/9 in humans (RELLING et al. 1990; VERONESE et al. 1991). As might be expected, these three isoforms, although sharing an ability to hydroxylate tolbutamide, are quite different with regard to other catalytic and inhibitory properties.

III. Reasons for Interspecies Differences

There are several mechanisms that underlie interspecies differences:

1. It is known that even quite subtle differences in protein structure can result in a profound change in substrate specificity (LINDBERG and NEGISHI 1989).
2. On the other hand, structurally quite dissimilar enzymes can catalyze the same reaction of the same substrate. The P-450 enzymes are notorious in having widely overlapping specificities. As an extreme example, 7-ethoxycoumarin O-deethylase is catalyzed by 10 out of 11 human P-450 isoforms studied (WAXMAN et al. 1991).
3. Duplication events after the divergence of two species lead to a situation whereby one of the species lacks one of the newly created genes (NEBERT and GONZALEZ 1987; GONZALEZ 1989, 1990). Gene duplications, deletions, and conversions are also possible. For example, the rat has four functional genes in the CYP2D family whereas man has only one, in addition to two mutated genes (GONZALEZ and MEYER 1991).

Our overall conclusion is that although animal experiments provide useful information about environmental effects on drug metabolism in general, detailed extrapolation is seldom possible and studies in humans are needed to procure definite information on humans.

Finally, animal experiments are not without considerable merit. They do offer a possibility to study a certain phenomenon in a controlled (even "idealized") situation, which is seldom possible in humans. Thereby they provide very useful background and mechanistic knowledge on drug-metabolizing enzyme regulation.

IV. Model Experiments in Animals

As is clear from the above discussion, interspecies extrapolation in pharmacokinetics is quite difficult even when P-450 isoforms in different species are strictly homologous. Consequently, it may be of relatively little use to provide detailed model experimental protocols, because their extrapolative value to the human situation may be limited. However, in Table 3 we list several model substances which have been studied in some detail and which may be useful for assessing the amount of some specific isoforms and revealing potential environmental conditions affecting kinetics in experimental animals. It should be noted that this list is not exhaustive. Another point to stress is that in animal experiments one can study the effect of environmental factors on drug-metabolizing enzymes in great detail in an in vitro situation, thus gaining very extensive background information relevant for planning in vivo studies, an approach which is very difficult or impossible in humans.

D. Important (Iso)enzymes in Man

I. P-450 Enzymes

Especially during the past decade, our knowledge on specific isoforms of P-450 enzymes in human tissues has increased enormously. Through purification, antibody production, immunoinhibition, use of panels of substrates and inhibitors, and, recently, cloning, sequencing, and heterologous expression, quite detailed knowledge on specific properties of isoforms has been acquired. For further information, see recent extensive reviews by Boobis and Davies (1984), Adesnik and Atchison (1986), Nebert and Gonzalez (1987), Beaune and Guengerich (1988), Nebert et al. (1989, 1991), Guengerich (1989, 1992a,b), and Gonzalez (1989, 1990), Wrighton and Stevens (1992), and Nelson et al. (1993).

A brief description of the biochemical and pharmacological characteristics of some major isoforms is given in Table 4 and below. This table and the following discussion serves as the background for the next section dealing with probe drugs, which are needed to detect the specificity of environmental effects on enzyme activity. Some isoforms, e.g., P-450 1A1, seem to be induced mainly (if not solely) in extrahepatic tissues and quantitatively may not be of great importance in pharmacokinetics. Also isoforms which

Table 3. Examples of model substrates useful in vivo for animal experiments, which may be of help in elucidating potential environmental influences

Probe substance	Inducer	Measured index	Species	Ref.[a]
Zozaxolamine	MC	Loss of righting reflex	Rat	1
Caffeine	MC, PB	Clearance	Mouse	2
Metronidazole	MC, PB	Salivary clearance	Rat	3
Antipyrine	MC, PB	Plasma/salivary clearance	Rat	4
Hexobarbital	MC, PB	Sleeping time, clearance	Rat, mouse	5
Aminopyrine	PB	Clearance	Rat	6
Coumarin	PB	7-Hydroxycoumarin in urine	Mouse	7
Theophylline	MC, PB	Clearance	Rat	8

MC, 3-methylcholanthrene; PB, phenobarbital
[a] References: 1, CONNEY et al. 1960; 2, APSELOFF et al. 1991; 3, LOFT et al. 1990; 4, LOFT et al. 1990; VAN DER GRAAFF et al. 1983; TEUNISSEN et al. 1986; 5, APPSELOFF et al. 1991; VAN DER GRAAFF et al. 1983; 6, PELKONEN et al. 1991; 7, LUSH and ANDREWS 1978; MÄENPÄÄ et al. 1993; 8, TEUNISSEN et al. 1986; APSELOFF et al. 1990

are regulated principally by polymorphic control, i.e., CYP2D6 and S-mephenytoin 4-hydroxylase, are treated rather briefly, because they are the subject of separate reviews in this volume. Two subfamilies, namely 2C and 3A, are somewhat problematic, because they contain several isoforms and there is still some uncertainty about the assignment of specific activities to specific isoforms.

From the point of view of this review, the most interesting characteristics of isoforms are substrate specificity and inhibitor selectivity, and in Table 4 several "specific" or "diagnostic" substrates and inhibitors are listed. It must be stressed here that specificity has in most cases only a relative meaning. The term "selectivity" would in principle be more appropriate. For example, substrates which were previously often regarded as "isoform-specific" (at the time when the dichotomy was principally between P-448 and P-450), such as benzo[a]pyrene or benzphetamine, are in fact not very specific (see LEVIN 1990; SOUCEK and GUT 1992). Later, the search was directed towards finding really isoform-specific substances, or series of homologous substances, e.g., alkoxycoumarins, alkoxyresorufins (BURKE and MAYER 1983), or alkoxyquinolines (MAYER et al. 1990), or compounds which are metabolized at specific positions by specific isoforms, e.g., testosterone (WAXMAN 1988; WAXMAN et al. 1983, 1991) or warfarin (KAMINSKY et al. 1984; RETTIE et al. 1989; see SUTCLIFF et al. 1987). Obviously the property of "isoform specificity" is not in itself sufficient for a probe to be used in vivo as well, but it is an important starting point.

With respect to inhibitors of enzyme activity, most substances are relatively nonspecific and even those claimed to be isoform-specific usually have affinity to other isoforms also, although at higher concentrations. One good example is cimetidine, a well-known inhibitor of P-450-linked reactions

Table 4. Human P-450 isoforms participating in the metabolism of drugs

Isoform	Level of characterization[a]	Tissues/organs where expressed[b]	Amount in liver	"Diagnostic" substrates[c]	"Diagnostic" inhibitors[c]	Environmental inducers
1A1	c,g	Extrahepatic	Negligible (smoking?)	Benzo[a]pyrene	7,8-Benzoflavone	Smoking, PCB
1A2	p,c,g	Liver	Major	Phenacetin, Ethoxyresorufin	Furafylline	Smoking, Charcoal-broiled meat, vegetables
2A6	p,c	Liver	Minor?	Coumarin (7) (Ethoxycoumarin)	8-Methoxypsoralen	?
2B6	c	Liver	Minor?		?	?
2C8–10	p,c	Liver	Major	Tolbutamide, hexobarbital, phenytoin	Sulfaphenazole	Rifampicin, Barbiturates
2Cmep	p	Liver	Major (polymorphic)	S-Mephenytoin	Teniposide	Rifampicin
2C17–19	C	Liver?	?	?	?	?
2D6	p,c,g	Liver	Major (polymorphic)	Debrisoquine, etc.	Quinidine	None known
2E1	p,c,g	Liver, Extrahepatic	Major	Chlorzoxazone, Demethylnitrosamine (Ethoxycoumarin)	Tetrahydrofurane	Ethanol, isoniazid
2F1	c	Lung	Not present		?	?
3A3–5	p,c	Liver, Extrahepatic	Major	Nifedipine, erythromycin, etc.	TAO, gestodene	Rifampicin, TAO, barbiturates, dexamethasone
4B1	c	Placenta, lung	Not present	?	?	?

PCB, polychlorinated biphenyls; TAO, triacetyloleandomycin

[a] Level of characterization: p, protein (purified); c, cDNA (cloned); g, gene (cloned, exon–intron stucture elucidation). See reviews by Gonzalez (1990), Gonzalez et al. (1991a), Guengerich (1989, 1992a,b), and Nebert et al. (1991)

[b] Based on the following reviews or original articles: D.E. Waziers et al. (1990), Forrester et al. (1992), Guengerich and Turvy (1991), Ketterer et al. (1991), and Morel et al. (1990)

[c] See especially reviews of Guengerich (1989, 1992), Guengerich and Shimada (1991), and Murray and Reidy (1990). P-450 inhibitors are notoriously nonspecific, e.g., cimetidine inhibits most of the isoforms at high concentrations

(PUURUNEN et al. 1980). It has been shown that cimetidine interacts with at least human hepatic 1A, 2C, 2D, 2E, and 3A isoforms, but with widely variable affinity (KNODELL et al. 1991). Further information on P-450 inhibitors can be found in reviews by TESTA and JENNER (1981) and MURRAY and REIDY (1990). Some important characteristics of human hepatic P-450 enzymes are presented in Fig. 2.

1. P-450 1A1

Although the nucleotide sequence of P-450 1A1 was the first among the P-450 isoforms to be elucidated in man (JAISWAL et al. 1985), there is still some uncertainty as to the role of this isoform in pharmacokinetics or toxicokinetics. There is evidence that it is expressed predominantly in extrahepatic tissues, such as placenta, and that its expression in liver may occur only in extreme inducing conditions (see BOOBIS et al. 1990). Much higher doses of inducers are needed to induce CYP1A1 in liver tissues as

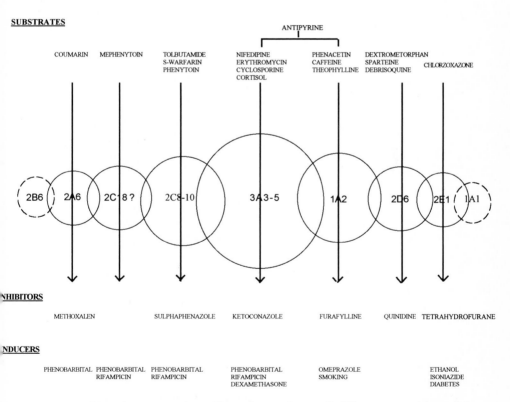

Fig. 2. A schematic presentation of hepatic cytochrome P-450 enzymes with model substrates, inhibitors, and inducers (modified from Breimer 1983). The size of *circles* is roughly proportional to relative amounts of enzymes in human liver. *Broken circles* indicate that the presence of enzymes is uncertain

compared with the induction of CYP1A2 (BOOBIS et al. 1990). Nevertheless, theoretical calculations and indirect experimental studies with perfused organs suggest that the induced CYP1A1 activity in extrahepatic tissues may contribute significantly to the overall elimination of drugs and environmental substances metabolized predominantly by this isoform (ROTH and WIERSMA 1979). As to specific substances potentially useful as probes, there are some compounds, such as ethoxyresorufin and benzo[a]pyrene, the metabolism of which is increased tremendously in placental microsomes of smoking mothers, presumably due to the increase in CYP1A1 (PASANEN and PELKONEN 1989/90; PASANEN et al. 1990), but none of these substrates seem to be specific to this isoform. However, there is a lot of interest in measuring this specific isoform in vivo because of its postulated role in chemical carcinogenesis (PELKONEN and NEBERT 1982; NEBERT and GONZALEZ 1987; NEBERT 1989; GUENGERICH 1988; GONZALEZ et al. 1991; KAWAJIRI and FUJII-KURIYAMA 1991; MILES and WOLF 1991). Recently, a restriction fragment length polymorphism has been uncovered, but the significance of this finding in terms of the regulation of inducibility of CYP1A1 is not known (KAWAJIRI et al. 1990).

2. P-450 1A2

Extensive experimental and human data on tissue localization and differential expression of CYP1A1/1A2 have been reviewed by BOOBIS et al. (1990). Human hepatic P-450 1A2 is inducible by exposure to cigarette smoke. This isoform is absent or present in extremely low quantities in extrahepatic tissues. On the basis of animal experiments one would expect that phenobarbital and presumably other phenobarbital-type inducers, as well as isosafrole, would have a modest effect on this isoform, but this has not been demonstrated convincingly in humans. On the basis of in vitro studies several substrates and pathways seem to be rather specific for this isoform, including phenacetin O-dealkylation, caffeine 3-demethylation, and theophylline 8-hydroxylation. Especially phenacetin O-dealkylation has been characterized in detail in vitro and it seems that both CYP1A1 and 1A2 are able to catalyze this reaction (SESARDIC et al. 1990; BOOBIS et al. 1990). Inhibitor selectivity of this isoform has been extensively characterized (MURRAY et al. 1992). Among primary oxidations of caffeine, only 3-demethylation is connected solely with P-450 1A2. It has been shown in in vitro studies on bacterial mutagenesis or DNA binding that this isoform is primarily responsible for catalyzing the metabolic activation of a number of potentially important procarcinogens (SHIMADA et al. 1989). This fact alone suffices to highlight the need for a specific in vivo probe, which may be caffeine 3-demethylation (see below). There is fairly wide agreement that properties of P-450 1A2 are rather strictly conserved across species and consequently quite detailed extrapolation is possible from animal experiments to the situation in man (BOOBIS et al. 1990).

3. P-450 2A6

The cDNA sequence of P-450 2A6, later shown to be a variant of CYP2A6, was elucidated at an early date (PHILLIPS et al. 1985). This isoform was subsequently cloned, sequenced, and expressed (YAMANO et al. 1990; MILES et al. 1990; CRESPI et al. 1990a) and the protein has been purified and partially characterized from human liver (YUN et al. 1991; MAURICE et al. 1991). Although on the basis of mouse experiments this isoform seems to be affected by numerous inducers (RAUNIO et al. 1988; ARVELA et al. 1991; see PELLINEN et al. 1993), there is limited information about its environmental sensitivity in man. It seems that coumarin 7-hydroxylation is relatively specific for this isoform, but the isoform is also able to catalyze the oxidative metabolism of other coumarin derivatives, including psoralens and aflatoxin B_1. The suitability of coumarin as a probe drug for this isoform is currently being investigated (RAUTIO et al. 1992).

4. P-450 2B6

The presence of isoforms in human liver similar to those induced by phenobarbital in experimental animals, i.e., CYP2B isoforms, has long been postulated, especially on the basis of the effect of antiepileptic drugs; direct evidence, however, has been lacking. Recently, an isoform belonging to this subfamily, CYP2B6, has been shown to be present in human liver, although its significance remains to be elucidated (MILES et al. 1988; YAMANO et al. 1989). Another relevant observation has been the induction of CYP3A isoforms in human liver by phenobarbital and antiepileptic drugs, which may be mainly responsible for the increased clearance of a number of drugs in "phenobarbital-type" induction in man (PERROT et al. 1989; MOREL et al. 1990; see WAXMAN and AZAROFF 1992). Consequently, it is not known how far one can extrapolate from experimental results on phenobarbital induction leading to the increase in CYP2B isoforms (among others, see Table 1) to the situation in man, in which principally CYP3A isoform(s) is (are) increased.

5. P-450 2C

The structure of the 2C subfamily in man is rather complex, consisting of three relatively well characterized members (2C8–10) (WILKINSON et al. 1989) and probably three members which have been studied only at the cDNA level thus far (ROMKES et al. 1991). Consequently it is difficult to discuss the individual members of this subfamily in any detail. The group of isoforms called 2C8–10 includes those which metabolize three important substrates, namely mephenytoin, phenytoin, and tolbutamide (RELLING et al. 1990; DOECKE et al. 1990; VERONESE et al. 1991). Both CYP2C8 and 2C9 have been purified from human liver and characterized with respect to some important substances. S-Mephenytoin 4-hydroxylation, and possibly also the metabolism of the other two above-mentioned substrates, is catalyzed by a polymorphic isoform. However, exact isoform assignment is not yet possible, because neither CYP2C8 nor 2C9 supports S-mephenytoin 4-hydroxylation. Tolbutamide methyl-hydroxylation is catalyzed by both CYP2C8 and 2C9, whereas R-mephenytoin 4-hydroxylation seems to be catalyzed only by CYP2C8 (RELLING et al. 1990). Although a lot is known about the rat 2C subfamily, this knowledge is not of much help for the elucidation of the human counterpart, because species differences are especially conspicuous in this subfamily (see examples in Table 2; also GUENGERICH 1992a,b; BANDIERA 1990). The rat P-450 2C subfamily has at least five expressed members. Three of these are sexually differentiated: 2C11 (16α) and 2C13 (g) are male-specific while 2C12 (15β) is female-specific (see BANDIERA 1990). Whether there are sexually differentiated members among human isoforms is not known at present.

Although S-mephenytoin 4-hydroxylation displays clear polymorphism (WILKINSON et al. 1989), which has been quite extensively studied in different populations (ALVAN et al. 1990b), there is still some evidence that its activity may be modulated by environmental factors, for example inducers and inhibitors (ATIBA et al. 1989; ZHOU et al. 1990).

6. P-450 2D6

P-450 2D6 displays the well-known and much researched polymorphic patterns of metabolism of debrisoquine, sparteine, dextromethorphan, and a number of other substrates (see ALVAN et al. 1990). The molecular basis of this polymorphism is known in great detail (MEYER et al. 1990; GONZALEZ and MEYER 1991). It is remarkable that the polymorphic enzyme seems to be resistant to almost all common environmental influences which tend to affect the activities of other P-450 enzymes. The only clear example of exogenous influence is the competitive inhibition of the isoform by a number of drugs, including quinidine and some neuroleptics (BROSEN and GRAM 1989). Thus, the study of environmental influences on P-450 2D6 is of interest, but mainly because of the possible interference with the phenotyping of the trait and clinically important drug interactions. Consequently, the probing of the activity of this isoform to reveal such influences is beyond the scope of this review. In any case the suitability of debrisoquine, sparteine, and dextromethorphan as in vivo probe drugs in man has been well established.

7. P-450 2E1

Once called MEOS (microsomal ethanol-oxidizing system; LIEBER and DECARLI 1968), P-450 2E1 has now been purified (WRIGHTON et al. 1986), cloned (SONG et al. 1986), and extensively characterized with respect to substrate specificity and capacity. More than 60 substances have been shown to be metabolized by this isoform (KOOP 1992; TERELIUS et al. 1992). Its activity is affected by numerous factors, including alcohol drinking, several drugs such as isoniazid, and some pathophysiological conditions such as diabetes, ketonemia, and obesity (see Koop 1992). Especially significant is the observation that CYP2E1 can be induced in considerable quantities in the human liver by chronic use of alcohol (Wrighton et al. 1986; Ekström et al. 1989; Perrot et al. 1989; Tsutsumi et al. 1990). This enzyme seems to be regulated at all levels, transcriptional as well as translational (Gonzalez et al. 1991). It seems probable that the isoform is also expressed and induced in some extrahepatic tissues, but the significance of extrahepatic activity for the kinetics of drugs in vivo is not clear (Shimizu et al. 1990). Although there are several in vitro substrates which have been claimed to be relatively specific for the isoform, including dimethylnitrosamine (at low concentrations) (Yang et al. 1990), p-nitrophenol (Koop 1986), and chlorzoxazone (Peter et al. 1990; see also Lucas et al. 1990), there are currently no specific and useful in vivo probes for the enzyme. For obvious reasons, substrates such as dimethylnitrosamine, a well-known carcinogen, are useless as in vivo probes. Several relatively specific inhibitors have been suggested, including isoniazid (also an inducer) and diethyldithiocarbamate (Guengerich et al. 1991). Obviously there is a great need for a specific probe drug, because CYP2E1 is of importance in hepatotoxicity and carcinogenesis caused by various chemicals such as benzene, other solvents, and nitrosamine carcinogens (Guengerich 1988; Miles and Wolf 1991).

8. P-450 3A

The human CYP3A subfamily consists of four members, one of which is expressed only in fetal liver (see Watkins 1990; Guengerich 1992a,b). Three adult isoforms display largely overlapping substrate specificity, although clear differences have also been observed. For example, erythromycin N-demethylation (as measured by the breath test) and cortisol 6β-hydroxylation have been shown to be catalyzed variably by different members of the subfamily, with the consequence that the correlation between these two substances is rather poor (Hunt et al. 1992). Nevertheless, the isoforms belonging to the CYP3A family seem to be quantitatively the most abundant ones in human liver and they have also been detected in substantial quantities in extrahepatic tissues, e.g., the gastrointestinal tract (see D.E. Waziers et al. 1990; Watkins 1990). The role of extrahepatic CYP3A isoform(s) in pharmacokinetics, and in particular in the first-pass phenomenon, is not known in great detail. The CYP3A isoforms are affected by a number of phenobarbital-type inducers, as well as rifampicin, macrolide antibiotics, and glucocorticoids. Extensive studies on substrate and product selectivity have been performed during recent years. Among the substrates and pathways which seem to be relatively specific for these isoforms in human liver are nifedipine oxidation (and possibly oxidation of some other dihydropyridines), lidocaine N-demethylation, and a number of others

(Soons et al. 1992). The 6β-hydroxylation of steroids seems to be predominantly catalyzed by these isoforms (Ged et al. 1989). Nevertheless, the presence of closely related isoforms not yet extensively compared and characterized with respect to substrates and inducers may lead to surprises in the use of probe drugs for extrapolative and correlative purposes. Currently most experience exists with nifedipine as a probe drug, the kinetics of which are very sensitive to environmental inducers and inhibitors (Soons et al. 1992). An interesting finding has been that grapefruit juice inhibits the metabolism of dihydropyridine calcium channel blocking agents, which may be related to certain flavonoids in grapefruit (Bailey et al. 1991; Soons et al. 1991).

II. Conjugative Enzymes

Due to the restricted space available, this review will not cover the current status of conjugative enzymes in human liver, although their role is certainly very important in the final elimination of foreign substances from the body. Furthermore, in some cases conjugating enzymes are "first-line" metabolizers, if a compound to be eliminated contains a suitable chemical group for conjugation. Paracetamol and oxazepam have even been suggested as suitable probes drugs for estimating the activity of these conjugation reactions, on the basis of their glucuronic acid and sulfate conjugation. Here were restrict ourselves to referring the reader to some of the most recent reviews dealing with the conjugation enzymes. Alvares and Pratt (1990) give a good overview of all drug-metabolizing enzymes with a number of basic references and Tukey and Johnson (1990) examine the molecular biology of the same enzymes. Extensive coverage of conjugation reactions can be found in a recent congress monograph (Mulder 1990). The nomenclature for glucuronyl transferases has been discussed by Burchell et al. (1991), and that for glutathione transferases by Mannervik et al. (1992).

III. Heterologous Expression Systems

Recent advances in molecular biology have yielded some novel approaches for the study of isoform-specific metabolism of drugs. The most promising is heterologous expression of cDNAs of P-450 isoforms in prekaryotic or karyotic cells (see Gonzalez et al. 1991). Several different vectors and host cells have been used, the most promising being vaccinia virus and the HepG2 human hepatoma cell line (Aoyama et al. 1989; see Gonzalez et al. 1991), extrachromosomal expression vectors having an Epstein-Barr virus origin of replication and suitable host cells, human B-lymphoblastoid AHH-1 cells (Davies et al. 1989; Crespi et al. 1990a,b, 1991), and retrovirus vector and human HeLa or mouse NIH 3T3 cells (Battula 1989; Battula et al. 1991). These engineered cells offer an experimental system in which the metabolic or inhibitor profile of a given isoform or the isoform dependence of the metabolism of a substance can be studied "in isolation." The battery of cells expressing a panel of human isoforms may help enormously in attempts to find isoform-specific probe substances. The "isozyme battery" approach has been applied for the study of the metabolism of aflatoxin B_1 (AOYAMA et al. 1990), nicotine (FLAMMANG et al. 1992), and warfarin (RETTIE et al. 1992).

E. Probe Drugs

I. The Probe Drug Concept

The term "probe drug," also called "marker drug" or "model drug," was introduced into clinical pharmacology during the 1970s, when considerable interest arose in the influence of genetic and environmental factors on drug-metabolizing enzyme activity (VESELL 1991; VESELL and PENNO 1983; PARK 1982, 1985). As the term "probe" implies, it is a drug or a chemical to search into, so as thoroughly to explore, or to discover or ascertain something (Oxford English Dictionary). As used nowadays, a probe drug is devised to provide information that exceeds information on the drug itself, i.e., that can be extrapolated to other important issues (enzyme activity, rate of metabolism of other compounds).

1. The "Ideal" Probe Drug

What is required of a probe to detect environmental influences in vivo? Ideally, it should be:

1. "Polyfunctional," i.e., able to detect the presence or absence of many different environmental and/or nongenetic host effects (e.g., cigarette smoke and polycyclic aromatic hydrocarbons, drugs, alcohol, diseases) on enzyme activity
2. "Poly-isozymic" and/or "isoform-specific", i.e., several P-450 isoforms can be quantitated simultaneously and several (polymorphic) pathways measured simultaneously by virtue of a specific metabolite
3. Not inhibitory to those (polymorphically) regulated isoforms that are probed simultaneously
4. Safe to be used in vivo in man and widely available
5. Easily and reliably assayed in suitable body fluids (including metabolites), i.e., the methodology ought not to be very complicated

In addition to the above features, the pharmacokinetics of the probe drug should be predominantly determined by metabolism (not by liver blood flow or protein binding) and be predictable, i.e., a limited number of samples should be able to provide quantitative information on the rate of metabolism and/or rate of metabolite formation.

It is very important to select the proper parameter to reflect the activity of the enzyme or enzymes under study (Wilkinson 1987; Breimer et al. 1984). The intrinsic clearance of a probe or of the metabolite(s) produced (formation clearance) is the most appropriate measure of activity. The elimination and metabolite formation rate constants are less suitable, but if the volume of distribution remains relatively constant they can also be used quite reliably in most situations. Under certain circumstances, i.e., one-compartment kinetics and reliable estimation of the volume of distribution, a single plasma concentration measurement may be sufficient for the estimation of plasma clearance, as has been shown for antipyrine (Poulsen and Loft 1988). Metabolic ratios (often used in metabolic phenotyping studies) are fairly sensitive to nonmetabolic factors and are thus less well suited for quantifying metabolic activities (Jackson et al. 1986). Nevertheless, in human studies ethical and practical considerations often dictate less than optimal solutions.

It is unlikely that one probe drug will be found that is able to reveal "all" or most relevant environmental or host conditions which affect oxidative drug metabolism and be poly-isozymic at the same time. Another approach is to find specific probes for each relevant condition, to be used selectively in appropriate settings, i.e., in situations when certain environmental influences or host conditions are expected to be of potential importance for the metabolism of an experimental drug under study.

2. "General" versus "Specific" Probe Drugs

One of the major shortcomings of probe drugs currently used to measure oxidative enzyme activity in vivo is that the results obtained with any one drug rarely possess predictive value for other drugs. Although this situation is very common, it is nevertheless useful to study correlations between different probes, if for no other purpose than to aid in the selection of probes for "cocktails" (see Sect. E.IV). It is important to identify the reasons behind poor correlations. Probe drugs may be metabolized by distinct isoforms, which are under different regulation. On the other hand, two probe drugs may both be metabolized by sets of isoforms with overlapping specificities, in which case a statistically significant but still rather poor correlation may be observed (Breimer 1990).

II. Importance of Enzyme Specificity

Studies on probe drugs for polymorphic isoforms have demonstrated the importance of isoform-specific probes. It also seems important to find isoform-specific probes for those isoforms which are regulated primarily by environmental factors. If a probe drug which is metabolized by several isoforms under different regulation is selected, one is bound to observe a "diluted" effect of an environmental factor, especially if that factor has a specific effect on one isoform only. If a strictly isoform-specific probe drug is used, detailed information will indeed be obtained on the behavior of that specific isoform, but not on potential changes of other isoforms. So, selection of an isoform-specific probe drug is appropriate only when it is warranted by the goal of the study. Otherwise a poly-isozymic probe or a combination of specific probes (cocktail) seems preferable.

III. Selected Probe Drugs

Against the background of the previous sections, some probe drugs that are currently widely applied will be briefly reviewed, together with some other candidate probe drugs/substances (Table 5). In-depth analysis of potential isoform specificity would need much more space than is available within the scope of this chapter; nevertheless, attention will be paid to probe substances that are claimed to be isoform-specific in vivo.

1. Antipyrine

Antipyrine has been used very extensively as a measure of in vivo oxidative drug metabolism (a Medline search revealed almost 3000 references between 1961 and 1990; Poulsen and Loft, personal communication) and has been dealt with in a large number of reviews (BREIMER 1983; SCHELLENS and BREIMER 1987; VESELL 1979; POULSEN and LOFT 1988, personal communication; see also SOTANIEMI and PELKONEN 1987). The elimination rate of antipyrine is enhanced by antiepileptic and other drugs and by cigarette smoking and is inhibited by various forms of liver disease and several concomitantly administered drugs. The measurement of urinary metabolites and thereby rates of formation of metabolites provides further information on the differential effects of substances with respect to different isoforms, but this issue has been investigated to only a limited extent (POULSEN and LOFT 1988). The claim that the production of the main primary metabolites is catalyzed by polymorphically regulated P-450 isoforms (PENNO and VESELL 1983) has not received complete acceptance. In most cases environmental and host factors influence overall antipyrine metabolism, which may hide any polymorphic pattern in metabolite formation. Antipyrine seems to be a quite useful and universal probe for detection of the influence of common environmental factors (including drug treatment) and disease processes on overall P-450 activity. An advantage is that the assay of the drug in one sample (saliva or plasma) seems to give a reliable estimate of antipyrine kinetics (see LOFT and POULSEN 1990). It may therefore be quite suitable for initial screening purposes, but does not detect effects on specific isoforms. Assessment of metabolite formation is of only limited value in this respect.

Thus far, little information is available on isoforms involved in antipyrine metabolism, except that classical inducers of 3-methylcholanthrene-type and phenobarbital-type affect metabolic pathways differentially. However, on the basis of studies with diagnostic inhibitors it seems probable that CYP2C (sulfaphenazole), CYP2D (debrisoquine, quinidine), and CYP3A (nifedipine) or at least certain isoforms belonging to these subfamilies do not participate in antipyrine metabolism.

Typically, the effect of environmental factors on antipyrine clearance is of the order of 10%–50% (POULSEN and LOFT 1988). This seems very modest and clinically insignificant. However, as discussed above, a general probe such as antipyrine may not be very efficient in revealing increases or decreases in specific isoforms. Consequently, the impact of an environmental factor on the elimination of a drug metabolized by a single isoform may be an order of magnitude larger than anticipated on the basis of information obtained using antipyrine.

2. Aminopyrine

Aminopyrine is principally demethylated and, if radiolabeled substrate is used, the subsequently formed CO_2 can be quantitated in the exhaled air (LAUTERBURG and BIRCHER 1973). It has been demonstrated that different exogenous and host factors affect the amount of exhaled radioactive CO_2 and consequently this parameter has been suggested to be useful for the investigation of liver function. An impressive amount of information is available on aminopyrine N-demethylation in the rat liver and the effects of all sorts of environmental and host conditions, but it is not known to what extent this information can be extrapolated to the human situation. In contrast to the situation in experimental animals, in which several isoforms N-demethylating aminopyrine have been claimed to be present, GARCIA-AGUNDEZ et al. (1990) interpret their in vitro studies in human liver biopsies as showing the presence of a single enzyme. However, its identity is not known.

3. Caffeine

Concise reviews on caffeine metabolism have recently appeared (KALOW and CAMPBELL 1988; KALOW and TANG 1993). Much interest has centered upon the measurement of caffeine metabolites because the formation of different metabolites seems to be catalyzed by various P-450 isoforms and acetyltransferase, and thus caffeine would in principle be a suitable probe drug for assessing the activity of several enzymes. However, recent studies on in vitro microsomal preparations and genetically engineered cells expressing human and animal P-450s have amply confirmed the primary role of CYP1A2 in caffeine metabolism (KALOW and CAMPBELL 1988; FUHR et al. 1992). CYP1A2 catalyzes the 3-demethylation of caffeine, which accounts for about 80% of primary caffeine degradation in man (BERTHOU et al. 1991). Furthermore, studies on in vitro systems have demonstrated that 1-demethylation is mainly and 7-demethylation partly catalyzed by CYP1A2 (FUHR et al. 1992). On this basis it seems that more than 90% of primary caffeine metabolism in man is due to CYP1A2, with other enzymes contributing very little. It has also been shown that furafylline, a specific CYP1A2 inhibitor (SESARDIC et al. 1990), retards caffeine elimination tremendously (TARRUS et al. 1987). In experimental situations, two measures of caffeine degradation are useful, the caffeine breath test, based on the 3-demethylation reaction and CO_2 exhalation, and the caffeine metabolite ratio for P-450 1A2, which is based on the urinary metabolite ratio of paraxanthine 7-demethylation products to a paraxanthine 8-hydroxylation product (KALOW and CAMPBELL 1988). Both of these measures are increased by cigarette smoking (WIETHOLZ et al. 1981; KOTAKE et al. 1982; GRANT et al. 1987; KALOW and TANG 1991), indicating an increase in the amount of P-450 1A2. Caffeine can also be used as a probe for acetyltransferase phenotyping (the ratio between the excretion of 5-acetylamino-6-formylamino-3-methyluracil and that of all products of the 7-demethylation pathway of paraxanthine shows complete concordance with acetylation polymorphism) and for xanthine oxidase activity. The widespread use of coffee and other caffeine-containing beverages in different parts of the world precludes any ethical considerations sometimes associated with the investigational use of medicinal substances. However, it is not known how "universal" a probe caffeine is with respect to environmental and host conditions. In the mouse, caffeine elimination is highly increased by both 3-methylcholanthrene and phenobarbital (APSELOFF et al. 1991), but in man, cigarette smoking seems to be the principal inducer of caffeine elimination, although some antiepileptic drugs may have an effect (WIETHOLTZ et al. 1989).

It is of interest that caffeine has been used to study the impact of environmental polybrominated biphenyl pollution in Michigan (LAMBERT et al. 1990). Caffeine clearance and metabolite formation were significantly increased as a function of body burden, indicating the usefulness of caffeine as a probe in human environmental toxicology.

4. Theophylline

The elimination and metabolic fate of theophylline in different clinical situations has been extensively studied (see OGILVIE 1978), the 8-hydroxylation pathway accounting for about 60% of total metabolites. Earlier in vitro studies seemed to indicate that two demethylations and 8-hydroxylation are catalyzed by different P-450 isoforms, the cigarette smoke-inducible isoform (presumably CYP1A2) being responsible for the 1- and 3-N-demethylations (ROBSON et al. 1987, 1988). However, recent results suggest that 3-N-demethylation is also catalyzed by a P-450 isoform different from, but closely related to, CYP1A2 (SARKAR et al. 1992). Furthermore, studies on expressed enzymes clearly demonstrate that human CYP1A2 is able to mediate 8-hydroxylation as a major metabolic pathway (FUHR et al. 1992). Consequently, there is still some controversy as to the isoforms catalyzing different primary oxidation pathways of theophylline. Nevertheless, theophylline is a useful compound for probing differential effects of environmental factors on P-450 isoforms if metabolite formation is taken into account, too. It is widely available and the small doses needed for screening purposes preclude any serious side-effects. The most striking environmental factor increasing theophylline clearance considerably is cigarette smoking in man and polycyclic aromatic hydrocarbons in experimental animals. In many respects theophylline resembles caffeine. A choice between the two compounds favors caffeine because it is a recreational substance, is more widely available, and is also able to reveal acetylation status. Compared to antipyrine, it has been shown that total theophylline metabolism is strongly correlated with the rate of formation of 4-hydroxyantipyrine (TEUNISSEN et al. 1985; SCHELLENS et al. 1988c). Therefore theophylline offers only a small amount of information over and above what can be obtained with antipyrine.

5. Nifedipine

The overall rate of oxidative metabolism of nifedipine was once thought to display polymorphic distribution (intrinsic clearance) (KLEINBLOESEM et al. 1984), but in recent years it has become clear that it is very sensitive to many different environmental and host influences (SCHELLENS et al. 1988b; BREIMER and SCHELLENS 1990; SOONS et al. 1992). The isoform(s) responsible for the major metabolic pathway of nifedipine has (have) been identified as belonging to the CYP3A subfamily, inducible by rifampicin, glucocorticoids, phenobarbital, and macrolide antibiotics (see Table 4). Consequently, nifedipine should be suitable for situations in which the changes in the activity of this isoform, with all its consequences, need to be elucidated. However, nifedipine is a high-extraction drug and liver blood flow therefore may be of considerable importance in its elimination, making it a less than ideal in vivo probe. Currently it is nevertheless the best available and understood probe drug for in vivo CYP3A activity.

6. Barbiturates

Hexobarbital and pentobarbital have been widely – almost routinely – used in animal studies, where changes in sleeping time are taken as indirect indications of changes in oxidative drug-metabolizing enzyme activity. Accordingly, several barbiturates have been used and suggested for in vivo drug metabolism studies: pentobarbital (RUBIN and LIEBER 1968), amobarbital (MAWER et al. 1972), and hexobarbital (VAN DER GRAAF et al. 1988). The elimination of each of these substances seems to be affected by environmental and nongenetic host factors. However, hexobarbital is the only compound studied more extensively thus far. The main metabolic pathway, 3'-oxidation, is catalyzed by a specific P-450 isoform (KNODELL et al. 1988) which is not known to display polymorphism and which may be influenced by exogenous and endogenous factors. It seems that there is a good correlation between antipyrine and hexobarbital metabolism, in particular if antipyrine metabolite formation is taken into account (SCHELLENS et al. 1988c). Hexobarbital therefore does not provide information additional to that obtained with antipyrine. Furthermore, the problem with barbiturates is that they are no longer widely used as drugs because of their relative lack of safety and their abuse potential.

7. Tolbutamide

Tolbutamide has been used as an in vivo measure of drug metabolism (SOTANIEMT et al. 1971; ZILLY et al. 1975; PAGE et al. 1991). These studies demonstrated that its elimination is affected by some environmental influences such as inducing substances and host factors, for example liver disease. The overall variability in the elimination half-life among a healthy population is more than tenfold, probably reflecting differences in metabolic clearance, but variability in volume of distribution cannot be excluded (SOTANIEMI and HUHTI 1974). There has been some controversy about the possible polymorphism in tolbutamide elimination. SCOTT and POFFENBERGER (1979) claimed that tolbutamide elimination is polymorphically controlled, but data from in vitro studies did not substantiate this claim (KNODELL et al. 1987). Tolbutamide seems to be quite safe when used as a single dose. However, it is highly bound to plasma proteins and this property complicates the unambiguous assessment of intrinsic clearance if only total drug is being measured and variability in protein binding is not taken into account.

8. Warfarin

Warfarin is oxidatively metabolized in vitro to several metabolites that display some isoform specificity, at least in rat and mouse liver microsomes (KAMINSKY et al. 1984; GUENGERICH et al. 1982). It is also of interest to note that it is a substrate for several P-450 isoforms purified from human liver (WANG et al. 1983; KAMINSKY et al. 1984b). Recent studies in expressed human P-450 isoforms have demonstrated that specific hydroxylations are at least partly catalyzed by specific isoforms, such as CYP2C9 and CYP3A4 (RETTIE et al. 1992). Thus warfarin would seem to be a promising compound for in vivo studies; however, it has been used only to a very limited extent. One of the reasons is that as an anticoagulant, warfarin has a potentially hazardous effect, although the use of a single, smaller than therapeutic dose may not cause prolongation of bleeding time. Another potential problem in the use of warfarin as a probe drug is its high protein binding, as has been discussed for tolbutamide. Furthermore, a complicating factor with warfarin is the stereochemical selectivity in its metabolism which requires stereoselective analysis of parent enantiomers and metabolites (see LAM 1988). It can currently only he hypothesized that the formation rate of some specific metabolites can be used as an index of the activity of specific P-450 isoforms in vivo.

9. Other Potential Probes

There are a number of other substances that have shown some promise as indices of drug metabolism, e.g., lidocaine, diazepam, trimethadione, and metronidazole (Table 5). For example, certain oxidative pathways of diazepam metabolism are catalyzed by the polymorphic mephenytoin hydroxylase and debrisoquine hydroxylase (in addition to nonpolymorphic pathways; see Bertilsson et al. 1990). Hence diazepam should in principle be an interesting candidate probe drug for measuring the influence of both environmental factors and certain hereditary factors on specific isoform activities. Trimethadione has been suggested as an alternative probe drug to antipyrine (Tanaka et al. 1989), but it is not clear whether it has any advantages over antipyrine. The same reservation applies with respect to

Table 5. Potential probe drugs/substances which are responsive to one or more environmental and/or host factors

Probe	Methods available	P-450	Responsive to	References[a]
Aminopyrine	p/b, m(r)/ex	NK	Many conditions	1
Antipyrine	p/b, p/s, pm/u	1A2, 3A?	Many conditions	2
Caffeine	m/u	1A2	Cigarette smoking	3
Diazepam	pm/b	2C, 2D	Many conditions	4
Erythromycin	m(r)/ex	3A	Many conditions	5
Hexobarbital	p/b, pm/u	2C?	Many conditions	6
Lidocaine	Adm i.v.; pm/b	3A	Many conditions	7
Metronidazole	p/b, pm/u	NK	Many conditions	8
Nifedipine	pm/b, pm/u	3A4	Many conditions	9
Pentobarbital	p/b	NK	Alcohol	10
Phenacetin	p/b, m(r)/ex	1A2	Cigarette smoking	11
Phenytoin	pm/b, pm/u	2C		12
Theophylline	p/b, pm/u	1A2	Cigarette smoking	13
Tolbutamide	p/b, pm/u	2C?	Many conditions	14
Trimethadione	p/b, pm/u	NK	Many conditions (like antipyrine)	15
Warfarin	p/b, pm/u	2C, others	?	16
6β-Hydroxycortisol	Endogenous	3A	Many conditions	17
D-Glucaric acid	Endogenous	NK	Phenobarbital inducers	18

p, parent drug; m, metabolite(s); b, blood (plasma, serum); u, urine; s, saliva; (r), radioactive label; ex, exhaled air; NK, not known

[a] References: 1, Lauterburg and Bircher 1973; Miotti et al. 1988; 2, Poulsen and Loft 1988, 1992; 3, Wietholtz et al. 1981; Grant et al. 1983; Campbell et al. 1987; Kalow and Campbell 1988; 4, Hepner et al. 1977; Bertilsson et al. 1990; 5, Watkins et al. 1989; 6, Van Der Graaff et al. 1988; 7, Oellerich et al. 1987, 1989, 1990; 8, Loft et al. 1988; 9, Breimer et al. 1989; Soons and Breimer 1992; 10, Rubin and Lieber 1968; 11, Schoeller et al. 1985; Inaba 1990; 12, Bachmann et al. 1985; 13, Miller et al. 1984; 14, Page et al. 1991; 15, Tanaka et al. 1989; 16, Sutcliff et al. 1987; 17, Ohnhaus et al. 1989; 18, Hunter et al. 1971; Sotaniemi and Huhti 1974. For a concise review on noninvasive methods see Loft and Poulsen (1990)

metronidazole (LOFT et al. 1988). Lidocaine has been used especially in connection with transplantation surgery as a liver function test (OELLERICH et al. 1989). The formation of MEGX, the main metabolite of lidocaine, has been shown to be catalyzed by CYP3A4 (BARGETZI et al. 1989). Erythromycin, as a breath test, has also been used as a probe for CYP3A4 (WATKINS et al. 1989). Although all these compounds have shown some promise and even potential advantages over existing probe drugs, it is still difficult to judge their utility in this respect, because of limited experience.

10. Endogenous Probes

The excretion of endogenous substances such as 6β-hydroxycortisol may sometimes also provide useful information on the influence of environmental factors on drug-metabolizing enzyme activity. The ratio between 6β-hydroxycortisol and corticosteroid excretion has been shown to be an index for CYP3A activity and has been the subject of recent investigations (GED et al. 1989; OHNHAUS et al. 1989). The excretion of D-glucaric acid is strongly enhanced by antiepileptic drug treatment and has been claimed to be a marker for phenobarbital-type induction in the liver (HUNTER et al. 1971; SOTANIEMI and HUHTI 1974). It has, however, not been proved to be useful for any other reason. Although endogenous probes are attractive for several obvious reasons, there is still insufficient information to decide on their place among exogenous probes. So far only 6β-hydroxycortisol has an established position among the probe canditates. Testosterone is theoretically an interesting compound because several hydroxylation reactions have been shown to be catalyzed by specific P-450 isoforms in vitro and in engineered cells (WAXMAN 1988; WAXMAN et al. 1991); however, there are major analytical difficulties in in vivo studies.

IV. Cocktail Approach

The principle behind the cocktail approach is clear: several model substrates, each reflecting the activity of different P-450 isoforms or other metabolizing enzymes, are administered simultaneously or during a relatively short time span (e.g., 1h), and the clearance and/or metabolite formation of each substance is assessed (BREIMER et al. 1988, 1990). Thereby, the activity of several isoforms is assessed in the context of one experiment. The kinetic parameters that most closely reflect enzyme activity in vivo are the intrinsic clearance of unchanged drug and the clearance for the production of metabolites (BREIMER et al. 1984, 1988).

There are in principle at least three major advantages of the cocktail approach (BREIMER and SCHELLENS 1990). It is obviously of great practical advantage when, for example, phenotyping for different types of polymorphism can be achieved in one session. Conceptually this approach is of advantage in metabolic correlation studies, because it excludes the influence of intraindividual variability in metabolizing activity with time. Furthermore the differential influence of environmental factors and host conditions on the activity of CYP isoforms can be assessed in the context of one experimental protocol. Although the basic strategy is relatively simple, there are certain prerequisites: (a) there should be no interactions between the different probes; (b) a high degree of selectivity and sensitivity of the analytical methodology is required for the determination of several drugs and metabolites in the same samples. The practical application of the cocktail approach includes studies designed to reveal the effects of sulfaphenazole, cimetidine, and primaquine on antipyrine and tolbutamide metabolism (Back et al. 1988), mutual relationships between antipyrine, hexobarbital, and theophylline (Tenuissen et al. 1985; Schellens et al. 1988c) and between nifedipine, sparteine, and phenytoin (Schellens et al. 1991), the influence of enzyme induction and inhibition on nifedipine, sparteine, mephenytoin, and antipyrine (Schellens et al. 1987, 1988a), the effect of diltiazem on antipyrine, trimethadione, and debrisoquine (Sakai et al. 1991), and the differential effect of quinidine on nifedipine, sparteine, and mephenytoin metabolism (Schellens et al. 1991).

Bachmann and Coworkers (1990, 1991) have developed a method in which they use multiple probes and single sample clearance estimates for the construction of a "handprint" for a given environmental influence. They have used antipyrine, phenytoin, quinidine, and carbamazepine to measure P-450 activities, lorazepam as a probe for UDP-glucuronosyl transferase activity, and valproic acid as a probe of both peroxisomal and microsomal β-oxidase activity. Phenobarbital administration in volunteers and smoking resulted in different fingerprints: phenobarbital increased the clearance of carbamazepine and also that of antipyrine, quinidine, and valproic acid to a certain extent, but had no effect on phenytoin, theophylline, or lorazepam (Bachmann et al. 1991). Cigarette smoking increased the clearance of theophylline in particular, but also that of antipyrine and carbamazepine (Bachmann et al. 1990).

Although the cocktail or multiple-probe approach has definite advantages as discussed, it is as yet too early to reach any conclusions on the "ideal" composition of a cocktail such that most of the different CYP isoform activities can be being estimated in the context of one experiment. In fact, the optimal composition may vary from experiment to experiment depending on the objective of the study in question.

F. Practical Considerations for Human Studies

What specific advice should be given to the clinical pharmacologist who is confronted with a problem like: How should I assess the activity of specific P-450 enzymes in my volunteers or patients without taking liver biopsies? The first consideration is whether there is any information from experimental animals or in vitro approaches about the situation that the clinical pharmacologist wants to investigate. If he – as is often the case – would like to study the effect of a specific drug on drug metabolism, i.e., induction and/or inhibition, it would be relatively simple to perform similar experiments in experimental animals. The information thus obtained should help to select proper probe drugs or a cocktail for the human study, although by no means would results obtained in animals necessarily be predictive of the human situation (as has been discussed earlier). The question of whether the clinical pharmacologist should perform the study in a longitudinal design in the same panel of subjects or patients, or in parallel groups, is beyond the scope of this review, but has been discussed previously (BREIMER 1983). If the effect of an environmental factor on the elimination of a new drug is to be investigated, it should be helpful to have a probe drug known to be affected by that environmental factor, so that the correlative approach can be taken. Probe drugs can also be applied in situations where information on the level and inducibility of enzymes is required, e.g., for the purpose of molecular epidemiological investigations on the relationship between metabolic activation and cancer.

One relatively difficult question concerns the selection of either a "general" or poly-isozymic probe or a cocktail. With the currently available knowledge – and if analytical methods are not limiting – the selection of a cocktail would yield more detailed and comprehensive information because hardly any poly-isozymic compound exists that can be used in man. The answer to this question is heavily dependent on the purpose of a particular study. Although antipyrine is rather nonspecific and may be insensitive, it still may be used as a first-line probe in many instances, and if interesting findings emerge, a more varied (cocktail) approach can be chosen.

If larger populations are to be studied, simplicity, ease, and (generally) noninvasiveness are in principle required to make such a study feasible. This often leads to a delicate balance between reliability and validity of results obtained (which are dependent on the methodology) and feasibility, including the resources available for the study. Careful judgement is required (preferably before launching the study or on the basis of a pilot study) on whether the use of less than optimal methodology will provide useful information or whether only spurious and confusing results will be the outcome.

G. Final Considerations

Current knowledge on environmental factors affecting drug-metabolizing enzyme activity is still rather fragmentary, in particular with regard to the assessment of specific environmentally regulated P-450 isoforms by means of probe substances. The success of mephenytoin and debrisoquine (or sparteine) as genetic probes is solely based on the fact that the isoforms involved in their metabolism are relatively stable and almost totally insensitive to environmental or host influences (except direct inhibition). However, as far as environmentally affected isoforms are concerned, fairly reliable information is available only for caffeine and CYP1A2 and several probes and CYP3A. Moreover the latter case is complicated by the fact that there are several members of this subfamily. On the other hand several "general" probes are available which have proved useful in situations not requiring such a degree of sophistication as those in which specific P-450 probing is attempted.

What about probe specificity in terms of specific environmental influences? Again, caffeine, CYP1A2, and cigarette smoking seems to be the clearest example. Otherwise the situation is much more complicated, perhaps because of the complex and nonspecific influences of environmental inducers and inhibitors. It should in principle, however, be possible to find probes which are more specific and informative in measuring, for example, the effect of alcohol consumption on CYP2E1, and more research should be devoted to this and similar issues.

What about important future developments? It seems probable that the use of various in vitro methods, including cells expressing single or a few enzymes, will enable the planning of in vivo experiments in a much more specific and detailed way than was previously possible. It is likely that the accumulated in vitro data will dictate in a very logical and natural way the in vivo experiments with the most suitable probe drug(s), and at that stage it will not be advisable to perform in vivo experiments without extensive coverage of in vitro approaches.

Apart from the great relevance of in vitro experiments, the importance of animal models and experiments should also finally be stressed. Although the foregoing discussion may sometimes have given the impression that animal experiments are of relatively limited significance with respect to the human situation, they are actually very important from a more basic point of view. Almost by necessity in human studies we have to concentrate upon the phenomenology of environmental influences. Nevertheless, it should always be kept in mind that a better understanding of the mechanisms involved may be even more important in our attempts to conceptualize the field and to predict the interactions between organism and environment.

Acknowledgements. Useful comments by Dr. Alan R. Boobis, Dr. Hannu Raunio, and Dr. Kirsi Vähäkangas are gratefully acknowledged. This review was written to contribute to the goals of the COST B1 Action Project. One of the authors (O.P.) was supported by The Academy of Finland Medical Research Council (contract no. 1051029).

References

Adesnik M, Atchison M (1986) Genes for cytochrome P-450 and their regulation. Crit Rev Biochem 19:247–305
Aitio A, Riihimäki V, Vainio H (eds) (1984) Biological monitoring and surveillance of workers exposed to chemicals. Hemisphere, Washington

Alvan G, Balant LP, Bechtel PR, Boobis AR, Gram LF, Pithan K (eds) (1990a) European Consensus Conference on Pharmacogenetics. EEC Directorate General Science, Research and Development, Luxemburg, pp 207

Alvan G, Bechtel P, Iselius L, Gundert-Remy U (1990b) The hydroxylation polymorphisms of debrisoquine and mephenytoin in European populations. Eur J Clin Pharmacol 39:533–537

Alvares AP, Pratt WB (1990) Pathways of drug metabolism. In: Pratt WB, Taylor P (eds) Principles of drug action. The basis of pharmacology, 3rd edn. Churchill Livingstone, Edinburgh, pp 365–422

Aoyama T, Korzekwa K, Nagata K, Gillette J, Gelboin HV, Gonzalez FJ (1989) cDNA-directed expression of rat testosterone 7α-hydroxylase using the modified vaccinia virus, T7-RNA-polymerase system and evidence for 6α-hydroxylation and D6-testosterone formation. Eur J Biochem 181:331–336

Aoyama T, Yamano S, Guzelian PS, Gelboin HV, Gonzalez FJ (1990) Five of 12 forms of vaccinia virus-expressed human hepatic cytochrome P450 metabolically activate aflatoxin B_1. Proc Natl Acad Sci USA 87:4790–4793

Apseloff G, Shepard DR, Chambers MA, Nawoot S, Mays DC, Gerber N (1990) Inhibition and induction of theophylline metabolism by 8-methoxypsoralen. In vivo study in rats and humans. Drug Metab Dispos 18:298–303

Apseloff G, Hilliard JB, Gerber N, Mays DC (1991) Inhibition and induction of drug metabolism by psoralens: alterations in duration of sleep induced by hexobarbital and in clearance of caffeine and hexobarbital in mice. Xenobiotica 21:1461–1471

Arvela P, Kraul H, Stenbäck F, Pelkonen O (1991) The cerium-induced liver injury and oxidative drug metabolism in DBA/2 and C57BL/6 mice. Toxicology 69:1–9

Atiba JO, Blaschke, Wilkinson GR (1989) Effects of ketoconazole on the polymorphic 4-hydroxylations of S-mephenytoin and debrisoquine. Br J Clin Pharmacol 28:161–165

Bachmann KA, Schwartz J, Forney R, Jauregui L (1985) Phenytoin as a probe of drug metabolism. Predicting clearance with a single salivary sample. Pharmacology 30:145–152

Bachmann KA, Nunlee M, Martin M, Schwartz J, Jauregui L, Forney R Jr (1990) The use of single sample clearance estimates to probe hepatic drug metabolism: handprinting the influence of cigarette smoking on human hepatic drug metabolism. Xenobiotica 20:537–547

Bachmann KA, Nunlee M, Martin M, Jauregui L (1991) The use of single sample clearance estimates to probe hepatic drug metabolism: handprinting the influence of phenobarbitone on human hepatic drug metabolism. Xenobiotica 21:1385–1392

Back DJ, Tjia J, Mönig H, Ohnhaus EE, Park BK (1988) Selective inhibition of drug oxidation after simultaneous administration of two probe drugs, antipyrine and tolbutamide. Eur J Clin Pharmacol 34:157–163

Bailey DG, Spence JD, Munzo C, Arnold JMO (1991) Interaction of citrus juices with felodipine and nifedipine. Lancet 337:268–269

Balant LP, Gundert-Remy U, Boobis AR, von Bahr C (1989) Relevance of genetic polymorphism in drug metabolism in the development of new drugs. Eur J Clin Pharmacol 36:551–554

Bandiera S (1990) Expression and catalysis of sex-specific cytochrome P450 isoforms in rat liver. Can J Physiol Pharmacol 68:762–768

Bargetzi MJ, Aoyama T, Gonzalez FJ, Meyer UA (1989) Lidocaine metabolism in human liver microsomes by cytochrome P450IIIA4. Clin Pharmacol Ther 46:521–527

Battula N (1989) Transduction of cytochrome P_3-450 by retroviruses: constitutive expression of enzymatically active microsomal hemoprotein in animal cells. J Biol Chem 2991–2996

Battula N, Schut HAJ, Thorgeirsson SS (1991) Cytochrome P4501A2 constitutively expressed from transduced DNA mediates metabolic activation and DNA-adduct formation of aromatic amine carcinogens in NIH 3T3 cells. Mol Carcinog 4:407–414

Beaune PH, Guengerich FP (1988) Human drug metabolism in vitro. Pharmacol Ther 37:193–211

Benford DJ, Bridges JW, Gibson GG (eds) (1987) Drug metabolism – from molecules to man. Taylor and Francis, London, p 787

Berthou F, Flinois J-P, Ratanasavanh D, Beaune P, Riche C, Guillouzo A (1991) Evidence for the involvement of several cytochromes P-450 in the first steps of caffeine metabolism by human liver microsomes. Drug Metab Dispos 19:561–567

Bertilsson L, Baillie TA, Reviriego J (1990) Factors influencing the metabolism of diazepam. Pharmacol Ther 45:85–91

Boobis AR, Davies DS (1984) Human cytochromes P-450. Xenobiotica 14:151–185

Boobis AR, Sesardic D, Murray BP, Edwards RJ, Singleton AM, Rich KJ, Murray S, Delatorre R, Segura J, Pelkonen O, Pasanen M, Kobayashi S, Zhiguang T, Davies DS (1990) Species variation in the response of the cytochrome P-450-dependent monooxygenase system to inducers and inhibitors. Xenobiotica 20:1139–1161

Breimer DD (1983) Interindividual variations in drug disposition. Clinical implications and methods of investigations. Clin Pharmacokinet 8:371–377

Breimer DD (1990) Potential clinical relevance of the interplay between genetic and environmental factors. In: Alvan G, Balant LP, Bechtel PR, Boobis AR, Gram LF, Pithan K (eds) Europen Consensus Conference on Pharmacogenetics. EEC Directorate General Science, Research and Development, Luxemburg, pp 69–80

Breimer DD, Schellens JHM (1990) A "cocktail" strategy to assess in vivo oxidative drug metabolism in humans. Trends Pharmacol Sci 11:223–225

Breimer DD, Vermeulen NPE, Danhof M, Teunissen MWE, Joeres RP, van der Graaff M (1984) Assessment and prediction of in vivo oxidative drug metabolizing enzyme activity. In: Benet LZ, Levy G (eds) Pharmacokinetics: a modern view. Plenum, New York, pp 191–216

Breimer DD, Schellens JHM, Soons PA (1988) Assessment of in vivo oxidative drug metabolizing enzyme activity in many by applying a cocktail approach. In: Miners JO, Birkett DJ, Drew R, May BK, McManus ME (eds) Microsomes and drug oxidations. Taylor and Francis, London, pp 232–240

Breimer DD, Schellens JHM, Soons PA (1989) Nifedipine: variability in its kinetics and metabolism in man. Pharmacol Ther 44:445–454

Brosen K, Gram LF (1989) Clinical significance of the sparteine/debrisoquine oxidation polymorphism. Eur J Clin Pharmacol 36:537–547

Burchell B, Nebert DW, Nelson DR, Bock KW, Iyanagi T, Jansen PLM, Lancet D, Mulder GJ, Chowdhury JR, Siest G, Tephly TR, Mackenzie PI (1991) The UDP glucuronosyltransferase gene superfamily: suggested nomenclature based on evolutionary divergence. DNA cell Biol 10:487–494

Burke MD, Mayer RT (1983) Differential effects of phenobarbitone and 3-methylcholanthrene induction on the hepatic microsomal metabolism and cytochrome P-450-binding of phenoxazone and a homologous series of its O-alkylethers (alkoxyresorufins). Chem Biol Interact 45:243–258

Campbell ME, Spielberg SP, Kalow W (1987) A urinary metabolite ratio that reflects systemic caffeine clearance. Clin Pharmacol Ther 42:157–165

Conney AH, Davison, C, Gastel R, Burns JJ (1960) Adaptive increases in drug metabolizing enzymes induced by phenobarbital and other drugs. J Pharmacol Exp Ther 130:1–8

Crespi CL, Steimel DT, Aoyama T, Gelboin HV, Gonzalez FJ (1990a) Stable expression of human cytochrome P450IA2 cDNA in a human lymphoblastoid cell line: role of the enzyme in the metabolic activation of aflatoxin B_1. Mol Carcinog 3:5–8

Crespi CL, Penman BW, Leakey JAE, Arlotto MP, Stark A, Parkinson A, Turner T, Steimel DT, Rudo K, Davies RL, Langenbach R (1990b) Human cytochrome

P450IIA3: cDNA sequence, role of the enzyme in the metabolic activation of promutagens, comparison to nitrosamine activation by human cytochrome P450IIE1. Carcinogenesis 11:1293–1300

Crespi CL, Penman BW, Steimel DT, Gelboin HV, Gonzalez FJ (1991) The development of a human cell line stably expressing human CYP3A4: role in the metabolic activation of aflatoxin B_1 and comparison to CYP1A2 and CYP2A3. Carcinogenesis 12:355–359

Davies RL, Crespi CL, Rudo K, Turner TR, Langenbach R (1989) Development of a human cell line by selection and drug-metabolizing gene transfection with increased capacity to activate promutagens. Carcinogenesis 10:885–891

Dawson GW, Vestal RE (1982) Smoking and drug metabolism. Pharmacol Ther 15:207–221

De Waziers I, Cugnenc PH, Yang CS, Leroux J-P, Beaune PH (1990) Cytochrome P450 isoforms, epoxide hydrolase and glutathione transferases in rat and human hepatic and extrahepatic tissues. J Pharmacol Exp Ther 253:387–394

Doecke CJ, Sansom LN, McManus ME (1990) Phenytoin 4-hydroxylation by rabbit liver P450IIC3 and identification of orthologs in human liver microsomes. Biochem Biophys Res Commun 166:860–866

Ekström G, von Bahr C, Ingelmann-Sundberg M (1989) Human liver microsomal cytochrome P-450 IIE1. Immunological evaluation of its contribution of microsomal ethanol oxidation, carbon tetrachloride reduction and NADPH oxidase activity. Biochem Pharmacol 38:689–693

Flammang AM, Gelboin HV, Aoyama T, Gonzales FJ, McCoy GD (1992) Nicotine metabolism by cDNA-expressed human cytochrome P450s. Biochem Arch 8:1–8

Forrester LM, Henderson CJ, Glancey MJ, Back DJ, Park BK, Ball SE, Kitteringham NR, McLaren AW, Miles JS, Skett P, Wolf CR (1992) Relative expression of cytochrome P450 isoforms in human liver and association with the metabolism of drugs and xenobiotics. Biochem J 281:359–368

Fuhr U, Doehmer J, Battula N, Wölfel C, Kudla C, Keita Y, Staib AH (1992) Biotransformation of caffeine and theophylline in mammalian cell lines genetically engineered for expression of single cytochrome P450 isoforms. Biochem Pharmacol 43:225–235

Garcia-Agundez JA, Luengo A, Benitez J (1990) Aminopyrine N-demethylase activity in human liver microsomes. Clin Pharmacol Ther 48:490–495

Ged C, Rouillon JM, Pichard L, Combalbert J, Bressot N, Bories P, Michel H, Beaune P, Marvel P (1989) The increase in urinary excretion of 6β-hydroxycortisol as a marker of human hepatic cytochrome P450IIIA induction. Br J Clin Pharmacol 28:373–387

Gonzalez FJ (1989) The molecular biology of cytochrome P450s. Pharmacol Rev 40:243–288

Gonzalez FJ (1990) Molecular genetics of the P-450 superfamily. Pharmacol Ther 45:1–38

Gonzalez FJ, Meyer UA (1991) Molecular genetics of the debrisoquine-sparteine polymorphism. Clin Pharmacol Ther 50:233–238

Gonzalez FJ, Crespi CL, Gelboin HV (1991a) cDNA-expressed human cytochrome P450s: a new age of molecular toxicology and human risk assessment. Mutat Res 247:113–127

Gonzalez FJ, Ueno T, Umeno M, Song BJ, Veech RL, Gelboin HV (1991b) Microsomal ethanol oxidizing system – transcriptional and posttranscriptional regulation of cytochrome P-450, CYP2E1. Alcohol Alcohol Suppl 1:97–102

Grant DM, Tang BK, Kalow W (1983) Variability in caffeine metabolism. Clin Pharmacol Ther 33:591–602

Grant DM, Campbell MP, Tang BK, Kalow W (1987) Biotransformation of caffeine by microsomes from human livers. Kinetics and inhibition studies. Biochem Pharmacol 36:1251–1260

Guengerich FP (ed) (1987a) Mammalian cytochromes P-450, vols I and II. CRC Press, Boca Raton

Guengerich FP (1987b) Enzymology of rat liver P450. In: Guengerich FP (ed) Mammalian cytochromes P450, vol 1. CRC Press, Boca Raton, pp 1–54

Guengerich FP (1988) Roles of cytochrome P450 enzymes in chemical carcinogenesis and cancer chemotherapy. Cancer Res 48:2946–2954

Guengerich FP (1989) Characterization of human microsomal cytochrome P-450 enzymes. Annu Rev Pharmacol Toxicol 29:241–246

Guengerich FP (1992a) Characterization of human cytochrome P450 enzymes. FASEB J 6:745–748

Guengerich FP (1992b) Human cytochrome P-450 enzymes. Life Sci 50:1471–1478

Guengerich FP, Shimada T (1991) Oxidation of toxic and carcinogenic chemicals by human cytochrome P-450 enzymes. Chem Res Toxicol 4:391–407

Guengerich FP, Turvy CG (1991) Comparison of levels of several human microsomal cytochrome P-450 enzymes and epoxide hydrolase in normal and disease states using immunochemical analysis of surgical liver samples. J Pharmacol Exp Ther 256:1189–1194

Guengerich FP, Dannan GA, Wright ST, Martin MV, Kaminsky LS (1982) Purification and characterization of liver microsomal cytochromes P450: electrophoretic, spectral, catalytic, and immunochemical properties and inducibility of eight isozymes isolated from rats treated with phenobarbital or β-naphthoflavone. Biochemistry 21:6019–6030

Guengerich FP, Kim D-H, Iwasaki M (1991) Role of human cytochrome P-450 IIE1 in the oxidation of several low molecular weight cancer suspects. Chem Res Toxicol 4:168–179

Hahnemann B, Salonpää P, Pasanen M, Mäenpää J, Honkakoski P, Juvonen R, Lang MA, Pelkonen O, Raunio H (1992) Effect of pyrazole, cobalt and phenobarbital on Cyp2a-4/5 (cytochrome P450 2a-4/5) expression in the liver of C57BL/6 and DBA/2 mice. Biochem J 286:289–294

Harris CC (1987) Tobacco smoke and lung disease: who is susceptible? Ann Intern Med 105:607–609

Hepner GW, Vesell ES, Lipton A, Harvey HA, Wilkinson GR (1977) Disposition of aminopyrine, antipyrine, diazepam and indocyanine green in patients with liver disease or on anticonvulsant drug therapy: diazepam breath test and correlations in drug elimination. Clin Pharmacol Ther 90:440–456

Honkakoski P, Auriola S, Lang MA (1992) Distinct induction profiles of three phenobarbital-responsive mouse liver cytochrome P450 isozymes. Biochem Pharmacol 43:2121–2128

Hunt CM, Watkins PB, Saenger P, Stave GM, Barlascini N, Watlington CO, Wright JT, Guzelian PS (1992) Heterogeneity of CYP3A isoforms metabolizing erythromycin and cortisol. Clin Pharmacol Ther 51:18–23

Hunter J, Carella M, Maxwell JD, Stewart DA, Williams R (1971) Urinary D-glucaric acid excretion as a test for hepatic enzyme induction in man. Lancet i:572–575

IARC (1986) Tobacco smoking. Monographs of the evaluation of carcinogenic risks to humans, vol 38

IARC (1988) Alcohol drinking. Monographs on the evaluation of carcinogenic risks to humans, vol 44

Idle JR (1990) Titrating exposure to tobacco smoke using cotinine – a minefield of misunderstandings. J Clin Epidemiol 43:313–317

Jackson PR, Tucker GT, Lennard MS, Woods HF (1986) Polymorphic drug oxidation: pharmacokinetic basis and comparison of experimental indices. Br J Clin Pharmacol 22:541–550

Jaiswal AK, Gonzalez FJ, Nebert DW (1985) Human dioxin-inducible cytochrome P450: complementary DNA and amino acid sequence. Science 228:80–83

Jenner P, Testa B (eds) (1980) Concepts in drug metabolism, parts A and B. Dekker, New York, pp 409, 582

Juchau MR (1990) Substrate specificities and functions of the P450 cytochromes. Life Sci 47:2385–2394

Jusko WJ (1979) Influence of cigarette smoking on drug metabolism in man. Drug Metab Rev 9:221–236

Kahn GC, Rubenfield M, Davies DS, Murray S, Boobis AR (1985) Sex and strain differences in hepatic debrisoquine 4-hydroxylase activity of the rat. Drug Metab Dispos 13:510–516

Kalow W, Campbell M (1988) Biotransformation of caffeine by microsomes. ISI Atlas Sci Pharmacol 2:381–386

Kalow W, Tang B-K (1991) Caffeine as a metabolic probe: exploration of the enzyme-inducing effect of cigarette smoking. Clin Pharmacol Ther 49:44–48

Kalow W, Tang B-K (1993) The use of caffeine for enzyme assays: a critical appraisal. Clin Pharmacol Ther 53:503–514

Kaminsky LS, Dannan GA, Guengerich FP (1984a) Composition of cytochrome P-450 isozymes from hepatic microsomes of C57BL/6 and DBA/2 mice assessed by warfarin metabolism, immunoinhibition, and immunoelectrophoresis with anti-(rat cytochrome P-450). Eur J Biochem 141:141–148

Kaminsky LS, Dunbar DA, Wang PP, Beaune P, Larrey D, Guengerich FP, Schnellman RG, Sipes IG (1984b) Human hepatic cytochrome P-450 composition as probed by in vitro microsomal metabolism of warfarin. Drug Metab Disp 12:470–477

Kawajiri K, Fujii-Kuriyama (1991) P450 and human cancer. Jpn J Cancer Res 82:1325–1335

Kawajiri K, Nakachi K, Imai K, Yoshii A, Shinoda N, Watanabe J (1990) Identification of genetically high risk individuals to lung cancer by DNA polymorphisms of the cytochrome P450IA1 gene. FEBS Lett 263:131–133

Ketterer B, Meyer DJ, Lalor E, Johnson P, Guengerich FP, Distlerath LM, Reilly PEB, Kadlubar FF, Flammang TJ, Yamazoe Y, Beaune PH (1991) A comparison of levels of glutathione transferases, cytochromes P450 and acetyltransferases in human livers. Biochem Pharmacol 41:635–638

Kleinbloesem CH, van Brummelen P, Faber H, Danhof M, Vermeulen NPE, Breimer DD (1984) Variability in nifedipine pharmacokinetics and dynamics: a new oxidation polymorphism in man. Biochem Pharmacol 22:3721–3724

Knodell RG, Hall SD, Wilkinson GR, Guengerich FP (1987) Hepatic metabolism of tolbutamide: characterization of the form of cytochrome P-450 involved in methyl hydroxylation and relationship to in vivo disposition. J Pharmacol Exp Ther 241:1112–1119

Knodell RG, Dubey RK, Wilkinson GR, Guengerich FP (1988) Oxidative metabolism of hexobarbital in human liver: relationship to polymorphic S-mephenytoin 4-hydroxylation. J Pharmacol Exp Ther 245:845–849

Knodell RG, Browne DG, Gwozdz GP, Brian WR, Guengerich FP (1991) Differential inhibition of individual human liver cytochromes P-450 by cimetidine. Gastroenterology 101:1680–1691

Koop DR (1986) Hydroxylation of p-nitrophenol by rabbit ethanol-inducible cytpochrome P-450 isoform 3a. Mol Pharmacol 29:399–404

Koop DR (1992) Oxidative and reductive metabolism by cytochrome P450 2E1. FASEB J 6:724–730

Kotake AN, Schoeller DA, Lambert GH, Baker AL, Schaffer DC, Josephs H (1982) The caffeine CO_2 breath test: dose response and route of N-demethylation in smokers and nonsmokers. Clin Pharmacol Ther 32:261–269

Lam YWF (1988) Stereoselectivity: an issue of significant inportance in clinical pharmacology. Pharmacotherapy 8:147–157

Lambert GH, Schoeller DA, Humphrey HEB, Kotake AN, Lietz H, Campbell M, Kalow W, Spielberg SP, Budd M (1990) The caffeine breath test and caffeine urinary metabolite ratios in the Michigan cohort exposed to polybrominated biphenyls: a preliminary study. Environ Health Perspect 89:175–181

Lane EA, Guthrie S, Linnoila M (1985) Effects of ethanol on drug and metabolite pharmacokinetics. Clin Pharmacokinet 10:228–247

Lauterburg B, Bircher J (1973) Hepatic microsomal drug metabolizing capacity measured in vivo by breath analysis. Gastroenterology 65:556–559

Levin W (1990) Functional diversity of hepatic cytochromes P-450. Drug Metab Dispos 18:824–830

Lieber CS (1988) Biochemical and molecular basis of alcohol-induced injury to liver and other tissues. N Engl J Med 319:1639–1650

Lieber CS (1991) Hepatic, metabolic and toxic effects of ethanol: 1991 update. Alcoholism: Clin Exp Res 15:573–592

Lieber CS, DeCarli LM (1968) Microsomal ethanol-oxidizing system. Science 162: 917–918

Lindberg RLP, Negishi M (1989) Alteration of mouse cytochrome P450$_{coh}$ substrate specificity by mutation of a single amino-acid residue. Nature 339:632–634

Loft S, Poulsen HE (1990) Prediction of xenobiotic metabolism by non-invasive methods. Pharmacol Toxicol 67:101–108

Loft S, Poulsen HE, Sonne J, Dossing M (1988) Metronidazole clearance: a one sample method and influencing factors. Clin Pharmacol Ther 43:420–428

Loft S, Nielsen AJ, Borg E, Poulsen HE (1990) Metronidazole and antipyrine metabolism in the rat: clearance determination from one saliva sample. Xenobiotica 20:185–198

Lucas D, Berthou F, Dreano Y, Floch HH, Menez JF (1990) Ethanol-inducible cytochrome P-450: assessment of substrates' specific chemical probes in rat liver microsomes. Alcoholism: Clin Exp Res 14:590–594

Lush IE, Andrews KM (1978) Genetic variation between mice in their metabolism of coumarin and its derivatives. Genet Res Camb 31:177–186

Mäenpää J, Sigusch H, Raunig H, Syngelmä T, Vuorela P, Vuorela H, Pelkonen O (1993) Differentiated inhibition of coumarin 7-hydroxylase activity in mouse and h liver microsomes. Biochem Pharmacol 45:1035–1042

Mannervik B, Awasthi YC, Board PG, Hayes JD, Di Ilio C, Ketterer B, Listowsky I, Morgenstern R, Muramatsu M, Pearson WR, Pickett CB, Sato K, Widersten M, Wolf CR (1992) Nomenclature for human glutathione transferases. Biochem J 282:305–308

Maurice M, Emiliani S, Dalet-Beluche I, Derancourt J, Lange R (1991) Isolation and characterization of a cytochrome P450 of the IIA subfamily from human liver microsomes. Eur J Biochem 200:511–517

Mayer RT, Netter KJ, Heubel F, Hahnemann B, Buchheister A, Klitschka Mayer G, Burke MD (1990) 7-Alkoxyquinolines: new fluorescent substrates for cytochrome P450 monooxygenases. Biochem Pharmacol 40:1645–1655

Mawer GE, Miller NE, Turnberg LA (1972) Metabolism of amylobarbitone in patients with chronic liver disease. Br J Pharmacol 44:549–560

Meyer UA, Skoda RC, Zanger UM (1990) The genetic polymorphism of debrisoquine/sparteine metabolism – molecular mechanisms. Pharmacol Ther 46:297–308

Miles JS, Wolf CR (1991) Developments and perspectives on the role of cytochrome P450s in chemical carcinogenesis. Carcinogenesis 12:2195–2195

Miles JS, Spurr NK, Gough AC, Jowett T, McLaren AW, Brook JD, Wolf CR (1988) A novel human cytochrome P450 gene (P450IIB): chromosomal localization and evidence for alternative splicing. Nucleic Acids Res 16:5783–5795

Miles JS, McLaren AW, Forrester LM, Glancey MJ, Lang MA, Wolf CR (1990) Identification of the human liver cytochrome P-450 responsible for coumarin 7-hydroxylase activity. Biochem J 267:365–371

Miller M, Opheim KE, Raisys VA, Motulsky AG (1984) Theophylline metabolism: variation and genetics. Clin Pharmacol Ther 35:170–182

Miotti T, Bircher J, Preisig R (1988) The 30-minute aminopyrine breath test: optimization of sampling times after intravenous administration of ^{14}C-aminopyrine. Digestion 39:241–250

Morel F, Beaune PH, Ratanasavanh D, Flinois J-P, Yang CS, Guengerich FP, Guillouzo A (1990) Expression of cytochrome P-450 enzymes in cultured human hepatocytes. Eur J Biochem 191:437–444

Mulder GJ (ed) (1990) Conjugation reactions in drug metabolism: an integrated approach. Taylor and Francis, London

Murray BP, Lennox SV, Murray S, Boobis AR (1992) Potent in vitro inhibition of human CYP1A2 by pharmacologically diverse agents. Br J Clin Pharmacol 33:233P–234P (abstr)

Murray M, Reidy GF (1990) Selectivity in the inhibition of mammalian cytochromes P-450 by chemical agents. Pharmacol Rev 42:85–101

Nebert DW (1989) The Ah locus: genetic differences in toxicity, cancer, mutation, and birth defects. Crit Rev Toxicol 20:153–174

Nebert DW, Gonzalez FJ (1987) P450 genes: structure, evolution, and regulation. Annu Rev Biochem 56:945–993

Nebert DW, Nelson DR, Adesnik M, Coon MR, Estabrook RW, Gonzales FJ, Guengerich FP, Gunsalus IC, Johnson EF, Kemper B, Levin W, Phillips IR, Sato R, Waterman MR (1989) The P450 superfamily: updated listing of all genes and recommended nomenclature for the chromosomal loci. DNA 8: 1–13

Nebert DW, Nelson DR, Coon MR, Estabrook RW, Feyereisen R, Fujii-Kuriyama Y, Gonzalez FJ, Guengerich FP, Gunsalus IC, Johnson EF, Loper JC, Sato R, Waterman MR, Waxman DJ (1991) The P450 superfamily: update on new sequences, gene mapping and recommended nomenclature. DNA Cell Biol 10:1–14

Nelson DR, Kamataki T, Waxman DJ, Guengerich FP, Estabrook RW, Feyereisen R, Gonzalez FJ, Coon MJ, Gunsalus IC, Gotoh O, Okuda K, Nebert DW (1993) The P450 superfamily: update on new sequences, gene mapping, accession numbers, early trivial names of enzymes, and nomenclature. DNA Cell Biol 12:1–51

Oellerich M, Raude E, Burdelski M, Schulz M, Schmidt FW, Ringe B, Lamesch P, Pichlmayr R, Raith H, Scheruhn M, Wrenger M, Wittekind CH (1987) Monoethylglycinexylidide formation kinetics: a novel approach to assessment of liver function. J Clin Chem Clin Biochem 25:845–853

Oellerich M, Burdelski M, Ringe B, Lamesch P, Gubernatis G, Bunzendahl H, Pichlmayr R, Herrmann H (1989) Lignocaine metabolite formation as a measure of pre-transplant liver function. Lancet i:640–642

Oellerich M, Burdelski M, Lautz H-U, Schulz M, Schmidt F-W, Herrmann H (1990) Lidocaine metabolite formation as a measure of liver function in patients with cirrhosis. Ther Drug Monitor 12:219–226

Ogilvie RI (1978) Clinical pharmacokinetics of theophylline. Clin Pharmacokinet 3:267–293

Ohnhaus EE, Breckenridge AM, Park BK (1989) Urinary excretion of 6β-hydroxycortisol and the time course measurement of enzyme induction in man. Eur J Clin Pharmacol 36:39–46

Okey AB (1990) Enzyme induction in the cytochrome P-450 system. Pharmacol Ther 45:241–298

Ortiz de Montellano PR (ed) (1986) Cytochrome P-450: structure, mechanism and biochemistry. Plenum, New York

Page MA, Boutagy JS, Shenfield GM (1991) A screening test for slow metabolisers of tolbutamide. Br J Clin Pharmacol 31:649–654

Park BK (1982) Assessment of the drug metabolism capacity of the liver. Br J Clin Pharmacol 14:631–651

Park BK (1985) Assessment of drug metabolising enzyme activity in man. Biochem Pharmacol Suppl 1:11–18

Pasanen M, Pelkonen O (1989/90) Human placental xenobiotic and steroid biotransformations catalyzed by cytochrome P450, epoxide hydrolase, and glutathione S-transferase activities and their relationships to maternal cigarette smoking. Drug Metab Rev 21:427–461

Pasanen M, Haaparanta T, Sundin M, Sivonen P, Vähäkangas K, Raunio H, Hines R, Gustafsson J-Å, Pelkonen O (1990) Immunochemical and molecular biological studies on human placental cigarette smoke-inducible cytochrome P-450-dependent monooxygenase activities. Toxicology 62:175–187

Pelkonen O, Nebert DW (1982) Metabolism of polycyclic aromatic hydrocarbons: etiologic role in carcinogenesis. Pharmacol Rev 34:189–222

Pelkonen O, Sotaniemi EA (1982) Drug metabolism in alcoholics. Pharmacol Ther 16:261–268

Pelkonen O, Sotaniemi EA (1987) Environmental factors of enzyme induction and inhibition. Pharmacol Ther 33:115–120

Pelkonen O, Puurunen J, Arvela P, Lammintausta R (1991) Comparative effects of medetomidine enantiomers on in vitro and in vivo microsomal drug metabolism. Pharmacol Toxicol 69:189–194

Pelkonen O, Raunio H, Rautio A, Mäenpää J, Lang MA (1993) Coumarin 7-hydroxylase: characteristics and regulation in mouse and man. J Irish Coll Physicians Surg 22 [Suppl 1]:24–28

Pellinen P, Stenbäck F, Rautio A, Pelkonen O, Lang M, Pasanen M (1993) Response of mouse liver coumarin 7-hydroxylase activity to hepatotoxicants: dependence on strain and agent and comparison to other monooxygenases. Naunyn-Schmiedebergs Arch Pharmacol 348:435–443

Penno MB, Vesell ES (1983) Monogenic control of variations in antipyrine metabolite formation. New polymorphism of hepatic drug oxidation. J Clin Invest 71: 1698–1709

Perrot N, Nalpas B, Yang CS, Beaune PH (1989) Modulation of cytochrome P450 isoforms in human liver, by ethanol and drug intake. Eur J Clin Invest 19: 549–555

Peter R, Bocker R, Beaune PH, Iwasaki H, Guengerich FP, Yang CS (1990) Hydroxylation of chlorzoxazone as a specific probe for human liver cytochrome P-450IIE1. Chem Res Toxicol 3:566–573

Phillips IR, Shephard EA, Ashworth A, Rabin BR (1985) Isolation and sequence of a human cytochrome P-450 clone. Proc Natl Acad Sci USA 82:983–987

Plaa GL, du Souich P, Erill S (eds) (1987) Interactions between drugs and chemicals in industrial societies. Esteve Foundation Symposia, vol 2. Excerpta Med Int Congr Series 734:274

Poland A, Mak I, Glover E (1981) Species differences in the action of 1,4-bis[2-(3,5-dichloropyridyloxy)]benzene, a potent phenobarbital-like inducer of microsomal monooxygenase activity. Mol Pharmacol 20:442–450

Poulsen HE, Loft S (1988) Antipyrine as a model drug to study hepatic drug metabolizing capacity. J Hepatol 6:374–382

Puurunen J, Sotaniemi EA, Pelkonen O (1980) Effect of cimetidine on microsomal drug metabolism in man. Eur J Clin Pharmacol 18:185–187

Raunio H, Kojo A, Juvonen R, Honkakoski P, Järvinen P, Lang MA, Vähäkangas K, Gelboin HV, Park SS, Pelkonen O (1988) Mouse hepatic cytochrome P-450 isozyme induction by 1,4-bis 2-(3,5-dichloropyridyloxy) benzene, pyrazole, and phenobarbital. Biochem, Pharmacol 37:4141–4147

Rautio A, Kraul H, Kojo A, Salmela E, Pelkonen O (1992) Interindividual variability of coumarin hydroxylation in healthy volunteers. Pharmacogenetics 2:227–233

Relling MV, Aoyama T, Gonzalez FJ, Meyer UA (1990) Tolbutamide and mephenytoin hydroxylation by human cytochrome P450s in the CYP2C subfamily. J Pharmacol Exp Ther 252:442–447

Renton KW, Knickle LC (1990) Regulation of hepatic cytochrome P-450 during infectious disease. Can J Physiol Pharmacol 68:777–781

Rettie AE, Eddy AC, Heimark LD, Gibaldi M, Trager WF (1989) Characteristics of warfarin hydroxylation catalyzed by human liver microsomes. Drug Metab Dispos 17:265–270

Rettie AE, Korzekwa KR, Kunze KL, Lawrence RF, Eddy AC, Aoyama T, Gelboin HV, Gonzalez FJ, Tragger WF (1992) Hydroxylation of warfarin by human cDNA-expressed cytochrome P-450: a rolefor P-4502C9 in the etiology of S-warfarin drug interactions. Chem Res Toxicol 5:54–59

Robson RA, Matthews AP, Miners JO, McManus ME, Meyer UA, Hall P de la M, Birkett DJ (1987) Characterization of theophylline metabolism in human liver microsomes: inhibition and immunochemical studies. Br J Clin Pharmacol 24:293–300

Robson RA, Miners JO, Matthews AP, Stupans I, Meller D, McManus ME, Birkett DJ (1988) Characterization of theophylline metabolism by human liver microsomes: inhibition and immunochemical studies. Biochem Pharmacol 37:1651–1659

Romkes M, Faletto MB, Blaisdell JA, Raucy JL, Goldstein JA (1991) Cloning and expression of complementary DNAs for multiple members of the human cytochrome P450IIC subfamily. Biochemistry 30:3247–3255

Roth RA, Wiersma DA (1979) Role of the lung in total body clearance of circulating drugs. Clin Pharmacokinet 4:355–367

Rubin E, Lieber CS (1968) Hepatic microsomal enzymes in man and rat: induction and inhibition by ethanol. Science 162:690–691

Sakai H, Kobayashi S, Hamada K, Iida S, Akita H, Tanaka E, Uchida E, Yasuhara H (1991) The effects of diltiazem on hepatic drug metabolizing enzymes in man using antipyrine, trimethadione and debrisoquine as model substrates. Br J Clin Pharmacol 31:353–355

Sarkar MA, Hunt C, Guzelian PS, Karnes HT (1992) Characterization of human liver cytochromes P-450 involved in theophylline metabolism. Drug Metab Dispos 20:31–37

Schellens JHM, Breimer DD (1987) Antipyrine and metabolite formation: influence of induction and application as a tool in cytochrome P-450 characterization. In: Sotaniemi EA, Pelkonen RO (eds) Enzyme induction in man. Taylor and Francis, London, pp 109–123

Schellens JHM, van der Wart JHF, Brugman M, Breimer DD (1987) Influence of enzyme induction and inhibition on the oxidation of nifedipine, sparteine, mephenytoin and antipyrine in humans as assessed by a "cocktail" study design. J Pharmacol Exp Ther 249:638–645

Schellens JHM, Edelbroek PM, Hilhorst M, van der Wart JHF, de Wolff FA, Breimer DD (1988a) Relationship between the oxidation of antipyrine, nortriptyline, sparteine and nifedipine in man. Bar J Clin Pharmacol 16:373–384

Schellens JHM, Soons PA, Breimer DD (1988b) Lack of bimodality in nifedipine plasma kinetics in a large population of healthy subjects. Biochem Pharmacol 37:2507–2510

Schellens JHM, van der Wart JHF, Danhof M, van der Velde EA, Breimer DD (1988c) Relationship between the metabolism of antipyrine, hexobarbital and theophylline in man as assessed by a "cocktail" approach. Br J Clin Pharmacol 26:373–384

Schellens JHM, Ghabrial H, van der Wart HHF, Bakker EN, Wilkinson GR, Breimer DD (1991) Differential effects of quinidine on the disposition of nifedipine, sparteine and mepheyntoin in humans. Clin Pharmacol Ther 50:520–528

Schoeller DA, Kotake AL, Lambert GL, Krager PS, Baker AL (1985) Comparison of the phenacetin and aminopyrine breath tests: effect of liver disease, inducers and cobaltous chloride. Hepathology 5:276–281

Scott J, Poffenberger PL (1979) Pharmacogenetics of tolbutamide metabolism in humans. Diabetes 28:41–51

Sesardic D, Pasanen M, Pelkonen O, Boobis AR (1990) Differential expression and regulation of members of the cytochrome P450IA gene subfamily in human tissues. Carcinogenesis 11:1183–1188

Shimada T, Iwasaki M, Martin MV, Guengerich FP (1989) Human liver microsomal cytochrome P450 enzymes involved in the bioactivation of procarcinogens detected by *umu* gene response in *Salmonella typhimurium* TA1535/pSK1002. Cancer Res 49:3218–3228

Shimizu M, Lasker JM, Tsutsumi M, Lieber CS (1990) Immunohistochemical localization of ethanol-inducible P450IIE1 in the rat alimentary tract. Gastroenterology 99:1044–1053

Sitar DS (1989) Human drug metabolism in vivo. Pharmacol Ther 43:363–375

Smith DA (1987) Species variations in pharmacokinetics. In: Benford DJ, Bridges JW, Gibson GG (eds) Drug metabolism – from molecules to man. Taylor and Francis, London, pp 330–351

Smith DA (1991) Species differences in metabolism and pharmacokinetics: are we close to an understanding? Drug Metab Rev 23:355–373

Song BJ, Gelboin HV, Park SS, Yang CS, Gonzalez FJ (1986) Complementary DNA and protein sequences of ethanol-inducible rat and human cytochrome P450s. J Biol Chem 261:16689–16697

Soons PA, Vogels BAPM, Roosemalen MCM, Schoemaker HC, Uchida E, Edgar B, Lundahl J, Cohen AF, Breimer DD (1991) Grapefruit juice and cimetidine inhibit stereoselective metabolism of nitrendipine in humans. Clin Pharmacol Ther 50:394–403

Soons PA, Schellens JHM, Breimer DD (1992) Variability in pharmacokinetics and metabolism of nifedipine and other dihydropyridine calcium entry blockers. In: Kalow W (ed) Pharmacogenetics of drug metabolism. Pergamon, New York, pp 769–789

Sotaniemi EA, Huhti E (1974) Half life of intravenous tolbutamide in the serum of patients in medicale wards. Ann Clin Res 6:146–154

Sotaniemi EA, Pelkonen O (eds) (1987) Enzyme induction in man. Taylor and Francis, London

Sotaniemi E, Arvela P, Huhti E (1971) Increased clearance of tolbutamide from the blood of asthmatic patients. Ann Allergy 29:139–141

Soucek P, Gut I (1992) Cytochromes P-450 in rats – structures, functions, properties and relevant human forms. Xenobiotica 22:83–104

Sutcliff FA, MacNicoll AD, Gibson GG (1987) Aspects of anticoagulant action: a review of the pharmacology, metabolism and toxicology of warfarin and congeners. Drug Metabol Drug Interact 5:225–272

Tanaka E, Kabayashi S, Nakamura K, Uchida F, Yasuhara H (1989) Simplified approach for determination of hepatic drug-oxidizing capacity using trimethadione metabolism as an indicator. Biopharm Drug Dispos 10:617–620

Tarrus E, Cami J, Roberts DJ, Spickett RGW, Celdran E, Segura J (1987) Accumulation of caffeine in healthy volunteers treated with furafylline. Br J Clin Pharmacol 23:9–18

Terelius Y, Lindros KO, Albano E, Ingelman-Sundberg M (1992) Isozyme-specificity of cytochrome P450-mediated hepatotoxicity. In: Ruckpaul K (ed) Frontiers in biotransformation, vol 9. Akademic, Berlin, pp 187–232

Testa B, Jenner P (1981) Inhibitors of cytochrome P-450s and their mechanism of action. Drug Metab Res 12:1–118

Teunissen MWE, de Leede LGJ, Boeijinga JK, Breimer DD (1985) Correlatioon between antipyrine metabolite formation and theophylline metabolism in man after simultaneous single dose administration and at steady-state. J Pharmacol Exp Ther 223:770–775

Tsutsumi R, Leo AM, Kim C, Tsutsumi M, Lasker J, Lowe N, Lieber CS (1990) Alcoholism. Clin Exp Res 14:174–179

Tukey RH, Johnson EF (1990) Molecular aspects of regulation and structure of the drug-metabolizing enzymes. In: Pratt WB, Taylor P (eds) Principles of drug action. The basis of pharmacology, 3rd edn. Churchill Livingstone, Edinburgh, pp 423–467

Upton RA, Thiercelin J-F, Guentert TW, Wallace SM, Powell JR, Sansom L, Riegelman S (1982) Intraindividual variability in theophylline pharmacokinetics: statistical verification in 39 of 60 healthy young adults. J Pharmacokinet Biochem 10:123–134 van der Graaff M, Vermeulen NPE, Breimer DD (1988) Disposition of hexobarbital. Fifteen years of an intriguing model substrate. Drug Metab Rev 19:109–164

Veronese ME, Mackenzie PI, Doecke CJ, McManus ME, Miners JO, Birkett DJ (1991) Tolbutamide and phenytoin hydroxylations by cDNA-expressed human liver cytochrome P4502C9. Biochem Biophys Res Commun 175:1112–1118

Vesell ES (1979) The antipyrine test in clinical pharmacology: conceptions and misconceptions. Clin Pharmacol Ther 26:275–286

Vesell ES (1982) On the significance of host factors that affect drug disposition. Clin Pharmacol Ther 31:1–7

Vesell ES (1991) The model drug approach in clinical pharmacology. Clin Pharmacol Ther 50:239–248

Vesell ES, Penno MB (1983) Assessment of methods to identify sources of inter-individual pharmacokinetic variations. Clin Pharmacokinet 8:378–409

Wang PP, Beaune P, Kaminsky LS, Dannan GA, Kadlubar FF, Larrey D, Guengerich FP (1983) Purification and characterization of six cytochrome P-450 isozymes from human liver microsomes. Biochemistry 22:5375–5383

Watkins PB (1990) Role of cytochromes P450 in drug metabolism and hepatotoxicity. Semin Liver Dis 10:235–250

Watkins PB, Murray SA, Winkelman LG, Heuman DM, Wrighton SA, Guzelian PS (1989) Erythromycin breath test as an assay of glucocorticoid-inducible liver cytochromes P-450. J Clin Invest 83:688–697

Waxman DJ (1988) Interactions of hepatic cytochromes P-450 with steroid hormones, regioselectivity and stereospecificity of steroid metabolism and hormonal regulation of rat P-450 enzyme expression. Biochem Pharmacol 37:71–84

Waxman DJ, Azaroff L (1992) Phenobarbital induction of cytochrome P-450 gene expression. Biochem J 281:577–592

Waxman DJ, Ko A, Walsh C (1983) Regioselectivity and stereoselectivity of androgen hydroxylations catalyzed by cytochrome P-450 isozymes purified from phenobarbital-induced rat liver. J Biol Chem 258:11937–11947

Waxman DJ, Lapenson DP, Aoyama T, Gelboin HV, Gonzalez FJ, Korzekwa K (1991) Steroid hormone hydroxylase specificities of eleven cDNA-expressed human cytochrome P450s. Arch Biochem Biophys 290:160–166

Wietholtz H, Vogelin M, Arnaud MJ, Bircher J, Preisig R (1981) Assessment of the cytochrome P-448 dependent liver enzyme system by a caffeine breath test. Eur J Clin Pharmacol 21:53–59

Wietholtz H, Zysset T, Kreiten K, Kohl D, Buchsel R, Matern S (1989) Effect of phenytoin, carbamazepine, and valproic acid on caffeine metabolism. Eur J Clin Pharmacol 36:401–406

Wilkinson GR (1987) Clearance approaches in pharmacology. Pharmacol Rev 39:1–47

Wilkinson GR, Guengerich FP, Branch RA (1989) Genetic polymorphism of S-mephenytoin hydroxylation. Pharmacol Ther 43:53–76

Wolf CR, Miles JS, Gough A, Spurr NK (1990) Molecular genetics of the human cytochrome P-450 system. Biochem Soc Trans 18:21–24

Wong G, Kawajiri K, Negishi M (1987) Gene family of male-specific testosterone 16Á-hydroxylase (C-P-45016Á) in mouse liver: cDNA sequences, neonatal imprinting, and reversible regulation by androgen. Biochemistry 26:8683–8690

Wrighton SA, Stevens JC (1992) The human hepatic cytohromes P450 involved in drug metabolism. Crit Rev Toxicol 22:1–21

Wrighton SA, Thomas PE, Molowa DT, Haniu M, Shively JE, Maines SL, Watkins PB, Parker G, Mendez-Picon G, Levin W, Guzelian PS (1986) Characterization of ethanol-inducible human liver N-nitrosodimethylamine demethylase. Biochemistry 25:6731–6735

Yamano S, Nhamburo PT, Aoyama T, Meyer UA, Inaba T, Kalow W, Gelboin HV, McBride OW, Gonzalez FJ (1989) cDNA cloning and sequence and cDNA-directed expression of human P450 IIB1: identification of a normal and two variant cDNAs derived from the CYP2B locus on chromosome 19 and differential expression of the IIB mRNAs in human liver. Biochemistry 28:7340–7348

Yamano S, Tatsuno J, Gonzales FJ (1990) The CYP2A3 gene product catalyzes coumarin 7-hydroxylation in human liver microssomes. Biochemistry 29:1322–1329

Yang CS, Yoo J-S, Ishizaki H & Hong J (1990) Cytochrome P450IIE1: roles in nitrosamine metabolism and mechanisms of regulation. Drug Metab Rev 22:147–159

Yun C-H, Shimada T, Guengerich FP (1991) Purification and characterization of human liver microsomal cytochrome P-450 2A6. Mol Pharmacol 40:679–685

Zhou HH, Anthony LB, Wood AJJ, Wilkinson GR (1990) Induction of polymorphic 4-hydroxylation of S-mephenytoin by rifampicin. Br J Clin Pharmacol 30:471–475

Zilly W, Breimer DD, Richter E (1975) Induction of drug metabolism in man after rifampicin treatment measured by increased hexobarbital and tolbutamide clearance. Eur J Clin Pharmacol 9:219–227

CHAPTER 11

Time Course of Drug Effect*

N.H.G. Holford and T.M. Ludden

A. Introduction

It has been recognized for many years (Sokolow and Edgar 1950; Swisher et al. 1954) that drug effect may on occasion be directly associated with the time course of drug or drug metabolites in the circulation. Subsequently it was also noted that the relationship between drug concentration and response could be quite complex such that the temporal relationship might be difficult to discern on first examination, e.g., warfarin (Nagashima et al. 1969). Wagner (1975) has provided a review of early work on this topic. Sheiner et al. (1979a) illustrated the usefulness of an effect compartment for linking the time course of d-tubocurarine effect to the time course of plasma concentrations. In this way the delay in onset of effect relative to concentration could be explained. Methods for describing the kinetic behavior of drug effects were further systematized by Holford and Sheiner (1981). This chapter will discuss the motivations for characterizing the time course of drug effect, outline some methodological concerns, and present the various mathematical approaches for modeling active drug and placebo effects.

In order to minimize confusion we use a specific terminology which helps to focus on the level of interaction of a drug with a living organism (Holford and Peck 1992). A drug *action* is expressed at a primary site, e.g., a receptor, which produces a response such as contraction of a muscle or inhibition of an enzyme. In an intact animal this action may be observable as a change in physiological function which is the drug *effect*, e.g., increased cardiac output or decreased anticoagulant activity. Finally, the effect (sometimes known as a *surrogate* effect) may be used to produce a therapeutic *response*, e.g., decreased mortality from heart failure or thromboembolic disease. When the context may refer to more than one level of interaction we use *effect* to encompass these phenomena.

---

* The views expressed in this paper are those of the authors and not necessarily those of the Food and Drug Administration.

I. Why Prediction of Effect Over Time Is Important

1. Drug Development

a) Preclinical

The quantitative description of the dose–concentration–effect–time relationship during preclinical drug development offers many advantages. The mathematical modeling activity stimulates the integration of both pharmacokinetic and pharmacodynamic behavior on a whole animal scale. Model failure often highlights areas of poor understanding or misapplied assumptions. Just as is true with chemical kinetics and the study of reaction mechanisms, pharmacokinetic–pharmacodynamic (PK/PD) models can lend substantial support to hypotheses of pharmacological mechanisms of action in complex biological systems. For example, Unadkat et al. (1986) developed an integrated model for the interaction of nondepolarizing neuromuscular blocking drugs and their antagonists based on canine data. Verotta et al. (1991) recently generalized the model to accommodate possible irreversible blockade and noninstantaneous reversal kinetics and illustrated its ability to describe the time courses of edrophonium and neostigmine in humans. Thus, PK/PD models can facilitate the cross-species comparisons of pharmacological activity.

Pharmacokinetic/pharmacodynamic modeling of several members of a pharmacological class throughout the sequence of drug development processes may yield valuable information about the predictive relationship of specific animal models to the quantitative behavior of the compounds in man. Knowledge that a specific test for pharmacological activity gives rise to exposure values predictive of, but not necessarily the same as, values in humans can facilitate initial dose-ranging studies (Collins et al. 1990).

b) Clinical

Early elucidation of the time course of drug effect and how it is influenced by formulation, environmental, and patient factors is essential for the efficient design of clinical studies and the eventual informed use in therapy. Collection of relevant dose–concentration–effect–time data during the earliest studies in humans, including dose titration tolerance studies in healthy volunteers, can often be accomplished. Subsequent focused, intensive studies in appropriate patient groups using dose titration or cross-over studies can often provide valuable information about individual dose–concentration–effect relationships (Sheiner 1989). For acute effects such as are seen with neuromuscular blockers and general anesthetics, the time course must be considered in order to obtain stable estimates of pharmacodynamic parameters. Estimates of inter- and intrapatient variability may also be acquired at this time and this knowledge of the sources of variability can be used to guide the choice of subsequent clinical trial designs (SANATHANAN and PECK 1991). A moderate to high level of intrasubject pharmacokinetic variability may underscore the importance of controlling for this variability in order to conduct an efficient study. A high degree of intersubject variability in pharmacodynamics would suggest that a stepwise individualization of dose might be required during eventual routine clinical use. A dose titration trial might then be undertaken to determine the most efficient escalation scheme. High, uncontrollable intrasubject variability in effect might suggest that the drug should not undergo further development. Even drugs that are know to develop their effects over weeks or months should have their time course of effect characterized so that clinical use can be continued long enough for there to be a legitimate opportunity for the drug to be effective but not so long as to deprive the patient of alternative, possibly beneficial, therapy.

Pharmacodynamic modeling can provide important clues about the complexities of drug effect that only emerge over time such as sensitization, tolerance (PORCHET et al. 1988), or the contributions of active metabolites (VOZEH et al. 1987). Early recognition of these characteristics can prevent irrational study designs that lead to inadequate demonstration of efficacy or excessive, unnecessary toxicity. More detailed discussions of the relevance of PK/PD modeling in drug development have been published recently (PECK et al. 1992; COLBURN and BLUE 1992).

2. Dosage Individualization

The total preclinical and clinical experience obtained during drug development should give rise to a reasonable understanding of the dose–concentration–effect–time relationship such that guidelines for individualization of dosage regimens can be based on patient characteristics, disease intensity, and other risk factors (SHEINER 1991). The power of PK/PD modeling to identify why important subpopulations of patients may respond differently has been illustrated for thiopental (STANSKI and MAITRE 1990), fentanyl, and alfentanil (SCOTT and STANSKI 1987). The elderly require lower doses of thiopental because of slower distribution of drug out of the central compartment while the need for lower doses of fentanyl and alfentanil is related to an increased pharmacodynamic sensitivity.

For a few drugs it may be found that "one dose fits all," but more likely some level of individualization will be required. Sometimes individualization can be accomplished by a priori adjustment of dose based on observed characteristics. In other cases, dose titration to a desired level of benefit may be needed. Finally, for a few drugs with relatively narrow therapeutic ranges and unpredictable individual responses, careful feedback-facilitated dosage adjustment, i.e., adaptive control, may be required (SHEINER et al. 1979b). This may involve simultaneous feedback of both pharmacokinetic and pharmacodynamic information as suggested for theophylline (PECK et al.

1985) or feedback of pharmacodynamic data alone, which is sufficient for individualization for warfarin therapy (Svec et al. 1985).

A thorough, quantitative understanding of pharmacokinetics and pharmacodynamics provides for the development of effective materials for communicating to the health care professional the specific characteristics of a therapeutic agent that make its use safer, more effective, and more efficient. This is illustrated by the simulations of the comparative pharmacodynamic profiles of fentanyl and alfentanil performed by Ebling et al. (1990) based on a PK/PD model. Graphical displays show that in spite of similar disposition curves during the initial 90 min after dosing, the hypothetical effect site concentrations are quite different and result in considerable differences in their time courses of effect.

B. Methodological Considerations Relevant to Measuring Effects

I. Standardization

Considerable attention has been directed to the development of quality control and validation procedures for chemical and immunological assays used in support of pharmacokinetic and drug metabolism studies (Shah et al. 1992). Levy (1985) has demonstrated that precision similar to that for many chemical assays can be obtained for pharmacodynamic measures when careful attention is given to the necessary details surrounding the measurement. Many pharmacodynamic measurements require analog signal processing which can be done with great precision once the instrumentation is properly calibrated. However, most procedures such as the EKG and the EEG still require the attention of a competent technician for quality data. In addition, pharmacodynamic measures are often influenced by the patient's recent and sometimes not so recent environmental experiences. For example, blood pressures must be obtained under controlled postural conditions in order to be reproducible and careful control of recent salt and fluid intake is necessary for urinary electrolyte excretion to be a useful indicator of response to a diuretic.

In many cases it is not practical to wait for episodic events in patients. Therefore, drug effects are often assessed by physiological or pharmacological challenge such as exercise-induced tachycardia, arrhythmias induced by electronic pacing, methacholine-induced bronchconstriction, or the isoproterenol test of β-adrenergic blocking drugs. The conditions of the challenge must be well standardized not only within a study but also across studies so that the results are comparable, as they would be for a properly standardized chemical assay.

Kelman et al. (1981) studied the use of incremental doses of atropine to increase heart rate and determined individual regression equations for systolic time intervals as a function of heart rate. Significant regressions between heart rate and both total electromechanical systole and left ventricular ejection time were obtained. There was considerable intersubject variability in the relationships but only modest intrasubject variability over a 3-week period. It was concluded that the individual regression equations were sufficiently stable to permit the detection of the small changes on the order of 5%–10% that were necessary for usefulness of the method.

Measurement of CNS drug effects can be particularly challenging (DINGEMANSE et al. 1988). Psychometric testing is susceptible to numerous variables that are difficult to control such as fatigue and motivation. In addition, there are often questions of clinical relevance. Neurophysiological measures such as the EEG are often use to measure CNS effects (GREEN-BLATT et al. 1989; STANSKI 1992) but the relationship to clinical effect is often uncertain. Studies of analgesic effects in humans are complicated by the subjective nature of pain and, in particular, extrapolations from animals to humans are often poor. For the evaluation of clinical pain, visual analog scales have been used with some success (INTURRISI et al. 1987).

Pharmacodynamic studies in cancer therapy have been focused more on relationships for toxicity than for remission and often the time course is not characterized, for example, correlation of white cell count nadir with exposure (area under the concentration–time curve). The difficulties associated with pharmacodynamic measurements in cancer therapy are often associated with the complexities of the mechanisms of action and the long periods required for clinical assessment (RATAIN et al. 1990).

ABERNETHY (1988) has discussed many of the common problems confronting pharmacodynamic studies, including the need to design pharmacokinetic sampling protocols such that the effect to be measured is not influenced. For example, it may be difficult to obtain blood samples during sleep laboratory studies without disturbing the observed polysomnographic effects.

II. Continuous Scale Versus Discrete Response

In a few situations it may be desirable to describe the time course of a discrete (bi- or multinomial or ordinal) response. Standard logistic regression has usually been used with steady-state data of this type as illustrated by the analysis of tricyclic antidepressant response as a function of plasma concentration reported by PERRY et al. (1987). This approach may also be useful in the non-steady-state situation using time and possibly concentration as the covariate(s). However, it may be more desirable to model the probability of outcome through a more traditional pharmacodynamic model such as the E_{max} model (see Sect. C.III). In this case, specialized software such as the NONMEM system (BEAL and SHEINER 1991) which has a user-definable objective function is needed to model the response as a nonlinear function of the covariates.

III. Baseline and Placebo Effect

Modeling of an unstable baseline such as occurs with many hormonal patterns may be required to obtain time-independent (stationary) estimates of pharmacodynamic parameters (Francheteau et al. 1991). Changes in underlying disease state can also contribute substantially to the difficulties in assessing drug effect. Often these problems can be addressed through the analysis of data from properly designed placebo studies (see Sect. C.V). However, when there are homeostatic changes that depend on the drug itself and are not evident with the placebo it may be necessary to understand and model these physiological complexities in order to describe accurately the interaction of the drug with the biological system (Fisher et al. 1992).

C. Pharmacokinetic–Pharmacodynamic Models

This section describes individual models that may be used to describe and explain the time course of drug action. Details of techniques for implementing pharmacodynamic models, model evaluation, and parameter estimation can be found elsewhere (Van Boxtel et al. 1992; Seber and Wild 1989; Bates and Watts 1988).

I. Pharmacokinetics

The relation between dose and drug concentration is the domain of pharmacokinetics. Most of the complexity of pharmacokinetics is concerned with the time course of the parent drug and metabolites in the body. Pharmacokinetic models are a necessary part of any description of the time course of drug action. They can be used to account for the input of drug into the body and the process of distribution to the site of action and subsequent elimination. Specific models are developed in detail in standard references such as Rowland and Tozer (1989), Gibaldi and Perrier (1982), and Wagner (1975). Much of the complexity of describing the time course of drug action can be embodied in these processes of pharmacokinetics.

II. Kinetics of Receptor Binding

The interaction of a drug molecule with its receptor may be formulated in terms of classical receptor theories (see Kenakin 1987, 1992 for reviews). Models relating binding to receptor activation are frequently nonlinear so that drug action is not directly proportional to receptor occupancy. This has been described as the phenomenon of *receptor reserve* but is probably more usefully interpreted as the consequence of a chain of processes from binding to eventual action with a limiting link beyond the initial binding step. In most cases drug actions can be described by assuming the equilibrium predictions because the time course of association and dissociation from a receptor is completed in a matter of seconds and can be ignored when describing in vivo phenomena which are studied over hours to years. However, the time course of binding may be the rate-determining factor for the expression of a drug effect. This will usually manifest itself as a delay in the onset and recovery of the effect in relation to the predictions of a steady-state pharmacodynamic model based on the time course of concentrations predicted from a pharmacokinetic model (see Sect. C.IV).

III. Steady-State Pharmacodynamic Models

The equilibrium relationship between concentration at the site of action, C_e, and effect, E, predicted by classical receptor theory, is known as the E_{max} model (HOLFORD and SHEINER 1981):

$$E(C_e) = E_0 + \frac{E_{max} \cdot C_e}{C_e + EC50}. \tag{1}$$

E_{max} is the maximum effect achievable by the drug, EC50 is the drug concentration producing 50% of E_{max}, and E_0 is the baseline effect without drug.

When drug concentration is much less than EC50, the E_{max} model reduces to a simpler linear model:

$$E(C_e) = E_0 + \beta \cdot C_e, \tag{2}$$

where β is the slope of the concentration–effect relationship.

The shape of the concentration–effect curve may not be a simple hyperbola but may be steeper or shallower than predicted by the E_{max} model. HILL (1910) proposed an empirical extension to the E_{max} model which is known as the sigmoid E_{max} model:

$$E(C_e) = E_0 + \frac{E_{max} \cdot C_e^N}{C_e^N + EC50^N}. \tag{3}$$

The steepness of the curve is modified by the Hill coefficient, N. When N is 1 (equivalent to the E_{max} model) a 16-fold change in concentration is required to go from 20% to 80% of E_{max} while only a fourfold change is required when N is 2. The use of this non-integer computational kludge often has no mechanistic interpretation but sometimes can be linked to allosteric cooperative phenomena. When the Hill coefficient is greater than 5, a small change in concentration may produce almost full effect from no detectable effect. This may be explained by the observed effect being dependent on a switch-like physiological mechanism, e.g., a reentry circuit as an arrhythmogenic focus which is blocked outside a critical conduction velocity range (HOLFORD 1992a). Agonist drug actions commonly have Hill coefficients greater than 1 while antagonist drug actions can usually be described with an inhibitory E_{max} model with a Hill coefficient of 1 (in cases where the agonist effect cannot be explicitly described).

More complex models of the steady-state effects of drugs and especially their interaction are beyond the scope of this chapter. Details can be found in recent monographs (Kenakin 1987; van Boxtel et al. 1992).

IV. Non-Steady-State Pharmacodynamic Models

When drug concentration is plotted against effect and the points joined in time sequence, the effects may not be the same at each concentration. The resulting loop exposes a time-related change in the apparent concentration–effect relationship. If the effect at later times is more pronounced at the same concentration then the loop reflects *hysteresis*, while if the effect is diminished the loop exhibits *proteresis* (Girard and Boissel 1989; Campbell 1990). An earlier terminology which equated an anticlockwise progression of the loop with hysteresis can be confusing because it assumes that increasing effects are plotted in the up direction, which may not be the case for an inhibitory effect.

The phenomena of hysteresis and proteresis can be explained by several mechanisms. The most common reflects the failure of the assumption that the concentration is in equilibrium with the site of drug action. If plasma concentration is used to predict effects then a hysteresis loop may arise because it takes time for the drug to distribute from plasma to a receptor biophase, bind to the receptor, and complete the chain of events required to express the observed effect. Conversely, if venous blood is used to measure concentration then proteresis may be observed because the drug is delivered to the site of action via the arterial circulation and the effect may be expressed before arteriovenous transit is completed (Sheiner 1989; Chiou 1991). Hysteresis may also be attributable to the accumulation of active metabolites of the parent drug and proteresis to antagonistic metabolites (see Sect. C.VII).

1. Effect Compartment

A pragmatic model for minimizing the apparent time dependence of the concentration–effect relationship can be obtained by the use of an *effect* compartment model (Segre 1968; Sheiner et al. 1979a). The concentration in this compartment, C_e, can be predicted from the time course of concentration, C_{pk}, predicted by a pharmacokinetic model:

$$\frac{dC_e}{dt} = K_{eq} \cdot (C_{pk} - C_e). \tag{4}$$

The rate constant K_{eq} [also known as K_{eo} (Sheiner et al. 1979a)] is assumed to determine the *exit rate* of drug from the site of drug effect. While this may be a reasonable explanation when the delay in observed effect is due to distribution of drug to the site of action or dissociation from a receptor binding site, a less mechanistic interpretation may be more generally appropriate (HOLFORD 1991). The rate constant K_{eq} can be directly related to an *equilibration half-time*, $T_{eq} = \ln(2)/K_{eq}$, which determines how long it takes for C_{pk} and C_e to reach equilibrium. With this meaning T_{eq} can be viewed as a measure of the rate-limiting step in the expression of the drug effect whether that is due to distribution to a receptor site or the kinetics of a physiological intermediate (see Sect. C.IV.2). One of the simplest integrated forms of Eq. 4 describes C_e following an increase in drug maintenance dose rate, MDR:

$$C_e(t) = \frac{\text{MDR}}{\text{CL}} \cdot [1 - e^{-K_{eq} \cdot t}]. \tag{5}$$

If the half-life of the drug is short in relation to T_{eq} then the average steady-state C_{pk} is simply MDR divided by clearance (CL). The effect will reach 50% of its final steady-state value after one T_{eq}.

Following a single bolus dose the time course of C_e rises to reach a peak and then declines:

$$C_e(t) = \frac{K_{eq} \cdot \text{Dose}}{(K_{eq} - K_{el}) \cdot \text{Vd}} \cdot [e^{-K_{el} \cdot t} - e^{-K_{eq} \cdot t}], \tag{6}$$

where K_{el} is the elimination rate constant (CL/Vd) and Vd is the volume of distribution. The peak C_e is reached at a time, $T_{e,max}$, predicted by:

$$T_{e,max} = \frac{\ln\left(\dfrac{K_{eq}}{K_{el}}\right)}{(K_{eq} - K_{el})}. \tag{7}$$

More extensive tabulations of effect compartment models can be found elsewhere (HOLFORD and SHEINER 1981; COLBURN 1981).

2. Physiological Mediator

Observable drug effects are usually not identical with the drug action. The binding of the drug to a receptor produces a local action at the target cell. Translation of the cellular action into a detectable effect involves a chain of further physiological processes. Each of these processes will have its own kinetics and may dominate the time course of the observed effect. A description of the time course of drug effect must also consider the time course of each physiological mediator.

The action of the drug may be to change synthesis of the mediator or to modify its elimination. If synthesis is altered, the time taken to reach a new steady-state effect will not be affected by the action of the drug. On the other hand, if the drug increases elimination of the mediator it will speed up the drug effect, while if it inhibits elimination it will slow it down.

a) Mediator Synthesis

This kind of physiological mechanism can be described by the following model, which can be solved to predict the concentration of the mediator, C_{PH}:

$$\frac{dC_{PH}}{dt} = R'_{syn,PH}[C_e(t)] - K_{PH} \cdot C_{PH}(t). \tag{8}$$

The rate of synthesis of the physiological mediator, $R'_{syn,PH}$, is a function of drug concentration, $C_e(t)$ (the' indicates the units of the synthesis rate are divided by the mediator's volume of distribution). The elimination of the mediator is described by a first-order rate constant, K_{PH}. Usually $R'_{syn,PH}$ cannot be measured directly but its baseline value when C_e is zero can be derived from Eq. 8:

$$R'_{syn,PH}(0) = K_{PH} \cdot C_{PH}(0). \tag{9}$$

The only parameters needed to predict the mediator concentration are then the baseline concentration of the mediator and its elimination rate constant. The time course of the observed drug effect can then be used to determine these parameters using a pharmacodynamic model describing how C_{PH} produces the drug effect.

The anticoagulant effect of warfarin provides a well-understood example of a drug which changes the synthesis of a physiological mediator (for review see HOLFORD 1986). The drug's action is to inhibit vitamin K epoxidase but the observable effect is a change in the activity of the prothrombin complex of anticoagulant factors in plasma. Inhibition of vitamin K recycling by the epoxidase reduces the synthesis rate of prothrombin complex factors by limiting the availability of vitamin K as a cofactor. The rate-limiting factor for the development of the anticoagulant effect is the time taken for the prothrombin complex to be eliminated from plasma. The half-time of the complex is about 14 h, so even if warfarin concentrations are constant it takes nearly 3 days to reach a new steady-state level of prothrombin activity.

b) Mediator Elimination

If a drug changes elimination of a mediator its action can be expressed using a model similar to Eq. 8:

$$\frac{dC_{PH}}{dt} = R'_{syn,PH} - K_{PH}[C_e(t)] \cdot C_{PH}(t). \tag{10}$$

In this case the rate constant describing elimination of the mediator, K_{PH}, changes as a function of C_e. Under this model it is not possible to define the delay in onset of effect in terms of a fixed parameter such as an equilibration half-time because this will change with drug concentration. However, the predrug baseline value of K_{PH} can be defined:

$$K_{PH}(0) = \frac{R'_{syn,PH}(0)}{C_{PH}(0)}.$$ (11)

$R'_{syn,PH}(0)$ is defined in exactly the same way as in Eq. 9.

JONKERS et al. (1989) used an effect compartment model to describe the delay in changes in potassium concentration produced by terbutaline. While this provided a description of the effects, the explanation of the delay in terms of equilibration of terbutaline with an effect compartment and subsequent immediate action of terbutaline to decrease potassium is not physiologically reasonable. β-Agonists are known to stimulate Na^+-K^+-ATPase-mediated potassium uptake by cells. The delay in changes in potassium concentration would then be determined by the half-life of potassium. The model shown in Eq. 10 has been applied to the data of JONKERS et al. (1989) and shown to describe the changes with an explanation based on enhanced clearance of potassium (HOLFORD et al. 1989).

V. Placebo Effect

The usual approach to the placebo effect is to examine the difference between measurements of effect after placebo and active drug treatment. This is a straightforward method when there are matching placebo and active drug observations. When the observations cannot be matched, e.g., placebo and active drug effects recorded at different times after starting treatment, then some kind of model for the placebo effect must be used.

1. Pharmacokinetics

A parametric approach to describing the placebo effect can be developed by assuming the start of treatment means a dose of a hypothetical placebo substance is given. This placebo substance equilibrates with a placebo effect compartment and is eliminated from the body. The concentration of placebo in its effect compartment can then be predicted using Eq. 6. This model allows the placebo concentration to reach a peak after some delay and then to decline and eventually disappear. The placebo effect compartment concentration can then be used with a pharmacodynamic model for the placebo effect. The pharmacokinetics of the placebo concentration will then be determined by its equilibration half-time, $T_{eq,P}$ [$\ln(2)/K_{eq}$] and elimination half-time, $T_{el,P}$ [$\ln(2)/K_{el}$].

2. Placebo Effect Model

A suitable model for the pharmacodynamics of a placebo must be determined empirically. However, if the active drug effect has a clearly defined maximum and the placebo effect is marked, e.g., analgesia, then an E_{max} model may be considered a priori. On the other hand, if the active drug effect appears to be linearly related to concentration and/or the placebo effect is small then a linear model may be appropriate.

3. Placebo Efficacy

Conventional analyses of the placebo effect assume that the placebo effect obtained from placebo treatment is the same as the placebo effect obtained from the active treatment. This assumption underlies the use of the difference between active and placebo treatment effects as a measure of the nonplacebo component of the active treatent effect. However, it is possible to imagine that the placebo effect associated with active treatment is not the same as placebo treatment. If an active drug has side-effects the patient may be given a clue that the treatment is not a placebo and the placebo component of the observed effect may be modified.

The effectiveness of an active treatment in producing a placebo effect can be compared with the effect from placebo treatment to define the placebo efficacy, ε, of the active treatment. If ε is less than 1 it means that the active treatment produces a smaller placebo effect than placebo treatment while if it is greater than 1 it means the active drug is more effective as a placebo than the placebo treatment itself.

Because the time course of the placebo effect is independent of the time course of the nonplacebo component of the active drug effect, it is possible to dissect out the placebo component from the total active drug effect and estimate the placebo efficacy under the assumption that the time course of the placebo effect is identical in placebo and active treatment groups.

$$E(C_{e_p}) = E_0 + \varepsilon \cdot \beta \cdot C_{e_p} \qquad\qquad (12)$$
$$if\ C_{e_A}\ = 0 \text{ then } \varepsilon = 1$$
$$else\ \varepsilon\ = \varepsilon_A.$$

VI. Disease Time Course and Drug Effects

The third component (after the active drug and placebo treatment effects) that contributes to the observed effect is the time course of the underlying disease.

1. Disease Time Course

a) None

When drug effects are studied over short periods or physiological stability of the measured effect can be assumed, the time course of the underlying disease may be ignored. Alternatively, the model used to describe the placebo effect may be indistinguishable from the progress of the disease. It is then a matter of personal preference how this component of the overall effect is described.

b) Linear Disease Progress

Over longer periods it may be assumed that there is a change in the disease, but its magnitude is small in relation to the effects of treatment and its progress can be approximated by a linear model. The progression of pain associated with cancer might be expected to increase linearly over a period of months associated with a clinical trial of an analgesic.

c) Nonlinear Disease Progress

Many acute illnesses will have a short course and a more complex model will be required. The pain after a surgical operation is expected to be short-lived and will go away after some days without pharmacological intervention. The time course of postoperative pain might reasonably be described by an exponential function.

2. Models of Drug Effect on Disease Progression

The prediction of the time course of disease progression and the way that it is influenced by drugs can be expressed by a direct action of the drug effect on a parameter of the disease progression model or by an autonomous effect of the drug.

a) Direct Action

Assuming a linear model for disease progression, the time course of the disease state, $DIS(t)$, is determined by its baseline value, S_0, and the rate of progression, α:

$$DIS(t) = S_0 + \alpha \cdot t. \tag{13}$$

α) Slope Model

The effect of treatment on the disease may be on the rate of progression, which will be a function of the time course of the drug effect, $E(t)$:

$$\frac{d\,DIS}{dt} = \alpha[E(t)]. \tag{14}$$

When the change in $E(t)$ is small from one observation of the disease state to the next it may be reasonable to approximate the solution of Eq. 14 by piecewise use of Eq. 15, which uses $E(t_{-1})$, the effect at the time of the preceding observation, to predict the effect from time t_{-1} to t:

$$DIS(t) = DIS(t_{-1}) + [E(t_{-1}) + \alpha] \cdot (t - t_{-1}). \tag{15}$$

β) Offset Model

Alternatively the effect of the drug may be to produce a shift of the disease progression curve so that beneficial responses would be reflected in a shift to the right, i.e., the time taken to reach a particular disease state would be delayed. This can be incorporated into a disease progress model by an offset added to or subtracted from the baseline:

$$\text{DIS}(t) = S_0 + E(t) + \alpha \cdot t. \tag{16}$$

The progress of the activity of Alzheimer's disease could be described and the delay in progress of the disease related to the daily dose of tacrine by using a linear model for tacrine's effect as an offset to the disease progress curve (HOLFORD and PEACE 1992a,b).

b) Autonomous

The interaction of disease progress and drug effect can be viewed as two independent processes. For instance, the effect of the drug may be simply subtracted from the current disease state:

$$\text{Response } (t) = \text{DIS}(t) - E(t). \tag{17}$$

But if the disease state must always be greater than the baseline value then it may be more pragmatic to constrain the magnitude of the drug effect by making it proportional to the current disease state:

$$\text{Response } (t) = \text{DIS}(t) \cdot E(t). \tag{18}$$

VII. Tolerance

Tolerance may be defined as a reduced effect of a drug in comparison with an earlier time, when all other factors are the same – especially concentration at the site of action. Recognition of tolerance requires a clear understanding of the factors that influence the time course of a drug effect. A diminished anticonvulsant response to the same dose of carbamazepine is more likely to reflect induction of carbamazepine metabolism and a lower concentration of active drug than the development of a change in responsiveness of the target cells.

The description of tolerance in terms of PK/PD models has largely been empirical because of the lack of identifiable mechanisms that might explain experimental observations.

1. Pharmacokinetics

The gradual development of tolerance suggests that it might be explained, at least in some instances, by the accumulation of an antagonist substance. Two approaches have been developed to account for the time course of an antagonist substance. The first uses the effect compartment model to predict concentrations of an antagonist as if it were a metabolite of the active drug while the second predicts the antagonist time course as if the antagonist were formed in response to a physiological mediator.

a) Effect Compartment

The time course of a tolerance-inducing substance, formed as if it were a metabolite, is predicted by the solution to the effect compartment model differential equation, where C_A is the concentration of active drug and C_{TOL} is the concentration of the tolerance-inducing substance:

$$\frac{dC_{tol}}{dt} = K_{eq_{tol}} \cdot (C_A - C_{tol}). \tag{19}$$

This model has been used by PORCHET et al. (1988) to describe tolerance to the cardiovascular effects of nicotine in humans (see also SHEINER 1989) and by CHENG and PAALZOW (1990) to describe time-dependent adaptation of dopaminergic activity produced by haloperidol in rats. Note, however, that C_A has been predicted from the time course of the parent compound. This is reasonable when tolerance is produced by a metabolite of the parent, but if it is the action of the active drug that induces the tolerance substance it may be more appropriate to use the effect compartment concentration of the active drug.

b) Physiological Mediator

When information about the physiological mechanisms associated with the action of the active drug is available then a more explanatory model can be developed. HOLFORD (1991) has proposed a physiological model for the development of tolerance to the euphoric effects of cocaine in humans. A major action of cocaine is to decrease the clearance of neurotransmitters (such as dopamine) from the synapse by blocking reuptake. This leads to an increase in the synaptic concentration of neurotransmitter which can be used to predict the degree of euphoria. Tolerance to the euphoric effects is modeled by the accumulation of a neurotransmitter release inhibitor whose formation is proportional to the synaptic concentration of neurotransmitter, C_{NT}. The time course of development of tolerance, at any constant C_{NT}, is then controlled by the half-life of the release inhibitor. The concentration of release inhibitor, C_{RI}, can be predicted by using a model similar to Eq. 8:

$$\frac{dC_{RI}}{dt} = R'_{syn,RI}[C_{NT}(t)] - K_{RI} \cdot C_{RT}(t). \tag{20}$$

C_{NT} is determined by neurotransmitter synthesis, $R'_{syn,NT}$, which is changed by C_{RI} and its elimination rate constant, K_{NT}, which is modified by the active drug concentration, C_A:

$$\frac{dC_{NT}}{dt} = R'_{syn,NT}/[C_{RI}(t)] - K_{NT}[C_A(t)] \cdot C_{NT}(t). \tag{21}$$

It is interesting to note that the effect of C_{RI} on neurotransmitter synthesis is independent of the effect of C_A on neurotransmitter elimination. A rapid decrease in C_A can lead to lower C_{NT} than existed before active drug exposure if the half-life of C_{RI} is longer than that of C_A. This is because synthesis of neurotransmitter will recover more slowly than the return of neurotransmitter clearance to the preexposure level. The physiological effect being observed will then be transiently less than before drug exposure and manifest as a withdrawal phenomenon.

2. Pharmacodynamics

a) Tolerance to Active Drug

Using a model for the time course of the concentration of a tolerance-inducing substance, C_{tol}, its influence on the nontolerant pharmacodynamics can be viewed as a direct action on the pharmacodynamics of the active drug or as an autonomous effect.

α) Direct Action

Models for direct action express the influence of C_{tol} as a modifier of the nontolerant parameters of the active drug pharmacodynamic model. For instance, tolerance may be due to an apparent decrease in the maximum (nontolerant) effect of the active drug, $E_{max,A}$:

$$E_{max,A,tol}(C_{tol}) = E_{max,A}\left(1 - \frac{C_{tol}}{C_{tol} + EC50_{tol}}\right). \tag{22}$$

The potency of the tolerance substance is described by $EC50_{tol}$. If the active drug pharmacodynamic model is linear then E_{max} in Eq. 22 can be replaced by β – the slope of the active drug concentration–effect curve.

A second model is similar to competitive antagonism and may be particularly appropriate if tolerance develops because of the accumulation of a metabolite that can compete with the active drug for a receptor binding site:

$$EC50_{A,tol}(C_{tol}) = EC50_A\left(1 + \frac{C_{tol}}{EC50_{tol}}\right). \tag{23}$$

Morphine-3-glucuronide is a metabolite of morphine which might be able to competitively antagonize morphine binding. It was reported recently that intravenous administration of morphine-3-glucuronide blunted the analgesic response to morphine in rats (Ekblom et al. 1993) but the time course of development of tolerance to morphine alone could not be explained by the observed concentrations of morphine-3-glucuronide.

The observation of a rebound phenomenon when the active drug is withdrawn is an indication that the direct effect model is not an adequate explanation for the time course of tolerance. This is because the direct effect model cannot predict an effect less than E_0.

β) Autonomous

CHENG and PAALZOW (1990) and PAALZOW (1992) have described a model for tolerance which proposes that C_{tol} works independently of the active drug. Tolerance is viewed as the net effect of opposing pharmacodynamic models for the active drug and the tolerance-inducing substance, e.g.:

$$E(C_A, C_{tol}) = E_0 + \frac{E_{max,A} \cdot C_A^{N_A}}{C_A^{N_A} + EC50_A^{N_A}} - \frac{E_{max,tol} \cdot C_{tol}^{N_{tol}}}{C_{tol}^{N_{tol}} + EC50_{tol}^{N_{tol}}}. \tag{24}$$

This model has greater flexibility in describing observations than the direct action models. Like the physiological mediator model, the independent time course of the active drug and the tolerance substance can be used to predict a withdrawal rebound phenomenon.

b) Tolerance to Placebo

Given that tolerance may develop to an active drug, it is also possible that tolerance may develop to a placebo treatment. If only one treatment is given, it is not possible to determine whether tolerance has developed, but if a patient in a clinical trial is assigned to a series of treatments which may include a placebo, the placebo effect associated with each treatment may diminish with time. One way of describing tolerance to a placebo is to propose that the placebo "dose" associated with each treatment decreases in an exponential fashion:

$$Dose_{P,tol}(t) = Dose_P \cdot e^{-K_{tol} \cdot t}. \tag{25}$$

D. Conclusion

> "All science is either stamp collecting or physics."
> Lord Rutherford

$$\text{stamp collecting} \rightarrow \text{MODEL} \rightarrow \text{physics} \tag{26}$$

The use of models to describe the time course of drug action provides a stepping stone between the complexity of observations of drug effects and the simplicity offered by as yet unstated comprehensive theory of the interaction between drugs and the biological organism.

The models described here are constructed from three mathematical building blocks – the straight line, the exponential, and the hyperbolic function. In general, when very little is known about the underlying mechanism, a linear model is used. When the time course of a substance must be defined, a first-order elimination process is defined by an exponential. Finally, if the equilibrium effect of the substance is to be described, the E_{max} family of hyperbolic functions is applied. The models we have elaborated are not definitive – they are just illustrations of how pharmacological phenomena can be reduced to a small number of basic concepts. Hypotheses can be tested by comparing alternative combinations of these building blocks and thereby lead to a more precise description and clearer understanding of the time course of drug effect.

References

Abernethy DR (1988) Problematic factors in pharmacodynamic studies. In: Kroboth PD, Smith RB, Juhl RP (eds) Pharmacokinetics and pharmacodynamics: 2. Current problems and potential solutions. Whitney, Cincinnati, p 60

Bates DM, Watts DG (1988) Nonlinear regression analysis and its applications. Wiley, New York

Beal SL, Sheiner LB (1991) NONMEM users guide. University of California, San Francisco

Campbell DB (1990) The use of kinetic-dynamic interactions in the evaluation of drugs. Psychopharmacology 100:433–450

Cheng YE, Paalzow (1990) A pharmacodynamic model to predict the time dependent adaptation of dopaminergic activity during constant concentrations of haloperidol. J Pharm Pharmacol 42:566–571

Chiou WL (1991) The significance of marked "universal" dependence of drug concentration on blood sampling site in pharmacokinetics and pharmacodynamics. In: D'Argenio DZ (ed) Advanced methods of pharmacokinetic and pharmacodynamic systems analysis. Plenun, New York, pp 37–54

Colburn WA (1981) Simultaneous pharmacokinetic and pharmacodynamic modeling. J Pharmacokinet Biopharm 9:367–388

Colburn WA, Blue JW (1992) Using pharmacokinetics and pharmacodynamics to direct pharmaceutical R&D. Appl Clin Trials 1:42–46

Collins JM, Grieshaber CK, Chabner BA (1990) Pharmacologically guided phase I clinical trials based upon preclinical drug development. J Natl Cancer Inst 82:1321–1326

Dingemanse J, Danhof M, Breimer DD (1988) Pharmacokinetic-pharmacodynamic modeling of CNS drug effects: an overview. Pharmacol Ther 38:1–52

Ebling WF, Lee EN, Stanski DR (1990) Understanding pharmacokinetics and pharmacodynamics through computer simulation: 1. The comparative clinical profiles of fentanyl and alfentanil. Anesthesiology 72:650–658

Ekblom M, Gårdmark, Hammarlund-Udenaes M (1993) Pharmacokinetics and pharmacodynamics of morphine-3-glucuronide in rats and its influence on the antinociceptive effect of morphine. Biopharm Drug Dispos (in press)

Fisher LE, Ludwig EA, Wald JA, Sloan RR, Middleton E Jr, Jusko WJ (1992) Pharmacokinetics and pharmacodynamics of methylprednisolone when administered at 8 AM versus 4 PM. Clin Pharmacol Ther 51:677–688

Francheteau P, Steimer J-L, Dubray C, Lavene D (1991) Mathematical model for in vivo pharmacodynamics integrating fluctuation of the response: application to the prolactin suppressant effect of the dopaminomimetic drug DCN 203-922. J Pharmacokinet Biopharm 19:287–309

Gibaldi M, Perrier D (1982) Pharmacokinetics, 2nd edn. Dekker, New York

Girard P, Boissel J-P (1989) Clockwise hysteresis or proteresis. J Pharmacokinet Biopharm 17:401–402

Greenblatt DJ, Ehrenberg BL, Gunderman J, Locniskar A, Scavone JM, Harmatz JS, Shader RI (1989) Pharmacokinetic and electroencephalographic study of intravenous diazepam, midazolam and placebo. Clin Pharmacol Ther 45:356–365

Hill AV (1910) The possible effects of the aggregation of the molecules of haemoglobin on its dissociation curves. J Physiol 40:iv–vii

Holford NHG (1986) Clinical pharmacodynamics of warfarin. Clin Pharmacokinet 11:486–504

Holford NHG (1991) Physiological alternatives to the effect compartment model. In: D'Argenio DZ (ed) Advanced methods of pharmacokinetics and pharmaco-dynamic systems analysis. Plenum, New York, pp 55–60

Holford NHG (1992a) Clinical pharmacokinetics and pharmacodynamics: the quantitative basis for therapeutics. In: Melmon KL, Morelli HF, Hoffman BB, Nierenberg DW (eds) Clinical pharmacology; basic principles in therapeutics, 3rd edn. McGraw-Hill, New York

Holford NHG (1992b) Parametric models of the time course of drug action: the population approach. In: Rowland M, Aarons L (eds) New strategies in drug development and clinical evaluation: the population approach. EUR 13775. Commission of the European Communities, Brussels, pp 193–206

Holford NHG, Peck CC (1992) Population pharmacodynamics and drug development. In: Van Boxtel CJ, Holford NHG, Danhof M (eds) The in vivo study of drug action. Elsevier, Amsterdam

Holford NHG, Peace KE (1992a) Methodologic aspects of a population pharmacodynamic model for cognitive effects in Alzheimer's disease treated with tacrine. Proc Natl Acad Sci USA 89:11466–11470

Holford NHG, Peace KE (1992b) Results and validation of a population pharmacodynamic model for cognitive effects in Alzheimer's disease treated with tacrine. Proc Natl Acad Sci USA 89:11471–11475

Holford NHG, Sheiner LB (1981) Understanding the dose–effect relationship: clinical application of pharmacokinetic-pharmacodynamic models. Clin Pharmacokinet 6:429–453

Holford NHG, Jonkers R, Van Boxtel CJ (1989) Comparison of a physiological pharmacokinetic-pharmacodynamic model with an effect compartment model describing the hypokalaemic effect of terbutaline with and without metoprolol. Proceedings of the 4th world congress on clinical pharmacology and therapeutics, Mannheim, July 1989

Inturrisi CE, Colburn WQ, Kaiko RF, Houde RW, Foley KM (1987) Pharmacokinetics and pharmacodynamics of methadone in patients with chronic pain. Clin Pharmacol Ther 41:392–401

Jonkers RE, Van Boxtel CJ, Koopmans RP, Oosterhuis B (1989) A nonsteady state agonist antagonist interaction model using plasma potassium concentrations to quantify the β_2-selectivity of β-blockers. J Pharmacol Exp Ther 249:297–302

Kelman AW, Sumner DJ, Whiting B (1981) Systolic time interval v. heart rate regression equations using atropine: reproducibility studies. Br J Clin Pharmacol 12:15–20

Kenakin T (1987) Pharmacologic analysis of drug-receptor interaction. Raven, New York

Kenakin T (1992) The study of drug-receptor interactions in in vivo systems. In: Van Boxtel CJ, Holford NHG, Danhof M (eds) The in vivo study of drug action. Elsevier, Amsterdam

Levy G (1985) Variability in animal and human pharmacodynamic studies. In: Rowland M, Sheiner LB, Steimer J-L (eds) Variability in drug therapy. Raven, New York, p 125

Nagashima R, O'Reilly RA, Levy G (1969) Kinetics of pharmacologic effects in man: the anticoagulant action of warfarin. Clin Pharmacol Ther 10:22–35

Paalzow LK (1992) Measurement and modeling of analgesic drug effect. In: Van Boxtel CJ, Holford NHG, Danhof M (eds) The in vivo study of drug action. Elsevier, Amsterdam

Peck CC, Nichols AI, Baker J, Lenert LL, Ezra D (1985) Clinical pharmacodynamics of theophylline. J Allergy Clin Immunol 76:292–297

Peck CC, Barr WH, Benet LZ et al. (1992) Opportunities for integration of pharmacokinetics, pharmacodynamics and toxicokinetics in rational drug development. Clin Pharmacol Ther 51:465–473

Perry PJ, Pfahl BM, Holstad SG (1987) The relationship between antidepressant response and tricyclic antidepressant plasma concentrations. Clin Pharmacokinet 13:381–392

Porchet HC, Benowitz NL, Sheiner LB (1988) Pharmacodynamic model of tolerance: application to nicotine. J Pharmacol Exp Ther 244:231–236

Ratain MJ, Schilsky RL, Conley BA, Egorin MJ (1990) Pharmacodynamics in cancer therapy. J Clin Oncol 8:1739–1753

Rowland M, Tozer TN (1989) Clinical pharmacokinetics: concepts and applications, 2nd edn. Lea and Febiger, Philadelphia

Sanaathanan LP, Peck CC (1991) The randomized concentration-controlled trial: an evaluation of its sample size efficiency. Controlled Clin Trials 12:780–794

Scott JC, Stanski DR (1987) Decreased fentanyl and alfentanil dose requirements with age. A simultaneous pharmacokinetic and pharmacodynamic evaluation. J Pharmacol Exp Ther 240:159–172

Seber GAF, Wild CJ (1989) Nonlinear regression. Wiley, New York

Segre G (1968) Kinetics of interaction between drugs and biological systems. Il Farmaco 23:907–918

Shah VP, Midha KK, Dighe S, McGilveray IJ, Skelly JP, Yacobi A, Layloff T, Viswanathan CT, Cook CE, McDowall RD, Pittman KA, Spector S (1992) Analytical methods validation: bioavailability, bioequivalence and pharmacokinetic studies. Pharm Res 9:588–592

Sheiner LB (1989) Clinical pharmacology and the choice between theory and empiricism. Clin Pharmacol Ther 46:605–615

Sheiner LB (1991) The intellectual health of clinical drug evaluation. Clin Pharmacol Ther 50:4–9

Sheiner LB, Stanski DR, Vozeh S, Miller RD, Ham J (1979a) Simultaneous modeling of pharmacokinetics and pharmacodynamics: application to d-tubocurarine. Clin Pharmacol Ther 25:358–371

Sheiner LB, Beal SL, Rosenberg B (1979b) Forecasting individual pharmacokinetic parameters. Clin Pharmacol Ther 26:294–305

Sokolow M, Edgar AL (1950) Blood quinidine concentration as a guide in the treatment of cardiac arrhythmias. Circulation 1:576–592

Stanski DR (1992) Pharmacodynamic modeling of anesthetic EEG drug effects. Annu Rev Pharmacol Toxicol 32:423–447

Stanski DR, Maitre PO (1990) Population pharmacokinetics and pharmacodynamics of thiopental: the effect of age revisited. Anesthesiology 72:412–422

Svec JM, Coleman RW, Mungall DR, Ludden TM (1985) Bayesian pharmacokinetics/ pharmacodynamic forecasting of prothrombin response to warfarin therapy: preliminary evaluation. Ther Drug Monit 7:174–180

Swisher WP, Wedell HG, Cheng JTO (1954) Studies of quinidine plasma levels and rate of decline following cessation of quinidine administration. Am Heart J 47:449–452

Unadkat JD, Sheiner LB, Hennis PJ, Cronnelly R, Miller RD, Sharma M (1986) An integrated model for the interaction of muscle relaxants with their antagonists. J Appl Physiol 61:1593–1598

Van Boxtel CJ, Holford NHG, Danhof M (1992) The in vivo study of drug action. Elsevier, Amsterdam

Verotta D, Kitts J, Rodriguez R, Coldwell J, Miller RD, Sheiner LB (1991) Reversal of neuromuscular blockade in humans by neostigmine and edrophonium: a mathematical model. J Pharmacokinet Biopharm 19:713–729

Vozeh S, Bindschedler M, Ha H-R, Kaufmann G, Guentert TW, Follath F (1987) Pharmacodynamics of 3-hydroxyquinidine alone and in combination with quinidine in healthy persons. Am J Cardiol 59:681–684

Wagner J (1975) Fundamentals of clinical pharmacokinetics. Drug Intelligence Publications, Hamilton

E. Future Trends in Pharmacokinetics

CHAPTER 12
Biotechnology Products

B.L. Ferraiolo, R.J. Wills, and M.A. Mohler

A. Introduction

This chapter is intended as an overview of the pharmacokinetics of biotechnology products. For the purposes of this chapter, biotechnology products
will be defined as proteins (polypeptides larger than 5 kDa) and antisense
oligonucleotides. The interested reader is referred to other chapters in this
volume (Chaps. 4 and 13) and other recent volumes and reviews (Ferraiolo
et al. 1992; Garzone et al. 1991; Kung et al. 1992; McMartin 1992) for
additional information.

B. Pharmacokinetic/Pharmacodynamic Studies

An important early goal of disposition studies for biotechnology products
should be an attempt to correlate the time course of the product-related
materials in the body with pharmacological (or toxicological) effects. This
may aid in the selection of new drug candidates based on their disposition
properties. In addition, these correlations may help identify and predict
optimum routes of administration, regimens, and doses, and thus optimal
therapy (Mazer 1990; Peck et al. 1992). However, correlations of effects
with concentrations have been limited for biotechnology products, perhaps
because the mechanisms and sites of action are often unknown (Gloff and
Benet 1990; Wills 1991).

I. Oligonucleotides

Antisense oligonucleotides bind to complementary messenger RNA or
DNA sequences that code for disease-causing proteins, thereby inhibiting
their production (Crooke 1991; Zon 1988). A few oligonucleotide pharmacokinetic studies have recently been reported (Agrawal et al. 1991;
Chem et al. 1990; Iversen 1991; Zendegui et al. 1992). These studies have
primarily used radioactivity (e.g., ^3H, ^{35}S, or ^{32}P) as a means of detection.
Table 1 summarizes selected pharmacokinetic parameters for antisense
oligonucleotides.

Phosphorothioate oligonucleotide analogs have been selected for development because of their resistance to degradation by a variety of nucleases.

Table 1. Oligonucleotide pharmacokinetic parameters

Oligonucleotide/ dose (mg/kg)	Species	Route	$t_{1/2a}$ (min)	$t_{1/2b}$ (h)	T_{max} (min)	AUC (mg min/ml)	Urinary excretion (% dose/time)
12-mer[a] (0.1 µmol)	Mouse	i.v.	6	0.28	NA	NR	70/1–2 h
20-mer[b] (30)	Mouse	i.v./i.p.	NR	NR	NR	NR	~30/24 h
27-mer[c] (NR)	Rat	i.v.	15–25	20–40	10	NR	~100/3 d
		i.p.	NR	NR	90	NR	
38-mer[d] (130)	Mouse	i.v.	<10	NR	NA	27[e]	25/4 h
		i.p.	NR	NR	30	30[e]	30/8 h

i.v., intravenous; i.p., intraperitoneal; NA, not applicable; NR, not reported
[a] Methylphosphonate (Chem et al. 1990)
[b] Phosphorothioate (Agrawal et al. 1991)
[c] Phosphorothioate (*rev*) (Iversen 1991)
[d] 3'-Phosphopropylamine (TFO-1) (Zendegui et al. 1992)
[e] AUC (0–240 min)

Single-dose studies in rats with a ^{35}S-labeled 27-mer complementary to the *rev* gene of HIV showed a time to peak plasma concentrations of 10 min after intravenous administration and 90 min after intraperitoneal administration (Iversen 1991). Clearance was linear with respect to dose (35–3500 µg) and elimination was biphasic, with a terminal half-life of 20–40 h. The radioactive dose was essentially completely eliminated in the urine over 3 days, predominantly as the parent compound. In this study, varying the oligonucleotide length and composition did not substantially influence plasma concentrations, tissue distribution, or excretion.

A similar study in mice with a ^{35}S-labeled 20-mer phosphorothioate oligonucleotide (Agrawal et al. 1991) (30 mg/kg) showed approximately 30% of the dose was excreted in urine within 24 h after intravenous or intraperitoneal administration. The oligonucleotide excreted in urine was more extensively degraded after intraperitoneal than after intravenous administration. Approximately 15% of the dose was excreted in feces within 48 h. Evidence of chain length extension of the oligonucleotide was observed in several tissues, although incorporation of liberated nucleoside ([35]thio)phosphate into endogenous nucleic acids is another possible explanation.

The pharmacokinetics of a ^{3}H-labeled methylphosphonate oligonucleotide (12-mer) have been determined in mice after intravenous administration (Chem et al. 1990). The biexponential plasma decline was characterized by half-lives of 6 and 17 min. Radioactivity was excreted primarily in the urine (70% of the dose in 60–120 min). Plasma protein binding was 16%–20%. The 11-mer metabolite was identified in plasma, urine, and tissues.

A ^{32}P-labeled 38-mer 3' phosphopropyl amine oligonucleotide (TFO-1) was used in pharmacokinetic studies in mice (Zendegui et al. 1992). After intravenous administration (130 mg/kg), the plasma level decline was biexponential. The initial half-life was less than 10 min. The time to maximum plasma concentrations after intraperitoneal administration was 30 min. Oligonucleotide remained largely intact in plasma for at least 8 h. Approximately 20%–30% of the dose was excreted in the urine over 8 h, apparently as intact compound.

II. Proteins

Proteins may show mono- or multiexponential profiles of decline in biological matrices. The shape of the profile depends in part on the assay sensitivity and the length of sampling (FERRAIOLO and MOHLER 1992). The calculated pharmacokinetic parameters may vary widely, since the physiological properties and structures of therapeutic proteins vary widely. Table 2 lists pharmacokinetic parameters for a variety of therapeutic proteins.

For many protein therapeutics, the pharmacokinetics in laboratory animals provide reasonable estimates of the human pharmacokinetics when analyzed as a function of body weight using allometric scaling techniques (GATTI et al. 1991; MORDENTI et al. 1991; YOUNG et al. 1990). Access to this predictive information during the drug development process can provide a rational basis for preclinical and clinical dose selection (MORDENTI and GREEN 1991; MORDENTI et al. 1991, 1992, 1994).

Table 2. Selected pharmacokinetic parameters for representative therapeutic proteins in humans

Protein	Mol. wt. (kDa)	Glycoprotein	CL (ml/min)	Vd (l)	$t_{1/2z}$ (min)
Relaxin[a]	6	No	175	17.4	NR
Insulin[b]	6	No	487	14.2	57.7
IFN-α[c]	18–23	Yes	81–350	12–40	240–960
IFN-γ[c]	20–25	No	211–540	12–40	25–35
GH[a]	22	No	152	4.1	31[f]
EPO[d]	36	Yes	4–15	2.8–6.3[g]	180–960
CD4[a]	41	Yes	57	4.9	~60[h]
t-PA[e]	59	Yes	687	8	26–36
CD4-IgG[a]	98	Yes	2.6	6.3	~2880[i]

CL, clearance; EPO, erythropoietin; GH, growth hormone; IFN, interferon; NR, not reported; t-PA, tissue plasminogen activator; $t_{1/2z}$, terminal half-life; Vd, volume of distribution
[a] MORDENTI et al. (1991)
[b] HOOPER et al. (1991)
[c] WILLS (1990)
[d] STOUDEMIRE (1992)
[e] TANSWELL et al. (1991)
[f] WILTON et al. (1988)
[g] 70 kg
[h] KAHN et al. (1990)
[i] HODGES et al. (1991)

A general discussion of the calculation of pharmacokinetic parameters for proteins has recently been published (Colburn 1991); numerous additional sources are available describing pharmacodynamic modeling (Holford and Sheiner 1981, 1982; Kroboth et al. 1988; Wills 1992). The application of a variety of approaches for acquiring and interpreting the information available from pharmacokinetic/pharmacodynamic studies with proteins is illustrated in the following examples.

1. Insulin

The relationship between the hypoglycemic effects of insulin therapies and plasma insulin concentrations has been well characterized (Bergman et al. 1985; Sorensen et al. 1982). Recently, the pharmacokinetics and pharmacodynamics of intravenous recombinant human insulin were studied in healthy male volunteers (Hooper et al. 1991). Insulin concentration versus time data were described by biexponential equations. The calculated pharmacokinetic parameters (Table 2) were used in a pharmacokinetic/pharmacodynamic model to estimate pharmacodynamic variables. A counterclockwise hysteresis was observed in the relationship between serum insulin concentration and glucose infusion rates necessary to maintain euglycemia after intravenous administration of insulin. There was a significant equilibrium delay between the serum compartment and the effect compartment (mean half-life of 2.7 h).

2. Relaxin

Relaxin is a two-chain protein hormone of pregnancy that is structurally analogous to insulin and insulin-like growth factor-I (Cronin et al. 1991; Sherwood 1988). Relaxin treatment induces lengthening of the pubic ligament in estrogen-primed mice. This effect is not observed unless relaxin is delivered in a repository vehicle (benzopurpurine) that results in sustained, prolonged elevated relaxin serum concentrations (Ferraiolo et al. 1989). Multiple doses of relaxin without benzopurpurine, administered by a regimen designed to emulate the pharmacokinetic profile achieved with benzopurpurine, result in pubic ligament lengthening, strongly supporting the hypothesis that sustained serum relaxin concentrations correlate with efficacy.

3. Interferon-α-2A

Acute adverse events associated with interferon-α-2A such as chills, headache, and myalgias have been observed to be more severe and of longer duration after intramuscular and subcutaneous administrations of interferon-α-2A than after intravenous administration. These effects are not a simple function of the serum concentrations attained, but appear to be related to exceeding and maintaining a threshold serum concentration (Wills 1990). These observations have been used to adjust and optimize clinical therapy.

C. Regimen-Dependent Effects

The regimen employed for biotechnology products may influence the pharmacodynamic effects observed. The route and rate of administration can be important treatment variables. In fact, the rate of delivery is an important aspect of the safety and pharmacodynamic profiles. This may be related in some cases to the natural pattern of presentation of the endogenous substance. For example, many protein hormones are secreted in a pulsatile fashion; in these cases, single bolus or continuous infusion delivery may not be optimal.

I. Growth Hormone

CLARK et al. (1985) showed the importance of regimen in the expression of growth hormone's effects. One intravenous dose of growth hormone per day in hypophysectomized rats caused significant gains in body weight and bone growth rate; however, the same total dose of growth hormone as nine pulses per day doubled the previous weight gain and increased the bone growth rate by more than 270% (CRONIN et al. 1991). Continuous intravenous delivery of the same daily growth hormone dose was less efficacious in increasing body weight than pulsatile delivery. Other investigators have confirmed and extended these observations in rats (ISGAARD et al. 1988; MAITER et al. 1988). These preclinical studies have been supported by clinical investigations showing that daily growth hormone administration promotes a greater growth rate in growth hormone-deficient children than three-times-a-week administration of the same total dose (ROSENBLOOM et al. 1990; SHERMAN and FRANE 1988; TUVEMO 1989).

II. Parathyroid Hormone

The effects of bovine parathyroid hormone (PTH) and its fragments administered by daily injections versus continuous infusions were compared in parathyroidectomized rats (TAM et al. 1982). Infusion of bovine PTH resulted in increased bone apposition and an increase in both bone formation and resorption surfaces, but there was a net decrease in trabecular bone. Equal doses by bolus injection increased bone apposition rate and bone formation surfaces, but did not increase resorption, so there was a net increase in bone volume. The bolus injection regimen provided a way to separate the resorptive effects of PTH from its effects on apposition rate. Intermittent bolus doses were more effective than continuous infusion in promoting anabolic skeletal effects. Supportive results have also been observed in dogs (PODBESEK et al. 1983).

III. Tissue Plasminogen Activator

The lytic efficacy of tissue plasminogen activator (t-PA) following different dosing regimens was studied in a dog model (KLABUNDE et al. 1990). Radiolabeled clots were inserted into an extracorporeal jugular loop and clot size was continuously recorded. t-PA was administered as an intravenous bolus, as multiple bolus injections, or as a bolus followed by a continuous intravenous infusion. Multiple injections of the same total dose of tPA resulted in 51%–76% greater clot lysis than a single bolus injection or a bolus followed by an infusion.

D. Binding Proteins/Inhibitors

As pharmacokinetic and metabolism studies for protein biotechnology products have matured, increasing numbers of examples of binding proteins for protein drugs have been reported. Binding proteins are known to have inhibitory or stimulatory effects on the pharmacodynamic responses to protein therapeutics; they may modulate efficacy at the cellular level and/or affect the protein's pharmacokinetics and metabolism. The relative importance of these binding proteins may be species or disease-state specific (MOHLER et al. 1992).

In addition to the specific examples described below, binding protein/inhibitor phenomena have recently been described for other proteins including nerve growth factor/α_2-macroglobulin (Koo and STACH 1989), transforming growth factor-β/α_2-macroglobulin (DANIELPOUR and SPORN 1990; LaMARRE et al. 1990; PHILIP and O'CONNOR-MCCOURT 1991), interleukin-4 (FERNANDEZ-BOTRAN and VITETTA 1990), interleukin-2 (LELCHUK and PLAYFAIR 1985), tumor necrosis factor (MALIK et al. 1991), and the interferons (HAVREDAKI and BARONA 1985).

I. Growth Hormone

Human growth hormone circulates in plasma in part bound to at least one plasma binding protein (BAUMANN et al. 1986; BAUMANN and SHAW 1990; HERINGTON et al. 1986; MOHLER et al. 1992). Based on the dissociation constant and concentration of the high-affinity growth hormone binding protein (which appears to be shed growth hormone receptor), a large proportion of endogenous growth hormone may be bound in the circulation between endogenous growth hormone pulses (CRONIN et al. 1991). In vitro studies have shown that growth hormone binding protein inhibits the biological effects and receptor binding of growth hormone (LIM et al. 1990; MANNOR et al. 1988). Bound growth hormone appears to show different clearance characteristics than unbound growth hormone (MOHLER et al. 1992). Recent studies indicate that coinjection of human growth hormone and the growth hormone binding protein prolongs growth hormone's half-life and reduces its clearance in rats (BAUMANN et al. 1987, 1988; MOORE et al. 1988, 1989). This effect may be a result of limited access of the growth hormone–binding protein complex to proximal tubule catabolic sites due to size restriction of glomerular filtration (BAUMANN et al. 1987; MOORE et al. 1988).

II. Tissue Plasminogen Activator

Tissue plasminogen activator circulates unbound and in complexes with various protease inhibitors. In most cases, protease inhibition is characterized by the formation of an irreversible complex between the active site on the protease and the protease inhibitor (MOHLER et al. 1992). Several inhibitors that react with and inhibit t-PA include (in order of importance) fast-acting plasminogen activator inhibitor (PAI-1), the protease nexin, plasminogen activator inhibitor-2 (PAI-2), α_2-antiplasmin, C_1-esterase inhibitor, and α_2-macroglobulin (HIGGINS and BENNETT 1990; MOHLER et al. 1988, 1992). While unbound t-PA is cleared rapidly, t-PA in protease inhibitor complexes persists in the circulation. It has been suggested that elevated PAI-1 activity associated with myocardial infarction could attenuate the fibrinolytic activity of t-PA postinfusion and contribute to the risk of reocclusion (LUCORE and SOBEL 1988).

III. Insulin-like Growth Factor-I

Insulin-like growth factor I (IGF-I) is extensively bound in plasma to multiple plasma carrier proteins (MOHLER et al. 1992; OOI 1990; ZAPF et al. 1990a). At least three classes of binding proteins have been characterized (BALLARD et al. 1990). The clearances of free IGF-I and IGF-I bound in the binding protein complexes differ; free IGF-I is cleared very rapidly compared to the clearances of the bound forms (COHEN and NISSLEY 1976; COOK et al. 1989; ZAPF et al. 1986). These binding proteins may modulate IGF-I actions by either inhibiting or potentiating its effects (CLEMMONS 1989; OOI 1990; ZAPF et al. 1990a,b). IGF-I's hypoglycemic effects in man appear to be related to free IGF-I concentrations (MANEVAL et al. 1990).

IV. Deoxyribonuclease

Deoxyribonuclease (DNase) is an endonuclease that hydrolyzes DNA to mono- and oligonucleotides. Recombinant human DNase is being developed as a potential mucolytic to treat respiratory conditions associated with cystic fibrosis and other suppurative diseases of the airways. Increasing clearance of DNase with increasing dose in preclinical studies suggested the presence of a saturable serum binding protein (MOHLER et al. 1993). To further characterize this phenomenon, rats were injected intravenously with ^{125}I-DNase or ^{125}I-DNase and excess unlabeled DNase. Serum samples analyzed by acid precipitation, size-exclusion high-performance liquid chromatography, and native polyacrylamide gel electrophoresis verified that there was a specific serum binding protein for DNase. The presence of excess unlabeled DNase decreased the ^{125}I-DNase–binding protein complex level relative to free ^{125}I-DNase.

E. Catabolism of Biotechnology Products

Catabolism of protein biotechnology products occurs primarily by the action of ubiquitous proteolytic enzymes (Bocci 1987, 1990; Colburn 1991; Lee 1988; Maack et al. 1985). However, preproteolytic modifications of proteins may render them much more susceptible to degradation (Daggett 1987).

Carbohydrates are known to regulate the in vivo survival time of glycoproteins (Ashwell and Harford 1982). Exposure of specific carbohydrate determinants for hepatic recognition by removal of terminal sialic acid residues is one mechanism proposed to explain this phenomenon. Other alterations of carbohydrate structure may have similar effects (Barbeau 1990; Hotchkiss et al. 1988). The importance of carbohydrate moieties in modulating the plasma clearance of proteins has been demonstrated for t-PA (Hotchkiss et al. 1988; Lucore et al. 1988), interferon-β (Bocci et al. 1982), and erythropoietin (Fukuda et al. 1989; Spivak and Hogans 1989).

Other determinants of in vivo protein degradation that have been suggested include the amino terminal residue (Bachmair et al. 1986), primary structure (Lombardo et al. 1988; Rogers et al. 1986), and tertiary structure (Kossiakoff 1988).

For reviews of the roles of the kidney and liver in the catabolism of protein therapeutics, the interested reader is referred to recent publications (Bocci et al. 1982; Colburn 1991; Ferraiolo and Mohler 1992; Maack et al. 1985).

I. Catabolism at Extravascular Sites of Administration

The bioavailability of proteins may vary widely (Table 3); this may be due in part to degradation during absorption at extravascular sites of injection (Lee 1988). Bioavailability data for proteins must be interpreted with caution, since assay limitations (lack of specificity) may contribute to artifactual results (viz. interferon-γ, Table 3) (Ferraiolo and Mohler 1992).

Catabolism of protein therapeutics at extravascular sites of administration has been described for insulin (Berger et al. 1979; Davies et al. 1980; Okumura et al. 1985), parathyroid hormone and calcitonin (Parsons et al. 1979), and interferon-β (Bocci et al. 1986a). This local degradation of therapeutic proteins has been prevented experimentally by coadministration of various protease inhibitors or alternate substrates for proteases including: collagen (Hori et al. 1989); benzyloxycarbonyl-Gly-Pro-Leu-Gly (Hori et al. 1983); bacitracin, leupeptin, and phosphoramidon (Komada et al. 1985); the enkephalinase inhibitor, thiorphan (Chipkin et al. 1984); ophthalmic acid and a bovine pancreatic proteinase inhibitor (Offord et al. 1979);

Table 3. Bioavailabilities of selected therapeutic proteins

Protein	Species	Route	Bioavailability (%)
Relaxin[a]	Mouse	s.c.	96
IFN-α[b]	Human	i.m./s.c.	>80
IFN-γ	Human	i.m./s.c.	30–70[b]
			161–575[c]
	Rhesus monkey	i.m./s.c.	20–297[d]
TNF-α[e]	Mouse	i.m.	12
GH[f]	Human	s.c.	71
EPO[g]	Human	s.c.	10–49
		i.p.	3–15
CD4[h]	Human	i.m./s.c.	45–51
CD4-IgG[i]	Human	i.m.	9–47

TNF, tumor necrosis factor; s.c., subcutaneous; i.m., intramuscular; i.p., intraperitoneal; see Table 2 for other definitions
[a] FERRAIOLO et al. (1989)
[b] WILLS (1990)
[c] MORDENTI et al. (1992)
[d] FERRAIOLO et al. (1988a)
[e] FERRAIOLO et al. (1988b)
[f] WILTON et al. (1987)
[g] STOUDEMIRE (1992)
[h] KAHN et al. (1990)
[i] HODGES et al. (1991)

albumin (BOCCI et al. 1986a); gelatin (BOCCI et al. 1986b); and aprotinin (BERGER et al. 1980, 1982; FREIDENBERG et al. 1981).

F. Drug Interactions

Proteins may directly or indirectly affect the elimination of concomitantly administered compounds. For example, interferons have been shown to alter the pharmacological effects of other drugs (MOORE et al. 1983; TAYLOR et al. 1985) and to depress cytochrome P-450 and alter drug metabolism activities (ANSHER et al. 1992; CRAIG et al. 1990; FRANKLIN and FINKLE 1985, 1986; PARKINSON et al. 1982; RUSTGI et al. 1987; SINGH et al. 1982; WILLIAMS and FARRELL 1986). However, conflicting results have been reported (ECHIZEN et al. 1990; SECOR and SCHENKER 1984). Treatment of mice with tumor necrosis factor caused a significant decrease in cytochrome P-450 levels and ethoxycourmarin deethylase activities (GHEZZI et al. 1986). Growth hormone appears to modulate the development and/or expression of the liver mixed function oxidase system (WILSON 1970; WILSON and FROHMAN 1974; YAMAZOE et al. 1986). Interleukin-1 has been reported to decrease cytochrome P-450 levels and drug metabolism activities in mice (SHEDLOFSKY et al. 1987). Interferons have been shown to affect the clinical pharmacokinetics and/or metabolism of other drugs (JONKMAN et al. 1989;

Nokta et al. 1991). Interleukin-2 has been shown to alter dacarbazine pharmacokinetics in melanoma patients (Chabot et al. 1990) and interferon-α has been shown to alter the disposition of a radiolabeled antibody in patients (Rosenblum et al. 1988).

References

Agrawal S, Temsamani J, Tang JY (1991) Pharmacokinetics, biodistribution and stability of oligodeoxynucleotide phosphorothioates in mice. Proc Natl Acad Sci USA 88:7595–7599

Ansher SS, Puri RK, Thompson WC, Habig WH (1992) The effects of interleukin-2 and alpha-interferon administration on hepatic drug metabolism in mice. Cancer Res 52:262–266

Ashwell G, Harford J (1982) Carbohydrate-specific receptors of the liver. Annu Rev Biochem 51:531–554

Bachmair A, Finley D, Varshavsky A (1986) In vivo half life of a protein is a function of its amino terminal residue. Science 234:179–186

Ballard FJ, Baxter RC, Binoux M, Clemmons DR, Drop SL, Hall K, Hintz RL, Rechler MM, Rutanen EM, Schwander JC (1990) Report on the nomenclature of the IGF binding proteins. J Clin Endocrinol Metab 70:817–818

Barbeau D (1990) Protein glycosylation and pharmacokinetics. Controlled Release Society Newsletter, pp 6–10

Baumann G, Shaw MA (1990) A second lower affinity growth hormone-binding protein in human plasma. J Clin Endocrinol Metab 70:680–686

Baumann G, Stolar MW, Amburn K, Barsano CP, DeVries BC (1986) A specific growth hormone binding protein in human plasma: initial characterization. J Clin Endocrinol Metab 62:134–141

Baumann G, Amburn KD, Buchanan TA (1987) The effect of circulating growth hormone-binding protein on metabolic clearance, distribution and degradation of human growth hormone. J Clin Endocrinol Metab 64:657–660

Baumann G, Shaw MA, Buchanan TA (1988) In vivo kinetics of a covalent growth hormone-binding protein complex. Metabolism 38:330–333

Berger M, Halban PA, Girardier L, Seydoux J, Offord RE, Renold AE (1979) Absorption kinetics of subcutaneously injected insulin. Diabetologia 17:97–99

Berger M, Cuppers HJ, Halban PA, Offord RE (1980) The effect of aprotinin on the absorption of subcutaneously injected regular insulin in normal subjects. Diabetes 29:81–83

Berger M, Cuppers HJ, Hegner H, Jorgens V, Berchtold P (1982) Absorption kinetics and biological effects of subcutaneously injected insulin preparations. Diabetes Care 5:77–91

Bergman RN, Finegood DT, Ader M (1985) Assessment of insulin sensitivity in vivo. Endocr Rev 6:45–86

Bocci V (1987) Metabolism of protein anticancer agents. Pharmacol Ther 34:1–49

Bocci V (1990) Catabolism of therapeutic proteins and peptides with implications for drug delivery. Adv Drug Del Rev 4:149–169

Bocci V, Pacini A, Bandinelli L, Pessina GP, Muscettola M, Paulesu L (1982) The role of the liver in the catabolism of human alpha- and beta-interferons. J Gen Virol 60:397–400

Bocci V, Muscettola M, Naldini A (1986a) The lymphatic route III pharmacokinetics of a human natural interferon-beta injected with albumin as a retarder in rabbits. Gen Pharmacol 17:445–448

Bocci V, Pacini A, Maioli E, Muscettola M, Paulesu L (1986b) Prolonged interferon plasma levels after administration of interferon with retarders. IRCS Med Sci 14:360–361

Chabot GG, Flaherty LE, Valdivieso M, Baker LH (1990) Alteration of dacarbazine pharmacokinetics after interleukin-2 administration in melanoma patients. Cancer Chemother Pharmacol 27:157–160

Chem T-L, Miller PS, Ts'o POP, Colvin OM (1990) Disposition and metabolism of oligodeoxynucleoside methylphosphonate following a single iv injection in mice. Drug Metab Dispos 18:815–818

Chipkin RE, Kreutner W, Billard W (1984) Potentiation of the hypoglycemic effect of insulin by thiorphan, an enkephalinase inhibitor. Eur J Pharmacol 102:151–154

Clark RG, Jansson J-O, Isaksson O, Robinson ICAF (1985) Intravenous growth hormone: growth responses to patterned infusions in hypophysectomized rats. J Endocrinol 104:53–61

Clemmons DR (1989) The role of insulin-like growth factor binding proteins in controlling the expression of IGF actions. In: LeRoith D, Raizada MK (eds) Molecular and cellular biology of the insulin-like growth factors and their receptors. Plenum, New York, p 381

Cohen KL, Nissley SP (1976) The serum half life of somatomedin activity: evidence for growth hormone dependence. Acta Endocrinol 83:243–258

Colburn WA (1991) Peptide, peptoid and protein pharmacokinetics/pharmacodynamics. In: Garzone PD, Colburn WA, Mokotoff M (eds) Pharmacokinetics and pharmacodynamics: 3. Peptides, peptoids and proteins. Whitney, Cincinnati, p 93

Cook JE, Ferraiolo BL, Mohler MA (1989) The role of binding proteins in the metabolism of IGF-I. Pharm Res 6:S30

Craig PI, Mehta I, Murray M, McDonald D, Astrom A, van der Meide PH, Farrell GC (1990) Interferon down regulates the male-specific cytochrome P450IIIA2 in rat liver. Mol Pharmacol 38:313–318

Cronin MJ, Ferraiolo BL, Moore JA (1991) Contemporary issues involving the activities of recombinant human hormones. In: Garzone PD, Colburn WA, Mokotoff M (eds) Pharmacokinetics and pharmacodynamics: 3. Peptides, peptoids and proteins. Whitney, Cincinnati, p 138

Crooke RM (1991) In vitro toxicology and pharmacokinetics of antisense oligonucleotides. Anticancer Drug Des 6:609–646

Daggett V (1987) Protein degradation: the role of mixed-function oxidases. Pharm Res 4:278–284

Danielpour D, Sporn MB (1990) Differential inhibition of transforming growth factor beta1 and beta2 activity by alpha2-macroglobulin. J Biol Chem 265:6973–6977

Davies JG, Offord RE, Halban PA, Berger M (1980) The chemical characterization of the products of the processing of subcutaneously injected insulin. In: Brandenburg D, Wollmer A (eds) Insulin – chemistry, structure and function of insulin and related hormones. De Gruyter, New York, p 517

Echizen H, Ohta Y, Shirataki H, Tsukamoto K, Umeda N, Oda T, Ishizaki T (1990) Effects of subchronic treatment with natural human interferons on antipyrine clearance and liver function in patients with chronic hepatitis. J Clin Pharmacol 30:562–567

Fernandez-Botran R, Vitetta ES (1990) A soluble, high-affinity, interleukin-4-binding protein is present in the biological fluids of mice. Proc Natl Acad Sci USA 87:4202–4206

Ferraiolo BL, Mohler MA (1992) Goals and analytical methodologies for protein disposition studies. In: Ferraiolo BL, Mohler MA, Gloff CA (eds) Protein pharmacokinetics and metabolism. Plenum, New York

Ferraiolo BL, Fuller GB, Burnett B, Chan E (1988a) Pharmacokinetics of recombinant human interferon-gamma in the rhesus monkey after intravenous, intramuscular and subcutaneous administration. J Biol Response Mod 7:115–122

Ferraiolo BL, Moore JA, Crase D, Gribling P, Wilking H, Baughman RA (1988b) Pharmacokinetics and tissue distribution of recombinant human tumor necrosis factor-alpha in mice. Drug Metab Dispos 16:270–275

Ferraiolo BL, Cronin M, Bakhit C, Roth M, Chestnut M, Lyon R (1989) The pharmacokinetics and pharmacodynamics of a human relaxin in the mouse pubic symphysis bioassay. Endocrinology 125:2922–2926

Ferraiolo BL, Mohler MA, Gloff CA (1992) Protein pharmacokinetics and metabolism. Plenum, New York

Franklin MR, Finkle BS (1985) Effect of murine gamma-interferon on the mouse liver and its drug metabolizing enzymes: comparison with human hybrid alpha interferon J Interferon Res 5:265–272

Franklin MR, Finkle BS (1986) The influence of recombinant DNA-derived human and murine gamma interferons on mouse hepatic drug metabolism. Fundam Appl Toxicol 7:165–169

Freidenberg GR, White N, Cataland S, O'Dorisio TM, Sotos JF, Santiago JV (1981) Diabetes responsive to intravenous but not subcutaneous insulin: effectiveness of aprotinin. N Engl J Med 305:363–368

Fukuda MN, Sasaki H, Lopez L, Fukuda M (1989) Survival of recombinant erythropoietin in the circulation: the role of carbohydrates. Blood 73:84–89

Garzone PD, Colburn WA, Mokotoff M (1991) Pharmacokinetics and pharmacodynamics: 3. Peptides, peptoids and proteins. Whitney, Cinicinnati

Gatti G, Kahn J, Gambertoglio J (1991) Interspecies pharmacokinetic scaling for GLQ223. Clin Pharmacol Ther 49:176

Ghezzi P, Saccardo B, Bianchi M (1986) Recombinant tumor necrosis factor depresses cytochrome P450-dependent microsomal drug metabolism in mice. Biochem Biophys Res Commun 136:316–321

Gloff CA, Benet LZ (1990) Pharmacokinetics and protein therapeutics. Adv Drug Del Rev 4:359–386

Havredaki M, Barona F (1985) Variations in interferon inactivators and/or inhibitors in human serum and their relationship to interferon therapy. Jpn J Med Sci Biol 38:107–111

Herington AC, Ymer S, Stevenson J (1986) Identification and characterization of specific binding proteins for growth hormone in normal human serum. J Clin Invest 77:1817–1823

Higgins DL, Bennett WF (1990) Tissue plasminogen activator: the biochemistry and pharmacology of variants produced by mutagenesis. Annu Rev Pharmacol Toxicol 30:91–121

Hodges TL, Kahn FO, Kaplan LD, Groopman JE, Volberding PA, Amman AJ, Arri CJ, Bouvier LM, Mordenti J, Izu AE, Allan JD (1991) Phase 1 study of recombinant human CD4-immunoglobulin G therapy of patients with AIDS and AIDS-related complex. Antimicrob Agents Chemother 35:2580–2586

Holford NHG, Sheiner LB (1981) Understanding the dose-effect relationship: clinical application of pharmacokinetic-pharmacodynamic models. Clin Pharmacokinet 6:429–453

Holford NHG, Sheiner LB (1982) Kinetics of pharmacologic response. Pharmacol Ther 16:143–166

Hooper SA, Bowsher RR, Howey DC (1991) Pharmacokinetics and pharmacodynamics of intravenous regular human insulin. In: Garzone PD, Colburn WA, Mokotoff M (eds) Pharmacokinetics and pharmacodynamics: 3. Peptides, peptoids and proteins. Whitney, Cincinnati, p 128

Hori R, Komada F, Okumura K (1983) Pharmaceutical approach to subcutaneous dosage forms of insulin. J Pharm Sci 72:435–439

Hori R, Komada F, Iwakawa S, Seino Y, Okumura K (1989) Enhanced bioavailability of subcutaneously injected insulin coadministered with collagen in rats and humans. Pharm Res 6:813–816

Hotchkiss A, Refino CJ, Leonard CK, O'Connor JV, Crowley C, McCabe J, Tate K, Nakamura G, Powers D, Levinson A, Mohler M, Spellman MW (1988) The influence of carbohydrate structure on the clearance of recombinant tissue-type plasminogen activator. Thromb Haemost 60:255–261

Isgaard J, Carlsson L, Isaksson OGP, Jansson J-O (1988) Pulsatile intravenous growth hormone (GH) infusion to hypophysectomized rats increases insulin-like growth factor I messenger ribonucleic acid in skeletal tissues more effectively than continuous GH infusion. Endocrinology 123:2605–2610

Iversen P (1991) In vivo studies with phosphorothioate oligonucleotides: pharmacokinetics prologue. Anticancer Drug Des 6:531–538

Jonkman JHG, Nicholson KG, Farrow PR, Eckert M, Grassmijer G, Oosterhuis B, De Noord OE, Guentert TW (1989) Effects of alpha-interferon on theophylline pharmacokinetics and metabolism. Br J Clin Pharmacol 27:795–802

Kahn JO, Allen JD, Hodges TL, Kaplan LD, Arri CJ, Fitch HF, Izu AE, Mordenti J, Sherwin SA, Groopman JE, Volberding PA (1990) The safety and pharmacokinetics of recombinant soluble CD4 (rCD4) in subjects with the acquired immunodeficiency syndrome (AIDS) and AIDS-related complex. Ann Intern Med 112:254–261

Klabunde RE, Burke SE, Henkin J (1990) Enhanced lytic efficacy of multiple bolus injections of tissue plasminogen activator in dogs. Thromb Res 58:511–517

Komada F, Okumura K, Hori R (1985) Fate of porcine and human insulin at the subcutaneous injection site: II. In vitro degradation of insulins in the subcutaneous tissue of the rat. J Pharmacobiodyn 8:33–40

Koo PH, Stach RW (1989) Interaction of nerve growth factor with murine alpha-macroglobulin. J Neurosci Res 22:247–261

Kossiakoff AA (1988) Tertiary structure is a principal determinant of protein deamidation. Science 240:191–194

Kroboth PD, Smith RB, Juhl RP (1988) Pharmacokinetics and pharmacodynamics: 2. Current problems/potential solutions. Whitney, Cincinnati

Kung AHC, Larrick JW, Baughman RA (1992) Protein therapeutics: pharmacokinetics and pharmacodynamics. Stockton, New York

LaMarre J, Wollenberg GK, Gauldie J, Hayes MA (1990) Alpha2-macroglobulin and serum preferentially counteract the mitoinhibitory effect of transforming growth factor-beta2 on rat hepatocytes. Lab Invest 62:545–551

Lee VHL (1988) Enzymatic barriers to peptide and protein absorption. Crit Rev Ther Drug Carrier Syst 5:69–97

Lelchuk R, Playfair JHL (1985) Serum IL-2 inhibitor in mice: I. Increase during infection. Immunology 56:113–118

Lim L, Spencer SA, McKay P, Waters MJ (1990) Regulation of growth hormone (GH) bioactivity by a recombinant human GH-binding protein. Endrocrinology 127:1287–1291

Lombardo YB, Morse EL, Adibi SA (1988) Specificity and mechanism of influence of amino acid residues on hepatic clearance of oligopeptides. J Biol Chem 263:12920–12926

Lucore CL, Sobel BE (1988) Interactions of tissue-type plasminogen activator with plasma inhibitors and their pharmacological implications. Circulation 77:660–669

Lucore CL, Fry ETA, Nachowiak DA, Sobel BE (1988) Biochemical determinants of clearance of tissue-type plasminogen activator from the circulation. Circulation 77:906–914

Maack T, Park CH, Camargo MJF (1985) Renal filtration, transport and metabolism of proteins. In: Seldin DW, Giebisch G (eds) The kidney: physiology and pathophysiology. Raven, New York, p 1773

Maiter D, Underwood LE, Maes M, Davenport ML, Ketelslegers JM (1988) Different effects of intermittent and continuous growth hormone (GH) administration on serum somatomedin-C/insulin-like growth factor I and liver GH receptors in hypophysectomized rats. Endocrinology 123:1053–1059

Malik S, Lantz M, Slevin M, Olsson I (1991) Infusion of recombinant human tumour necrosis factor (rhTNF) causes an increase in circulating TNF-binding protein in man. Int J Exp Pathol 72:A6

Maneval DC, Chen SA, Ferraiolo BL, Mordenti J, Clark R, Cook J, Mohler MA (1990) Pharmacokinetic/pharmacodynamic modeling of the hypoglycemic response to recombinant human insulin-like growth factor-I (rhIGF-I). American Association of Pharmaceutical Scientists 5th Annual Meeting, Symposium Abstract

Mannor DA, Shaw MA, Winer LM, Baumann G (1988) Circulating growth hormone-binding proteins inhibit growth hormone (GH) binding to GH receptors but not in vivo GH action. Clin Res 36:870A

Mazer NA (1990) Pharmacokinetic and pharmacodynamic aspects of polypeptide delivery. J Control Rel 11:343–356

McMartin C (1992) Pharmacokinetics of peptides and proteins; opportunities and challenges. Adv Drug Res 22:39–106

Mohler MA, Tate K, Bringman TS, Fuller G, Keyt B, Vehar G, Hotchkiss AJ (1988) Circulatory metabolism of recombinant tissue type plasminogen activator in monkeys and rabbits. Fibrinolysis 2:17–23

Mohler MA, Cook J, Baumann G (1992) Binding proteins of protein therapeutics. In: Ferraiolo BL, Mohler MA, Gloff CA (eds) Protein pharmacokinetics and metabolism. Plenum, New York, pp 35–71

Mohler M, Cook J, Moore J, Lewis D, Sinicropi D, Championsmith A, Ferraiolo B (1993) Altered clearance of recombinant human deoxyribonuclease in rats due to the presence of a binding protein. Drug Metab Dispos 21:71–75

Moore JA, Marafino BJ, Stebbing N (1983) Influence of various purified interferons on effects of drugs in mice. Res Commun Chem Pathol Pharmacol 39: 113–125

Moore JA, Vandlen R, McKay P, Spencer SA (1988) Serum clearance of human growth hormone bound to growth hormone binding protein. Endocrinology 122 [Suppl]:121

Moore JA, Celniker A, Fuh G, Light D, McKay P, Spencer S (1989) Cloned human growth hormone binding protein effects on disposition of human growth hormone in rats. Proc US Endocrine Soc 71:435

Mordenti J, Green JD (1991) The role of pharmacokinetics and pharmacodynamics in the development of the therapeutic proteins. In: Rescigno A, Thakur A (eds) New trends in pharmacokinetics. Plenum, New York, p 411

Mordenti J, Chen SA, Moore JA, Ferraiolo BL, Green JD (1991) Interspecies scaling of clearance and volume of distribution data for five therapeutic proteins. Pharm Res 8:1351–1359

Mordenti J, Shaieb D, Chow P, Cossum P, Ferraiolo B, Lewandowski M, Moore J, Green JD (1994) Preclinical safety evaluation strategy for biomacromolecules – a perspective. In: Gad SC (ed) Safety assessment for pharmaceuticals. Van Nostrand Reinhold, Princeton (in press)

Mordenti J, Chen SA, Ferraiolo BL (1992) Pharmacokinetics of interferon-gamma. In: Kung AHC, Larrick JW, Baughman RA (eds) Therapeutics: protein pharmacokinetics and pharmacodynamics. New York, Freeman, pp 187–199

Nokta M, Loh JP, Douidar SM, Ahmed EA, Pollard RB (1991) Metabolic interaction of recombinant interferon-beta and zidovudine in AIDS patients. J Interferon Res 11:159–164

Offord RE, Philippe J, Davis JG, Halban PA, Berger M (1979) Inhibition of degradation of insulin by ophthalmic acid and a bovine pancreatic proteinase inhibitor. Biochem J 182:249–251

Okumura K, Komada F, Hori R (1985) Fate of porcine and human insulin at the subcutaneous injection site: I. Degradation and absorption of insulin in the rat. J Pharmacobiodyn 8:25–32

Ooi GT (1990) Insulin-like growth factor-binding proteins (IGFBPs): more than just 1,2,3. Mol Cell Endocrinol 7:C39–C43

Parkinson A, Lasker J, Kramer MJ, Huang M-T, Thomas PE, Ryan DE, Reik LM, Norman RL, Levin W, Conney AH (1982) Effects of three recombinant human leukocyte interferons on drug metabolism in mice. Drug Metab Dispos 10:579–585

Parsons JA, Rafferty B, Stevenson RW, Zanelli JM (1979) Evidence that protease inhibitors reduce the degradation of parathyroid hormone and calcitonin injected subcutaneously. Br J Pharmacol 66:25–32

Peck CC, Barr WH, Benet LZ, Collins J, Desjardins RE, Furst DE, Harter JG, Levy G, Ludden T, Rodman JH, Sanathanan L, Schentag JJ, Shah VP, Sheiner LB, Skelly JP, Stanski DR, Temple RJ, Viswanathan CT, Weisinger J, Yacobi A (1992) Opportunities for integration of pharmacokinetics, pharmacodynamics and toxicokinetics in rational drug development. Clin Pharmacol Ther 51:465–474

Philip A, O'Connor-McCourt MD (1991) Interaction of transforming growth factor-beta1 with alpha$_2$-macroglobulin. J Biol Chem 266:22290–22296

Podbesek R, Edouard C, Meunier PJ, Parsons JA, Reeve J, Stevenson RW, Zanelli JM (1983) Effects of two treatment regimes with synthetic human parathyroid hormone fragment on bone formation and the tissue balance of trabecular bone in greyhounds. Endocrinology 112:1000–1006

Rogers S, Wells R, Rechsteiner M (1986) Amino acid sequences common to rapidly degraded proteins: the PEST hypothesis. Science 234:364–368

Rosenbloom AL, Knuth C, Shulman D (1990) Growth hormone by daily injection in patients previously treated for growth hormone deficiency. South Med J 83:653–655

Rosenblum MG, Lamki LM, Murray JL, Carlo DJ, Gutterman JU (1988) Interferon-induced changes in pharmacokinetics and tumor uptake of [11]In-labeled anti-melanoma antibody 96.5 in melanoma patients. J Natl Cancer Inst 80:160–165

Rustgi VK, Suou T, Jones DB, Lisker-Melman M, Vergalla J, Jones EA, Hoffnagle JH (1987) The effect of rat gamma interferon on antipyrine metabolism by the isolated perfused rat liver. Clin Res 35:414A

Secor J, Schenker S (1984) Effect of recombinant alpha-interferon on in vivo and in vitro markers of drug metabolism in mice. Hepatology 4:1081

Shedlofsky SI, Swim AT, Robinson JM, Gallicchio VS, Cohen DA, McClain CJ (1987) Interleukin-1 (IL-1) depresses cytochrome P450 levels and activities in mice. Life Sci 40:2331–2336

Sherman B, Frane J (1988) Optimizing treatment of growth hormone deficiency (GHD): influence of growth hormone (GH) schedule and dose. The Endocrine Society 70th annual meeting, program and Abstracts, Abstract 406

Sherwood OD (1988) Relaxin. In: Knobil E, Neill J (eds) The physiology of reproduction. Raven, New York, p 585

Singh G, Renton KW, Stebbing N (1982) Homogeneous interferon from E. coli depresses hepatic cytochrome P450 and drug biotransformation. Biochem Biophys Res Commun 106:1256–1261

Sorensen JT, Colton CK, Hillman RS, Soeldner JS (1982) Use of a physiologic pharmacokinetic model of glucose homeostasis for assessment of performance requirements for improved insulin therapies. Diabetes Care 5:148–157

Spivak JL, Hogans BB (1989) The in vivo metabolism of recombinant human erythropoietin in the rat. Blood 73:90–99

Stoudemire JB (1992) Pharmacokinetics and metabolism of hematopoietic proteins. In: Ferraiolo BL, Mohler MA, Gloff CA (eds) Protein pharmacokinetics and metabolism. Plenum, New York, pp 189–222

Tam CS, Heersche JNM, Murray TM, Parsons JA (1982) Parathyroid hormone stimulates the bone apposition rate independently of its resorptive action: differential effects of intermittent and continuous administration. Endocrinology 110:506–512

Tanswell P, Seifried E, Stang E, Krause J (1991) Pharmacokinetics and hepatic catabolism of tissue-type plasminogen activator. Arzneimittelforschung/Drug Res 41II:1310–1319

Taylor G, Marafino BJ, Moore JA, Gurley V, Blaschke TF (1985) Interferon reduces hepatic drug metabolism in vivo in mice. Drug Metab Dispos 13:459–463

Tuvemo T (1989) What is the best mode of growth hormone administration. Act Paediatr Scand Suppl 362:44–49

Williams SJ, Farrell GC (1986) Inhibition of antipyrine metabolism by interferon. Br J Clin Pharmacol 22:610–612

Wills RJ (1990) Clinical pharmacokinetics of interferons. Clin Pharmacokinet 19:390–399

Wills RJ (1991) A kinetic/dynamic perspective of a peptide and a protein: GRF and rHuIFN-alpha2a. In: Garzone PD, Colburn WA, Mokotoff M (eds) Pharmacokinetics and pharmacodynamics: 3. Peptides, peptoids and proteins. Whitney, Cincinnati, p 116

Wills RJ (1994) Basic pharmacodynamic concepts and models. In: Cutler N, Narang PK (eds) Pharmacodynamics: perspectives in clinical pharmacology. Raven, New York (in press)

Wilson JT (1970) Alteration of normal development of drug metabolism by injection of growth hormone. Nature 225:861–863

Wilson JT, Frohman LA (1974) Concomitant association between high plasma levels of growth hormone and low mixed-function oxidase activity in the young rat. J Pharmacol Exp Ther 189:255–270

Wilton P, Widlund L, Guilbaud O (1987) Bioequivalence of Genotropin and Somatonorm. Acta Paediatr Scand Suppl 337:118–121

Wilton P, Widlund L, Vangbo B (1988) Pharmacokinetics of recombinant human growth hormone in healthy volunteers (in press)

Yamazoe Y, Shimada M, Kamataki T, Kato R (1986) Effects of hypophysectomy and growth hormone treatment on sex-specific forms of cytochrome P-450 in relation to drug and steroid metabolism in rat liver microsomes. Jpn J Pharmacol 42:371–382

Young JD, Bell DP, Luo ZP, Marian M, Bauer R (1990) Comparative pharmacokinetics of lymphokines, cytokines and antibodies from mouse to man. Drug Information Association Workshop, nonclinical development isues for biotechnology-derived products, San Diego

Zapf J, Hauri C, Waldvogel M, Froesch ER (1986) Acute metabolic effects and half lives of intravenous insulin like growth factor I and II in normal and hypophysectomized rats. J Clin Invest 77:1768–1775

Zapf J, Kiefer M, Merryweather J, Masiarz F, Bauer D, Born W, Fischer JA, Froesch ER (1990a) Isolation from adult human serum of four insulin-like growth factor (IGF) binding proteins and molecular cloning of one of them that is increased by IGF I administration and in extrapancreatic tumor hypoglycemia. J Biol Chem 265:14892–14898

Zapf J, Schmid C, Binz K, Guler HP, Froesch ER (1990b) Regulation and function of carrier proteins for insulin-like growth factors. In: Sara VR (ed) Growth factors: from genes to clinical application. Raven, New York, p 227

Zendegui JG, Vasquez KM, Tinsley JH, Kessler DJ, Hogan ME (1992) In vivo stability and kinetics of absorption and disposition of 3' phosphopropyl amino oligonucleotides. Nucleic Acids Res 20:307–314

Zon G (1988) Oligonucleotide analogues as potential chemotherapeutic agents. Pharm Res 5:539–549

CHAPTER 13
Peptide and Protein Drugs

C. McMartin

A. Introduction

Peptide and protein hormones and transmitters play a wide variety of extremely important regulatory roles in the body. A large number of these molecules have been isolated and shown to act as very potent messengers carrying specific signals between cells in the body. They frequently have valuable therapeutic properties. For some diseases the natural peptide may be used but often analogs of the peptides are used. An example of the first type of application is replacement therapy with insulin for diabetes or with growth hormone for pituitary deficiency. Where the natural peptide is not administered it may serve as a lead for products modified to improve biological specificity, to produce a receptor antagonist, or to optimize pharmacokinetic properties. Whether the peptide is administered as a natural or a modified product, understanding of the pharmacokinetics can be helpful in a variety of ways.

As with other drugs, frequency of administration and dose depend on pharmacokinetic properties as well as on the time course of the biological response. Frequently the short half-life and high clearance of peptides render pharmacokinetic considerations of prime importance. An understanding of the unique processing of peptides in the body is essential for the design and interpretation of pharmacokinetic and metabolism and excretion studies. Finally, knowledge of factors leading to rapid clearance can also be helpful for the design of compounds with improved properties.

I. Differences Between the Pharmacokinetics of Peptides/Proteins and Other Drugs

As shown in Table 1 and Fig. 1, peptides have a large number of properties which differentiate them from most other drugs.

Unlike many drugs, peptides and proteins, because of their polarity and size, do not passively cross cell membranes. They tend to be confined to the extracellar space at least during the distribution phase. Circulating peptides are often rapidly degraded by extracellular peptidases. Receptor-mediated clearance (see Sect. B.II.3) can also result in short half-lives. A short half-life is not, however, inevitable and arises from specific sequences or secondary structural features of the molecule.

Table 1. Differences between the pharmacokinetics of peptides/proteins and the majority of conventional drugs

Property	Typical values or behavior[a]	
	Peptides and proteins	Low-molecular-weight drugs
Plasma half-life	1–5 min	30 min–24 h
Volumes of distribution	0.04–0.20 l/kg	1–20 l/kg
Elimination mechanisms	Peptidolysis, receptor-mediated clearance	Oxidation, conjugation, active secretion
Tissues of clearance	Multiple, can include lungs muscle, skin, and brain	Liver, gut, kidneys
Cellular sites of clearance	Cell surface enzymes and receptors	Intracellular enzymes

[a] Listed are the types of properties the investigator should be prepared to find; significant exceptions occur (see Bennet and McMartin 1979b; McMartin 1992)

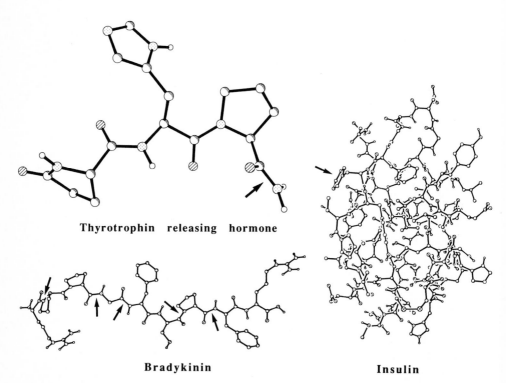

Thyrotrophin releasing hormone

Bradykinin

Insulin

Fig. 1. Three peptide hormones illustrating wide differences in complexity of structure and in mechanisms of inactivation in vivo. *Thyrotrophin releasing hormone* is inactivated by a plasma amidase which cleaves the bond indicated by the *arrow* with a half-time of around 3 min (Nair et al. 1971). *Bradykinin* is very rapidly degraded by cleavage of many peptide bonds indicated by the *arrows* (Ryan et al. 1970). It is degraded in plasma but even more rapidly in tissue beds so that its half-life is probably of the order of a few seconds. *Insulin* also has a short half-life of approximately 3 min. Mutation of the residue Phe-B25, shown by the *arrow*, results in a substantial increase in half-life and a reduction in receptor binding (Kobayashi et al. 1985)

Table 2. Roles of various tissues in pharmacokinetic processing of peptides and proteins. A few of these mechanisms are likely to dominate the pharmacokinetics of a given peptide or protein. For further details see text and McMartin (1989, 1992)

Tissue or organ	Pharmacokinetic functions
Plasma	Rapid cleavage of specific peptides; formation of inactive complexes with specific inactivator proteins
Lungs	Extensive inactivation or conversion of certain peptides in the capillary bed
Kidneys	Glomerular filtration; post-filtration brush-border degradation and/or resorption; cleavage and/or receptor-mediated clearance in peritubular capillaries
Liver	Receptor-mediated clearance; biliary excretion
Muscle/skin	Large extracellular distribution volume; extensive single-passage degradation of certain peptides
Brain	Blood-brain barrier impermeable to most peptides; several ectopeptidases with highly individual distribution patterns line the intracellular space

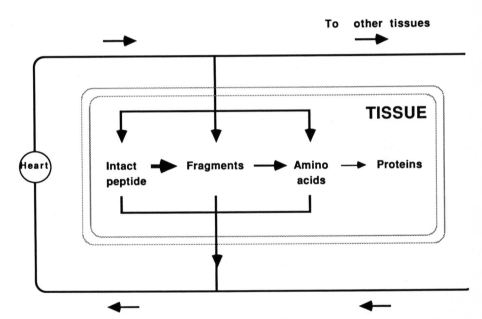

Fig. 2. Processing of circulating intact peptide and peptide fragments during passage through a metabolically active tissue bed. Usually several tissue beds will be involved in catabolism as a result of which a very complex mixture of peptide fragments appears in the circulation within 1 or 2 min after administration (Bennett and McMartin 1979a; Hudson and McMartin 1980). Also shown is conversion of liberated amino acid into protein. This process usually occurs more slowly than initial degradation but makes it impossible to carry out simple mass balance elimination studies for most peptides. It can also lead to artifacts in whole-body autoradiography studies. Typically at early times bone marrow and the gut mucosa, which have a high intrinsic rate of protein synthesis, incorporate liberated labeled amino acids

Peptides and proteins typically have multiple mechanisms of inactivation giving rise to a large number of primary and secondary products (Table 2, Fig. 2).

Although the properties summarized above make the study of pharmacokinetics of peptides and proteins challenging, a considerable amount can be learnt from careful interpretation of suitably designed experiments.

II. Scope of This Review

A number of reviews on peptide pharmacokinetics are available (broad coverage: HUMPHREY and RINGROSE 1986; McMARTIN 1989; BENNETT and McMARTIN 1979b; specific topics: RABKIN and KITAJI 1983; MAACK et al. 1985). A more recent review covers mechanisms of distribution and clearance of peptides and proteins in considerable detail (McMARTIN 1992). The main part (Sect. C) of the present survey, therefore, concentrates on experimental aspects of the subject and especially on the design and interpretation of experiments. This section is preceded by background information on major mechanisms of distribution and clearance.

B. Pharmacokinetic Mechanisms

When a drug is administered its subsequent concentration at any specific point in the body depends on two quite distinct types of phenomenon, namely, transport and elimination. Since these processes are usually occurring at the same time it can be difficult to separate them experimentally, especially for molecules where elimination is rapid and strongly influences the observed distribution even at very early times. It is useful, however, to consider the properties of these individual processes separately.

I. Distribution in the Body

Once a molecule has reached the circulation it will be transported through all the capillary beds of all the tissues in the human body within 1 min (a shorter time in smaller animals). Studies with stable water-soluble molecules show that these leave the blood vessels and enter the interstitial space (the fluid lying between the cells of the tissue) at a rate depending on molecular weight and permeability of the specific tissue (LANDIS and PAPPENHEIMER 1963; CRONE and LEVITT 1984; TAYLOR and GRANGER 1984). The exchange process is passive and reversible. For small molecules the rate of exchange is so rapid that distribution into the tissue occurs at the rate of supply through the blood and takes only a few minutes.

For higher molecular weight products the rate of entry into the interstitial space may be lower than the rate of exit through lymphatic drainage so that tissue concentration may never reach the plasma value even if no degradation takes place. Factors other than molecular weight, such as charge and lipophilicity, may modify distribution but there is no evidence to suggest that they have large effects. It may be necessary to take selective transport processes into account for some peptides. However, a reasonable if approximate model for the kinetics of many peptides does not appear to require such mechanisms (McMARTIN 1992).

II. Inactivation and Elimination

A large number of mechanisms can operate to eliminate active peptides from the circulation or extracellular space. Although there are obviously opportunities for multiple clearance processes to act simultaneously, for certain peptides it is clear that one or two processes play a dominant role.

1. Glomerular Filtration

Molecules of molecular weight less than 20 000 readily pass the glomerular barrier. The process is usually slow compared to other mechanisms of clearance. When it is the major mechanism it gives rise to plasma half-lives of 20–40 min. Peptides are often resorbed and degraded extensively once filtered so that urinary excretion of products is an unreliable guide to clearance by filtration (MAACK et al. 1985).

2. Peptidolysis

Proteins and especially peptides of lower molecular weight are often inactivated by peptidases. These may be present as soluble enzymes in plasma or as ectoenzymes, i.e., enzymes bound to the plasma membranes of specific cells in an orientation which presents the catalytic site to molecules in extracellular fluid bathing the cell (KENNY et al. 1987). Peptidases are very efficient at hydrolyzing peptide bonds of appropriate specificity. They are of high selectivity but it is difficult to predict which bonds in a peptide sequence will be susceptible to cleavage. Proteins with well-formed tertiary structures present fewer targets for peptidase action.

3. Receptor-Mediated Clearance

The rate-limiting step for elimination is formation of a noncovalent complex between peptide and cell surface receptor (MAACK et al. 1987; SATO et al. 1988). The complex is internalized inside the cell and transported to the lysosome, where degradation to amino acids occurs. A similar process can occur where the complex is formed with a soluble circulating protein (BACHMANN and KRUITHOF 1984).

III. Uptake from Site of Administration

A comprehensive recent review of this topic is available (MACKAY 1990).

1. Subcutaneous or Intramuscular Injection

As a rule small peptides enter the bloodstream over a 10- to 30-min period after subcutaneous or intramuscular injection. Depot or controlled-release formulations can be used to produce tailored plasma concentration–time profiles (MACKAY 1990).

2. Intranasal Administration

Intranasal administration is an efficient route of administration for products of up to 1 kDa. Uptake occurs within 10–15 min of administration (CHIEN and CHANG 1985; McMARTIN et al. 1987; FISHER 1990). Uptake of larger molecular weight substances can be enhanced with adjuvant (LEE and LONGENECKER 1988).

3. Oral or Rectal Administration

Uptake following oral or rectal administration is usually poor unless adjuvants are used. A considerable amount of work has been carried out in this area (MACKAY 1990).

IV. Pharmacokinetic Behavior Resulting from the Distribution and Elimination Processes

When a peptide is administered intravenously the blood levels typically drop very rapidly to rather low concentrations. At this time both distribution and degradation are likely to make major contributions to the rate of decline.

If the peptide is measured with a sensitive assay, a second slower period of decline will often be observed. The peptide continues to be degraded but now redistribution is occurring from the interstitial spaces of tissues that have become equilibrated with peptide which survived degradation or elimination during the early phase (McMARTIN 1992).

Where clearance is by glomerular filtration or peptidolysis, linear pharmacokinetics can be expected over a wide range of concentrations. Receptor-mediated clearance may become saturated at low concentrations, making it essential to work in the physiological range to obtain reliable information.

C. Experimental Approaches

The study of the pharmacokinetics of peptides and proteins is complicated by two factors: (a) a lack of totally specific analytical methods to assay pure substance and to separate and identify the large numbers of metabolites that may be formed (see Fig. 1); (b) a complex, rapidly changing pattern of peptides, peptide fragments, and amino acids (see Table 2 and Fig. 2).

I. Analytical Methods

There is usually no single assay method which will resolve and measure exactly the small amounts of all the molecular species involved in a peptide metabolism study in vivo. It is important to bear in mind the limitations of each method and to use the method most appropriate to the questions under investigation.

1. Ex Vivo Bioassay

Samples removed from the animal are subjected to an in vitro bioassay. If the functional basis for the bioassay is related to the desired therapeutic effect, bioassay can give very useful information on the plasma kinetics of bioactive material. The limitation of this technique is that bioactive fragments may be included in the measurement so the results cannot be used to establish absolute information about pharmacokinetic parameters such as clearance or volume of distribution.

2. Radioimmunoassay

Specificity can be a major problem with radioimmunoassays. It is necessary to make sure that the assay is specific for the peptide being studied and essential to make sure that partially or completely inactive metabolic products of the peptide being studied do not cross-react. If inactive fragments cross-react the assay can be misleading.

3. Radiolabeling

Tritium and carbon-14 labeling require moderately large doses of material which must be specially synthesized. High specific activity iodine labeling is often used since the labeling is easy to perform and very small amounts of material can be detected. Iodination, however, may modify metabolic behavior and where possible this should be tested [e.g., by measuring the bioactivity of labeled product, comparing plasma decay curves of bioactivity versus radiolabel separated by high-performance liquid chromatography (HPLC) after intravenous administration].

4. High-Performance Liquid Chromatography

The discovery that peptides could be rapidly separated at high resolution and in high yield on reversed-phase HPLC columns has proved to be very helpful for peptide metabolism studies (BENNETT et al. 1977). This method can be combined with the use of radiolabel to measure fragment profiles in plasma and other tissues. It can also be used to investigate the specificity of other assay methods, e.g., to find out whether a radioimmunoassay or bioassay method is measuring products other than intact peptide.

5. Radiosequencing

An interesting and potentially powerful approach to metabolite identification is radiosequencing of complex mixtures of unseparated products which have been specifically labeled in a known position (CONDRA et al. 1988).

II. Plasma Pharmacokinetics

Before carrying out in vivo or tissue perfusion studies, the stability of peptide in plasma or whole blood should be tested. When collecting blood samples the use of anticoagulant is essential since many peptides are degraded as soon as the clotting cascade is activated. If the peptide is unstable in plasma, then addition of acid or effective peptidase inhibitors will be necessary during sample collection.

1. Intravenous Bolus and Infusion Studies

The simplest type of whole animal experiment is to study plasma concentrations of peptide and peptide fragments after intravenous bolus administration or infusion. A variety of types of assay can be used for such studies.

2. Methods of Assaying Samples

Where bioassay or radioimmunoassay has been used it may be possible to introduce an HPLC step to ascertain whether fragments are being formed which are positive in the assay. For radiolabeling studies a chromatographic step is essential.

3. Information That Can Be Derived from Plasma Pharmacokinetic Studies

If intact peptide can be measured the plasma concentrations can be analyzed using compartmental analysis to obtain estimates of half-lives, clearance rates, and volumes of distribution (McMARTIN 1992). This can be useful for comparing peptide analogs to find out exactly how modifications of structure affect pharmacokinetic properties.

Where radiolabeling and HPLC are used, the rates of formation of fragments and appearance of free amino acids can also be observed. Usually this process occurs very rapidly. It may be possible to isolate products from the plasma, identify them, and in this way characterize the likely cleavage steps leading to inactivation in vivo (HUDSON and McMARTIN 1992).

Where inhibitors of the relevant enzymes are available it may be possible to assess their effect on the clearance rate of the peptide in vivo and thus the quantitative significance of a particular enzymatic process for clearance.

4. Use of Organ Ablation to Locate Clearance Sites

When experiments are performed under anesthesia it is possible to observe the effect of removal of organs on plasma pharmacokinetic parameters.

Caution is needed in interpreting the results. Ligation or ablation will result in a redistribution of cardiac output to other tissues and thus alter clearance rates.

III. Distribution, Metabolism, and Elimination

1. Typical Experiments and Results

Labeled material is usually injected rapidly by the intravenous route and the animal killed during the 30s to 1h range. Blood and tissues are removed and processed as rapidly as possible. Where the peptide is unstable in plasma, acidification or trichloracetic acid (TCA) treatment may be required. The tissues must be rapidly homogenized in a medium which totally inactivates peptidases. Failure to do this may result in the conversion of the peptide to multiple fragments or amino acids. The extracts are analyzed by HPLC. The outcome of such experiments is usually to find a large number of fragments within 1 min of injection and virtually complete conversion of the dose to free amino acids within a few minutes (BENNETT and McMARTIN 1979a).

2. Difficulties in Interpreting Results

The speed of degradation to free amino acids and redistribution of labeled products throughout the body makes it hard to interpret the data from such experiments. These experiments initially were of interest because they demonstrated convincingly the extremely rapid and thorough inactivating mechanisms for peptides which are present in the body. They are less useful for locating specific mechanisms of inactivation for a peptide.

Once a fragment has been formed it can rapidly distribute throughout the body. However, some tissues are observed to accumulate intact peptide or fragments and this has proved of interest for elucidation of clearance mechanisms (MAACK et al. 1985). Ultrastructural studies of uptake in the kidney reveal a powerful resorption mechanism in the proximal tubule (BAKER et al. 1977).

A caveat is necessary concerning the interpretation of urinary excretion data. The appearance of a specific fragment in the urine does not mean that this occurs in plasma. Renal tubules are rich in peptidases, allowing degradation to take place post-filtration (BENNETT and McMARTIN 1979b).

3. Problems in Carrying Out Drug Elimination Studies

For a new product studies are usually required to show that accumulation of drug or metabolites does not occur. For a labeled peptide a balance study is not possible because the amino acids in the peptide rapidly become incorporated into endogenous protein. To quantitate accumulation requires an approach which either prevents incorporation of amino acids into protein or measures the extent of incorporation. Where products contain nonnatural molecular features it may be desirable to specifically label these parts and study the distribution and elimination of radiolabel.

IV. Organ Clearance

The contribution of an organ to clearance can be estimated directly by measurement of the arteriovenous difference of peptide across the organ while arterial blood concentration remains constant. These investigations are often carried out in animal models (SINGER et al. 1972) and can sometimes be carried out in man (CROZIER et al. 1986). This is a very powerful method for quantitatively determining the clearance role of various tissues.

V. Receptor-Mediated Clearance Kinetics

With the demonstration using isolated cell systems that peptides and proteins can be internalized and degraded once bound to receptors, it became clear that in addition to the possibility of inactivation by peptidases a major alternative mechanism must be considered.

Detailed studies of receptor-mediated peptide clearance have been carried out with isolated perfused liver (SATO et al. 1988) and kidney (SUZUKI et al. 1987) and in the intact animal (MAACK et al. 1987; KIM et al. 1988).

VI. Absorption (Bioavailability) Measurement

The assessment of the effectiveness of routes of administration other than the intravenous route is often an important experimental requirement. The standard method for doing this is to compare the area under a plasma time curve obtained after intravenous dosage with that obtained by the test route of administration. For these studies the precautions mentioned in Sect. C.II clearly also apply. Inclusion of an inactive fragment in the assay result will tend to lead to overestimation of the bioavailability since the fragment may form before the drug can enter the circulation. In addition care should be taken to work, if possible, with doses where pharmacokinetics are linear. This can be assessed using intravenous doses to investigate the relationship between the area under the curve and dose. The doses used must give plasma concentrations in the range found using the test route of administration.

1. Oral Route

A number of animal models can be used to investigate oral bioavailability. Care should be taken to ensure that the mucosa is not damaged by the operation or by any adjuvants that are used. In man different regions of the intestine can be accessed by use of endoscopy to place a delivery cannula in the appropriate region.

2. Nasal Route

Sample can be placed in the nasal cavity by spray or as a measured volume in conscious man and larger animals. An anesthetized rat model developed by HIRAI et al. (1981) is useful for comparing bioavailability of experimental compounds under controlled conditions.

D. Conclusions

Although the mechanisms for processing peptides are diverse and the spectrum of products of metabolism is large, it is possible to obtain answers to many of the more important questions concerning their distribution and fate in the body. It is important to realize at the outset of such a study that the assumptions made about low-molecular-weight drugs may not apply so that questions may need to be carefully defined if meaningful answers are to be obtained.

Pharmacokinetic procedures can be used to determine plasma concentration profiles of peptides and peptide analogs. It has also proved possible to identify critical steps in the processing of a peptide and to design resistant molecules or inhibitors. It is not clear at present exactly how to evaluate products derived from proteins or peptides for safety. Perhaps some of the results of the extensive investigations summarized and reviewed briefly in this chapter will help to provide a solution.

References

Bachmann F, Kruithof EKO (1984) Tissue plasminogen activator: chemical and physiological aspects. Semin Thromb Haemost 10:6–17

Baker JRJ, Bennett HPJ, Christian RA, McMartin C (1977) Renal uptake and metabolism of adrenocorticotrophin analogues in the rat: an autoradiographic study. J Endocr 74:23–35

Bennett HPJ, McMartin C (1979a) Distribution and degradation of two tritium-labelled corticotrophin analogues in the rat. J Endocr 82:33–42

Bennett HPJ, McMartin C (1979b) Peptide hormones and their analogues: distribution, clearance from the circulation and inactivation. Pharmacol Rev 30:247–292

Bennett HPJ, Hudson AM, McMartin C, Purdon GE (1977) Use of octadecasilyl-silica for the extraction and purification of peptides in biological samples. Biochem J 168:9–13

Chien YW, Chang SF (1985) Historic development of transnasal systemic medications. In: Chien YW (ed) Transnasal medications. Elsevier, Amsterdam, pp 1–99

Condra CL, Leidy EA, Bunting P, Colton CD, Nutt RF, Rosenblatt M, Jacobs JW (1988) Clearance and early hydrolysis of atrial natriuretic factor in vivo. J Clin Invest 81:1348–1354

Crone C, Levitt DG (1984) Capillary permeability of small solutes. In: Hamilton WF (ed) Handbook of physiology, vol VI. American Physiological Society, Washington, pp 411–466

Crozier IG, Nicholls MG, Ikram H, Espiner EA, Yandle TG, Jans S (1986) Atrial natriuretic peptide in humans. Production and clearance by various tissues. Hypertension 8[Suppl II]:11–15

Fisher AN (1990) Absorption across the nasal mucosa of animal species: compounds applied and mechanisms involved. In: Gibson GG (ed) Progress in drug metabolism, vol 12. Taylor and Francis, London, pp 87–145

Hirai S, Yashiki T, Matsuzawa T, Mima H (1981) Absorption of drugs from the nasal mucosa of rat. Int J Pharm 7:317–325

Hudson AM, McMartin C (1980) Mechanisms of catabolism of corticotrophin-(1–24)-tertacosapeptide in the rat in vivo. J Endocr 85:92–103

Humphrey MJ, Ringrose PS (1986) Peptides and related drugs: a review of their absorption, metabolism and excretion. Drug Metab Rev 17:283–310

Kenny AJ, Stephenson SL, Turner AJ (1987) Cell surface peptidases. In: Kenny AJ, Turner AJ (eds) Mammalian ectoenzymes. Elsevier, Amsterdam, pp 169–210

Kim DC, Sugiyama T, Satoh H, Fuwa T, Iga T, Hanano M (1988) Kinetic analysis of in vivo receptor-dependent binding of human epidermal growth factor by rat tissues. J Pharm Sci 77:200–206

Kobayashi M, Ishibashi O, Takata Y, Haneda M, Maegawa H, Watanabe N, Shigeta Y (1985) Prolonged disappearance rate of a structurally abnormal mutant insulin from the circulation in humans. J Endocr Metab 61:1142–1144

Landis EM, Pappenheimer JR (1963) Exchange of substances through the capillary wall. In: Hamilton WF (ed) Handbook of physiology, sect 2, vol 2. American Society of Physiology, Washington, pp 961–1003

Lee WA, Longenecker JP (1988) Intranasal delivery of proteins and peptides. Biopharmacology 1:30–37

Maack T, Park CH, Camargo MJ (1985) Renal filtration, transport, and metabolism of peptides. In: Selin DW, Giebisch G (eds) The kidney: physiology and pathophysiology. Raven, New York, pp 1773–1803

Maack T, Suzuki M, Almeida FA, Nussenzveig D, Scarborough RM, McEnroe GA, Lewicki JA (1987) Physiological role of silent receptors of atrial natriuretic factor. Science 238:675–678

Mackay M (1990) Delivery of recombinant peptide and protein drugs. Biotech Protein Eng Rev 8:251–278

McMartin C (1989) Molecular seiving, receptor processing and peptidolysis as major determinants of peptide pharmacokinetics in vivo. Biochem Soc Trans 17:931–934

McMartin C (1992) Pharmacokinetics of peptides and proteins: opportunities and challenges. In: Testa B (ed) Advances in drug research. Academic, London, p 40

McMartin C, Hutchinson LEF, Hyde R, Peters GE (1987) Analysis of structural requirements for the absorption of drugs and macromolecules from the nasal cavity. J Pharm Sci 76:535–540

Nair RMG, Redding TW, Schally AV (1971) Site of inactivation of thyrotrophin releasing hormone by human plasma. Biochemistry 10:3621–3624

Rabkin R, Kitaji J (1983) Renal metabolism of peptide hormones. Miner Electrolyte Metab 9:212–226

Ryan JW, Roblero J, Stewart JM (1970) Inactivation of bradykinin in rat lung. Adv Exp Med Biol 8:263–271

Sato H, Sugiyama Y, Sawada Y, Iga T, Sakamoto S, Fuwa T, Hanano M (1988) Dynamic determination of kinetic parameters for the interaction between polypeptide hormones and cell-surface receptors in the perfused rat liver by the multiple indicator dilution method. Proc Natl Acad Sci USA 85:8355–8359

Singer FR, Habener JF, Greene E, Godin P, Potts JT (1972) Inactivation of calcitonin by specific organs. Nature New Biol 237:269–270

Suzuki M, Almeida FA, Nussenzweig DR, Sawyer D, Maack T (1987) Binding and functional effects of atrial natriuretic factor in isolated rat kidney. 253:F917–F928

Taylor AE, Granger DN (1984) Exchange of macromolecules across the microcirculation. In: Hamilton WF (ed) Handbook of physiology, vol VI. American Physiological Society, Washington, pp 467–520

CHAPTER 14

Toxicokinetics

J. Kantrowitz and A. Yacobi

A. Introduction

Toxicokinetics is defined as the application of pharmacokinetics to doses used in toxicology testing. As part of the safety evaluation of a new chemical entity (NCE), acute, range-finding, and pivotal toxicity studies are conducted to characterize the safety and target organ toxicity in two or three animal species. Doses employed in these studies are often 10- to 1000-fold greater than the doses used to assess the pharmacology in the preclinical testing of NCEs. Until recently, most pharmacokinetic evaluation of NCEs was conducted at pharmacologically relevant doses, often using different species or strains of animals, vehicles, fed/fasting conditions, sexes, and age of the animals than are used in the safety evaluation studies.

Extrapolation of the pharmacokinetics from pharmacology doses to the high doses and experimental conditions employed in the safety evaluation studies are often not meaningful. Thus, the need to establish toxicokinetic programs to characterize the pharmacokinetics unique to the high doses used in toxicology studies has become readily apparent. Investigational new drug (IND) applications for NCEs now routinely include toxicokinetic data. These data are utilized to support exposure level and safety claims at different dose levels.

B. Principles of Toxicokinetics

The implementation of a toxicokinetics program can be done in a manner which will facilitate protocol design, dosing regimen selection, and interpretation of safety findings by toxicologists without compromising the primary objectives of the study. For example, a sufficient number of blood samples should be collected in order to determine appropriate pharmacokinetic parameters – usually C_{max}, t_{max}, AUC, and $t_{1/2}$ after oral dosing and also Vd_{ss} and CL_T after intravenous dosing – without jeopardizing the health of the animals and proper interpretation of the toxicity data.

The primary goals of the toxicokinetic studies are: (a) to ensure "adequate" exposure to the NCE in the pivotal toxicity studies; (b) to determine the time course of this exposure; (c) to determine the relationship between the extent of absorption of the NCE and the dose; (d) to evaluate the changes in the pharmacokinetics of the NCE upon multiple dosing; and (e) to determine a possible relationship between exposure (C_{max} and/ or AUC) and toxicity findings. This information can be extremely important to toxicologists to allow proper design of safety studies (SMYTH and HOTTENDORF 1980). Also, these findings are important as they provide information for the development of a proper dosing regimen, under which no untoward accumulation of toxic parent or metabolite compound occurs. Thus, a rapid turnaround time for the toxicokinetic data, discussions of relevant findings between pharmacokineticist and toxicologist, and collaborative planning for the successive study designs are all necessary components if the goals of these studies as outlined above are to be achieved.

The types of toxicology study usually supported by toxicokinetic data include acute, 2-week range-finding, and pivotal chronic studies in two species, usually a rodent (rat) and a large animal (dog or monkey). For the acute studies, the doses are often very high and the dosing schedule is so irregular that pharmacokinetic support for these studies may not always be required at this early stage. The range-finding studies, therefore, are often the first studies supported with toxicokinetic data and are sometimes the only studies which provide information on the dose-relativeness of absorption and effects of multiple dosing on the pharmacokinetics of an NCE provided in an IND submission. The availability of dose proportionality data prior to the start of the 2-week studies can contribute to the optimum design of these studies.

Long-range toxicology studies, including 1-month, 3-month, 6-month, and 1-year studies may be routinely supported with toxicokinetic data, usually for the first and final days of dosing, and sometimes 1 or 2 days in between. Other toxicology studies for which toxicokinetic information has become a necessary and useful component are the range-finding and pivotal carcinogenicity studies in mice and rats and the reproduction and fertility studies conducted in mice, rats, and rabbits.

Different approaches are often used to support the toxicokinetic program. In most instances, pharmacokinetic aspects of these studies are integrated into the toxicology study design. For rodent studies, satellite groups of animals may be used. For the large species, the same animals evaluated by the toxicologists may be used for pharmacokinetic purposes. In these studies, as many as five or six samples/day from several animals per timepoint may be taken. Alternatively, independent toxicokinetic studies may be conducted in order to characterize further the pharmacokinetics of the NCE. If the assay sensitivity to measure the NCE in plasma is inadequate or if sample volume is insufficient for quantitation of the NCE in the biological sample, the use of radiolabeled compound may become necessary.

C. Bioanalytical Procedures to Support Toxicokinetic Studies

Once an NCE has been selected for further development as a clinical lead, a preclinical program is developed to support an IND package and subsequent initiation of dosing in man. Among the highest priorities is the development of methodologies for the quantitation of drug (and possibly drug metabolite) concentrations in biological fluids to support preclinical and, hopefully, eventual clinical pharmacokinetic studies (MONRO 1976). These methodologies should be specific, sensitive, and reproducible. If accurate quantitation is in question, then all results and conclusions derived from the analytical data will be in doubt (GRAVES et al. 1989). These methods should also be rugged and able to handle the large volume of samples generated from these preclinical studies. The methods often employed to handle routine sample analyses are high-performance liquid chromatography with either UV or fluorescence detection; other methodologies, such as gas chromatography and radioimmunoassay are used, as well as other detection systems, but less frequently.

During the initial stages of a preclinical drug development program, it is possible that sample analyses may potentially become rate limiting, thereby delaying the conduct of these studies, which may include the toxicokinetic studies. Careful planning and consideration of the following points may ensure a smoother path to the IND: (a) the availability of specific methodologies; (b) quality assurance and methods validation (to assure ruggedness of the assay); (c) revalidation of the assay at each site of analysis prior to utilization of these methods; (d) feedback and adjustments when needed on the assay sensitivity requirements (during different stages of drug development); (e) fine tuning and modification of the assay conditions due to endogenous interfering substances resulting from different species or populations; and (f) timing for sample analysis turnaround (which could influence the pace of drug development).

Special consideration must be given to the bioanalytical support of the toxicokinetic studies. While the initial acute toxicity studies are exploratory and "non-GLP" (non-good laboratory practices), the pivotal multiple dose toxicity studies which require the bulk of pharmacokinetic support are GLP studies and therefore require validated analytical methods. Furthermore, these methods must be validated in the biological matrices of the species to be evaluated in these toxicology studies, usually rodent (rat) and dog (or monkey) plasma. Stability of drug in the biological matrices, for short durations at room temperature and long durations in the freezer, should be established and communicated to the appropriate study personnel prior to the start of these studies to ensure analysis of nondegraded sample. In these studies, dosing solutions are also analyzed for drug content and stability to ensure proper dosing of the animals.

Assay parameter requirements are unique for the toxicokinetic studies. While assay sensitivity is usually not as critical in these studies due to the very high doses given, the concentration range of the validated assay method should be wide enough to support the anticipated high plasma concentrations from these studies. The volume of sample required for analysis may become an issue, particularly in the rodent studies, due to the volume constraints associated with using satellite animals for the toxicology studies. Therefore, consideration of these issues should be enlisted during assay development.

Preliminary pharmacokinetic information may also influence the bioanalytical methodology employed for the toxicokinetic studies. If a compound has been observed to partition into red blood cells, then the development of an assay for measuring drug in whole blood may be warranted for these studies. If early metabolism work suggests significant metabolism, particularly formation of an active metabolite(s), methods to measure both unchanged drug and primary metabolite(s) should be developed. Early pharmacokinetic information is vital in order to develop a meaningful toxicokinetic profile of a compound.

Finally, bioanalytical support of a toxicokinetic program should include the handling of a large number of samples generated from these studies and the analysis of these samples in a timely fashion to ensure that a study's findings are properly evaluated prior to the start of the subsequent studies.

D. Dose–Plasma Concentration Relationship (Linear–Nonlinear Kinetics)

In safety evaluation studies, doses are selected to represent increasing multiples of the intended dose to be targeted in the clinic, the rationale being that these doses will reflect a certain margin of safety for the human trials. Toxicological doses are relatively large and usually much greater than the pharmacologically active dose. Unless there is a linear relationship between these doses and the achieved plasma concentrations of the NCE, the actual margin of safety may be much different than that anticipated by inspection of the doses alone. Therefore, it is essential to know what the relative bioavailability is at all dose levels (Hawkins and Chasseaud 1985). Since absorption process(es) may become saturated at higher doses, it is critical to ascertain the relationship between the extent of bioavailability and the dose. This information may prove to be very important in substantiating the safety claims for each given dose.

An example of an NCE showing linear drug exposure after oral dosing is illustrated in Fig. 1. As shown, increasing the dose from 10 to 40 mg/kg results in dose proportional increases in plasma drug concentrations (Fig. 1a) and a linear increase in the extent of absorption, as reflected in the area under the plasma concentration vs time curve (AUC) (Fig. 1b). In certain cases, the extent of exposure will remain the same but the rate of absorption

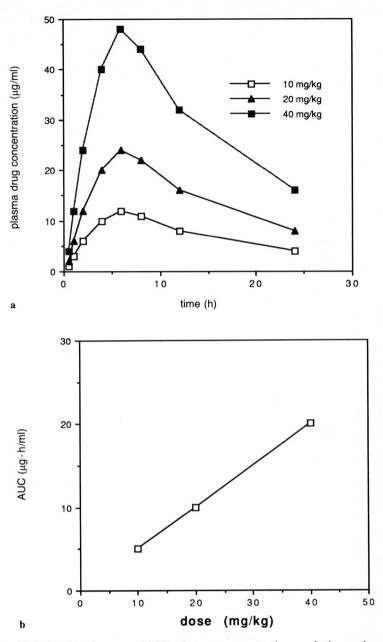

Fig. 1. a Relationship between NCE plasma concentration and time when the absorption is linear. **b** Relationship between area under the plasma concentration-time curve and dose when the absorption is linear

may change with increasing dose (Fig. 2). In this case, there is a change in both the peak concentration (C_{max}) and time to peak (t_{max}) with increasing dose. This may be of importance if either the pharmacological or the toxicological threshold concentration is being achieved.

When absorption processes are saturated, increases in the dose do not result in a proportional increase in drug exposure. This is depicted in Fig. 3. As can be seen, at the highest dose, there is no further increase in plasma concentrations (Fig. 3a) or in the AUC (Fig. 3b). Many factors can influence the absorption of a compound, including the gastrointestinal (GI) motility, the presence of food, gastric emptying, disease state, blood flow, and age. In many instances, saturable absorption is observed in a particular species due to the physiochemical properties of the NCE. In other words, at high doses, solubility constraints of the NCE in the dosing vehicle or degradation of the NCE due to pKa/pH factors in the GI tract most often play a role (Welling 1984). In this case, the exposure level will be dependent on the rate and extent of absorption and the safety claim will be governed by the plasma concentrations of the NCE and not the dose.

Alternatively, a situation may occur in which greater than proportional increases in the extent of drug exposure are observed with increasing dose (Fig. 4). An example would be compounds which are subject to extensive first-pass metabolism in the liver after oral administration. Another example would be an NCE which has saturable binding to either plasma proteins or red blood cells, resulting in increasing concentrations of free drug at these higher doses. In either case, a greater extent of exposure is observed, resulting in an increase in effect proportional to plasma concentrations of the NCE (total or free) and not proportional to the dose.

When nonlinear kinetics are observed in the safety evaluation studies, it is incumbent upon the toxicokineticist to communicate the data promptly. The findings may have important implications in the design of the subsequent toxicity studies since they will influence how high the doses should be in these studies and in the clinical studies, which are dependent on exposure levels in animals. In addition, the toxicokineticist can suggest ways in which the absorption may be enhanced at the higher doses if deemed necessary. Recommendations would include: (a) determining the effect of food, (b) changing the drug delivery vehicle, (c) using enteric-coated capsules to bypass acidic gastric medium, and (d) in extreme cases, using different routes of administration.

Thus, the role of toxicokinetics is important since it assists in the selection of a dosing regimen and an optimum drug delivery vehicle or route of administration based on both achieved toxicity and adequate drug exposure, including dose-related exposure. In addition, the toxicokinetic data will offer the opportunity to determine a more accurate safety margin of an NCE based on observed exposure level instead of on dose, an assessment often made inaccurately when absorption is either incomplete or saturable.

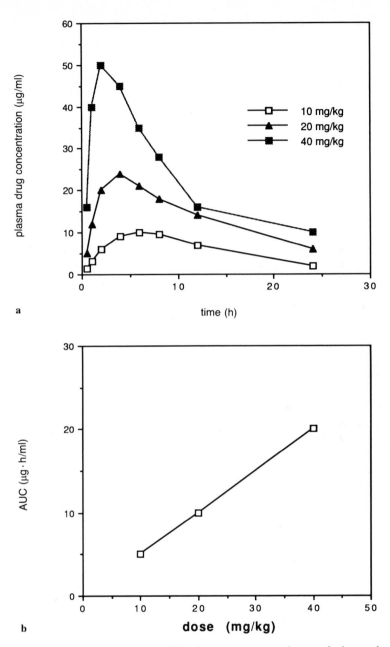

a

b

Fig. 2. a Relationship between NCE plasma concentration and time when the absorption rate changes with increasing dose. **b** Relationship between area under the plasma concentration-time curve and dose showing no change in exposure concurrent with a change in the rate of absorption

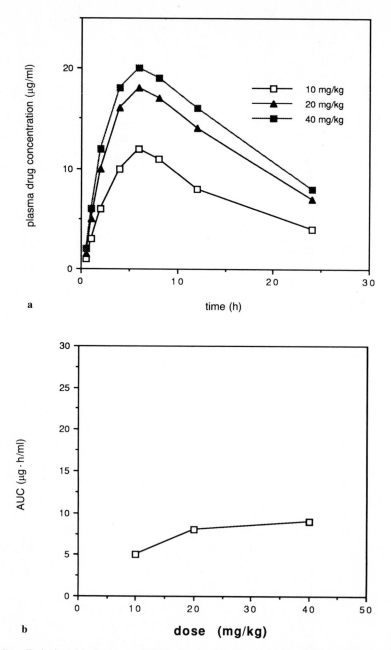

Fig. 3. a Relationship between NCE plasma concentration and time when nonlinear absorption results in smaller than proportional increases in drug concentrations at higher doses. **b** Relationship between area under the plasma concentration-time curve and dose showing nonlinear (less than proportional) absorption with increasing dose

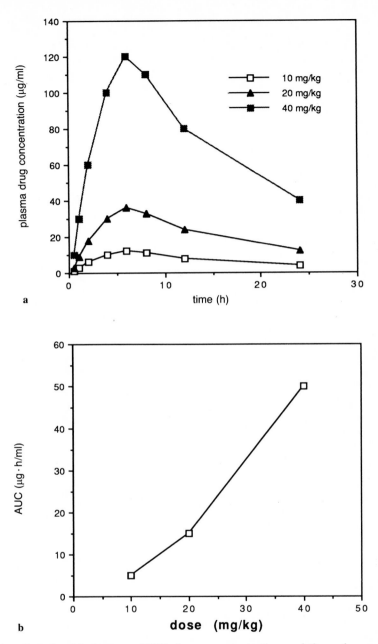

Fig. 4. a Relationship between NCE plasma concentration and time when nonlinear exposure results in greater than proportional increases in drug concentrations at higher doses. **b** Relationship between area under the plasma concentration-time curve and dose showing nonlinear (greater than proportional) drug exposure with increasing dose

E. Changes in Concentrations upon Multiple Dosing

In safety evaluation studies, where eliciting severe toxicity and mortality is not the intended endpoint, monitoring plasma concentrations may be useful to avoid unexpected accumulation of and excessive exposure to an NCE or its metabolites in the body (YACOBI et al. 1982). Assuming linear kinetics, the extent to which this accumulation will occur can be predicted based on the equation:

$$R_{ac} = \frac{1}{(1 - e^{-k\tau})}$$

where R_{ac} is the accumulation ratio, k is the elimination rate constant, and τ is the dosing interval. Thus, accumulation is based on the half-life of a compound and the frequency of dosing. For example, for an NCE with a 24-h half-life ($k = 0.0289\,h^{-1}$) dosed once a day ($\tau = 24\,h$), the R_{ac} value will equal 2 (Fig. 5a). Whenever a compound is dosed once every half-life, the expected accumulation will be a twofold increase in plasma concentrations. If, however, the half-life greatly exceeds the dosing interval, more significant accumulation can occur (Fig. 5b). For example, if an NCE has a half-life of 24 h but is dosed every 6 h, an accumulation ratio greater than 6 would be expected. As can be seen, accumulation occurs because drug from previous doses has not been completely removed. An important consideration, then, in the design of safety evaluation studies is defining a dosing frequency which does not result in excessive drug and/or metabolite accumulation and exposure. It should be kept in mind, however, that if the absorption or elimination of an NCE is nonlinear, a different approach to calculating the accumulation factor must be employed.

Ideally, the dosing frequency should mimic that intended in the clinic. However, due to physical and sometimes practical limitations, this may not always be possible. Knowledge of toxicokinetic parameters should allow a dosing regimen and dosing frequency which will produce the most reliable safety evaluation data under the desired study conditions. Also, understanding the relationship between the pharmacological or toxicological effect, AUC, and/or C_{max} may be critical for dosing regimen design in a safety evaluation study. Since the extent and duration of exposure are governed by both AUC and C_{max}, it may be critical to determine prospectively the effective and toxic plasma concentration range, which in turn may aid in the planning and designing of the subsequent safety evaluation studies.

The pharmacokinetics of an NCE may be altered during the repeated dosing regimens used in the safety evaluation testing, resulting in unexpected accumulation ratios, which could have profound effects on the outcome and interpretation of these studies. Repeated drug administration can influence the toxicity of an NCE by induction or inhibition of its own metabolism (BATRA and YACOBI 1989). Examples of both are given in Fig. 6, in which the effects of enzyme inhibition (Fig. 6a) and induction (Fig. 6b) on plasma

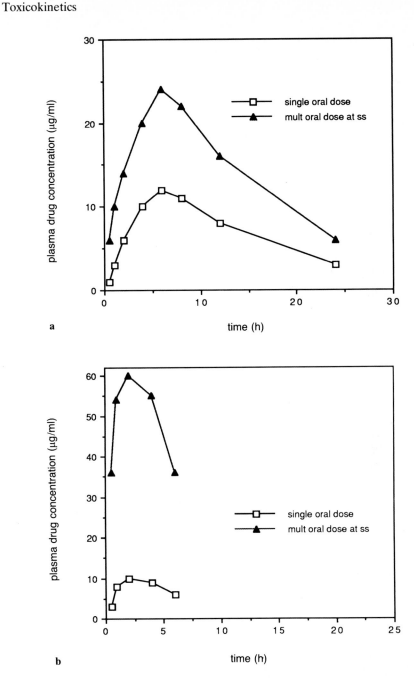

Fig. 5. a Relationship between NCE plasma concentration and time showing two-fold accumulation at steady state. In this example, the dosing interval and the half-life are the same (24 h). **b** Relationship between NCE plasma concentration and time showing marked accumulation at steady-state. In this example, the half-life (24 h) is much longer than the dosing interval (6 h), resulting in a accumulation ratio of 6

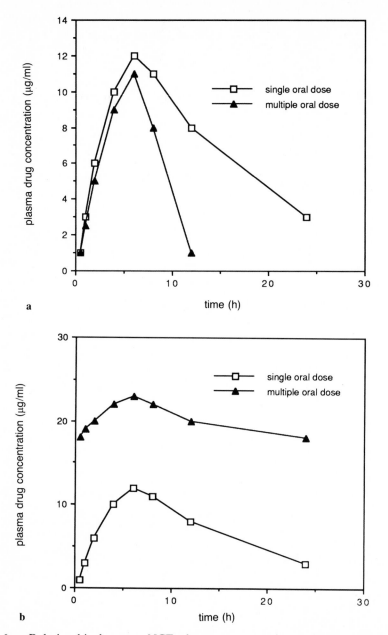

Fig. 6. a Relationship between NCE plasma concentration and time depicting the impact of enzyme induction on the anticipated accumulation ratio of an NCE. **b** Relationship between NCE plasma concentration and time depicting the impact of enzyme inhibition on the anticipated accumulation ratio of an NCE

drug concentrations upon multiple dosing are shown. Thus, enzyme induction will enhance drug elimination and reduce toxicity caused by the parent compound. If toxicity is due to the formation of a metabolite, toxicity may in fact be enhanced. Conversely, enzyme inhibition will result in accumulation of and therefore enhance the toxicity due to the parent compound and reduce the toxicity resulting from potential metabolites. Unexpected drug accumulation ratios may also occur due to changes in drug absorption, pharmacological effects of the NCE, or physiological factors (e.g., age and sex) in the animal. It is important to determine, if possible, the mechanism of these changes and their possible impact on the understanding of safety and toxicity data. Prospective studies to delineate possible changes in drug exposure may provide data for a more rational protocol design and possible dosage adjustments in the long-term toxicology studies.

F. Designing Troubleshooting Studies to Explain Aberrant Data

Often in toxicology studies, issues arise which require further information and explanation outside the realm of the toxicology support studies. Thus, studies are designed to address specific issues related to the toxicology findings and are conducted separately by the toxicokinetics group. Some actual examples of problems encountered in a typical toxicokinetics program related to absorption or metabolism and how they were resolved are indicated below.

I. Absorption Issues

1. Dose Proportionality

The most effective way to initiate a toxicokinetic program, even prior to the dose range-finding studies, is to conduct a dose proportionality study to determine a dose range at which exposure is not saturated; such studies have recently become more routine. A typical example follows.

In a 2-week range-finding study in the dog, no target organ toxicity was observed. Evaluation of pharmacokinetic data indicated similar achieved plasma concentrations of parent compound following oral administration of 100, 300, or 1000 mg/kg (Table 1). A separate pharmacokinetic study was designed at lower doses to support dose selection for the pivotal long-range studies. The data (Table 2) indicated reasonable dose proportionality between doses of 1 and 30 mg/kg, with minimal increases in AUC above this range. As a result, these doses were selected for the chronic toxicity studies. However, to support phase I clinical trials, it was deemed essential to document a higher exposure level in rats, necessitating an additional safety study where the drug was administered parenterally.

Table 1. Pharmacokinetics of an NCE following a single oral dose in the dog[a]

Dose (mg/kg)	C_{max} (μg/ml)	AUC_{0-24} (μg $\cdot$ h/ml)
100	3.1	28.1
300	3.4	43.9
1000	2.2	33.4

[a] Vehicle: Methocel/Tween suspension

Table 2. Pharmacokinetics of an NCE following a single oral dose in the dog[a]

Dose (mg/kg)	C_{max} (μg/ml)	AUC_{0-24} (μg $\cdot$ h/ml)
1	0.4	0.9
3	0.6	2.0
10	1.4	8.9
30	3.0	20.9

[a] Vehicle: Methocel/Tween suspension

2. Effect of Diet

Preliminary studies conducted with another NCE indicated very low bioavailability in the dog following dosing in methylcellulose/Tween 80 or as neat encapsulated powder in the fasted state (Table 3). As a result, a study was conducted to evaluate the bioavailability in the fed state. The data (Table 3) indicated a fivefold increase in the bioavailability at equivalent doses, which was sufficient for conducting the long-term toxicity studies under these conditions.

3. Effect of Vehicles

Initial assessment of an NCE in the rat indicated an absorption of 23% from drug-diet. Various vehicles were evaluated to determine whether absorption could be enhanced. Rats received radiolabeled compound in either a triolein emulsion, oleic acid, or methylcellulose/Tween 80 (Table 4). The results indicated the highest absorption was from triolein emulsion; however, since this vehicle could confound the results of a toxicity study, methylcellulose/Tween 80 was the vehicle of choice for the 1-year toxicity study in the rat.

II. Metabolism Issues

1. Enzyme Induction

Following chronic dosing of an NCE in the rat, some hepatotoxicity, including increased liver weights and morphological changes, was observed.

Table 3. Comparison of pharmacokinetics of an NCE in fed[a] versus fasted dogs receiving drug orally as neat encapsulated powder

Dose (mg/kg)	C_{max} (μg/ml)	AUC_{0-24} (μg · h/ml)
Fasted dogs		
250	4.4	29.9
500	3.1	14.5
Fed dogs		
250	20.0	144
500	29.3	208

[a] Animals were offered food for 1 h prior to dosing

Table 4. Absorption of ^{14}C-NCE following oral administration of 20 mg/kg in the rat

Vehicle	% absorption
0.05% drug in diet	23
Triolein emulsion	50
Oleic acid	11
0.5% methylcellulose/0.01% Tween 80 suspension	39

Although there were no decreases in plasma concentrations upon multiple dosing, it was decided that the induction potential of this compound should be investigated. In a separate pharmacokinetic study, rats received oral doses of the compound for 5 days, were killed, and the potential of the hepatic mixed function oxidase system for induction evaluated. The results (Table 5) indicated moderate (less than phenobarbital) induction, suggesting that this mechanism may be a component of the compound's hepatotoxic potential.

2. Effect of Age

A pharmacokinetic study was conducted to assess the effect of age on the pharmacokinetics of an NCE when given in combination with an antibiotic to beagle dogs. For both compounds, when administered alone or in combination, the half-life was longer (40%–45% increase) in 3-day-old dogs than in 5- or 13-week-old dogs and was reflected in a lower systemic clearance (Table 6). The pharmacokinetics of both compounds were similar in dogs between the ages of 5 and 13 weeks.

In older animals, a diminution of excretory organ function can cause a reduction in the clearance of an NCE, which could potentially lead to drug

Table 5. The effects of an NCE on the levels of the mixed function oxidase system in the livers of adult rats[a]

Parameters analyzed	Percent of control ± standard deviation	
	Male	Female
Body weight	93 ± 7	92 ± 4
Liver weight	122 ± 16*	141 ± 8**
Liver/body weight	129 ± 8**	151 ± 14**
Microsomal protein/gram liver	104 ± 4	122 ± 10**
Total microsomal protein	127 ± 19*	178 ± 13**
Cytochrome P-450[b]	216 ± 33**	326 ± 57**
Cytochrome b_5[b]	67 ± 8**	165 ± 30**
Cytochrome P-450 reductase[b]	181 ± 18**	196 ± 30**
Aminopyrine-N-demethylase[b]	113 ± 31	369 ± 145**
Aniline hydroxylase[b]	227 ± 38**	299 ± 175*

[a] Eight rats/group dosed orally (gavage) for 5 consecutive days, at 100 mg/kg per day
[b] Corrected to total capacity of the total liver (that is, activity/microsomal protein × mg microsomal protein/g liver × liver weight)
*,** Significantly different from control using Student's t-test: * $P < 0.05$; ** $P < 0.01$

Table 6. Mean (CV%) pharmacokinetic parameters of an NCE and antibiotic in young dogs following single intravenous doses

Dose (mg/kg) antibiotic/NCE	Age	$AUC_{0 \to \infty}$ (μg · h/ml)	C_0[a] (μg/ml)	$t_{1/2}$ (min)	CL (ml/min per kg)
Pharmacokinetic parameters for NCE					
0:80	3 days	262 (18)	176 (24)	84 (7)	5.2 (17)
	5 weeks	134 (13)	199 (16)	45 (11)	10.1 (13)
	13 weeks	159 (13)	220 (13)	44 (11)	8.5 (13)
160:20	3 days	61 (15)	43 (17)	81 (29)	5.6 (16)
	5 weeks[b]	46 (0)	47 (14)	47 (1)	7.2 (11)
	13 weeks	43 (12)	68 (15)	46 (13)	7.9 (11)
640:80	3 days	235 (17)	191 (19)	75 (4)	5.8 (17)
	5 weeks	191 (6)	263 (23)	49 (16)	7.0 (7)
	13 weeks	199 (8)	210 (12)	49 (3)	6.7 (9)
Pharmacokinetic parameters for antibiotic					
640:0	3 days	2233 (16)	1621 (8)	67 (16)	4.9 (18)
	5 weeks	1736 (18)	2558 (31)	43 (12)	6.3 (22)
	13 weeks	1556 (10)	2378 (26)	40 (13)	6.9 (10)
160:20	3 days	540 (18)	463 (16)	64 (28)	5.1 (20)
	5 weeks	236 (43)	379 (25)	34 (29)	13.2 (43)
	13 weeks	292 (13)	677 (28)	30 (10)	9.3 (14)
640:80	3 days	2415 (9)	1966 (4)	61 (5)	4.4 (9)
	5 weeks	1572 (10)	2666 (32)	42 (10)	6.8 (10)
	13 weeks	1477 (4)	2005 (17)	33 (6)	7.2 (6)

[a] C_0 extrapolated from available data
[b] $n = 2$; $n = 4$ in all other groups

accumulation (YACOBI et al. 1982). Therefore, changes in clearance should be monitored in these older animals to avoid unanticipated toxicity findings. This variable is critical in the design of and interpretation of the results of long-term toxicity studies, particularly in rodents.

3. Sex Dependency

Pharmacokinetic differences between males and females are usually not evaluated in the initial pharmacokinetic studies, since a sufficient population size of each sex would be required to discern a difference. Another consideration, particularly if differences are due to metabolism, is that an analytical procedure to measure metabolite concentrations in biological fluids must be in place. For another NCE following 3 months of oral dosing in the rat, sex differences in the metabolism to its primary desethyl metabolite (Tables 7 and 8) were observed, with females showing higher unchanged compound and lower metabolite concentrations as compared to males. These differences may have been related to the sex-related toxicity profiles, in which females showed greater toxicity at equivalent doses.

G. Species Comparisons and Interspecies (Allometric) Scaling

Once the pharmacokinetics have been characterized in a number of animal species, the information can be used to predict possible human exposure in the early clinical trials and whether it relates to the desired pharmacological actions or toxicological side-effects observed in the animal species. Pharmacokinetic parameters such as the maximum concentration (C_{max}), the extent of exposure (AUC), and the duration of exposure (time during which

Table 7. Pharmacokinetics[a] in the rat following oral gavage dosing of an NCE for 3 months: data for parent compound (cf. Table 8)

Dose (mg/kg)	Sex	Day 0		Day 28/29		Day 91/92	
		C_{max} (μg/ml)	AUC $0 \rightarrow 24$ (μg · h/ml)	C_{max} (μg/ml)	AUC $0 \rightarrow 24$ (μg · h/ml)	C_{max} (μg/ml)	AUC $0 \rightarrow 24$ (μg · h/ml)
5	Male	0.7	2.06	0.8	1.9	1.3	4.13
	Female	0.9	1.67	0.7	1.5	1.3[b]	3.01[b]
50	Male	6.8	53.0	10.0	45.2	8.9	35.2
	Female	9.7	72.3	10.6	61.8	9.1[b]	36.9[b]
100	Male	11.5	90.4	13.4[b]	76.7[b]	12.9[b]	68.3[b]
	Female	16.2	125	13.9[b]	101[b]	11.1[b]	82.1[b]
200	Male	17.6	168	10.3	82.1	13.2[b]	131[b]
	Female	18.7	220	16.0[b]	167[b]	30.1[b]	194[b]

[a] Calculated from mean ($n = 3$) plasma concentrations
[b] Calculated from samller population, due to mortalities

Table 8. Pharmacokinetics[a] in the rat following oral gavage dosing of an NCE for 3 months: data for primary desethyl metabolite of compound in Table 7

Dose (mg/kg)	Sex	Day 0		Day 28/29		Day 91/92	
		C_{max} (μg/ml)	AUC $0 \to 24$ (μg · h/ml)	C_{max} (μg/ml)	AUC $0 \to 24$ (μg · h/ml)	C_{max} (μg/ml)	AUC $0 \to 24$ (μg · h/ml)
5	Male	0.4	1.42	0.8	2.56	1.2	5.15
	Female	0.4	0.92	0.4	1.13	0.8[b]	2.24[b]
50	Male	7.8	79.5	10.4	84.2	11.2	103
	Female	5.6	52.9	9.4	66.6	10.2[b]	53.5[b]
100	Male	11.9	140	17.7[b]	154[b]	15.0[b]	153[b]
	Female	7.5	92.8	12.7[b]	122[b]	10.0[b]	109[b]
200	Male	15.4	291	19.2	210	23.6[b]	316[b]
	Female	12.0	171	15.6[b]	205[b]	32.5[b]	259[b]

[a] Calculated from mean ($n = 3$) plasma concentrations
[b] Calculated from samller population, due to mortalities

detectable plasma concentrations are observed) should be compared across species to determine whether the exposure observed in the animals, particularly at doses with no overt toxicity, exceeds the anticipated exposure level in man (Campbell and Ings 1988). Such comparisons are more likely to equate to real safety margins than extrapolations based solely on dosages. These types of comparisons provide a level of comfort in the design of the early clinical trials, helping to ensure that toxic plasma concentrations of an NCE are avoided.

When assessing the appropriateness of extrapolating data from animals to man, factors such as protein binding and metabolic differences must be kept in mind. Therefore, it is critical that this type of pivotal information is available before species comparisons are made. If the extent of protein binding varies significantly across species, it may be essential to assess the pharmacokinetics across species in terms of unbound plasma concentrations. If metabolism studies suggest little or no metabolism of the NCE and/or similar metabolites across species, then extrapolating the data to man will be meaningful and can provide key information for the design of the initial clinical studies in man. If, however, the metabolic profiles are qualitatively or quantitatively different across species, then the predictive value of the data to man may be minimal. In fact, if extensive metabolism occurs, it may be more relevant to compare metabolite concentrations across species, particularly if it is an active or toxic metabolite, rather than parent compound. In this way, it can be documented that animals will be exposed to higher concentrations of a metabolite than those anticipated in man.

Predictions of human drug exposure based on the appropriately selected (see above) animal data have had some successes recently with the use of interspecies (allometric) scaling (Mordenti 1985). This is a method of interpolation and extrapolation based on the underlying anatomical, physiological, and biochemical similarities in mammals. Allometric scaling is based on the concept that small animals are performing the same physiological functions as larger animals but at much faster rates. These functions include oxygen consumption, energy metabolism, chemical metabolism, cardiac output and heart rate, oxygen function, and chemical excretions. The relationship of these functions to body weight have been applied to pharmacokinetics as described in the following equation:

$$Y = aW^b,$$

where Y is the pharmacokinetic variable of interest, W is the body weight, $\log a$ is the y-intercept and b is the slope obtained from the plot of $\log Y$ versus $\log W$. This power equation accurately scales pharmacokinetic parameters (clearance, volume of distribution, half-life) between animals and man (BOXENBAUM 1984), as shown in the example for methotrexate in Fig. 7. Use of allometric scaling must take into account that a minimum of three animal species are required and the appropriateness of the species comparisons (i.e., protein binding and metabolite differences) as described above. Prospective incorporations of these concepts into study designs can

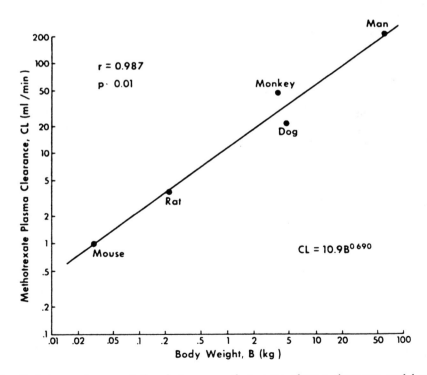

Fig. 7. Interspecies correlation between methotrexate plasma clearance and body weight. Linear regression analysis was performed on logarithmically transformed data. Intercept and slope values were used to calculate coefficient and exponent, respectively (by permission, BOXENBAUM 1982)

result in more meaningful data from animal studies, resulting in an enhanced ability to predict the activity, efficacy, and toxicity of NCEs in man with greater accuracy.

H. Utilization of Pharmacokinetic/Toxicokinetic Data in the Design of Early Clinical Trials

The strategy for the selection of doses for phase I clinical trials is to target a dose range which will likely result in efficacy in man. The process is often a haphazard one and has been traditionally based on doses resulting in efficacy in animal studies. As already mentioned, interspecies differences in pharmacokinetics, such as differences in absorption or metabolism, can result in poorly designed clinical trials if only dosages are considered and preclinical pharmacokinetic information is ignored. The impact of improper selection of doses in the clinical phase I trials can be enormous. Finding a safe starting dose is only the initial step. A balance needs to be struck between escalating doses too rapidly, which could result in unwanted toxicity, and escalating too slowly, which could result in patients being treated at subtherapeutic doses and overall increasing the costs of drug development enormously.

A rational approach to the design of phase I trials would incorporate sufficient preclinical pharmacokinetic and pharmacodynamic data early in drug development to more accurately target an efficacious and nontoxic dosing regimen in man (VOISIN et al. 1990). One means of achieving this goal is to monitor plasma concentrations of an NCE in an animal disease model that has relevance to the clinical situation. While preclinical pharmacokinetic/pharmacodynamic studies are not routinely conducted as part of a preclinical drug development program, information derived from these studies would be very useful for targeting efficacious concentrations in man.

Recently, it has been shown that animal toxicokinetic data can offer a reliable measure for predicting toxicity of an NCE in man, thus allowing for dose escalation strategies that are both safe and substantially more rapid than the often used Fibonacci scheme (COLLINS et al. 1986). The basic concept is that toxic effects of oncology agents in different species are similar for similar drug exposure levels or AUC. In retrospective analyses, it was shown that the ratio of the AUCs at the mouse LD_{10} and the human maximum tolerated dose (MTD) are close to 1 for a number of anticancer agents. These observations formed the basis of a proposal that phase I oncology trials be pharmacokinetically guided by targeting a maximum plasma AUC for man equivalent to the AUC achieved at the LD_{10} in the mouse (EORTC PHARMACOKINETICS and METABOLISM GROUP 1987). The subsequent reduction in the number of dose levels would decrease the demand on clinical resources and improve the individual patient's chances of receiving a therapeutic dose. Subsequent to the proposal, successful application of its principles has been shown for a number of oncology agents, including an analog of doxorubicin (GIANNI et al. 1990). Thus, the benefits of prospective planning to incorporate mouse LD_{10} pharmacokinetic studies as part of the preclinical development of an oncology agent should be apparent.

References

Batra VK, Yacobi A (1989) An overview of toxicokinetics. In: Yacobi A, Skelly JP, Batra VK (eds) Toxicokinetics and new drug development. Pergamon, New York

Boxenbaum H (1982) Interspecies scaling, allometry, physiological time, and the ground plan of pharmacokinetics. J Pharmacokin Biopharm 10(2):201–227

Boxenbaum H (1984) Interspecies pharmacokinetic scaling and the evolutionary-comparative paradigm. Drug Metab Rev 15:1071–1121

Campbell DB, Ings RMJ (1988) New approaches to the use of pharmacokinetics in toxicology and drug development. Human Toxicol 7:469–479

Collins JM, Zaharko DS, Dedrick RL, Chabner BA (1986) Potential roles for preclinical pharmacology in phase I clinical trials. Cancer Treat Rep 70/1:73–80

EORTC Pharmacokinetics and Metabolism Group (1987) Pharmacokinetically guided dose escalation in phase I clinical trials. Commentary and proposed guidelines. Eur J Cancer Clin Oncol 23:1083–1087

Gianni L, Vigano L, Surbone A, Ballinari D, Casali P, Tarella C, Collins JM, Bonadonna G (1990) Pharmacology and clinical toxicity of 4'-iodo-4'-deoxydoxorubicin: an example of successful application of pharmacokinetics to dose escalation in phase I trials. J Natl Cancer Inst 82/6:469–477

Graves DA, Locke CS Jr, Muir KT, Miller RP (1989) The influence of assay variability on pharmacokinetic parameter estimation. J Pharm Biopharm 17/5:571–592

Hawkins DR, Chasseaud LF (1985) Reasons for monitoring kinetics in safety evaluation studies. Arch Toxicol [Suppl] 8:165–172

Monro AM (1976) The role of metabolism studies in drug safety evaluation. Drug Dev Commun 2:377–392

Mordenti J (1985) Pharmacokinetic scaleup: accurate prediction of human pharmacokinetic profiles from animal data. J Pharm Sci 74:1097–1099

Smyth RD, Hottendorf GH (1980) Application of pharmacokinetics and biopharmaceutics in the design of toxicological studies. Toxicol Appl Pharmacol 53:179–195

Voisin EM, Ruthsatz M, Collins JM, Hoyle PC (1990) Extrapolation of animal toxicity to humans: interspecies comparisons in drug development. Regul Toxicol Pharmacol 12:107–116

Welling PG (1984) Effects of gastrointestinal disease on drug absorption. In: Benet LZ, Massoud N, Gambertoglio JG (eds) Pharmacokinetic basis for drug treatment. Raven, New York

Yacobi A, Kamath BL, Lai CM (1982) Pharmacokinetics in chronic animal toxicity studies. Drug Metab Rev 13/6:1021–1051

CHAPTER 15

The Population Approach: Rationale, Methods, and Applications in Clinical Pharmacology and Drug Development*,**,***

J.-L. STEIMER, S. VOZEH, A. RACINE-POON, N. HOLFORD, and R. O'NEILL

A. Introduction

Variation in the response of individual patients to drugs is a matter of major concern in drug evaluation and therapy (ROWLAND et al. 1985). Since the seminal paper in 1972 (SHEINER et al. 1972), followed by its first application to digoxin 5 years later (SHEINER et al. 1977) and the release of software (BEAL and SHEINER 1980), "population pharmacokinetics" has been an area of active research in clinical pharmacology, despite scepticism among many pharmacokineticists, most clinicians, and, with rare exceptions, general indifference or even antagonism within the pharmaceutical industry. Over the last 10 years, publications on the subject have included:

1. Extensive reviews of the statistical methodology (BEAL and SHEINER 1982, 1985; STEIMER et al. 1985; RACINE-POON and SMITH 1990)
2. Reviews of the applications of population pharmacokinetics to drug therapy (WHITING et al. 1986, 1990; PECK and RODMAN 1986, 1992; SHEINER and LUDDEN 1992)
3. Special issues of journals with primary emphasis on theoretical and practical aspects of population pharmacokinetics (DI CARLO 1984; ANTAL and GRASELA 1991)
4. Discussions on its advantages and limitations in comparison with classical approaches (SHEINER and BEAL 1981; STEIMER et al. 1984b; ENDRENYI 1985; COLBURN and OLSON 1988; COLBURN 1989; AARONS 1991a, 1992a,b; THOMSON and TUCKER 1992)
5. International symposia with sponsorship from academic societies (American Society of Clinical Pharmacology and Therapeutics, American

---

* Opinions expressed in this chapter are those of the authors and do not implicate the institutions with which they are associated.
** Parts of this work have been presented at the COST-B1 conference "New Strategies in Drug Development and Clinical Evaluation: The Population Approach," Manchester, 21–23 September 1991.
*** This chapter is based largely on discussions held in Basel (Switzerland) within a "Population Pharmacokinetics Working Group," during sabbatical leave of R. O'Neill at the Department of Research, Kantonsspital, University of Basel, and N. Holford at the Department of Clinical Pharmacology, Hoffmann-La Roche, from August 1989 to December 1990.

Association of Pharmaceutical Scientists, etc.), pharmaceutical manufacturers (Pharmaceutical Manufacturers Association, Interpharma, etc.), and regulatory bodies [Food and Drug Administration (FDA: US regulatory authority), Bundesgesundheitsamt (German regulatory authority), etc.] (DI CARLO 1984; ROWLAND et al. 1985; ANTAL and GRASELA 1991)

This chapter will not be restricted solely to population *pharmacokinetics* in its early meaning (JUSKO 1980; RIEGELMAN et al. 1980; SHEINER and BEAL 1981) but rather will embrace the *"population approach"* (including pharmacokinetics and pharmacodynamics) considered as a general conceptual framework for drug evaluation (ROWLAND and AARONS 1992). The authors will try to illustrate the integrating role of the population approach within the multidisciplinary environment of drug research, in an attempt to bridge the existing gap between clinicians, clinical pharmacologists, pharmacokineticists, and biometricians in this area.

In Sect. B, the population approach is introduced as a natural link between studies in large samples of patients and extensive studies in small groups of volunteers. In Sect. C, the nonlinear mixed effects model (which is at the core of current concepts of population data analysis) and the related statistical methodology for parameter estimation are briefly introduced. Current applications of the population approach for drug evaluation and therapy are presented in Sect. D. A discussion of some problems and issues is given in Sect. E, emphasizing the need for validation of results of any population analysis. A prospective view is taken in Sect. F, with concrete thoughts on integration of the population approach into the drug development process. Concluding remarks are given in Sect. G.

B. Rationale

The goal of pharmacokinetic and pharmacodynamic investigations is to establish a rational basis for the therapeutic use of a drug. Specifically, clinical trials aim at determining the dose and the dosage regimen of the new drug that will produce therapeutic benefit in patients while minimizing the inconvenience of side-effects and risks of adverse drug reactions. This is particularly true in the clinical evaluation of new chemical and biological entities during drug development.

The object of drug treatment is to produce a therapeutic benefit in an individual patient. Clinical evaluation is based on the principle that results obtained in selected subgroups of healthy volunteers and patients can be generalized to other patients. Each individual is viewed as a member of a patient population, which is usually quite heterogeneous. Identical doses may produce effects which differ markedly in nature, extent, and duration in different individuals. As a consequence, successful drug development should end up not only with therapeutic advances but also with guidelines for the optimal use of the drug in each patient. To reach this goal, insight into the dose–effect or, more precisely, the dose–concentration–effect relationship throughout clinical evaluation is required (TEMPLE 1989).

The subjects of pharmacokinetic and pharmacodynamic studies are often healthy volunteers or highly selected patients. Traditionally interest has focused on the average behavior of a group, i.e., the *mean* response (plasma concentration profile, pharmacodynamic response). Interindividual *variability* in pharmacokinetics, pharmacodynamics, or clinical outcomes is viewed as a nuisance that has to be overcome, often through complex study designs and control schemes, and reduced through restrictive inclusion criteria. Rigid standardization of study design and selection of volunteers so they are as homogeneous as possible are thus frequently encountered as typical features of pharmacokinetic/pharmacodynamic investigations. These studies are therefore often performed under quite artificial conditions which are not representative of the intended clinical use of the drug.

In contrast to this currently employed approach, the population approach to pharmacokinetic/pharmacodynamic evaluation in man encompasses the following aspects:

1. It aims at obtaining relevant pharmacokinetic and pharmacodynamic information in subjects (usually patients) who are representative of the target patient population to be treated with the drug.
2. It recognizes variability as an important feature that should be identified and measured during drug evaluation.
3. It aims at explaining variability by identifying factors of environmental, demographic, pathophysiological, or drug-related origin that may influence the pharmacokinetic and pharmacodynamic behavior of the drug.
4. It aims at a quantitative estimation of the unexplained part of the variability in the patient population.

Resolving issues 1–4 provides a framework for defining optimum dosing strategies in a population, in a subgroup, or for the individual patient (see Sect. D). These issues have been addressed in the past in different ways, not necessarily with the population approach. Also, past emphasis has been largely put on pharmacokinetics, with efforts aimed at the identification of influential factors and/or the detection of subgroups with deviant behavior. It therefore seems worthwhile to present the concept of the population approach within the context of the current practice. Before detailing the population approach, the key features of two currently used methodologies will be presented. This will be done with respect to both data *collection* and data *analysis*.

I. "Population Studies" in Large Samples of Subjects

When a given influential factor is suspected, then a *focused* population study can be based on the measurement of a single pharmacokinetic characteristic (e.g., the plasma level 24 h after drug intake, or a steady-state level after chronic administration, or a drug/metabolite ratio of amounts excreted in urine). The data analysis can take the form of simple descriptive statistical estimates of the measured quantity because it is the parameter of interest. The investigation of the statistical characteristics of its empirical probability distribution can provide clinically useful insight into the frequency and magnitude of specific pharmacokinetic problems. An example related to the acetylation polymorphism of isoniazid is given as Fig. 1. Successful reports on this simplest form of a population study suggest that it may be adequate in selected instances (PRICE EVANS et al. 1960; FEELY et al. 1981; RENWICK et al. 1988; SCAVONE et al. 1988).

This idea has been improved upon (in an exploratory/observational rather than confirmatory/controlled context) with the concept of the "pharmacokinetic screen" in clinical trials (TEMPLE 1983, 1987; FDA 1989). In its most simple version, the "trough" pharmacokinetic screen, it relies upon the collection of blood samples just before the next dose in patients undergoing chronic dosing. There is an expectation for serendipitous detection of unexpected influential factors and/or patient groups associated with extreme or outlying drug concentrations, which reflect an altered dose–concentration relationship. The data collection procedure which the trough screen relies

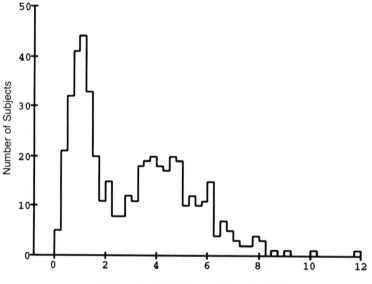

Fig. 1. An example of a population study based on a single plasma level measurement: the distribution of the 6-h plasma concentration of isoniazid in 483 subjects after 9.8 mg/kg isoniazid orally. In this case, the display of the raw data as a histogram suffices to suggest that the distribution is bimodal, as a consequence of acetylation polymorphism. (From PRICE EVANS et al. 1960)

upon mimics the standard practice of collection of plasma concentration data for drug monitoring purposes (see, e.g., HUNDT et al. 1983). A priori, data analysis techniques from the machinery of linear statistics (e.g., analysis of variance, multivariate regression) can be used for investigating associations between plasma levels and, for instance, laboratory data and/or adverse events. Preliminary pharmacokinetic evaluation of the data is useful for guiding statistical analysis, especially when both drug and metabolite(s) have been assayed (GEX-FABRY et al. 1990). The traditional approach to the analysis of the pharmacokinetic screen based on measurement of trough values has two main disadvantages compared to the population methods described later. Both arise from the fact that it does not explicitly implement a pharmacokinetic model: (a) it is limited to studies in which the same dosing regimen is used in all patients; (b) the results cannot usually be used for designing dosing regimens in future patients. An extension of the trough pharmacokinetic screen which is of general interest is a data collection scheme in which timing of samples is flexible (or "random") within a dosing interval rather than restricted to predose sampling (STEIMER et al. 1984; SHEINER and BENET 1985). Subject-specific timing is the usual design in population pharmacokinetic studies. It does not impede model-based analysis of the data (see Sects. C and D) and has been shown to be of advantage over standard sampling when data are sparse (MALLET and MENTRE 1988). The main differences between such a "full" kinetic screen (SHEINER and BENET 1985) and the "trough" screen reside in the richness of the data, in the complexity of the model, and in the level of sophistication of the statistical methodology (see Sect. C), and consequently in the power of the results. In this sense the traditional analysis of trough pharmacokinetic screen data can be considered as a poor man's population analysis. After substantial debate in the academic, industrial, and regulatory community (JENNINGS 1984; REIDENBERG and ABRAMS 1984; COLBURN 1989), the concept of the screen was explicitly recognized by the FDA as one acceptable design for assessment of kinetics and dynamics of drugs in the elderly (FDA 1989). The full screen design provides a framework for implementation of the population approach in large-scale clinical trials.

II. Controlled Experimental Studies in Small Groups

Experimental pharmacokinetic data arise from studies carried out specifically for pharmacokinetic investigations, under controlled conditions of drug dosing and extensive blood sampling. The investigation of the influence of external factors like age, renal function, and comedications is often achieved by means of such intervention studies in selected groups of volunteers (for a detailed description of studies carried out during new drug development, see COLBURN and OLSON 1988; BALANT et al. 1990).

With respect to data analysis, the raw data, usually in the form of profiles of plasma concentration or urinary excretion of drug/metabolite versus time, are "converted" into pharmacokinetic parameters (e.g., clearance, volume) which account for the drug's absorption, distribution, and elimination characteristics. The evaluation of such parameters either by noncompartmental methods (e.g., an estimate of clearance from the area under the plasma concentration–time curve) or through nonlinear regression techniques involving the fitting of parametric models to each individual's data has become routine practice in pharmacokinetic and pharmacokinetic/pharmacodynamic data analysis. Regarding assessment of variability, this procedure builds the first stage of the so-called standard two-stage (STS) method. In the second stage, the individual's estimates serve as input data for calculation of descriptive summary statistics on the sample (typically mean and variance–covariance) or for comparisons across groups. This latter stage can also include the analysis of dependencies between parameters and covariates (e.g., age, creatinine clearance) using classical statistical approaches (linear stepwise regression, cluster analysis, analysis of covariance, etc.).

With respect to statistical methodology, several refinements of the simplest STS approach have been proposed (STEIMER et al. 1984a; RACINE-POON 1985; AMISAKI and TATSUHARA 1988). They improve STS within the framework of the statistical EM algorithm (DEMPSTER et al. 1977) by some sort of weighting according to the respective quality of the individual estimates. STS and other two-stage methods provide calculation schemes for statistical summary ("pooling" or "aggregation") of parameter estimates in a sample of subjects. Recently, a technique was suggested in the special case of multiple studies with identically replicated experiments (LYNE et al. 1992). It performs the estimation of population parameters based on model fits with the software SAAM. However, while all these methods belong to the general methodology for population modeling and estimation, they are applicable only to a restricted class of experimental designs because they require the number of observations from an individual to be larger than the number of parameters in the model (see Table 1 for details).

At present, full profile pharmacokinetic studies are mostly comparative in that they are used to see whether important differences in the plasma concentration are to be expected between groups. In these studies the pharmacokinetic parameters in a group of subjects with potentially altered kinetic behavior (kidney, liver, heart failure) are compared with those of healthy young persons or patients without the feature or insufficiency in question. Such studies are performed to test for a statistically significant difference between groups or, if not, to establish their equivalence with respect to the pharmacokinetic parameters of the drug. This study-by-study approach can be complemented by a "meta-analysis" where the pooled statistical analysis of parameters and covariate data across successive studies serves for integration of the results at a "population" level. Such meta-analysis may be carried out with traditional methods (BLYCHERT et al. 1991) or with the methodology of population analysis (see Sect. C).

Table 1. A contrasting view of some methods for estimating population characteristics of parameters: STS, NONMEM, and NPML

Method	Data	Model			Results			
	Ability to analyze sparse data?	Postulated population distribution	Assumption about structure of residual error	Incorporation of covariates	Population parameters	Exploratory and confirmatory diagnostics	Quality of estimates of population parameters
STS	NO Model must be identifiable for each individual		As in usual nonlinear regression, e.g., least squares	Separate second-stage analysis of parameter estimates. Generally parametric too	Histogram of estimates. Generally first two moments (mean, variance)	Usual model testing procedures for regression diagnostics (linear and nonlinear)	Inherently inflated variance estimates. Bias in practice probably not very large
NONMEM	Yes	Defined by its two first moments (usually normal or log-normal)	Variance model with parameters to be estimated	Nonlinear multivariate models of parameter on covariates (one-stage estimation)	First two moments	Population residual plots. Standard error of estimates, covariance matrix	A function of adequacy of first-order approximation. Generally good for predictive purposes
NPML	Yes	None	Error structure fully specified	Nonparametric estimation of joint distribution of parameters and covariates (one-stage estimation)	Nonparametric probability density function, as a set of spikes ("atomic distribution")	Limited smoothing of conditional or univariate distributions	Shares good and bad properties of maximum likelihood reliance on error model being properly specified. No standard error of estimates
Comment	NONMEM and NPML implement the one-stage population approach					Not good yet. Needs improvement for one-stage methods especially	All are approximate but in different ways. Sensitivity to misspecification of model assumptions not documented but can probably be substantial

STS, standard two-stage method; NONMEM, nonlinear mixed effects model, currently with first-order approximation; NPML, nonparametric maximum likelihood

Although representing the present standard for detecting patient groups with different pharmacokinetic behavior, such comparative intervention studies have the current important drawback that the subjects are not a sample from the population to be treated with the drug (see, e.g., SHEINER and BENET 1985).

III. The Population Approach

The "population approach" in the specific context of the evaluation of a drug in its pharmacokinetic and pharmacodynamic aspects arose from the recognition that, if pharmacokinetics/pharmacodynamics is to be investigated in patients, pragmatic considerations dictate that the data ought not be collected under too stringent and restrictive design conditions. The consequent design recognizes that: the dosing history is subject-specific, the amount of data collected from each subject is variable, the timing with respect to drug administration differs, and the number of measurements per patient may be small (with only one value from some patients). These are, among others, some of the essential characteristics of *observational* (population) data, where the data may be collected as a supplement to a clinical study designed and carried out for another primary purpose.

In application to pharmacokinetics, such a data collection scheme has been called a "full" kinetic screen (SHEINER and BENET 1985), i.e., an extension of the so-called trough screen (TEMPLE 1983). The nature of the drug-dosing regimen affects the way the data can be analyzed. In the case of concentration- and time-invariant kinetics and constant chronic dosing frequency (e.g., twice a day), the data still have a fairly simple underlying structure (see Fig. 2 for an example). This allows the use of "exploratory" data analysis methods (CHAMBERS et al. 1983), essentially a mix of graphical and statistical techniques, in order to take a first look at the data in a way which conforms to the goal of the study, which is exploratory by nature. Sometimes, data sets derived from several distinct clinical studies may be analyzed together. An example based on phase III pharmacokinetic data for the drug isradipine has been published (LAPLANCHE et al. 1991). For a general survey on graphical exploratory methods, see POLLAK (1990).

However, more commonly, dosing and timing of doses will be subject-specific. In this case, a direct plot of the plasma concentrations versus time provides an uninterpretable picture, which arises from the lack of rigidity in the design as well as patient variability in response (Fig. 3). The analysis of such data requires an explicit mathematical model, including both pharmacokinetic and statistical features, in order to describe variability and to detect the influential factors mentioned above. Model-based statistical methodology for analyzing sparse kinetic data from a population is intimately linked to the whole population approach idea. Indeed, the first description of the nonlinear mixed effects model (SHEINER et al. 1972) proposed a general solution intended to cope with the features of routinely collected

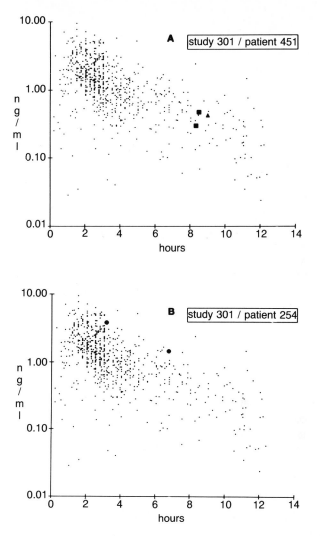

Fig. 2A,B. The scatterplot of 697 isradipine plasma concentrations in 252 hypertensive patients under long-term chronic b.i.d. dosage regimen. All data have been normalized with respect to dose (from 2.5 to 10 mg) and displayed within one unique dosing interval regardless of week of therapy. Concentration values for two individuals are superimposed. Different symbols refer to different doses. (From LAPLANCHE et al. 1991)

clinical data, in particular, sparse individual pharmacokinetic data with subject-specific dosing. The use of a mathematical model allows the population approach to go far beyond the sole description of variability or the comparison of pharmacokinetics across subgroups, as will be shown in Sect. D.

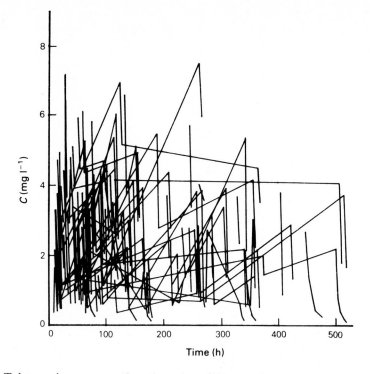

Fig. 3. Tobramycin concentration time data (322 levels) from 97 patients treated with the drug. In addition to between-patient pharmacokinetic variability, the apparent chaotic picture of the data is a consequence of subject-specific dosage regimen, varying duration of therapy, and heterogeneity in number of blood samples (one to nine) and in timing of the samples. A model-based population analysis is required in order to interpret such data. (From Aarons et al. 1989)

C. An Overview of Statistical Methodology for Model-Based Population Analysis

In this section, we focus on one major aspect of the population approach, the statistical methodology for analysis of sparse data from nonexperimental (observational) designs. The population analysis of pharmacokinetic and pharmacokinetic/pharmacodynamic data relies on a population statistical model (for details, see Sheiner and Grasela 1991; Grasela and Sheiner 1991) and on specific population methods for estimation of the unknown parameters (for details see Beal and Sheiner 1982, 1985; Steimer et al. 1985; Peck and Rodman 1986; Racine-Poon and Smith 1990).

I. Population Model

In order to deal with sparse kinetic data of the observational type, an elaborate statistical model is needed. In the formulation of the model, it is recognized that the overall variability in the measured response data in a sample of individuals that cannot be explained by the pharmacokinetic/pharmacodynamic model reflects both intersubject variation in kinetics and residual variation, the latter including intraindividual variability and measurement error. The observed response of an individual within the framework of a population nonlinear mixed-effects regression model can be described as:

$$y_{ij} = f_{ij} (\phi_i, x_{ij}) + \varepsilon_{ij},$$

where y_{ij} for $j = 1, \ldots, n_i$ are the observed data (e.g., n_i plasma concentration levels measured at time points x_{ij}) of the i-th subject. An appropriate model of this type is defined for all $i = 1, \ldots, N$, where N is the number of subjects in the sample. f_{ij} is a specified function for predicting the response in the i-th subject (e.g., one or several exponentials for pharmacokinetic data), ϕ_i is the vector (i.e., the collection) of unknown subject-specific parameters (e.g., clearance and volume), and ε_{ij} accounts for the error between the "true" (unknown) value and the corresponding measurement.

It should be clear from the above notation that the *population* model is, indeed, a collection of models for *individual* observations. In routine clinical practice as well as in clinical trials, various doses and/or dosage regimens and/or application routes (e.g., oral, intravenous, intramuscular) will generally be used in different patients and in the same patient at different stages of therapy. Also several responses might be measured (e.g., drug plasma concentration, arterial blood pressure), and diverse administration schedules (single dose and chronic dosing) might be considered. Accordingly, the functions f_{ij} will generally differ within and across individuals. In contrast, it is realistic to assume that the set of underlying structural parameters (in this case pharmacokinetic or pharmacodynamic parameters) is qualitatively the same for all individuals and that the parameters values differ between one individual and another (e.g., total body clearance and volume of distribution of the drug in a pharmacokinetic investigation).

The individual parameter ϕ_i is assumed to arise from some (multivariate) probability distribution $F(\theta)$, where θ is the vector (or collection) of so-called hyperparameters or "population characteristics." In the mixed-effects formulation, according to a recent terminology (PECK and RODMAN 1986, 1992), the collection of population hyperparameters θ is composed of population "typical values" (generally the mean vector) and of population "variability values" (generally the variance–covariance matrix). Herein, the notation θ embraces all above-mentioned unknown population characteristics, as well the fixed effects as the variance of random effects. Mean and variance characterize the location and dispersion of the probability distribution of ϕ in statistical terms. This minimal set of hyperparameters is "sufficient" (in the statistical sense) when F is a normal or log-normal distribution.

To assist clinical decision-making, it is of importance to relate differences among individuals to readily identifiable and routinely measurable individual attributes or "covariates" like age, sex, body weight, renal or liver function, or other demographic or laboratory data. Knowing the value of an influential covariate in a new patient before starting therapy increases the predictive power and therefore makes the choice of dose more reliable. The probability distribution can then be written as $F(\theta; z_i)$ where z_i is the set of covariate data of the i-th patient. For a dichotomous or *categorical* covariate (e.g., gender or presence of a disease), this notation expresses that the population distribution is, in fact, a mixture of two or more component distributions, each of which characterizes one subgroup of subjects. In order to express the dependency of a parameter on one or more *continuous* covariates (e.g., age, weight, creatinine clearance), a regression model of ϕ on z can be defined, which involves additional population parameters. This approach is used in the estimation method implemented in the software NONMEM (see Sect. C.II). A typical example in population pharmacokinetics is the search for a linear relationship between total body drug clearance and creatinine clearance, which may exist especially for drugs with significant renal excretion (Fig. 4). A "nonparametric" method for including the covariates in the analysis can also be envisaged. The unknown to be estimated is then the joint probability distribution of parameters and covariates, which are all treated (statistically) in the same way. No particular functional relationship needs to be postulated a priori. This approach is used in the nonparametric maximum likelihood method (see below). The mapping of the overall population distribution into component subpopulations in relation to categorical and continuously quantitative covariates is illustrated in Fig. 5.

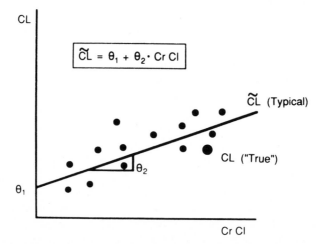

Fig. 4. An example of a simple tentative statistical "model" between a pharmacokinetic parameter and a covariate within the population: a linear relationship between the drug's total body clearance (CL), and creatinine clearance ($Cr\ CL$). Such a relationship can be tested for statistical significance with the software NONMEM. (From GRASELA and SHEINER 1991)

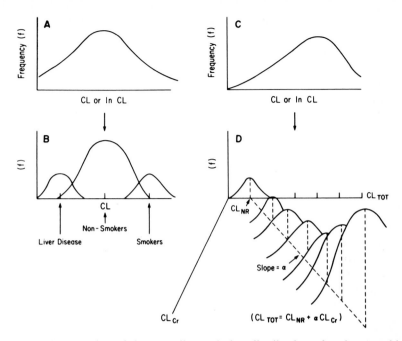

Fig. 5A-D. The mapping of the overall population distribution of a pharmacokinetic parameter (here total drug clearance of a fictive drug) into component subpopulations in relation to categorical covariates (e.g., smoking or liver disease status for a drug like theophylline) and a continuously quantitative covariate (e.g., creatinine clearance for a drug like gentamicin). (From PECK and RODMAN 1986)

The full set of assumptions and models on the structural relationships for pharmacokinetics and pharmacodynamics (via the function f), on interindividual variation (via the probability distribution F, the relationships with covariates, and the corresponding θ), and on residual error variance (via ε) build a so-called pharmacostatistical population model.

II. Population Methods for Data Analysis

A population approach analysis aims to estimate the probability distribution of the parameters and their relationships with covariates by considering the complete sample (rather than the individual) as the unit of analysis. Accordingly, the full collection of individual response values is used in a global estimation step. This formulation allows the use of population pharmacokinetic data of the observational type, which are unbalanced and fragmentary, in addition to or instead of conventional experimental data arising from a rigid and extensive design.

The nonlinear mixed-effects model provides, as population characteristics, estimates of the hyperparameters that define the population distribution of the pharmacokinetic/pharmacodynamic parameters (as defined in Sect. C.I) (Sheiner et al. 1972, 1977; Beal 1984). This parametric model is implemented in the software NONMEM (Beal and Sheiner 1989). Despite the approximation involved in the current derivation of the likelihood (the "first-order method"), NONMEM has shown overall good performance on simulated data (for review, see Beal and Sheiner 1985; Steimer et al. 1985). However, biased estimates were found in some cases (Beal and Sheiner 1985; Rodman and Evans 1991). Solutions have been worked out and are available in the new release (version IV) of the software NONMEM (Beal and Sheiner 1992). In parallel, there have been numerous successful applications of NONMEM to real pharmacokinetic data (for details see Sect. D and also Whiting et al. 1986; Antal and Grasela 1991). These achievements have triggered further developments in statistical methodology for population analysis. The nonparametric maximum likelihood approach (NPML), in contrast to NONMEM, provides a discrete estimate of the probability distribution F as a set of "spikes" whose number is less than or equal to the number of subjects in the sample (Mallet 1986). The number of applications of this complex methodology is still small, but the existing reports for cyclosporin (Mallet et al. 1988a), gentamicin (Mallet et al. 1988b) and zidovudine (Mentre and Mallet 1992) highlight its potential. A contrasting view of NONMEM and NPML regarding the specific assumptions involved in the modeling and the dedicated features of the results is given in Table 1.

In addition, there have been some recent statistical developments with relevance for population analysis of kinetic data: a stochastic approximation method (Mentre et al. 1988), the Gibbs sampler (Gelfand et al. 1990; Wakefield et al. 1992), a nonparametric version of the "expectation-maximisation" algorithm (Schumitzky 1991; Kisor et al. 1992), and a maximum likelihood procedure with a smooth random effects density (Davidian and Gallant 1992). Also the general area of nonlinear mixed effects modeling is attracting increasing interest in the biometric literature (Lindstrom and Bates 1990; Vonesh and Carter 1992). The emergence of these methods reflects the rapid evolution of the field at the statistical and algorithmic levels. They are likely to gain wider audiences as more successful applications are reported.

III. Synthesis

It should be recognized that, beyond pharmacokinetics and pharmacodynamics, population modeling and parameter estimation represent a particular instance of a statistical model which has general validity, the nonlinear mixed effects model. The model has wide applicability in all areas, in the biomedical sciences and elsewhere, where a parametric functional relationship between some input and some response is studied and where random variability across experimental units (in our case individuals) is of concern.

D. Current Experience with the Population Approach and Its Applications to Drug Therapy

I. Introduction

The population approach has been applied up to the present mainly in the field of pharmacokinetics, with the goal of estimating parameters that describe the dose–concentration relationship and its variability in patients. Although in principle pharmacodynamics bears more relevance to therapeutic response, past interest has focused on pharmacokinetics because of its particular relevance for drugs with a narrow therapeutic index and also because concentration–time data and well-understood compartmental models were available. The main goals of the different studies in which population pharmacokinetics have been successfully applied can be summarized as follows:

1. Detection of patient groups who are at increased risk of over- or underdosing because of different kinetics (Sect. D.II), with subsequent design of optimum dosage regimen recommendations (Sect. D.III). This type of application has been the most popular in the past. The statistical analysis was performed in most cases with the NONMEM program, which is still the only widely available software. A selection of population pharmacokinetic studies carried out since the emergence of the population approach in patients undergoing routine drug treatment is given in Table 2. Similarly, pertinent results about more than 40 studies have been reported recently (SHEINER and LUDDEN 1992).
2. Use of population characteristics for estimation of individual pharmacokinetic parameters using Bayesian regression (Sect. D.IV). These individual estimates were used to (a) individually adjust the dose both in clinical studies during drug development and later in patients receiving the drug, and (b) investigate the relationship between the predicted plasma concentration profile and the therapeutic effect.

Applications are currently expanding out of pharmacokinetics per se, especially into pharmacodynamics (AARONS et al. 1991; SCHMITH et al. 1992) and dose–response investigations (SHEINER et al. 1989; SAMBOL and SHEINER 1991; HOLFORD 1992). Recent extensions of nonlinear mixed effects models to population analysis of other drug-related issues are given in Sect. D.V.

Although the listed examples mostly originate from studies carried out after introduction of the drug in routine clinical use, they illustrate that the approach should also be applicable during drug development. This point will be detailed in Sect. F.

II. Detection of Patient Groups with Altered Kinetics

One of the important questions to be answered for a drug is its pharmacokinetic behavior in different patient populations. Of particular interest are

Table 2. A selection of population analyses of pharmacokinetics in patients for drugs in clinical use

Drug	Subjects		ntot / n	Covariates	Method	Authors
	N	Type				
Digoxin	141	In- and outpatients, Two hospitals	586(P) 46(U) 4.2	5	NONMEM	Sheiner et al. 1977
Phenytoin	49	32 in- and outpatients from Basel Hospital 17 from literature	124 2.5	0	NONMEM	Vozeh et al. 1981
Phenytoin	322	Adults and children 3 countries	780 2.4	5	NONMEM	Grasela et al. 1983
Gentamicin	143	Neonates Young children	482 3.4	4	NONMEM	Kelman et al. 1984
Lidocaine	42	Patients 22 with CHF	327 7.8	5	NONMEM	Vozeh et al. 1984
Procainamide	39	Patients 24 with CHF	116(P) 14(U) 3.0	5	NONMEM	Grasela and Sheiner 1984
Warfarin	163	32 hospitalized 131 outpatients	613 3.8	7	NONMEM	Mungall et al. 1985
Phenobarbital	59	Preterm infants	160 2.7	4	NONMEM	Grasela and Donn 1985
Phenytoin	37	Black patients	99 2.7	1	NONMEM	Miller et al. 1987
Metoclopramide	47	Cancer patients	? 8 to 10	6	NONMEM	Grevel et al. 1988
Cyclosporin	188	Bone marrow transplants age 1 mo to 44 yrs	1487 7.9	1	NPML	Mallet et al. 1988
Gentamicin	113	Neonates	270 2.4	11	NONMEM	Thomson et al. 1988
Gentamicin	113	Neonates	? $1 < n < 3$	3	NPML	Mallet et al. 1988

Drug	n	Patients	Values		Method	Reference
Phenytoin (intravenous)	49	Adults and elderly	122 2.5	5	NONMEM	Vozeh et al. 1988
Midazolam	12	Patients after cardiac surgery	Many	2	NONMEM	Maitre et al. 1989
Phenytoin	220	Japanese patients (steady state)	505 $18 < n < 23$	3	NONMEM	Yukawa et al. 1989
Midazolam Thiopental	40	Neonates (and mothers)	? 2.3	?	NONMEM	Bach et al. 1989
Teophylline	108	Neonates and young infants	$3 < n < 6$ 391 3.6	9	NONMEM	Moore et al. 1989
Mitoxantrone	21	Cancer patients	>300	0	APIS (NLMEM)	Launay et al. 1989
Theophylline	84	Hospitalized children	$7 < n < 20$ 314 3.7	8	NONMEM	Driscoll et al. 1989
Tobramycin (intravenous)	97	Heterogeneous group Hospitalized patients	322 3.3	4	NONMEM	Aarons et al. 1989
Zidovudine	72	HIV-infected patients	305 $1 < n < 14$	1	NONMEM	Gitterman et al. 1990
Thiopental	64	26 surgical patients 11 "heavy" drinkers	2325 36.3	3	NONMEM	Stanski and Maitre 1990
Gentamicin	18	Neonates: ExtraCorp. Membrane Oxygenation	? 2 to 8(?)		NONMEM	Cohen et al. 1990
Phenytoin	334	Japanese patients (ss, different doses)	756 2.3	4	NONMEM	Yukawa et al. 1990
Netilmicin	74	Neonates 27-42 weeks	258 3.5	5	NONMEM	Fattinger et al. 1991b
Carbamazepine	45	Psychiatric patients (trough samples)	159 3.5	10–12	NONMEM	Martin et al. 1991
Quinidine	60	Adults above 40 yrs	260 4.3	6	NONMEM	Fattinger et al. 1991a
Flurbiprofen	26	Rheumatoid arthritis patients	237(P) 23(syn)	0	NONMEM	Aarons 1991b

Table 2. *Continued*

Drug	Subjects		ntot / n	Covariates	Method	Authors
	N	Type				
Indomethacin (intravenous)	83	Neonates 25–36 weeks	665 / 8.0	9	NONMEM	Wiest et al. 1991
Lithium	79	Psychiatric inpatients	266 / 3.4	9	NONMEM	Jermain et al. 1991
Theophylline	35	Neonates treated with suppositories	138 / 3.9	7	NONMEM	Karlsson et al. 1991
Digoxin (plus quinidine)	94	Patients treated with digoxin 37 with quinidine	230 / 2.4	7	NONMEM	Williams et al. 1992
Quinidine	139	Male hospitalized patients up to 92 yrs	391 / 2.8	>10	NONMEM	Verme et al. 1992

N, total number of individuals; $ntot$, total number of (blood) samples; n, number of samples per subject (average = $ntot/N$); (P), drug level in plasma; (U), drug level in urine; (syn), drug level in synovial fluid; CHF, congestive heart failure; HIV, human immuno-deficiency virus; NONMEM, software which implements a nonlinear mixed-effects model; NPML, nonparametric maximum likelihood estimation method; NLMEM, nonlinear mixed-effects model patients who have an altered function of the drug-eliminating organs due to a pathological disorder (for example, patients with liver disease or renal failure), age (e.g., old patients and neonates), or a drug–drug interaction. These patients may be at increased risk of over- or underdosing.

As an example, in a recent study with the antiarrhythmic agent quinidine (FATTINGER et al. 1991a), a population analysis with NONMEM was performed on data from 60 patients (one to ten concentration values per individual). It could be shown that the pharmacokinetics in patients with moderate liver dysfunction did not substantially differ from those in patients with a normal liver function on the same dosing regimen. This means that dose adjustment in these patients is not needed. Different results were obtained in that study for patients with severe impairment of either liver or heart function. Although this group comprised only five patients, a clear trend for higher serum concentrations was detected. This subgroup deserves, therefore, further study.

To detect factors that influence pharmacokinetic parameters represents part of every population pharmacokinetic analysis. Most published studies listed in Table 2 investigated widely used drugs in special populations, with the goal of detecting patient subgroups with different kinetics. The list emphasizes the increasing focus on neonates and children who, obviously, represent a target group for use of the population approach. Also, several reports have documented the ability of population analysis of sparse plasma level data to detect the influence of concomitant administration of pharmacokinetically interacting drugs (GRASELA et al. 1987; YUKAWA et al. 1990; WILLIAMS et al. 1992).

Among the studies listed in Table 2, the 322-patient study on phenytoin (GRASELA et al. 1983), based on a compilation of three data sets, was exceptional in size. Most studies in which the influence of one or more factors on pharmacokinetics could be established and quantitated relied on less than 100 patients. This sample size is far less than the typical recruitment in multicenter phase III clinical trials with new drugs. Apart from a few exceptions in surgery (MAITRE et al. 1987; STANSKI and MAITRE 1990) and cancer patients (LAUNAY et al. 1989), the studies listed in Table 2 all relied on sporadic blood sampling, typically three to four or even less blood samples per subject. As a consequence, the total number of blood samples (300–600 in most cases) in each study was typically of the same order as in a comparative cross-over or parallel group pharmacokinetic study in 12–18 volunteers.

This compilation brings strong evidence that with suitable statistical methodology, only a few blood samples suffice to take advantage of each subject's data within a study. This illustrates the power of the population approach. Data from patients receiving a drug for therapeutic reasons during clinical studies can help to investigate/discover the influence of different factors on the pharmacokinetics of the drug. The full kinetic screen for data collection together with a traditional analysis (if feasible) or a population analysis (always possible) of the corresponding data provides an ethical approach for investigation of drug kinetics, for instance in extreme age classes such as the elderly (TEMPLE 1989; THOMSON and TUCKER 1992) and the neonate. Most drugs listed in Table 2 have a narrow therapeutic index. All applications share in common the ultimate goal of providing rationale for optimum dosing in a population (Sect. III) or the individual patient (Sect. IV).

III. Design of Optimum A Priori Dosage Regimen

As soon as possible during drug development, a rational choice of dose or dosing regimen to be tested is desirable, in particular in studies investigating the concentration–effect relationship. The inclusion of considerations on pharmacokinetic/pharmacodynamic variability in the a priori selection of dose and dosage regimen will increase the chances for the efficacy trial to be successful.

In the past, thoughts on dosing regimens have been based largely on pharmacokinetic considerations. An optimum a priori dosing regimen can be defined as that dosage which will maximize the number of patients having plasma (or serum or blood) concentrations within a desired range. That range will depend on several factors, such as the concentration–effect relationship, the severity of toxic effects, and the prognosis of the disease without treatment. Since the population pharmacokinetic parameters describe the average dose–concentration relationship and its variability in a patient population, these estimates can be used to predict the fraction of patients whose concentration is expected to lie within a given range under a given dosing regimen. Scenarios can be as simple as standard dosing across individuals or, also, involve dosage regimen adjusted for the covariates (e.g., weight, APGAR score, smoking status, race) which were found to be significant in the corresponding population analysis (see examples in Table 2). Methods have been described that derive a clinically relevant optimum dosing strategy by minimizing an associated mathematically suitable "cost" function (GAILLOT et al. 1979; VOZEH and STEIMER 1985). However, for practical purposes, a simple "trial and error" method based on Monte Carlo computer simulations for predicting mean ($\pm$ confidence limits) plasma concentration profile under different dosing schemes may suffice in many cases (Fig. 6). Different scenarios regarding dosing regimen can be investigated, allowing post hoc decision-making by the clinician in view of his/her knowledge and understanding of the relationship between concentration and therapeutic effect. This approach has been successfully applied in several studies (VOZEH et al. 1982a,b, 1988; AARONS et al. 1989; FATTINGER 1991b).

Figure 7 illustrates the results of a prospective evaluation in patients of a dosing scheme based on a population analysis of the antiepileptic agent phenytoin. It shows an excellent agreement between the Monte Carlo simulation and the results of the subsequent clinical study with respect to the fraction of patients having serum concentrations in the desired range (BLASER

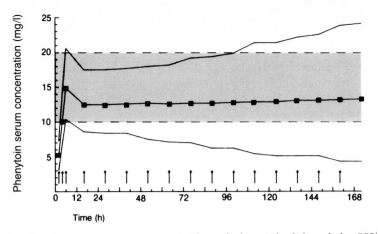

Fig. 6. Predicted average serum concentration of phenytoin (■) and the 90% confidence interval (*solid lines*) after the loading scheme consisting in three intravenous bolus doses of 5 mg/kg administered 2 h apart. The *arrows* indicate the times a dose was given. The expected concentration–time course (trough levels) on a maintenance dose (150 mg intravenously every 12 h in a 70-kg patient) following the initial loading is also shown. Pharmacokinetic parameters for the predictions during maintenance therapy (V_{max}, K_m) were obtained from the literature. Monte Carlo simulations ($n = 1000$) were used to predict average concentration and interindividual variability. Note that 6 h after starting therapy almost the entire 90% confidence interval lies within the recommended therapeutic range for phenytoin (10–20 mg/l). (From Vozeh et al. 1988)

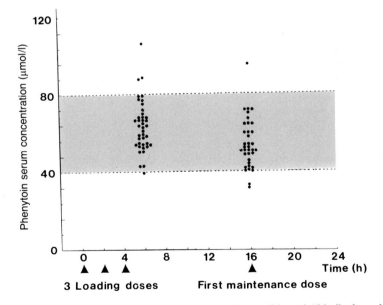

Fig. 7. Serum concentration of phenytoin in 40 patients, 2 h and 12 h (before the first maintenance dose) after intravenous loading. The loading scheme was three doses of 5 mg/kg/body weight each, given 2 h apart (*arrows*). The serum concentrations in 36 of 40 patients were within the recommended therapeutic range (*shaded area*). (From Blaser et al. 1989)

et al. 1989). This is an example of a population a priori dosage regimen in which, as in most other applications to date, the target is of a pharmacokinetic type. The underlying concepts are applicable to pharmacodynamic targets as well, provided a suitable mathematical model for the dose–effect relationship is available.

IV. Bayesian Estimation of Individual Pharmacokinetic Parameters

One primary interest in population parameter estimates derives from their usefulness for *individual* decision-making. The parameter estimates obtained in a population analysis can be used as prior distribution for Bayesian estimation of the individual pharmacokinetic parameters in a patient treated with the drug. This is the so-called Bayesian feedback procedure. An a priori (before treatment) standard dosing regimen can then be improved in a given patient using feedback on the basis of limited plasma concentration data (one or two measurements) (Sheiner et al. 1979; Vozeh et al. 1981; Vozeh and Steiner 1987). With this information the dose can be adjusted to achieve in each patient a concentration within a narrow range. This tool has been applied for individual dosage optimization of several drugs with a narrow therapeutic range (for a review, see Vozeh and Steimer 1985), with special emphasis on gentamicin, theophylline, and phenytoin (Table 2). For phenytoin, several comparative studies against nomograms have all shown superiority of Bayesian feedback (Vozeh et al. 1981; Yukawa et al. 1991). Some clinical pharmacokinetics groups have gained early and broad experience with drug dosing feedback techniques relying on population parameters (Kelman et al. 1982), which lead to substantial improvement in cost-effectiveness of therapeutic drug monitoring (Vozeh 1987). A recent review documents the widespread application of Bayesian parameter estimation in the area of drug monitoring (Thomson and Whiting 1992).

There has been recent emphasis on concentration-controlled randomized clinical trials during drug development (Sanathanan and Peck 1991; Sanathanan et al. 1991). Patients are randomized with respect to several levels of drug concentration rather than doses. The principle has been shown to be feasible and useful in dedicated clinical studies (Kragh-Sorensen et al. 1976; Vozeh et al. 1982b; Gelenberg et al. 1989). Clinical efficacy in relationship to plasma level can be evaluated without Bayesian feedback. For instance, successful applications in cancer pharmacodynamics have been reported for predicting the area under the plasma concentration–time curve, as a measure of exposure to the drug, through a weighted linear combination of two to three plasma levels collected according to a "limited sampling" procedure (Ratain et al. 1990). However, Bayesian feedback can be applied in concentration-monitored studies as an efficient tool for adjusting the individual dosage, insofar as reasonable estimates of population pharmacokinetic characteristics are available at the start. Experience from therapeutic drug monitoring suggests that the corresponding target value will be achieved quicker and more reliably than with less elaborate methods (VOZEH 1987).

Bayesian estimation can also considerably facilitate the evaluation of the concentration–effect relationship in clinical studies. Often, an appropriate investigation of the concentration–effect relationship is not possible because the information on the concentration of the drug in individual patients is limited. The use of Bayesian estimates of the individual parameters within the associated pharmacokinetic model has been shown to yield accurate and precise predictions of the concentration time course in individual patients (VOZEH et al. 1985). The fact that information about the full concentration profile is available for each patient substantially increases the probability that important connections between plasma concentration and drug effects will be detected. An example of applying this approach is a clinical study that investigated the relationship between the recurrence of the disturbances of the heart rhythm and the lidocaine serum concentration in patients after acute myocardial infarction (VOZEH et al. 1987).

One major output of the population approach is that it allows an estimate of the complete individual concentration profile to be calculated for every patient according to his/her personal dosing history. In a drug-monitoring perspective, this information is used for ad hoc titration of the patient. In an investigational context, the information can be used to look for the presence and the form of the relationship between the therapeutic effect or side-effects and different concentration-related values (area under the curve, average steady-state value, trough or peak levels). It should be noted that Bayesian estimation has a filtering effect towards the population mean. The less data will be available within an individual, the more the Bayesian estimate may deviate from the true value, until further collection causes the individual data to outweigh the population information.

A global synthetic scheme of the population approach, with the combined use of population and individual data for prediction of population response and (Bayesian) estimation of individual parameters is given as Fig. 8.

V. Recent Novel Applications of Nonlinear Mixed Effects Models to Other Drug-Related Areas

The general formulation of the population model offers great potential in diverse drug-related areas, which is receiving increased recognition. Among recent novel applications, we shall cite:

1. *The use of population analysis methodology for pooled analysis of a set of conventional pharmacokinetic studies* in drug development (Table 3). Recent studies, especially on alfentanyl (MAITRE et al. 1987), bisoprolol (GREVEL et al. 1989) and felbamate (GRAVES et al. 1989), have shown the usefulness of population methods for such meta-analyses. However, most studies to date (Table 3) had been restricted to the straightforward application of one population method (NONMEM), as a statistical tool, to

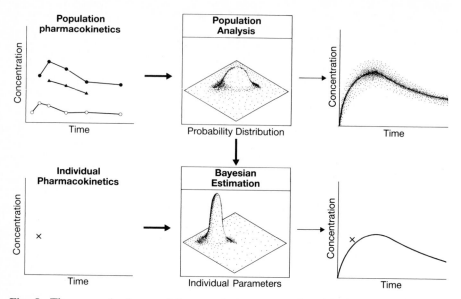

Fig. 8. The general scheme of the population approach, with the example of pharmacokinetic data. *Top*: Population analysis of (sparse) kinetic data (*left panel*) aims at estimating the probability distribution of the parameters (*center panel*) which, through the kinetic model, allows MonteCarlo calculation of predicted profiles in response to drug administration (*right panel*). *Bottom*: The combination of subject-specific data, e.g., one single measurement (*left panel*) with the population distribution which serves as "prior" information (*top center panel*) allows Bayesian estimation of a "posterior" probability distribution (*bottom center panel*); its mode (maximum) can serve as an estimate of the individual's parameters which, through the kinetic model, allows reconstruction of the corresponding profile (*right panel*) and therefore prediction of concentration versus time for any tentative dosing regimen

pharmacokinetic profiles of the conventional experimental type with more than ten points per subject (see GRASELA et al. 1986 for an extreme example). In several cases, the category of volunteers was healthy subjects, not patients, the number of individuals was small, not large, and blood sampling was extensive, not sparse. Also, further applications where population analysis with NONMEM was used as a substitute or complement to classic statistical analysis include assessment of bioavailability (GRAVES and CHANG 1990; KANIWA et al. 1990) and sustained-release characteristics of oral dosage forms (MURATA et al. 1989). The comparison of Table 2 (based on drug studies carried out in routine clinical practice) and Table 3 shows a clear discrepancy between several such applications and the regular claims in favor of the population approach, especially with regard to the number and type of subjects, as well as to the number of samples. This practice had led over some time to ambiguity, confusion, and even misunderstanding regarding the application of the population approach to pharmacokinetics or even its meaning. Also, several reports of premarketing studies focused

Table 3. Some reported applications of population kinetics during new drug development

Drug	Subjects N	Subjects Type	n_{tot}	n	Covariates	Method	Authors
Mexiletine (antiarrhythmic)	58	Patients 27 with CHF 8 liver abnormal	452	7.8	4	NONMEM	VOZEH et al. 1982a
Maprotiline (antidepressant)	99	Healthy subjects	1095	11.1	0	NONMEM	FLUEHLER et al. 1984
Alprazolam (antianxiety)	10	Healthy volunteers	480	48	0	NONMEM	GRASELA et al. 1986
	28	Interaction with imipramine	255	9.1	2 +1	NONMEM	GRASELA et al. 1987
	61	Patients (prospective)	249	4.1	1	NONMEM	ANTAL et al. 1989
	248	Patients (retrospective)	445	1.8	1		
Alfentanil (analgesic)	45	Patients undergoing surgery	614	13.6	6	NONMEM	MAITRE et al. 1987
Lisinopril (ACE inhibitor)	60	Elderly (40) Renal dis. (20)	381	6.4	6	NONMEM	THOMSON et al. 1989
Bisoprolol (β-antagonist)	84	Patients (all types)	1158	13.8	10	NONMEM	GREVEL et al. 1989
Felbamate (antiepileptic)	29	Resistant patients	300	$8 < n < 13$	7	NONMEM	GRAVES et al. 1989
Felodipine (calcium antagonist)	140	Hypertensive (67) Healthy volunteers (73)	?	$n > 10$	4	STS	BLYCHERT et al. 1991
Isradipine (calcium antagonist)	252	Hypertensive patients	697	2.8	22	EDA	LAPLANCHE et al. 1991
Imazodan (cardiotonic)	42	Patients with CHF	439	10.5	10	NONMEM	OLSON 1991
Didanosine (anti-HIV)	69	AIDS patients	?	>15	3	NONMEM	PAI et al. 1992

ACE, angiotensin-converting enzyme; STS, standard two-stage estimation method; EDA, exploratory data analysis; other abbreviations as in Table 2 solely on the quantification of variability, without an attempt to relate it to influential covariates. Attempts have been made to clarify these issues (COLBURN 1989; ANTAL and GRASELA 1991). Indeed, population analysis as a statistical tool for handling sparse data is also applicable to extensive data. This property just reflects the power and the broad applicability in clinical pharmacology of the nonlinear mixed-effects model, the statistical methodology which underlines the population approach (SAMBOL 1992). Recent reports (ANTAL et al. 1989, 1991; LAPLANCHE et al. 1991) illustrate the trend towards prospective population studies in phase III multicenter clinical trials, with extensive discussion of the corresponding issues. The study on isradipine (LAPLANCHE et al. 1991) was the first one to focus on a widespread exploratory effort associated with a high-dimensional set of covariates.

2. *The analysis of dose–response escalation trials* (e.g., tolerability or efficacy studies) where individual volunteers are titrated in dose, e.g., up to some response (SHEINER et al. 1989; SAMBOL and SHEINER 1991). The fact that repeated measurements are carried out on each subject is handled within the framework of a statistical mixed-effects regression analysis with a dose–response model (e.g., a hyperbolic one). The methodology suggests superiority of cross-over in comparison with standard parallel-group designs. One major difference with respect to classical analysis resides in the point of view to be taken for clinical investigation: modeling and estimation (model fitting, regression, and parameter estimation) rather than testing hypotheses (treatment group comparison). In clinical pharmacology, the need for such a change in emphasis has been recently advocated (SHEINER 1989, 1990, 1991). If pursued, it would have substantial consequences for many aspects of clinical trials, far below statistical analysis per se (SHEINER 1992).

3. *The longitudinal analysis of clinical response data* (e.g., mental scores in Alzheimer's patients during drug treatment) in relationship to dosing rate in long-term phase III efficacy studies. One suggested model included the role of placebo associated with treatment changes and the deleterious influence arising from disease progression (HOLFORD 1992). The a priori superiority of nonlinear mixed-effects modeling over the conventional endpoint analysis at completion of the study is its ability to cope with changing dosing histories across as well as within subjects. A model-based population analysis allowed all data at repeated visits during the trial to be included in the analysis. Another example was the study of the association between average plasma level of zidovudine and the occurrence of either opportunistic infection or toxicity in 34 chronically treated AIDS patients, including intraindividual pharmacokinetic changes within patients (MENTRÉ and MALLET 1991).

4. *The use of "few-point" designs and population analysis in animal studies* for data collected under severe blood sampling constraints, e.g., sparse or even destructive sampling (LINDSTROM and BIRKES 1984). Specific applications to data in rats have been reported in the areas of physiological pharmacokinetics (LUDDEN et al. 1991) and pharmacokinetics/pharmacodynamics (AARONS et al. 1991). In the future, mixed-effects modeling may

also be useful for assessment of exposure to drug of animals participating in long-term and/or high-dose toxicology investigations, with minimal physiological disturbance since few-point sampling can be adopted.

Other specific applications of the software NONMEM to situations where kinetics are difficult to study have been reported, including pharmacokinetics of flurbiprofen in synovial fluid of rheumatoid arthritis patients (AARONS 1991b), the comparison in chimpanzees of the pharmacokinetics of two types of recombinant human tissue-type plasminogen activator (TANIGAWARA et al. 1991), the pharmacokinetics of subcutaneous cyclosporine over 18 weeks in rabbits (SHAH et al. 1992), and a proposal for pharmacokinetic study design under microgravity conditions (DRUSANO 1991).

Forthcoming methodological developments in the handling of categorical (e.g., binary) outcome variables in addition to graded responses are likely to have a major impact since, quite often, side-effects and adverse drug reactions or toxic events are of the categorical type. Such a feature has been announced in the version IV of NONMEM, released in late 1992 (BEAL and SHEINER 1992). It can be anticipated that further developments and applications of the population approach will occur in the near future in relationship with ongoing progress in methodology and software.

E. Problems and Issues?

The population approach relies on principles for data collection and data analysis which gave rise to extensive debate in the past (ENDRENYI 1985; SHEINER and BENET 1985; COLBURN and OLSON 1988; COLBURN 1989; AARONS 1991a). However, one should clearly distinguish between misconceptions and real problems.

I. Misconceptions

1. Misconception 1 (from some clinicians): "We are not interested in *population* kinetics, we have to focus on the *individual* patient."

This statement contrasts the individual and the population. As detailed in Sect. C.I and as outlined in the title of the seminal paper on the methodology (SHEINER et al. 1972), there should be no ambiguity: the population approach is based explicitly on the modeling of each individual's data. Each subject is recognized and identified as such all along the calculation steps. Only the necessity to cope with sparse individual data forces the focus on the estimation of *population* parameters, which can be achieved in one stage based on all data. In addition, the population parameters serve the ultimate goal of group-specific or subject-specific dosing, as illustrated in previous sections. They clearly represent relevant and useful information for the choice of drug dose and regimen in an *individual* patient.

2. Misconception 2 (from some data analysts): "You claim that you estimate a set of (pharmacokinetic) parameters with only one to three plasma levels per subject. . . . This is impossible! At least 3 to 5 times more points than parameters are needed."

The latter statement indeed may apply when separate (individual) analysis of plasma concentration profiles is performed. In the conventional approach the attempt is made to estimate the parameters of each individual separately. When data are sparse, the model is not identifiable and precise estimates cannot be obtained. In contrast, the population analysis is a global one. Under appropriate modeling assumptions, each individual borrows strength from the others. It is the very nature of the data which requires the analyst to adopt a "population" point of view so as to take advantage of similarities across subjects. The accuracy of the resulting estimates is governed by the number of subjects more than by the number of points per subject.

3. Misconception 3 (from some investigators): "Thank God! . . . We now have statistical methodology for deriving meaningful estimates from badly collected data in poorly designed studies."

Indeed, the population approach can cope with sparse data, observational data, routine data characterized by lack of control, and few design restrictions. This claim, however, should not be subject to overinterpretation. Population modeling and estimation offers a meaningful solution for analyzing unbalanced data with a complex underlying structure. But, just as any other statistical methodology, it is unable to rescue poor-quality data (e.g., when dosing history is poorly recorded in a clinical study or when dosing data is false due to poor compliance). It is likely that occasional failures in the analysis of retrospective data with population methods have their origin in poor data collection and/or overoptimistic belief in accuracy of the data.

II. Some Practical Problems

1. Reliability of Data and Analysis

Data collection can be prone to errors, especially in outpatients. A full pharmacokinetic screen design in phase III trials, although allowing flexibility regarding administration and timing of the sample, requires adequate logistics for drawing of blood, collection of plasma, recording of sampling information, shipment and storage of samples, assay for drug/metabolite(s), etc. In general, such practical problems can be solved through suitable organization according to good clinical practice requirements. Evidence from real studies exists that these difficulties can be overcome (Antal et al. 1989; Laplanche et al. 1991) and that pharmacokinetic screening during clinical trials is feasible at a reasonable cost and effort. Also, noncompliance is a well-known source of variability, especially in outpatients. Close monitoring of the patients' dosing behavior enhances the reliability of the data and of the pharmacokinetic extrapolations, avoiding variations of the input (drug administration) to be counted as changes in the pharmacokinetic process. For that purpose, devices like medication event monitoring systems (URQUHART and CHEVALLEY 1988) may be of help to deliver precise information about systematic or episodic noncompliance (CRAMER et al. 1989) and to provide insight into the actual rather than the prescribed dosing scheme in each patient (RUBIO et al. 1992)

Because of the complexity and the volume of the data, the creation of a data base suitable for population analysis requires substantial effort (GREVEL et al. 1987). The data analysis itself can also be a time-consuming process. The sequential nature of the statistical model-building and -testing process requires extensive model coding and reviewing of computer outputs in the form of tables and graphs. Even with a skilled data analyst, this can become a rate-limiting and time-critical factor for completion of a study. Although some strategies for detecting relationships between parameters and covariates have been suggested (MAITRE et al. 1987, 1991) and formalized recently (MANDEMA et al. 1992), success in model-building heavily relies upon the skill, experience, and intuition of the analyst. It requires a substantial number of iterative runs and/or models on a given data set for the data interpretation to be achieved. Over 60 analyses (i.e., "NONMEM runs") were performed in the model-building phase in two recent publications (WILLIAMS et al. 1992; VERME et al. 1992). In addition to the time required for reviewing of outputs, speed may also depend on numerical capabilities. All methods for population analysis are computer-intensive. A typical NONMEM or NPML run (e.g., on data from 100–200 subjects with about five plasma levels per individual) might well take several minutes of CPU time on a mainframe computer or a workstation, even with "reasonable" initial estimates. The use of "supercomputers" may be considered (SHAH et al. 1992).

Despite these concerns about the reliability of the data and the current lack of trained analysts familiar with population model-building, a recent survey within the European pharmaceutical industry indicated that 30 among 33 companies are interested in the population approach and that 14 (roughly one-half of them) already devote resources to it (JOCHEMSEN 1992). A coordinated data collection program in clinical pharmacokinetics is successfully ongoing in Japan for creation of a nationwide data base on selected drugs (TANIGAWARA and HORI 1992). This joint effort in more than 50 hospitals is largely based on the availability of the software NONMEM for data analysis (HORI 1988).

2. Methodological Issues

Even with good-quality data, the population approach raises methodological issues.

a) Investigations with Simulated Data

Computer simulation studies showed that population methods, primarily NONMEM (which is best documented) and NPML, work well when the assumptions made for analysis reflect the choices made for generating the simulated data (for a review, see STEIMER et al. 1985). More recently, simulation studies were also employed for comparing population study designs for pharmacokinetic and pharmacokinetic/pharmacodynamic investigations. These studies yielded further evidence that sparse data, when analyzed with (population) model-based statistical tools, are adequate for meaningful pharmacokinetic parameter estimation (AL-BANNA et al. 1990; WANG and ENDRENYI 1992) and comparison (WHITE et al. 1992), and pharmacokinetic/pharmacodynamic assessment (HASHIMOTO and SHEINER 1991).

b) Some Issues of General Concern

Besides study design, several statistical issues should be mentioned, including: the overlooking of an important covariate; the erroneous detection as being statistically influential of a factor which is in fact of no clinical relevance; the absence of knowledge about the actual level of the significance testing; the difficulty in assessing confidence intervals for the estimates; the impact of model misspecification at any level (kinetics, covariates, error); and the existence of bias in parameter estimates. Most of these issues are common to all nonlinear regression situations (BATES and WATTS 1988). They are not specific to population analysis with mixed-effects models but are indeed of concern in any model-based statistical analysis. A broader discussion of the statistical issues in population models, including regulatory considerations, has been given recently (O'NEILL 1992).

c) An Issue Specific to NONMEM up to Version III

NONMEM up to version III (BEAL and SHEINER 1980, 1989) has relied solely upon the "first-order" algorithm. Depending on the magnitude of between individual variation and on the degree of (parametric) non-linearity in the model, the approximation involved (a first-order Taylor expansion) might turn out to be poor. When inclusion of explanatory co-variates or identification of "homogeneous" subgroups in the regression analysis leads to substantial reduction of residual (unexplained) variation, this limitation of the first-order method becomes of less concern. Simulation studies indeed pinpoint the need for caution regarding the quality of NONMEM point and interval estimates when variability increases (WHITE et al. 1991). Improvements in the calculation scheme of NONMEM are foreseen in the near future, which will alleviate this issue (BEAL and SHEINER 1992).

III. Validation of the Results

Population analysis of drug-related data is inherently a difficult statistical problem. Therefore, despite ongoing methodological progress, the "unexplored areas" are not likely to be fully clarified soon. They are, however, of special concern in drug-related applications because of the potential impact of the findings, which are likely to influence the therapeutic drug dosing practice in patients, one major aspect of health care. In order to gain acceptance especially by regulatory authorities, there is a need to explicitly state the assumptions underlying the population data analysis and to provide a complete inventory of the multiple steps involved (PECK 1992). Also, it is essential that the quality of the results of a population study/analysis be evaluated in terms of robustness and/or sensitivity, and that evidence be provided for the results to be reasonable and independent of the analyst. Beyond pharmacokinetic applications per se, this remark holds for most applications which can be envisioned in the context of drug evaluation and therapy, also at the pharmacodynamic and clinical levels. Accordingly, some evaluation/validation scheme of the population model should be built into any pharmacokinetic or pharmacokinetic/pharmacodynamic population study (MAITRE et al. 1988; VOZEH et al. 1990). Among 30 studies published between 1977 and the end of 1989, we found 14 which included a validation step. Given the novelty of the population approach in this period, this figure can be considered satisfactory. Of concern is the fact that in recent years, which have seen a significant rise in the number of published studies, we observed a slight decline in the proportion of those which were validated. Among the 20 studies which were issued between 1990 and mid-1992, eight included a validation scheme. In the future, this trend should be corrected and validation should become a systematic practice in population analysis.

As already mentioned, the complexity of the population models and the fact that only sparse data are available in each individual increases the possibility of biased results. For instance, the nonlinearity of the statistical model and the ill-conditioning of a given problem can produce numerical difficulties and force the estimation algorithm into a false minimum. However, the most crucial issue is the diversity among data analysts. In population analysis, the quality and reliability of the results depend on the level of expertise of the data analyst to a greater extent than is the rule for other more classical statistical approaches (see, e.g., RODDA et al. 1988 for general statistical issues related to clinical trials). Due to the exploratory nature of the data analysis, unique solutions often do not exist. Different scientists will use different models and make different technical decisions. One pragmatic approach to solve this problem "within the study" is to divide the available data into a learning sample (e.g., two-thirds of the data) and a test sample (e.g., one-third of the data). The former is used for the analysis, whereas the latter serves for validation purposes. This idea is, of course, not new, nor does it represent a unique feature of the population approach. Such data splitting for empirical validation of the final model and its predictive performance was recommended for linear multiple regression many years ago (see, e.g., NETER and WASSERMAN 1974). However, this issue of statistical validation is still open. Recent work in the area of linear regression suggests that, in order to maximize predictive accuracy, the entire sample be used rather than a subset of it for both development and assessment of the statistical model (ROECKER 1991).

Within the context of population analysis, the actual procedure how this validation is performed (choice of the response variable, choice of the test sample, validation criteria) should be governed primarily by the ultimate goal of the population study. It is recommended that a "pragmatic approach" be used showing as directly as possible that the model derived in the analysis performs satisfactorily when it is used for the intended purpose. Such a pragmatic approach has the advantage of being relatively independent of model and distributional assumptions and not requiring complex statistical methodology. This increases the probability of convincing an independent reviewer that the data analysis is reasonable, which is particularly important if the results are used within the context of a regulatory authorization procedure. For example, if the estimates of the population pharmacokinetic parameters are used in a Bayesian estimation scheme to predict individual plasma concentration–time profiles in order to demonstrate that a relationship between the drug concentration and effect exists, the investigator would be well-advised to present data that show that the population parameter estimates, when used in the Bayesian estimation, in fact reliably predict the individual concentration profile. This has been done in the example of the lidocaine concentration–effect relationship mentioned above in Sect. D.IV (VOZEH et at. 1985, 1987). If, on the other hand, the estimates of the population pharmacokinetic parameters in otherwise healthy patients are used as a basis to see whether patients with a concomitant disease of the eliminating organs are expected to attain different concentration levels and therefore need different dosing recommendations, convincing evidence has to be presented that the estimates reliably predict both the mean response and the variability of the plasma concentration in these otherwise healthy patients. This can be done, for example, by comparing the point prediction and the estimate of the variability with the serum concentration data in the test sample (FATTINGER et al. 1991a). Finally, if the parameter estimates are used to generate dosing recommendations, it has to be shown that they reliably describe the dose–concentration relationship in the patient population of interest (see Fig. 7). The pragmatic approach to validation of the results is fairly straightforward in cases like plasma concentration monitoring. It is not yet clear how the validation can be carried out when the aim of the (population) analysis is to confirm or deny drug efficacy.

F. Integration of the Population Approach into Clinical Drug Development

I. Introduction

Currently, there is increasing focus on the role of pharmacokinetics in pharmaceutical research and regulation (BALANT et al. 1990; SALMONSON and RANE 1990), and on implementation of pharmacokinetic/pharmacodynamic investigation and modeling as a core tool for drug development (PECK et al. 1990; CAMPBELL 1990; KROBOTH et al. 1991; SALE and BLASCHKE 1992). The consensus reached by scientists from the FDA, academia, and industry is outlined in a recent conference report (PECK et al. 1992). The general integration of strategies involving specifically the population approach has also been advocated (SHEINER 1992) and its potential contribution was discussed from a regulatory perspective, both European (GUNDERT-REMY 1992) and American (PECK 1992). In this section, we formulate a proposal on how the population approach can be implemented within the framework of studies that are currently performed during clinical drug development. The suggestions consider the advantages and limitations as highlighted in earlier papers (COLBURN and OLSON 1988; BALANT et al. 1990). They represent a consensus of the authors reached at the discussions within the "Population Pharmacokinetics Working Group" in Basel in 1990. It is conceivable that other experts in this field would suggest a broader application of the population approach in the drug development program. However, one of the primary goals of this section is to make recommendations that are supported by both theoretical considerations and some practical experience. Since up to the present most experience has been collected in studies concerning pharmacokinetics, the proposal is largely devoted to the application of population *pharmacokinetics*. There is, however, as already mentioned, a clear trend towards broader use of population concepts regarding study design, data analysis, and especially estimation of population and individual parameters in clinical research, towards expanding *pharmacodynamic investigation*, and also towards refining *dose–response analysis*. These aspects also will be touched upon. A further promising dimension is the application of population concepts to animal preclinical research, for instance in toxicokinetics as a support to safety assessment in toxicological studies. The related issues will not be discussed herein.

Although the advantages of the population approach will be most apparent in clinical trials in patients, the concept also can be implemented in early human studies. In the following sections, the opportunities for application of the population approach to pharmacokinetics/pharmacodynamics will be discussed separately for the different phases of drug development research. The primary objectives of the studies are discussed briefly. We focus on the new aspects associated with implementation of the population approach.

II. Early Human Studies (Phase I)

In these studies, the drug is administered under well-defined and controlled experimental conditions to a limited number of subjects (usually healthy volunteers), in order to establish the tolerance profile of the new chemical entity. First information about the pharmacokinetics and the pharmaco-dynamics of the compound in man is obtained. It can be strongly recom-mended to assess pharmacokinetics via extensive concentration–time profiles and pharmacodynamics, if possible, using an outcome that can be relatively immediately observed and quantified. Phase I studies then deliver as much information as possible about pharmacokinetics (such as linearity and major pathways of elimination) and the concentration–effect relationship (such as identification of pharmacodynamic endpoints that show dose–concentration–effect dependency). These data serve to define the (mathematical) model(s) which will serve for later analyses and predictions, and assist in the design of an optimum research strategy in the later phases of development. If a relatively large number of samples is obtained in each subject (full profile pharmacokinetic/pharmacodynamic studies), the statistical methodology to analyze these data can in most cases involve individual fitting using standard nonlinear regression models. The individual estimates of the pharmacokinetic and pharmacodynamic parameters then can be used to obtain estimates of the mean and variability of the parameters in the studied population according to the two-stage approach (Sect. B.II).

III. Early Clinical Studies (Phase II)

Phase II studies examine whether the compound has the expected clinical effect and aim at defining the possible clinical dose range in patients. The most important role of the population approach at this stage is to help examine the dose–concentration–effect relationships in patients for both clinical efficacy and safety. Of course, the identification of a dose–response relationship will depend upon the ability to observe a clinically useful outcome or at least a surrogate endpoint in a temporal relationship with the dosing history. The presence (or absence) of a detectable and, possibly, quantifiable relationship between concentration and the clinical outcome (safety and efficacy) will strongly influence the research strategy in later phases. The relationships of fixed dose to concentration level and of con-centration level to clinical outcome can be explored.

The application of population pharmacokinetics here requires that several timed blood samples are obtained in each patient together with accurate information on each subject's relevant dosage history. The number of blood samples and the sampling design (time points) will depend on the pharmacokinetics of the drug (information obtained in phase I studies) and on the pharmacokinetic model expected to be used by the population analysis. It should be noted that the latter model need not be identical to the pharmacokinetic model identified in phase I studies. Depending on the expected concentration–effect relationship and technical and ethical considerations, a less complex model can be implemented for the population analysis than the model established in phase I studies. This use of a less complex or "incomplete" model has been described in the literature in another context as the "minimal model" approach (BERGMAN and COBELLI 1980). Although not explicitly stated, this idea was present in the first paper describing the population analysis of pharmacokinetics of a drug in patients (SHEINER et al. 1977). In that study, although digoxin pharmacokinetics are known to be described by a multicompartment model, the authors chose to use a one-compartment model. All concentration measurements had been obtained in the "postdistribution" phase, as concentration values taken early after the dose were considered to be of little clinical relevance.

The goal of the population analysis at this stage is to obtain a first set of estimates of the (patient) population pharmacokinetic parameters which can be obtained by analyzing the plasma concentration data using one of the global model-based population methods (see Sect. C). These analyses and estimates form the basis to explore the concentration–effect relationship for both toxicity and efficacy. The estimates of the population pharmacokinetic parameters and an estimated individual complete drug concentration profile for the whole duration of the study can be calculated for every patient for whom concentration measurements and accurate information about the dosing history are available (see Sect. D.IV). This information may then be used to explore associations between different concentration-related values used as indices of exposure to the drug (e.g., area under the curve, concentration at trough or at peak) and the effect endpoints. Besides providing important information for the rational design of the clinical trials including fixed-dose designs (see Sect. F.IV), the investigation of the concentration–effect relationship may support the claim for drug efficacy by demonstrating the existence of a relationship between the desired therapeutic effect and the plasma concentration of the drug. This may be achieved with the full pharmacokinetic/pharmacodynamic model or, as indicated above, using some integrated measure of exposure to the drug. Current results in the field of cancer chemotherapy appear promising (RATAIN et al. 1990).

IV. Clinical Trials (Late Phase II, Phase III)

The design strategy for confirmatory clinical trials to establish the efficacy of a drug in a therapeutic setting will be influenced by the results of the analysis described in the previous section, i.e., the population pharmacokinetic parameters and the information about the dose–concentration–effect relationship in the efficacy and toxicity domain. For example, for a compound for which the dose–clinical effect relationship does not show substantially larger interindividual variability compared to the relationship between concentration and effect (be it because of low pharmacokinetic variability or because of a shallow concentration–effect curve resulting in similar intensity of the drug effects over a wide range of concentration values), the collection of pharmacokinetic data can be quite limited. Here the goal is to see, in patient groups with known risk factors (e.g., renal failure), whether different recommendations for the initial (a priori) dosage are needed because the estimates of pharmacokinetic parameters are sufficiently different among subgroups to warrant such initial dosing changes. On the other hand, if a compound shows very large variability of the pharmacokinetic parameters between patients and there is a relationship between concentration and effect, a design that controls for this variability by randomizing patients to different plasma concentration intervals (instead of doses) may be appropriate to increase the power of the study to demonstrate that increasing doses of drug are effective and safe. If the desired concentration range can be established, individual dose adjustment to achieve the target window in most patients may be the optimum strategy. In studies in which a concentration target is to be achieved for each patient, estimates of population pharmacokinetic parameters derived from prior studies are needed in conjunction with the concentration measurements in patients during the course of study in order to adjust efficiently the dose individually for each subject.

For drugs in routine clinical use (Table 2), valuable results could be obtained with patient numbers of about 100 or sometimes less. In some cases, less than ten patients in a disease subgroup proved sufficient to deliver a strong enough signal for detection of a clinically relevant alteration in kinetics. In the prospective context of drug development, however, it would be unwise to take these figures for granted. Ideally, the sample for population analysis should include all patients foreseen in the clinical study. Also, independent of whether a dose-or concentration-based design is used, it would be of benefit for patients belonging to potential risk groups (e.g., elderly, liver failure or renal failure patients) to be included at this relatively early stage in the studies in order to obtain a full-range picture of variability in the population. In this way, the influence of different factors on the pharmacokinetics of the compound and on the clinical outcomes can be investigated in actual therapeutic settings (see Sect. D), with the expectation of detecting some predictive covariates among the set of recorded individual attributes. Differential efficacy or toxicity observed in some subgroups may then be related to the pharmacokinetics. This strategy may, however, pose problems concerning the power of the clinical trials to demonstrate efficacy. By including patient groups with possibly different pharmacokinetics and/or response, the variability in clinical outcome response may increase, which results in lower power to demonstrate differences in efficacy versus reference therapy or placebo. In addition, ethical considerations can arise from the fact that severely ill patients may receive an inactive treatment in placebo-controlled trials. Our proposal in order to avoid these problems is that these risk group patients, who would normally be excluded from an efficacy trial, be included in the study in parallel or more precisely *in addition* to the group that fulfills the stringent inclusion criteria, with a different study design. These patients would all receive the active compound and be closely monitored with respect to the achieved plasma concentrations and the drug effects (including undesirable adverse effects). Thus, they would not be included in the data base used for efficacy assessment. The results (pharmacokinetic and pharmacodynamic) in these additional groups would then be combined with the results in the patients who were included in the controlled part of the trial to see whether important differences are present. Regarding, for instance, the effect of age, disease states, and comedications, such an approach would yield results representative for patients who will be treated with the drug, and it would allow the evaluation of the effect (and side-effects) in addition to the pharmacokinetic parameters. Also it would avoid the ethical problems of giving a new compound to and performing a pharmacokinetic study in patients who do not need the drug for therapeutic reasons.

V. Late Clinical Trials (Late Phase III, Phase IV)

Late clinical trials that are mainly performed to assess the safety profile of a compound that has been shown to be effective also can be used to elucidate further the pharmacokinetic/pharmacodynamic characteristics of a new compound and its dosing requirements in different subpopulations of patients, for instance ethnic groups which may be underrepresented in earlier trials. The implementation of the population approach during these studies will depend on the state of knowledge of the pharmacokinetic and pharmacodynamic properties of the compound and, of course, on the relevance of plasma levels or pharmacodynamic markers for optimal drug therapy. As the catalogue of applications listed in Sect. D shows, phase IV studies are closest to the studies that have so far been analyzed using population approaches. Also, the growing experience in the Japanese drug monitoring program suggests that large-scale multicenter drug surveillance in outpatients in feasible and useful (TANIGAWARA and HORI 1992).

G. Concluding Remarks

The "population approach" is a new point of view in clinical drug evaluation and therapy. It emphasizes the *estimation* of parameters describing the dose–concentration–response relationship both within and between patients (including its variability), in addition to making between-groups comparisons for efficacy/safety assessment. The population approach has been shown to hold the promise of providing meaningful analyses of data from nonstringent designs, provided the data are of good quality. Accordingly, for successful implementation, it should take advantage of the rigorous study design, data collection logistics, and methodologies of clinical trials and not be opposed to existing clinical trials. The population approach can be a valuable complement to conventional approaches for collection of pharmacokinetic/ pharmacodynamic data, for assessment of efficacy/safety in relationship to drug plasma levels (defining the "therapeutic window"), and for building of knowledge for drug dosing (at both the pharmacokinetic and the clinical level) in the target population, including special subgroups. Ideally, activity should start in phase I tolerability trials at the very first administration in humans. It should continue with pharmacokinetic/pharmacodynamic investigation in phase II for providing guidance on dosing to be used in confirmatory trials. In phase III, a full pharmacokinetic screen is a potential alternative to selected pharmacokinetic investigations in subgroups and for the examination of drug–drug interactions. We have emphasized the need for a validation step in order to ascertain the results of a population analysis in a prospective context. The population approach employs the statistical methodology of mixed-effects modeling, which is of special value when the number of blood samples is limited for practical and/or ethical reasons (e.g., in extreme age classes). While continuing to evolve and be evaluated, the level of development of the mathematical/statistical methodology is sufficient regarding both methods and software to justify efforts for data collection in volunteers and patients. But the required time and capacity for data analysis and validation of results of a given study, along with the present lack of expertise and of skilled personnel needed for data analysis (for all methods with the possible exception of NONMEM, where training courses do exist), may be limiting factors.

The population approach is still in its infancy in drug development. Before its implementation can be envisaged as a routine practice even for drugs with a narrow therapeutic index, the logistics and methodologies need to be further carefully evaluated on a broad basis in clinical trials. The responsibility lies within both the research-based industry and the regulatory bodies. Within industry, which has the obligation to carry out presubmission clinical trials, there is still a general fear that additional delays in drug development, submission of registration files, and ultimately approval will result from the implementation of novel approaches. Regulatory authorities have the opportunity to be open-minded and to give credit to scientifically and clinically innovative approaches in new drug applications with an obvious potential to improve the efficiency of drug development in the long run. This process has started, as shown by recent approvals in the United States (PECK 1992) and by the efforts of the FDA to provide guidance to industrial investigators. The authors are confident that the benefits of the population approach should favorably counterbalance its costs and risks for all parties involved in drug development, evaluation, and therapy.

Acknowledgements. The authors acknowledge the constructive contributions made by members of the European COST-B1's subcommittee on "Population Approaches in Drug Development and Use" (L. AARONS, L.P. BALANT, M. ROWLAND). J.-L. STEIMER is grateful to M.-E. EBELIN, H. ECKERT, R. LAPLANCHE, W. NIEDERBERGER, B. VON WARTBURG, and other colleagues from Sandoz Pharma for input and support.

References

Aarons L (1991a) Population pharmacokinetics: theory and practice. Br J Clin Pharmacol 32:669–670

Aarons L (1991b) The kinetics of flurbiprofen in synovial fluid. J Pharmacokinet Biopharm 19:265–269

Aarons L (1992a) Population pharmacokinetics. Int J Clin Pharmacol Ther Toxicol 30:520–522

Aarons L (1992b) Population pharmacokinetics: a Trojan horse? Pharm Med 6:359–366

Aarons L, Vozeh S, Wenk M, Weiss PH, Follath F (1989) Population pharmacokinetics of tobramycin. Br J Clin Pharmacol 28:305–314

Aarons L, Mandema J, Danhof M (1991) A population analysis of the pharmacokinetics and pharmacodynamics of midazolam in the rat. J Pharmacokinet Biopharm 19:485–496

Al-Banna MK, Kelman AW, Whiting B (1990) Experimental design and efficient parameter estimation in population pharmacokinetics. J Pharmacokinet Biopharm 18:347–360

Amisaki T, Tatsuhara T (1988) An alternative tow-stage method via the EM-algorithm for the estimation of population pharmacokinetic parameters. J Pharmacobiodyn 11:335–348

Antal EJ, Grasela TH (eds) (1991) The application of population pharmacokinetics to drug development and utilization. J Pharmacokinet Biopharm 19 [Suppl]: 1S–113S

Antal EJ, Grasela TH, Smith RB (1989) An evaluation of population pharmacokinetic trials: III. Prospective data collection versus retrospective data assembly. Clin Pharmacol Ther 46:552–559

Antal EJ, Grasela TH, Ereshefsky L, Wells BG, Evans RL, Smith RB (1991) A multi-center study to evaluate the pharmacokinetic and clinical interactions between alprazolam and imipramine. J Pharmacokinet Biopharm [Suppl]19: 93S–100S

Bach V, Carl P, Ravlo O, Crawford ME, Jensen AG, Mikkelsen BO, Crevoisier C, Heizmann P, Fattinger K (1989) A randomized comparison between midazolam and thiopental for elective cesarean section anesthesia: III. Placental transfer and elimination in neonates. Anesth Analg 68:238–242

Balant LP, Roseboom H, Gundert-Remy UM (1990) Pharmacokinetic criteria for drug research and development. Adv Drug Res 19:1–138

Bates DM, Watts DG (1988) Nonlinear regression analysis and its applications. Wiley, New York

Beal SL (1984) Population pharmacokinetic data and parameter estimation based on their first two statistical moments. Drug Metab Rev 15:173–193

Beal SL, Sheiner LB (1980) The NONMEM system. Am Stat 34:118–119

Beal SL, Sheiner LB (1982) Estimating population kinetics. Crit Rev Biomed Eng 8:195–222

Beal SL, Sheiner LB (1985) Methodology of population pharmacokinetics. In: Garrett ER, Hirtz J (eds) Drug fate and metabolism, vol 5. Dekker, New York, pp 135–183

Beal SL, Sheiner LB (eds) (1989) NONMEM users guides, version III. NONMEM Project Group, University of California, San Francisco

Beal SL, Sheiner LB (eds) (1992) NONMEM users guides, version IV. NONMEM Project Group, University of California, San Francisco

Bergman RN, Cobelli C (1980) Minimal modeling partition analysis and the estimation of insulin sensitivity. Fed Proc 39:110–115

Blaser KU, Vozeh S, Landolt H, Kaufmann G, Romppainen J, Gratzl O (1989) Intravenous phenytoin: a loading scheme for desired concentrations. Ann Intern Med 110:1029–1031

Blychert E, Edgar B, Elmfeldt D, Hedner T (1991) A population study of the pharmacokinetics of felodipine. Br J Clin Pharmacol 31:15–24

Campbell DB (1990) The use of kinetic–dynamic interactions in the evaluation of drugs. Psychopharmacology 100:43–450

Chambers JM, Cleveland WS, Kleiner B, Tukey PA (1983) Graphical methods for data analysis. Wadsworth, Belmont

Cohen P, Collart L, Prober CG, Fischer AF, Blaschke TF (1990) Gentamicin pharmacokinetics in neonates undergoing extracorporeal membrane oxygenation. Pediatr Infect Dis J 9:562–566

Colburn WA (1989) Controversy IV: population pharmacokinetics, NONMEM and the pharmacokinetic screen; academic, industrial and regulatory perspectives. J Clin Pharmacol 29:1–6

Colburn WA, Olson SC (1988) Classic and population pharmacokinetics. In: Welling PG, Tse FLS (eds) Pharmacokinetics: regulatory, industrial, academic perspectives. Dekker, New York, pp 337–384

Cramer JA, Mattson RH, Prevey ML, Scheyer RD, Ouellette VL (1989) How often is medication taken as prescribed? A novel assessment technique. JAMA 261:3273–3277

Davidian M, Gallant RA (1992) The nonlinear mixed effects model with a smooth random effects density. Institute of Statistics MS No. 2206, North Carolina State University, Raleigh

Dempster AP, Laird NM, Rubin DB (1977) Maximum likelihood from incomplete data via the EM algorithm. J R Stat Soc B 39:1–38

Di Carlo FJ (ed) (1984) Special symposium on frontiers in pharmacokinetic data analysis. Drug Metab Rev 15:1–400

Driscoll MS, Ludden TM, Casto DT, Littlefield LC (1989) Evaluation of theophylline pharmacokinetics in a pediatric population using mixed effects model. J Pharmacokinet Biopharm 17:141–168

Drusano GL (1991) Optimal sampling theory and population modeling: application to determination of the influence of the microgravity environment on drug distribution and elimination. J Clin Pharmacol 31:962–967

Endrenyi L (1985) Principles and evaluation of variability in drug therapy (discussion). In: Rowland M, Sheiner LB, Steimer JL (eds) Variability in drug therapy: description, estimation and control. Raven, New York, pp 219–233

Fattinger K, Vozeh S, Ha HR, Borner M, Follath F (1991a) Population pharmacokinetics of quinidine. Br J Clin Pharmacol 31:279–286

Fattinger K, Vozeh S, Olafsson A, Vlcek J, Wenk M, Follath F (1991b) Netilmicine in the neonate: population pharmacokinetics analysis and dosing recommendations. Clin Pharmacol Ther 50:55–65

Feely J, Crooks J, Stevenson IH (1981) The influence of age, smoking and hyperthyroidism on plasma propranolol steady state concentrations. Br J Clin Pharmacol 12:73–78

FDA (Food and Drug Administration) (1989) Guideline for the study of drugs likely to be used in the elderly. Center for Drug Evaluation and Research, Food and Drug Administration. DHHS, Washington

Fluehler H, Huber H, Widmer E, Brechbuehler S (1984) Experiences in the application of NONMEM to pharmacokinetic data analysis. Drug Metab Rev 15(1&2):317–339

Gaillot J, Steimer JL, Mallet A, Thebault JJ, Bieder A (1979) A priori lithium dosage regimen using population characteristics of pharmacokinetic parameters. J Pharmacokinet Biopharm 7:579–628

Gelenberg AJ, Kane JM, Keller MB, Lavori P, Rosenbaum JF, Cole K, Lavelle J (1989) Comparison of standard and low serum levels of lithium for maintenance treatment of bipolar disorder. N Engl J Med 321:1489–1493

Gelfand AE, Hills SE, Racine-Poon A, Smith AFM (1990) Illustration of Bayesian influence in normal data models using Gibbs sampling. J Am Stat Assoc 85: 972–985

Gex-Fabry M, Balant-Gorgia AE, Balant LP, Garrone G (1990) Clomipramine metabolism: model-based analysis of variability factors from drug monitoring data. Clin Pharmacokinet 19:241–255

Gitterman SR, Drusano GL, Egorin MJ, Standiford HC (1990) Population pharmacokinetics of zidovudine. Clin Pharmacol Ther 48:161–167

Grasela TH, Donn SM (1985) Neonatal population pharmacokinetics of phenobarbital derived from routine clinical data. Dev Pharmacol Ther 8:374–383

Grasela TH, Sheiner LB (1984) Population pharmacokinetics of procainamide from routine clinical data. Clin Pharmacokinet 9:545–554

Grasela TH, Sheiner LB (1991) Pharmacostatistical modeling for observational data. J Pharmacokinet Biopharm 19:25S–36S

Grasela TH, Sheiner LB, Rambeck B, Boenigk HE, Dunlop A, Mullen PW, Wadsworth J, Richens A, Ishisaki T, Chiba K, Miura H, Minagawa K, Blain PG, Mucklow JC, Bacon CT, Rawlins M (1983) Steady-state pharmacokinetics of phenytoin from routinely collected patient data. Clin Pharmacokinet 8: 355–364

Grasela TH, Antal EJ, Townsend RJ, Smith RB (1986) An evaluation of population pharmacokinetics in therapeutic trials: I. Comparison of methodologies. Clin Pharmacol Ther 39:605–612

Grasela TH, Antal EJ, Ereshefsky L, Wells BG, Evans RL, Smith RB (1987) An evaluation of population pharmacokinetics in therapeutic trials: II. Detection of a drug–drug interaction. Clin Pharmacol Ther 42:433–441

Graves DA, Chang I (1990) Application of NONMEM to routine bioavailability data. J Pharmacokinet Biopharm 18:145–160

Graves NM, Ludden TM, Holmes GB, Fuerst RH, Leppik IE (1989) Pharmacokinetics of felbamate, a novel antiepileptic drug: application of mixed-effect modeling to clinical trials. Pharmacotherapy 9:372–376

Grevel J, Whiting B, Kelman AW, Kutz K (1987) Compilation of a clinical pharmacokinetic database for population analysis during drug development. Pharm Med 2:127–136

Grevel J, Whiting B, Kelman AW, Taylor WB (1988) Population analysis of the pharmacokinetic variability of high-dose metoclopramide in cancer patients. Clin Pharmacokinet 14:52–63

Grevel J, Thomas P, Whiting B (1989) Population pharmacokinetic analysis of bisoprolol. Clin Pharmacokinet 17:53–63

Gundert-Remy U (1992) Population approach in pharmacokinetics and pharmacodynamics–views within regulatory agencies: Europe. In: Rowland M, Aarons L (eds) New strategies in drug development and clinical evaluation: the population approach. Commission of the European Communities, Luxembourg, pp 153–156

Hashimoto Y, Sheiner LB (1991) Designs for population pharmacodynamics: value of pharmacokinetic data and population analysis. J Pharmacokinet Biopharm 19:333–353

Holford NHG (1992) Parametric models for the time course of drug action: the population approach. In: Rowland M, Aarons L (eds) New strategies in drug development and clinical evaluation: the population approach. Commission of the European Communities, Luxembourg, pp 193–206

Hori R (1988) Population pharmacokinetics for therapeutic drug monitoring (in Japanese). Yakugyoujihousya, Tokyo

Hundt HKL, Aucamp AK, Mueller FO, Potgieter MA (1983) Carbamazepine and its major metabolites in plasma: a summary of eight years of therapeutic drug monitoring. Ther Drug Monit 5:427–435

Jennings J (1984) Response to "Discussion paper on testing of drugs in the elderly". Pharmaceutical Manufacturers Association, Washington

Jermain DM, Crismon ML, Martin III ES (1991) Population pharmacokinetics of lithium. Clin Pharm 10:367–381

Jochemsen R (1992) Current experience of population pharmacokinetics within the pharmaceutical industry: an introduction. In: Rowland M, Aarons L (eds) New strategies in drug development and clinical evaluation: the population approach. Commission of the European Communities, Luxembourg, pp 127–130

Jusko WJ (1980) Concepts for population pharmacokinetics of theophylline. In: Gladtke E, Heimann G (eds) Pharmacokinetics. Fischer, Stuttgart, pp 181–189

Kaniwa N, Aoyagi N, Ogata H, Ishii M (1990) Application of the NONMEM method to evaluation of the bioavailability of drug products. J Pharm Sci 79:1116–1120

Karlsson MO, Thomson AH, McGovern EM, Chow P, Evans TJ, Kelman AW (1991) Population pharmacokinetics of rectal theophylline in neonates. Ther Drug Monit 13:195–200

Kelman AW, Whiting B, Bryson SM (1982) OPT: a package of computer programs for parameter optimisation in clinical pharmacokinetics. Br J Clin Pharmacol 14:247–256

Kelman AW, Thomson AH, Whiting B, Bryson SM, Steedman DA, Mawer GE, Samba-Donga LA (1984) Estimation of gentamicin clearance and volume of distribution in neonates and young children. Br J Clin Pharmacol 18:685–692

Kisor DF, Watling SM, Zarowitz BJ, Jelliffe RW (1992) Population pharmacokinetics of gentamicin: use of the nonparametric expectation maximisation (NPEM) algorithm. Clin Pharmacokinet 23:62–68

Kragh-Sorensen P, Eggert Hansen C, Baastrup PC, Hvidberg EF (1976) Self-inhibiting action of nortriptylin's antidepressive effect at high plasma levels. Psychopharmacologia 45:305–312

Kroboth PD, Schmith VD, Smith RB (1991) Pharmacodynamic modeling: application to new drug development. Clin Pharmacokinet 20:91–98

Laplanche R, Fertil B, Nüesch E, Jais JP, Niederberger W, Steimer JL (1991) Exploratory analysis of population pharmacokinetic data from clinical trials with application to isradipine. Clin Pharmacol Ther 50:39–54

Launay MC, Iliadis A, Richard B (1989) Population pharmacokinetics of mitoxantrone performed by a NONMEM method. J Pharm Sci 78:877–880

Lindstrom MJ, Bates DM (1990) Nonlinear mixed effects models for repeated measures data. Biometrics 46:673–687

Lindstrom FT, Birkes DS (1984) Estimation of population pharmacokinetic parameters using destructively obtained experimental data: a simulation study of the one-compartment open model. Drug Metab Rev 15:195–264

Ludden T, Allerheiligen SRB, Burk RF (1991) Application of population analysis to physiological pharmacokinetics. J Pharmacokinet Biopharm [Suppl] 19: 101S–113S

Lyne A, Boston R, Pettigrew K, Zech L (1992) EMSA: a SAAM service for the estimation of population parameters based on model fits to identically replicated experiments. Comput Methods Programs Biomed 38:117–151

Maitre PO, Vozeh S, Heykants J, Thomson DA, Stanski DR (1987) Population pharmacokinetics of alfentanil: the average dose-plasma concentrations relationship and interindividual variability in patients. Anesthesiology 66:3–12

Maitre PO, Ausems M, Vozeh S, Stanski DR (1988) Evaluating the accuracy of using population pharmacokinetic data to predict plasma concentrations of alfentanil. Anesthesiology 68:59–67

Maitre PO, Funk B, Crevoisier C, Ha HR (1989) Pharmacokinetics of midazolam in patients recovering from cardiac surgery. Eur J Clin Pharmacol 37:161–166

Maitre PO, Bührer M, Thomson D, Stanski DR (1991) A three step approach combining Bayesian regression and NONMEM population analysis: application to midazolam. J Pharmacokinet Biopharm 19:377–384

Mallet A (1986) A maximum likelihood estimation method for random coefficient regression models. Biometrika 73:645–656

Mallet A, Mentre F (1988) An approach to the design of experiments for estimating the distribution of parameters in random models. In: Vichnevetsky R, Borne P, Vignes J (eds) Proc 12th IMACS World Congr 5:134–137

Mallet A, Mentre F, Steimer JL, Lokiec F (1988a) Nonparametric maximum likelihood estimation for population pharmacokinetics, with application to cyclosporine. J Pharmacokinet Biopharm 16:311–327

Mallet A, Mentre F, Gilles J, Kelman AW, Thomson AH, Bryson SM, Whiting B (1988b) Handling covariates in population pharmacokinetics, with an application to gentamicin. Biomed Meas Inf Cont 2:138–146

Mandema JW, Verotta D, Sheiner LB (1992) Building population pharmacokinetic-pharmacodynamic models. J Pharmacokinet Biopharm (in press)

Martin III ES, Crismon ML, Godley PJ (1991) Postinduction carbamazepine clearance in an adult psychiatric population. Pharmacotherapy 11:296–302

Mentre F, Mallet A (1991) Relationships between intra- or interindividual variability and biological covariates: application to zidovudine pharmacokinetics. In: D'Argenio DZ (ed) Advanced methods of pharmacokinetic and pharmacodynamic systems analysis. Plenum, New York, pp 119–128

Mentre F, Mallet A (1992) Experiences with NPML–application to dosage individualisation of cyclosporine, gentamicin and zidovudine. In: Rowland M, Aarons L (eds) New strategies in drug development and clinical evaluation: the population approach. Commission of the European Communities, Luxembourg, pp 75–88

Mentre F, Mallet A, Steimer JL (1988) Hyperparameter estimation using stochastic approximation with application to population pharmacokinetics. Biometrics 44:673–683

Miller R, Rheeders M, Klein C, Suchet I (1987) Population pharmacokinetics of phenytoin in South African black patients. S Afr Med J 72:188–190

Moore ES, Faix RG, Banagale RC, Grasela TH (1989) The population pharmacokinetics of theophylline in neonates and young infants. J Pharmacokinet Biopharm 17:47–66

Mungall DR, Ludden TM, Marshall J, Hawkins DW, Talbert RL, Crawford MH (1985) Population pharmacokinetics of racemic warfarin in adult patients. J Pharmacokinet Biopharm 13:213–227

Murata K, Yamahara H, Kobayashi M, Noda K, Samejima M (1989) Pharmacokinetics of an oral sustained-release diltiazem preparation. J Pharm Sci 78: 960–963

Neter J, Wasserman W (1974) Applied linear statistical models. Irwin, Homewood, p 388

Olson SC (1991) A population pharmacokinetic profile of imazodan in congestive heart failure patients. J Pharmacokinet Biopharm [Suppl] 19:47S–58S

O'Neill RT (1992) Statistical issues in population models. In: Rowland M, Aarons L (eds) New strategies in drug development and clinical evaluation: the population approach. Commission of the European Communities, Luxembourg, pp 99–105

Pai SM, Shukla UA, Grasela TH, Knupp CA, Dolin R, Valentine FT, McLaren C, Liebman HA, Martin RR, Pittman KA, Barbhaiya RH (1992) Population pharmacokinetic analysis of didanosine (2′,3′-dideoxyinosine) plasma concentrations obtained in phase I clinical trials in patients with AIDS or AIDS-related complex. J Clin Pharmacol 32:242–247

Peck CC (1992) Population approach in pharmacokinetics and pharmacodynamics: FDA view. In: Rowland M, Aarons L (eds) New strategies in drug development and clinical evaluation: the population approach. Commission of the European Communities, Luxembourg, pp 157–168

Peck CC, Rodman JH (1986) Analysis of clinical pharmacokinetic data for individualizing drug dosage regimens. In: Evans WE, Schentag JJ, Jusko WJ (eds) Applied pharmacokinetics, 2nd edn. Applied Therapeutics Inc, Vancouver, pp 55–82

Peck CC, Rodman JH (1992) Analysis of clinical pharmacokinetic data for individualizing drug dosage regimens. In: Evans WE, Schentag JJ, Jusko WJ (eds) Applied pharmacokinetics, 3rd edn. Applied Therapeutics Inc, Vancouver, pp 3.1–3.31

Peck CC, Harter J, Sanathanan L, Collins J (1990) Simultaneous pharmacokinetic-pharmacodynamic modeling in drug development and registration. Proceedings of IUPHAR satellite symposium "Measurement and kinetics of in vivo drug effects", 28–30 June 1990, Noordwijk, pp 28–29

Peck CC, Barr WH, Benet LZ, Collins J, Desjardins RE, Furst DE, Harter JG, Levy G, Ludden T, Rodman JH, Sanathanan L, Schentag JJ, Shah VP, Sheiner LB, Skelly JP, Stanski DR, Temple RJ, Viswanathan CT, Weissinger J, Yacobi A (1992) Conference report: opportunities for integration of pharmacokinetics, pharmacodynamics, and toxicokinetics in rational drug development. Clin Pharmacol Ther 51:465–473

Pollak T (1990) The exploration of pharmacokinetic and pharmacodynamic data using interactive three-dimensional graphs, a tool borrowed from particle physics. Eur J Clin Pharmacol 39:525–532

Price Evans DA, Manley KA, McKusick VA (1960) Genetic control of isoniazid metabolism in man. BMJ 2:485–491

Racine-Poon A (1985) A Bayesian approach to non-linear random effects models. Biometrics 41:1015–1024

Racine-Poon A, Smith AFM (1990) Population models. In: Berry DA (ed) Statistical methodology in the pharmaceutical sciences. Dekker, New York, pp 139–162

Ratain MJ, Schilsky RL, Conley BA, Egorin MJ (1990) Pharmacodynamics in cancer therapy. J Clin Oncol 8:1739–1753

Reidenberg MM, Abrams WB (1984) Report of the workshop on proposed FDA guidelines for clinical evaluation of drugs being developed for use in the elderly. American Society of Clinical Pharmacology and Therapy workshop report, 13–14 September 1984, Rockville

Renwick AG, Robertson DRC, Macklin B, Challenor V, Waller DG, George CF (1988) The pharmacokinetics of oral nifedipine–apopulation study. Br J Clin Pharmacol 25:701–708

Riegelman S, Sheiner LB, Beal SL (1980) Population based approach to pharmacokinetic and bioavailability studies in patients. In: Gladtke E, Heimann G (eds) Pharmacokinetics. Fischer, Stuttgart, pp 83–95

Rodda BE, Tsianco MC, Bologness JA, Kersten MK (1988) Clinical development. In: Peace K (ed) Biopharmaceutical statistics for drug development. Dekker, New York

Rodman JH, Evans WE (1991) Targeted systemic exposure for pediatric cancer therapy. In: D'Argenio DZ (ed) Advanced methods of pharmacokinetic and pharmacodynamic systems analysis. Plenum, New York, pp 177–183

Roecker EB (1991) Prediction error and its estimation for subset-selected models. Technometrics 33:459–468

Rowland M, Aarons L (eds) (1992) New strategies in drug development and clinical evaluation: the population approach. Commission of the European Communities, Luxembourg

Rowland M, Sheiner LB, Steimer JL (eds) (1985) Variability in drug therapy: description, estimation and control. Raven, New York

Rubio A, Cox C, Weintraub M (1992) Prediction of diltiazem plasma concentration curves from limited measurements using compliance data. Clin Pharmacokinet 22:238–246

Sale ME, Blaschke TF (1992) Incorporating pharmacokinetic/pharmacodynamic modeling in drug development – are we ready? Drug Inf J 26:119–124

Salmonson T, Rane A (1990) Clinical pharmacokinetics in the drug regulatory process. Clin Pharmacokinet 18:177–183

Sambol NC (1992) The population approach: applications to experimental data. In: Rowland M, Aarons L (eds) New strategies in drug development and clinical evaluation: the population approach. Commission of the European Communities, Luxembourg, pp 183–191

Sambol NC, Sheiner LB (1991) Population dose versus response of betaxolol and atenolol: a comparison of potency and variability. Clin Pharmacol Ther 49: 24–31

Sanathanan L, Peck CC (1991) The randomized concentration controlled trial: an evaluation of its sample size efficiency. Controlled Clin Trials 12:780–794

Sanathanan L, Peck CC, Temple R, Lieberman R, Pledger G (1991) Randomization, pharmacokinetic-controlled dosing, and titration: an integrated approach for designing clinical trials. Drug Inf J 25:425–431

Scavone JM, Greenblatt DJ, Blyden GT, Harmtz JS, Graziano PJ (1988) Simplified approaches to the determination of anti-pyrine pharmacokinetic parameter. Br J Clin Pharmacol 25:695–699

Schmith VD, Fiedler-Kelly J, Abou-Donia M, Huffman CS, Grasela TH (1992) Population pharmacodynamics of doxacurium. Clin Pharmacol Ther 52:528–536

Schumitzky A (1991) Nonparametric EM algorithms for estimating prior distributions. Appl Math Comput 45:143–157

Shah AK, Brundage RC, Gratwohl A, Sawchuk RJ (1992) Pharmacokinetic model for subcutaneous absorption of cyclosporine in the rabbit during chronic treatment. J Pharm Sci 81:491–495

Sheiner LB (1989) Clinical pharmacology and the choice between theory and empiricism. Clin Pharmacol Ther 46:605–615

Sheiner LB (1990) Implications of an alternative approach to dose-response trials. J AIDS 3 [Suppl 2]:S20–S26

Sheiner LB (1991) The intellectual health of clinical drug evaluation. Clin Pharmacol Ther 50:4–9

Sheiner LB (1992) Population approach in drug development: rationale and basic concepts. In: Rowland M, Aarons L (eds) New strategies in drug development and clinical evaluation: the population approach. Commission of the European Communities, Luxembourg, pp 13–29

Sheiner LB, Beal SL (1981) Estimation of pooled pharmacokinetic parameters describing populations. In: Endrenyi L (ed) Kinetic data analysis. Plenum, New York, pp 271–284

Sheiner LB, Benet LZ (1985) Premarketing observational studies of population pharmacokinetics of new drugs. Clin Pharmacol Ther 38:481–487

Sheiner LB, Grasela TH (1991) An introduction to mixed effect modeling: concepts, definitions and justification. J Pharmacokinet Biopharm 19:11S–24S

Sheiner LB, Ludden TM (1992) Population pharmacokinetics/pharmacodynamics. Annu Rev Pharmacol Toxicol 32:185–209

Sheiner LB, Rosenberg B, Melmon KL (1972) Modeling of individual pharmacokinetics for computer-aided drug dosage. Comp Biomed Res 5:441–459

Sheiner LB, Rosenberg B, Marathe VV (1977) Estimation of population characteristics of pharmacokinetic parameters from routine clinical data. J Pharmacokinet Biopharm 5:445–479

Sheiner LB, Beal SL, Rosenberg B, Marathe VV (1979) Forecasting individual pharmacokinetics. Clin Pharmacol Ther 26:294–305

Sheiner LB, Beal SL, Sambol NC (1989) Study designs for dos-ranging. Clin Pharmacol Ther 46:63–77

Stanski DR, Maitre PO (1990) Population pharmacokinetics and pharmacodynamics of thiopental: the effect of age revisited. Anesthesiology 72:412–422

Steimer JL, Mallet A, Golmard JL, Boisvieux JF (1984a) Alternative approaches to estimation of population pharmacokinetic parameters: comparison with the nonlinear mixed-effect model. Drug Metab Rev 15/1–2:265–292

Steimer JL, Mentre F, Mallet A (1984b) Population studies for evaluation of pharmacokinetic variability: Why? How? When? In: Aiache JM, Hirtz J (eds) 2nd European congress on biopharmaceutics and pharmacokinetics, vol 2. Experimental pharmacokinetics. Lavoisier, Paris, pp 40–49

Steimer JL, Mallet A, Mentre F (1985) Estimating interindividual pharmacokinetic variability. In: Rowland M, Sheiner LB, Steimer JL (eds) Variability in drug therapy: description, estimation and control. Raven, New York, pp 65–111

Tanigawara Y, Hori R (1992) Population approach in post-marketing dose adjustment. In: Rowland M, Aarons L (eds) New strategies in drug development and clinical evaluation: the population approach. Commission of the European Communities, Luxembourg, pp 223–232

Tanigawara Y, Hori R, Okumura K, Tsuji JI, Shimizu N, Noma S, Suzuki J, Livingston DJ, Richards SM, Keyes LD, Couch RC, Erickson MK (1991) Pharmacokinetics in chimpanzees of recombinant human tissue-type plasminogen activator produced in mouse C127 and Chinese ovary cells. Chem Pharm Bull 38:517–522

Temple R (1983) Discussion paper on the testing of drugs in the elderly. Memorandum of the Food and Drug Administration (September 30). DHHS, Washington DC

Temple R (1987) The clinical investigation of drug use by the elderly: food and drug guidelines. Clin Pharmacol Ther 42:681–685

Temple R (1989) Dose–response and registration of new drugs. In: Lasagna L, Erill S, Naranjo CA (eds) Dose–response relationships in clinical pharmacology. Elsevier, New York

Thomson AH, Tucker GT (1992) Gerontokinetics – a reappraisal. Br J Clin Pharmacol 33:1–2

Thomson AH, Whiting BW (1992) Bayesian parameter estimation and population pharmacokinetics. Clin Pharmacokinet 22:447–467

Thomson AH, Way S, Bryson SM, McGovern GM, Kelman AW, Whiting B (1988) Population pharmacokinetics of gentamicin in neonates. Dev Pharmacol Ther 11:173–179

Thomson AH, Kelly JG, Whiting B (1989) Lisinopril population pharmacokinetics in elderly and renal disease patients with hypertension. Br J Clin Pharmacol 27:57–65

Urquhart J, Chevalley C (1988) Impact of unrecognized dosing errors on the cost and effectiveness of pharmaceuticals. Drug Inf J 22:363–378

Verme CN, Ludden TM, Clementi WA, Harris SC (1992) Pharmacokinetics of quinidine in male patients: a population analysis. Clin Pharmacokinet 22:468–480

Vonesh EF, Carter RL (1992) Mixed-effects nonlinear regression for unbalanced repeated measures. Biometrics 48:1–17

Vozeh S (1987) Cost-effectiveness of therapeutic drug monitoring. Clin Pharmacokinet 13:131–140

Vozeh S, Steimer JL (1985) Feedback control methods for drug dosage optimisation: concepts, classification and clinical application. Clin Pharmacokinet 10:457–476

Vozeh S, Steiner C (1987) Estimates of the population pharmacokinetic parameters and performance of Bayseian feedback: a sensitivity analysis. J Pharmacokinet Biopharm 15:511–528

Vozeh S, Muir KT, Sheiner LB, Follath F (1981) Predicting individual phenytoin dosage. J Pharmacokinet Biopharm 9:131–146

Vozeh S, Katz G, Steiner V, Follath F (1982a) Population pharmacokinetic parameters in patients treated with oral mexiletine. Eur J Clin Pharmacol 23:445–451

Vozeh S, Kewitz G, Perruchoud A, Tschan M, Kopp C, Heitz M, Follath F (1982b) Theophylline serum concentration and therapeutic effect in severe acute bronchial obstruction: the optimal use of intravenously administered aminophylline. Am Rev Respir Dis 125:181–184

Vozeh S, Wenk M, Follath F (1984) Experience with NONMEM: analysis of serum concentration data in patients treated with mexiletine and lidocaine. Drug Metab Rev 15:305–315

Vozeh S, Uematsu T, Hauf GF, Follath F (1985) Performance of Bayesian feedback to forecast lidocaine serum concentration: evaluation of the prediction error and the prediction interval. J Pharmacokinet Biopharm 13:203–212

Vozeh S, Uematsu T, Ritz R, Schmidlin O, Kaufman G, Scholer A, Follath F (1987) Computer-assisted individualized lidocaine dosage: clinical evaluation and comparison with physician performance. Am Heart J 113:928–933

Vozeh S, Uematsu T, Aarons L, Maitre P, Landolt H, Gratzl O (1988) Intravenous phenytoin loading in patients after neurosurgery and in status epilepticus: a population pharmacokinetic study. Clin Pharmacokinet 14:122–128

Vozeh S, Maitre PO, Stanski DR (1990) Evaluation of population (NONMEM) pharmacokinetic parameter estimates. J Pharmacokinet Biopharm 18:161–173

Wakefield JC, Smith AFM, Racine-Poon A, Gelfand AE (1992) Bayesian analysis of linear and nonlinear population models using the Gibbs sampler. Appl Stat (in press)

Wang J, Endrenyi L (1992) A computationally efficient approach for the design of population pharmacokinetic studies. J Pharmacokinet Biopharm 20:279–294

White DB, Walawander CA, Tung Y, Grasela TH (1991) An evaluation of point and interval estimates in population pharmacokinetics using NONMEM analysis. J Pharmacokinet Biopharm 19:87–112

White DB, Walawander CA, Liu DY, Grasela TH (1992) Evaluation of hypothesis testing for comparing two populations using NONMEM analysis. J Pharmacokinet Biopharm 20:295–313

Whiting B, Kelman AW, Grevel J (1986) Population pharmacokinetics. Theory and clinical application. Clin Pharmacokinet 11:387–401

Whiting B, Kelman AW, Grevel J (1990) Population pharmacokinetics. In: Taylor JB (ed) Comprehensive medicinal chemistry, vol V. Pergamon, Oxford, pp 297–304

Wiest DB, Pinson JB, Gal PS, Brundage RC, Schall S, Ransom JL, Weaver RL, Purohit D, Brown Y (1991) Population pharmacokinetics of intravenous indomethacin in neonates with symptomatic patent ductus arteriosus. Clin Pharmacol Ther 49:550–557

Williams PJ, Lane J, Murray W, Mergener MA, Kamigaki M (1992) Pharmacokinetics of the digoxin-quinidine interaction via mixed-effect modeling. Clin Pharmacokinet 22:66–74

Yukawa E, Higuchi S, Aoyama T (1989) Population pharmacokinetics of phenytoin from routine clinical data in Japan. J Clin Pharmacol Ther 14:71–77

Yukawa E, Higuchi S, Aoyama T (1990) Population pharmacokinetics of phenytoin from routine clinical data in Japan: an update. Chem Pharm Bull 38:1973–1976

Yukawa E, Higuchi S, Aoyama T (1991) One-point feedback control method for phenytoin dosage adjustment. J Pharm Pharmacol 43:499–503

F. Impact of New Methods on Pharmacokinetics

CHAPTER 16

Contribution of Positron Emission Tomography to Pharmacokinetic Studies

B. Mazière and J. Delforge

A. Introduction

Pharmacokinetics, whose aim is to explain and predict drug action in the human body, describes the processes that determine the concentration of the active substance at its site of action.

Radioisotopes are conventionally utilized in two different types of pharmacokinetic study:

1. In direct radiotracer applications, the drug itself is labeled with a radio-isotope which is used to determine the drug tissue distribution and fate.
2. In indirect radioactive indicator applications, the radioisotope is used to label a specific probe and it is the interaction of the drug with the radiolabeled probe which is observed.

In these applications, the noninvasive measurement of the tissular kinetics of a drug (or a probe) requires the intravenous injection of a very small amount (tracer dose) of a drug (or a probe) labeled with an isotope emitting a signal that can be externally detected. The necessary condition in such a pharmacokinetic investigation is that the radioisotope incorporated into the drug (or the probe) does not modify the biochemical properties of the original molecule. Practically, this means that the radiotracer must be a radioisotope of one of the chemical elements constituting the drug, usually carbon, hydrogen, nitrogen, or oxygen (isotopic labeling). ^{14}C and ^{3}H, which are largely used in animal pharmacokinetic studies, cannot be used for external detection measurements because the negative electrons emitted during their radioactive decay are rapidly absorbed by the surrounding tissues. The only radioisotopes of carbon, oxygen, and nitrogen emitting externally detectable gamma rays are positron (positively charged electron) emitters. As there is no such radioactive isotope of hydrogen, positron-emitting isotopes of halogens (fluorine, bromine, or iodine) are often substituted for the hydrogen of a hydroxyl group (analogic labeling).

With positron emission tomography (PET), a safe noninvasive visualization technique, serial quantitative images of the spatial distribution of a drug labeled with such positron-emitting radionuclides can be obtained in any desired transverse section of the body.

Positron-emitting isotopes are usually produced relatively free of stable or radioactive contamination (very high specific activity) by means of trans-

Table 1. Positron-emitting radioisotopes used in PET clinical investigations

Isotope	Half-life (min)	Target (reaction)	Available forms
^{15}O	2	$^{14}N(d,n)^{15}O$	$^{15}O_2$, $C^{15}O$
^{13}N	10	$^{16}O(p,\alpha)^{13}N$	^{13}N, $^{13}NH_3$
^{11}C	20	$^{14}N(p,\alpha)^{11}C$	^{11}CO, $^{11}CO_2$
^{18}F	110	$^{20}Ne(d,a)^{18}F$	$H^{18}F$, $^{18}F_2$
^{76}Br	972	$^{75}As(He3,2n)^{76}Br$	$^{76}Br_2$

mutation nuclear reactions using beams of cyclotron-accelerated charged particles.

B. Positron Emitters

Some common positron-emitting radioisotopes used in PET studies are listed in Table 1.

These radioisotopes have short half-lives and consequently production and incorporation into molecules have to be extemporaneously carried out "on site." Short half-lives also mean that repeated studies can be performed in humans without excessive absorbed radiation.

C. Drug Labeling – Radiochemistry

For pharmacokinetic studies, the isotopes produced in a cyclotron in very simple molecular forms, such as $^{11}CO_2$, $^{13}NH_3$, or $H^{18}F$, have to be incorporated into a drug (or a probe). Due to the rapid decay of the isotope, the radiochemical synthesis must be fast to allow the desired radiolabeled molecule to be isolated, purified, and formulated as a sterile, isotonic, pyrogen-free radiopharmaceutical solution within two or three half-lives of the isotope (Comar et al. 1982). This constraint has promoted the development of new methods of remote-controlled rapid chemistry (Mazière et al. 1977; Crouzel et al. 1993). As an example, starting from 1–2 Ci (37–74 GBq) of ^{11}C, 100–200 mCi (3.7–7.4 GBq) of ^{11}C-labeled compounds is usually obtained after 30–40 min synthesis.

Owing to the short half-lives of the radioisotopes used, radiolabeled drugs are produced with very high specific activities (500–4000 mCi/μmol or 18.5–148 GBq/μmol, i.e., 20–200 times the specific activity of tritiated molecules). High activities (required to obtain good images) are carried by very small masses of drugs (a few nanomoles) and then can be administered safely to subjects without any risk of pharmacological activity and, a fortiori, of chemical toxicity.

D. Positron Emission Tomography

Radioisotopes that decay by emitting positrons are detectable from outside the body thanks to the photons emitted after annihilation of the positrons. In fact, the positron travels a very short path in the tissue (2–5 mm) before eventually combining with an ambient negative electron. This interaction results in the annihilation of both original electrons with electromagnetic annihilation radiation released in the form of two high-energy (511 keV) photons (Fig. 1). These two simultaneously emitted photons travel nearly 180° apart, and can be detected by scintillators placed on opposite sides of the subject. These detectors are electronically connected to a coincidence circuit so that detected radiations will only be recorded if both scintillators register the events within a brief time window. Using this electronic collimation (the annihilation process is assumed to have occurred somewhere within the tissue volume located between the two detectors) and an accurate correction of the scatter and attenuation of the gamma rays in the body, PET cameras with several rings of detectors have been designed. Using computer-applied filtered retroprojection algorithms (identical to those developed for conventional computed tomography x-ray scanners), the PET tomograph produces images that show up the quantitative, regional, and temporal distribution of the administered radiolabeled compound in slices throughout the body (number of slices: 5–35) (Fig. 2). Multiple, simultaneously obtained slices allow a three-dimensional reconstruction of the distribution of the radiolabeled compound. The resolution is 4–8 mm and successive images can be produced at intervals of a few seconds (4–10 s).

A PET image, then, can be considered an accurate map of radioactive concentrations in a tomographic slice. These radioactive concentrations can easily be determined in regions of interest (ROIs). These ROIs can be

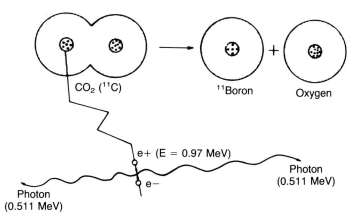

Fig. 1. Positron emitter decay: the disintegration of an ^{11}C-labeled molecule is illustrated ($T = 20.4$ min)

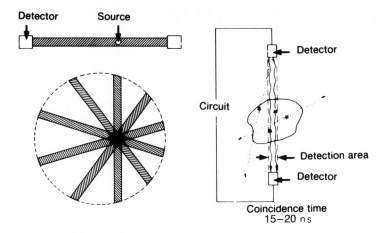

Fig. 2. Principle of PET

delineated directly on the PET image using the anatomical information inherent in the functional images. However, this information is limited by the spatial resolution of the PET camera. When the PET study requires measurements on accurately determined structures, ROIs have to be localized on an anatomical image obtained using MRI (retrospectively matched with the PET image using surface landmarks) before being copied on the PET image.

Regional drug concentrations (nmol/cm^3) can easily be computed from regional radioactive concentrations (nCi/cm^3) by taking into account the specific radioactivity of the radiolabeled drug and the possible metabolism of the drug (in the blood and the tissues) during the time course of the PET scans. The results obtained in vivo in humans by PET are then similar to those obtained in animals by quantitative autoradiography with the drawback of a much lower resolution but with the advantage, for pharmacokinetic studies, of allowing the acquisition of time course sequential images in a single subject. Moreover the duration of a PET investigation is limited (by the short physical half-lives of the radioisotopes used) to 90–120 min for ^{11}C and a few hours for ^{18}F or ^{76}Br studies.

The PET studies are safe, noninvasive, and, due to the short half-lives of the radioisotopes used, weakly irradiating. The values of various radiation dose estimations show that, with the activity usually injected [10–20 mCi (740 GBq) for ^{11}C, 5–10 mCi (185–370 GBq) for ^{18}F, and 1–1.5 mCi (37–55 GBq) for ^{76}Br ligands], the total body doses are around 2 mGy/study while the resultant doses of radiation absorbed by the critical target organs (i.e., liver, lower larger intestine, bladder) remain within the accepted 50 mGy per organ limit per single study (Harvey et al. 1985; Kilbourn et al. 1989; Herzog et al. 1990; Blin et al. 1990; Crawley et al. 1984; B. Mazière et al. 1985).

By allowing in vivo noninvasive sequential measurements of regional drug concentrations, with sensitivity and specificity equivalent to those of plasma radioimmunoassays (nanomolar to picomolar differences can be detected), PET provides, in animals and humans, a unique opportunity to ascertain the kinetics of drugs in various tissues (by measuring either the biodistribution of radiolabeled drugs in direct studies or the interaction of cold drugs with radiolabeled probes in indirect studies).

E. Direct Radiolabeled Drug Studies

Pharmacokinetic studies describe the time course of the fate of drugs (absorption, distribution, metabolism, elimination) in the body. Many pertinent data from animal or human studies are listed in the scientific literature.

However, most of the time, human pharmacokinetic studies examine the fate of the drug only from a transport perspective (absorption and excretion processes). In contrast, using PET, which allows measurement in vivo of the concentrations of a radiolabeled molecule in any organs (HERZOG et al. 1990) and particularly in the target organ, it is possible to study the time course of the regional biodistribution in human. During the course of various diseases, organ impairment may alter the pharmacokinetics of drugs in the body; PET also allows one to compare the drug kinetics in physiological and pathological conditions.

The PET approach does, however, suffer from some limitations as various barriers are present between the site of administration (usually a brachial vein) and the target itself. The first barrier is the pulmonary filter. In a single passage through the lung circulation, lipophilic molecules can be totally extracted by the pulmonary endothelial or epithelial cells; then, the amount of drug which will reach the investigated organ will depend on its clearance from the lungs. The second barrier is the capillary barrier and this problem is very acute in the brain, where the intercellular junctions are very tight. The last limitation comes from the binding of the labeled molecule to plasma proteins, the free fraction of the drug being available for uptake by the target tissue.

Another complication with PET investigations derives from the fact that PET measures only the global radioactivity of the tissue and makes no distinction between the unchanged and metabolized or free and bound forms of the radiolabeled drug.

I. Drug Distribution

After administration of the radiolabeled drug itself, drug tissue concentrations can be measured in vivo in organs such as liver, kidney, heart, or brain, supplementing the data available from plasma and urine. This unique ability of PET to determine the actual drug tissular concentrations will be illustrated by reference to some applications.

The brain pharmacokinetics of imipramine labeled with ^{11}C were studied in the baboon as early as 1977 (Mazière et al. 1977). PET tissue pharmacokinetics of antibiotics labeled with ^{11}C (erythromycin) or ^{18}F (fleroxacin) have been described in infected lungs of humans (Wollmer et al. 1982) and in infected rabbits (Fischman et al. 1992), respectively. Brain concentrations of 5,5-diphenylhydantoin (DPH), an antiepileptic drug, have been measured in humans using DPH labeled with ^{11}C (Baron et al. 1983).

Using an analog (ethyl spiperone) labeled with ^{18}F, the brain and whole-body distribution of spiperone, a neuroleptic drug, was studied in man. Only 1% of the total administered drug was found in the brain 2 h following injection, while urinary bladder, gallbladder, and liver were the organs with the highest drug concentration (from 6% to 25% of the dose) (Herzog et al. 1990).

In oncology, the use of PET in pharmacokinetics is expanding. To determine the selective tumor uptake of antineoplastic agents used for chemotherapy, BCNU, for example, has been labeled with ^{11}C. The PET pharmacokinetic studies have shown that [^{11}C] BCNU specific penetration in the tumor was 50 times higher after intracarotid than after intravenous administration (Tyler et al. 1986). Recent experience using ^{18}F-labeled drugs has shown how it is possible to achieve high spatial and temporal resolution of the uptake of an anticancer drug within the abdominal area. Following administration of ^{18}F-labeled 5-fluorouracil (5FU), it was possible to identify renal secretion, uptake within the liver and liver metastasis, and transport into the gall bladder and the kidneys (Jones et al. 1992).

Analysis of PET tracer kinetics of [^{11}C]melatonin has shown that this hormone secreted by the pineal gland readily crosses the blood-brain barrier (Le Bars et al. 1991).

The uptake rate and distribution volume of [^{11}C]methionine measured during PET pharmacokinetic studies were found to represent a useful tool for better diagnosing and grading the biological malignancy of brain tumors (Derlon et al. 1989; Leskinen-Kallio et al. 1992; Sato et al. 1992).

II. Drug–Drug and Drug–Nutrient Interactions

Positron emission tomography allows in vivo study in humans of the modification in the kinetics of the transport through the blood-brain barrier induced by the presence in the body fluids of various substances such as drugs or nutritients. Thus, entry of many amino acids across the blood-brain barrier into the brain is known to occur via a carrier-mediated process known as the large neutral amino acid (LNAA) carrier system. The various substrates for the LNAA transport system all compete for the same binding site and the carrier operates near saturation in normal biological conditions. Thus it was shown, using PET, that the ingestion of large doses of aspartame, which induced an increase in the plasma levels of phenylalanine, induced small but measurable decreases (11.5%) in the amino acid transport rate constant k_1

(KOEPPE et al. 1991). In the same way, PET allows investigation of the possible effects of elevation of the plasma amino acid level on the uptake of various synthetic amino acid drugs such as L-dopa, using as tracer the radiofluorinated analog 6-[^{18}F]-fluoro-L-dopa (^{18}F-L-DOPA). Thus it could be demonstrated that the cerebral uptake (k_1) of ^{18}F-L-DOPA in the striatum was considerably reduced (by a factor of 3.6) when the concentrations of eight dietary LNAAs were increased (by a factor of 2.4) by means of an intravenous infusion (LEENDERS et al. 1986; GJEDDE 1988).

Furthermore, PET kinetic studies using ^{18}F-L-DOPA have shown that L-dopa uptake is not modified during the course of systemic treatment with an aromatic amino acid decarboxylase inhibitor (such as carbidopa). It is possible to assume that the increase in the measured striatal tomographic activity that can be recorded after such a treatment is probably secondary to an increase in plasma 6-[^{18}F]-fluoro-L-dopa (and then L-dopa) levels and not related to a modification in the influx rate constant (HOFFMAN et al. 1992).

III. Drug–Receptor Interactions

Positron emission tomography is well suited for quantitating the availability and the affinity of receptor sites. Consequently PET makes it possible to examine in the various organs of living humans the kinetics and effects of drugs which block (antagonists) or stimulate (agonists) recognition sites.

Complexities in PET receptor studies are partly due to the nonspecific binding of the radioligand (the higher the lipophilicity, the higher the nonspecific to specific concentration ratio) and to its removal process within the tissue by various mechanisms such as uptake by different (neuronal and nonneuronal) cells, binding to different receptors or receptor subtypes, possible enzymatic or chemical degradation, and possible intracellular trapping.

The binding of a drug by a receptor exhibits two unique properties: *molecular specificity* and *saturability*. Molecular specificity describes the behavior of ligand binding in terms of affinity and ability to recognize a particular receptor while saturability is related to receptor density. For example, brain tissue contains a minute concentration of receptors (approximately 10^{-12} mol/g) and if a specific drug is delivered in excess, the receptors will be saturated. Only very low masses of specific drugs may then be injected, which implies the preparation of radioligands or drugs labeled with very high specific activities (curies per nanomole).

Receptor-mediated localization of a ligand (drug) in an organ or a structure can be demonstrated in vivo on the basis of the following criteria:

1. *Specific regional distribution*: The radiolabeled drug must be found in higher amounts in structures known for their high recognition site densities.

2. *Saturability*: Competition experiments (displacement and presaturation) are used to demonstrate this property (Fig. 3):

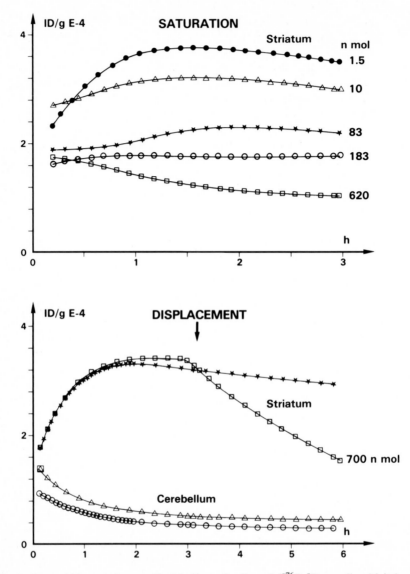

Fig. 3. Saturability of the specific binding of a ligand ([^{76}Br]Bromolisuride) for the receptor (dopamine D2 receptors). [^{76}Br]Bromolisuride is an antagonist of the D2 receptors. *Above*: When the mass of unlabeled bromolisuride coinjected with the radiotracer increased from 0 to 620 nmol, the percentage of injected dose measured in vivo in the striatum of a baboon brain, 2 h post injection, decreased from $3.8 \cdot 10^{-2}$ to $1 \cdot 10^{-2}$. *Below*: When a load of unlabeled bromolisuride (700 nmol) was injected 3 h after the administration of the radiotracer, in a baboon, it induced a rapid decrease in the specifically bound radioactivity (in the striatum) but did not induce any changes for the nonspecifically bound ligand (in the cerebellum)

a) In displacement experiments, an excess of "cold" (nonradioactive) agonists or antagonists, preferably belonging to different chemical classes, is intravenously administered at a time when the tissue radioligand concentration reaches its maximum. The inhibitive competition between the tracer and the excess of unlabeled drug induces a rapid decrease in the specific binding.

b) In presaturation experiments, the specific binding sites are blocked by an excess of unlabeled ligand administered prior to the administration of the radioligand. In this case, the regional tracer radioactive concentration remains lower than that measured in the absence of the cold drug. All these saturability experiments are dose dependent. However, the possibility of applying this characterization technique in humans is often limited by the pharmacological or the toxicological effects of the large amounts of drug that have to be administered.

3. *Stereospecificity*: Stereoselectivity is a powerful tool for the characterization of specific binding. When a drug possesses an asymmetrical carbon, its two enantiomers have to be labeled. In the presence of specific binding, the isomer with the pharmacological activity (the eutomer) displays a higher specific accumulation than the one without pharmacological activity (the distomer) (FOWLER et al. 1987; FARDE et al. 1988). When the two isomers of a drug are available but have not been radiolabeled, the displacement of a radiolabeled probe from the specific binding site is mostly obtained with the eutomer (HANTRAYONE et al. 1984).

4. *High affinity* of the radiolabeled drug for the specific binding site. Receptors generally have lower affinity for endogenous transmitters or exogenous agonists $(10^{-6}M)$ than for antagonists $(10^{-9}M)$. Therefore, In PET pharmacokinetic studies, better results are often obtained with drugs possessing antagonist properties than with drugs possessing agonist properties (MAZIÈRE et al. 1983).

5. *Biological effect*: To distinguish between the binding of the drug to an acceptor site, with no signal transmission, or to a receptor (or an enzyme) site, associated with a pharmacological response, a correlation between binding affinity or binding site occupancy and potency of biological effect has to be demonstrated.

When it has been demonstrated in vivo that the drug actually binds to receptors, the parameters governing the fate of the drug in vivo, i.e., equilibrium constant (K_d), association and dissociation rate constants, and maximum concentration of available receptors (B'_{max}), still have to be measured.

Taking into account the individual characteristics of the radiolabeled drugs, suitable quantitative approaches have been applied to interpret the local concentration data or the regional uptake kinetic curves in terms of physiologically significant parameters:

1. For drugs which dissociate rapidly from the receptors, allowing equilibrium of binding to be established in vivo within the time span of a

PET experiment (Farde et al. 1986, 1989; Huang et al. 1986; Mazière et al. 1990), an equilibrium analysis of specific binding can be performed. A regional time-activity curve is used to define a point in time that represents equilibrium of specific binding to receptors. Series of PET scans are then performed in the same individual using the drug labeled with various specific activities. On the basis of regional radioactivity at equilibrium time, B'_{max} and K_d values can be calculated from a saturation curve or a Scatchard plot.

2. For drugs with a slow dissociation rate from the receptor, a kinetic analysis according to a compartmental model provides more valuable information. Under these circumstances, the chosen mathematical model will attempt to simulate the variations of the tissue radioactivity versus time (cf. Sect. G).

To illustrate the ability of PET to directly image the binding of drugs to neuroreceptors, some applications will be reviewed.

1. Tranquilizers

The first PET in vivo imaging study of the binding of a drug to brain receptors was performed in a baboon more than a decade ago using the benzodiazepine flunitrazepam labeled with [11]C. In this pioneer investigation, it was possible to show that a trace amount of the labeled drug could be specifically displaced from the baboon's brain by a therapeutic load of competing unlabeled benzodiazepine (Comar et al. 1979).

The pharmacokinetic properties of the benzodiazepine antagonist flumazenil (RO 15 1788) labeled with ^{11}C have been extensively studied in baboons (Mazière et al. 1983) and in humans (Samson et al. 1985; Persson et al. 1985; Pappata et al. 1988; Delforge et al. 1993) with PET. These studies have shown that this antagonist:

1. Crosses the blood-brain barrier easily and intensively
2. Is for the major part (90%) rapidly, specifically, and selectively bound to receptors from which it can be stereoselectively displaced by the eutomer of enantiomeric benzodiazepines
3. Is rapidly eliminated from the brain (the biological half-life in humans is about 50 min)

Pharmacokinetic properties of tranquilizers such as suriclone, a cyclopyrrolone (Frost et al. 1986), or triazolam, a triazolobenzodiazepine (Bottlaender et al. 1992), have been studied by PET using ^{11}C-labeled tracers. The cerebral distribution of ^{11}C suriclone and of ^{11}C]triazolam, observed by PET in baboons and humans, were found to be similar to that of ^{11}C]RO 15 1788.

2. Neuroleptics

Positron emission tomography investigations of chlorpromazine (Comar et al. 1979) and pimozide (Crouzel et al. 1980) labeled with ^{11}C showed that the drug distributions were essentially in the gray matter and in structures such as the caudate nucleus. However, the in vivo nonspecific binding of these drugs was too high to enable identification of their supposed sites of action, the D2 dopamine receptors.

The methodology which is used in PET pharmacokinetic studies to validate the specific binding of drugs to receptors can be used to demonstrate the binding of a drug to an enzyme. Thus, the kinetics of deprenyl, an inhibitor of the enzyme monoamine oxidase B (MAO B) that is used to treat Parkinson's disease, was studied in the human brain using as a tracer [^{11}C]deprenyl. In this study, comparison of the magnitude of brain uptake and retention of the ^{11}C-labeled inactive (D-) and active (L-) enantiomers of deprenyl exemplified the stereospecificity effect: (a) L-deprenyl is bound by sites containing MAO B to a degree 25 times that of D-deprenyl; (b) rapid clearance of the inactive enantiomer and retention of the active enantiomer are observed within MAO B-rich brain structures such as the corpus striatum and thalamus (FOWLER et al. 1987).

F. Indirect Radioactive Pharmacokinetic Studies

For technical reasons, it can be tedious, expensive, or impossible to label a drug with a positron emitter. In these cases, it is still possible to study in vivo the kinetics of the possible interaction of the drug with certain classes of receptors. The strategy then consists in performing an "in vivo radio-receptor assay," using a specific positron-emitting radioligand to label the receptors (a radiolabeled probe) and testing the cold drug as a competing agent on this binding. Specific radiolabeled ligands for every type of receptor are not yet available, but quite a number of new drugs can be tested using this approach (Table 2).

Blockade of the central dopamine receptors is held to be the essential mechanism in the pharmacological action of neuroleptics. Hence, in patients treated with neuroleptics, measurement in vivo of the actual dopamine D2 receptor blockade (receptor occupancy) by the treatment should provide an estimate of the effective neuroleptic tissue concentration. Treatment of schizophrenic patients with conventional doses of chemically distinct classical antipsychotic drugs (haloperidol, flupenthixol, sulpiride, clozapine, levopromazine, thioproperazine, propericiazine, thiethylperazine) almost completely abolished the imaging of dopamine D2 receptor binding by specific radioligands labeled with ^{11}C, such as spiperone (WONG et al. 1986b) or raclopride (FARDE et al. 1986), or with ^{76}Br, such as spiperone (CAMBON et al. 1987) or bromolisuride (MARTINOT et al. 1990).

Positron emission tomography "in vivo radioreceptor assays" indicate that during conventional clinical treatments with such neuroleptics the D2 receptor occupancy is total or subtotal, rapidly induced, and dose related; following drug withdrawal, recovery to normal or supranormal receptor

Table 2. Labeled probes for "in vivo radioreceptor assays"

Receptors	Probes	Subtypes	References
Dopaminergic			
D1	[^{11}C]SCH 23390	D1	FARDE et al. (1986)
D2	[^{11}C]Methylspiperone	D2, 5HT2	WAGNER et al. (1983)
	[^{76}Br]Bromospiperone	D2, 5HT2	MAZIÈRE et al. (1984)
	[^{11}C]Raclopride	D2	FARDE et al. (1986)
	[^{76}Br]Bromolisuride	D2	MAZIÈRE et al. (1986)
Serotoninergic	[^{18}F]Setoperone	5HT2	BLIN et al. (1988)
	[^{11}C]MethylbromoLSD	5HT2	WONG et al. (1987)
Opioid	[^{11}C]Carfentanyl		FROST et al. (1987)
	[^{11}C]Diprenorphine		JONES et al. (1988)
	[^{18}F]Acetylcyclofoxy		PERT et al. (1984)
Benzodiazepine	[^{11}C]Flumazenil	BZ1, BZ2	M. MAZIÈRE et al. (1985)
	[^{11}C]PK 11195	"Périph"	CHARBONNEAU et al. (1986)
Muscarinic	[^{11}C]MQNB	M1, M2	SYROTA et al. (1984)
	[^{11}C]Levetimide	M1, M2	DANNALS et al. (1988)
	[^{11}C]Scopolamine	M1, M2	FREY et al. (1988)
	[^{11}C]Cogentin	M1, M2	DEWEY et al. (1990)
Adrenergic	[^{11C}]CGP 12177		SYROTA (1989)

availability appears to require only a matter of days. Using [^{11}C]SCH-23390 as a specific probe for the dopaminergic D1 receptor, it has been shown that these conventional neuroleptics do not cause any evident D1 blockade, while atypical neuroleptics like clozapine induce, in addition to blockade of the D2 receptor, D1 receptor occupancy in a dose-dependent manner (FARDE et al. 1992).

As another example of this indirect strategy for the measurement of the duration of a drug action, one may cite a study done with naltrexone. This drug is a long-acting antagonist of opiate receptors used in the treatment of opiate dependence. For this investigation, the opioid receptors were labeled with a potent mu-type agonist, [^{11}C]carfentanil. The results of the PET studies showed that the half-time of the duration of blockade by naltrexone in the brain ranged from 72 to 108 h, which is greater than the fast component of clearance of the drug and its principal metabolite from plasma (LEE et al. 1988).

By combining the PET investigations with EEG recordings, it has been shown that the convulsant or anticonvulsant actions of drugs such as β-carbolines or diazepam acting on the GABA receptor complex is mediated by the [^{11}C]flumazenil binding sites (HANTRAYE et al. 1988).

The kinetics of the binding of various parent drugs or metabolites to benzodiazepine receptors have also been studied using this indirect strategy. A first example concerns triazolam, a benzodiazepinic tranquilizer, which, in baboon brain, was found to have a very high potency for inhibiting [^{11}C]RO

15 1788 binding and a high positive intrinsic efficacy (BOTTLAENDER et al. 1992) (Fig. 4). Another example is the tranquilizer suriclone, which is known to be mainly metabolized in demethylated and sulfoxide derivatives. A PET kinetic study, using [^{11}C]RO 15 1788 for the labeling of the benzodiazepine receptors, demonstrated that unlike the parent drug, the suriclone metabolites have only a low potency for inhibiting the probe binding and thus should not seriously affect the in vivo GABAergic transmission (BROUILLET et al. 1990).

G. Kinetic Modeling with PET

Mathematical modeling is an important tool for the analysis of dynamic series of images obtained by PET because physiological parameters, such as local blood flow, glucose metabolism, or receptor concentration, can be extracted from experimental data (time course of the labeled molecule tissue

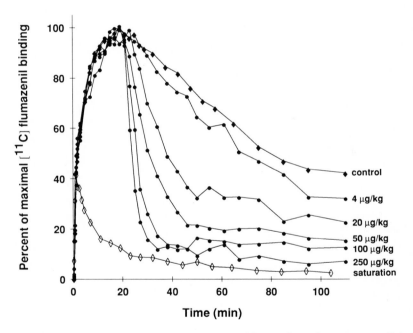

Fig. 4. In vivo interaction of triazolam with central benzodiazepine receptors (labeled with the probe [^{11}C]RO 15 1788) in the baboon brain. The radiolabeled probe was injected at time T_0. Typical kinetics under control conditions showed that the maximal binding of [^{11}C]RO 15 1788 obtained at time $T_0 + 20$ min was followed by a slow decrease in the brain-bound radioactivity (control). When unlabeled triazolam was administered at $T_0 + 20$ min, the wash-out of the radioligand was dramatically accelerated; the intensity of the displacement was dose dependent. When unlabeled flumazenil (1 mg/kg) was injected 5 min before the radiotracer [^{11}C]RO 15 1788 (saturation), the specific binding of the radiolabeled probe was totally prevented

concentrations). To estimate these physiological parameters a mathematical model must be devised to simulate the kinetics of the labeled molecule in the tissue. The physiological parameters will appear as model parameters which have to be identified from the experimental PET data curves simultaneously with the other model parameters (usually local kinetic rate constants).

The estimation of model parameters from experimental data is a well-known problem and many numerical identification methods (usually using nonlinear least-squares fitting procedure) are now available (Eykhoff 1974; Kagiwada 1977; Beck and Arnold 1977). However, evaluation of the parameter uncertainties is equally essential in any complete identification procedure. Usually, the information matrix and the measure of residual errors between experimental data and model-predicted values are used to generate an approximation of the parameter covariance matrix. An estimation of this standard deviation of each parameter and a description of an asymptotic confidence region can then be deduced from this matrix (Beck and Arnold 1977; Carson 1986; Delforge et al. 1989).

The complexity of the model, that is to say of the simulated physiological process, varies a great deal, depending on the tracer used, the process studied, and the available experimental data. When the number of parameters is too large in comparison with the experimental information, the parameter uncertainties can be very large and as a result the identification procedure can be disappointing. Two difficulties may appear. First, the parameter uncertainties may be so large that the identified values are meaningless. Second, the identification problem may have several solutions, i.e., several very distinct sets of parameter values lead to similar theoretical curves. In both cases, the identification procedure may not lead to a valid solution. Such a risk is not negligible with PET data since usually only one experimental curve is obtained whereas the nature of the problems leads to complex models. The necessary balance between the respective complexities of the model structure and experimental data is related to the general identifiability problem (Cobelli and DiStefano 1980; Delforge et al. 1990).

To illustrate the interest and the complexity of modeling PET kinetic data, the compartmental model used to study some kinetic phenomena such as blood flow, glucose consumption, and drug receptor binding will be briefly reviewed.

I. A Two-Compartment Model: the [^{15}O]Water Model

The determination of the local blood flow using oxygen-15 labeled water as a tracer gives an example of a very simple model. It includes only two compartments (i.e., the concentration of [^{15}O]water in the blood and in the studied tissue) and two kinetic parameters, k_1 and k_2. This is a relatively simple configuration due to the absence of any biochemical reaction in the tissue, the only phenomenon being the transport across the capillary wall and the cell membranes. The two parameters are estimated by fitting the PET concentration data using a weighted least-squares method and the regional blood flow is estimated using the k_1 parameter.

II. A Three-Compartment Linear Model: the [^{18}F]Fluorodeoxyglucose Model

The determination of the regional metabolic rate of glucose, using [^{18}F]fluoro-deoxyglucose (FDG) as a tracer, is an example of a more complex model (the main advantage of using FDG, instead of labeled natural glucose, is the absence of any measurable loss of tracer during the time of measurement). The three-compartment model was originally developed by SOKOLOFF et al. (1977) to study the kinetics of [^{14}C]deoxyglucose. For the last 15 years, this model has been employed by many authors to mark metabolic activity mainly in the brain (see review in MAZZIOTTA and PHELPS 1986) and heart (see review in SCHELBERT and SCHWAIGER 1986).

The usual model is illustrated in Fig. 5. The three compartments represent respectively the FDG concentration in the plasma, the FDG concentration in the tissue, and the concentration of [^{18}F]fluorodeoxyglucose-6-phosphate. All transfers between these compartments are linear. The parameters k_1 and k_2 correspond to the exchanges between the tissue and the plasma; the parameters k_3 and k_4 correspond to the FDG phosphory-lation and dephosphorylation respectively.

The identification of these model parameters is difficult from only one PET experiment and usually some parameters (such as k_4) have to be set using normal values. The estimated model parameters provide an estimate of the regional metabolic rate of glucose (rMRglu) in a region of interest which is given by the following equation:

$$rMRglu = (C_p/LC) \cdot (k_1 \cdot k_3)/(k_2 + k_3),$$

where C_p is the FDG concentration in the plasma and LC is a correcting factor, the lumped constant, which takes into account the difference between FDG and glucose in the kinetics of transport across the blood-brain barrier and in phosphorylation rate. This constant LC can differ between patients and regions of interest. It can be estimated via relations using the respective properties of FDG and glucose (volumes of distribution, maximal velocities

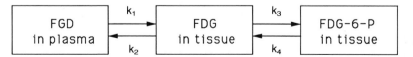

Fig. 5. A three-compartment linear model used to study the [^{18}F]FDG kinetics. The rate constants k_1, k_2, k_3, k_4 identified from the PET data, allow estimation of the regional metabolic rate of glucose (rMRglu)

of phosphorylation) or it can be selected so that the calculated average value for global MRglu in normal subjects equals that determined by earlier investigators using more invasive techniques (Phelps et al. 1979).

III. A Multicompartment Nonlinear Model:
the Ligand–Receptor Model

It is now possible to characterize various receptors using specific antagonists labeled with positron-emitting isotopes. To investigate the affinity of drugs for these receptors and/or the possible alterations in the status of these receptors in various diseases, a method for quantitatively measuring their binding parameters has been devised.

Several models have recently been proposed as a framework for the analysis and quantification of drug (ligand)–receptor interactions investigated in vivo with PET (Syrota et al. 1984; Frey et al. 1985; Farde et al. 1986; Perlmutter et al. 1986; Wong et al. 1986a,b). In these models, the reactions are considered to include at least two steps: a free ligand is first transported from blood to tissue where binding sites are located and the ligand–receptor complex is then formed. However, the model structure may differ depending on the organ, the molecule, or the experimental protocol used. For example, the binding of ligands can be reversible or not, or a nonspecifically bound ligand compartment may or may not have to be introduced.

Figure 6 shows an example of a model structure including nonspecific binding. The flux of free ligand that crosses the capillary barrier is equal to $p \cdot V_R \cdot C_a^*(t)$, where $C_a^*(t)$ is the plasma radioactive concentration at time t, p is an unknown rate constant (permeability), and V_R is defined as the fraction of the region of interest delineated by PET in which the ligand can react with the receptors. With a hydrophilic ligand, V_R should correspond approximately to the fraction of extracellular fluid. The free ligand $M_f^*(t)$ can either bind directly to a free receptor site or to a nonspecific site (parameter k_{+ns}) or escape with rate constant k. The binding probability depends on the rate constant (k_{+1}/V_R) and on the local concentration of available free receptors which is equal to $[B_{max}' - M_b^*(t)]$ where B_{max}' is the unknown concentration of available receptor sites and $M_b^*(t)$ is the bound ligand concentration. The rate constant for the dissociation of bound ligand is represented by k_{-1}, and that for the nonspecifically bound ligand by k_{-ns}.

The PET experimental data correspond to the sum of the labeled ligand concentration in the extravascular compartment and a fraction of the blood concentration. F_V represents the fractional volume including the fraction of blood present in the tissue volume.

If the experimental protocol includes injections of unlabeled ligand, it is necessary to simulate the kinetics of this unlabeled ligand that affect the local concentration of free receptors and must therefore be taken into

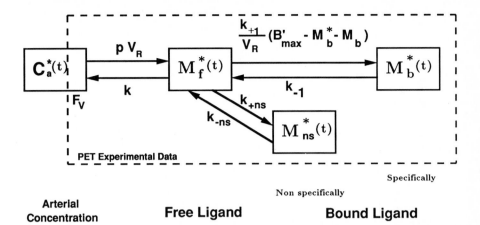

Fig. 6. The usual compartmental ligand–receptor model. It includes four compartments corresponding to labeled ligand concentrations: the ligand in the arterial blood, the free ligand in the tissue, and the ligand nonspecifically and specifically bound to receptors. All transfer probabilities of drug between compartments are linear except for the binding probability, which depends on the bimolecular association rate constant and on the local concentration of free receptors. If the protocol used includes injections of unlabeled ligand, the kinetics of this unlabeled ligand are simulated using the same model. The unlabeled ligand concentrations are not directly observable from PET data, but the concentration of the unlabeled specifically bound ligand [$M_b(t)$] has an effect on the local concentration of free receptors and consequently on the binding probability of free labeled ligand. See text for further definitions

account. Thus, the model shown in Fig. 6 includes two parts having the same structure and the same parameters: the labeled and unlabeled ligand kinetics. With this approach all types of PET ligand–receptor studies may be described. However, some more simple approaches have been proposed. For example, the coinjection of unlabeled ligand together with the labeled ligand has been interpreted by some authors (HUANG et al. 1989; FARDE et al. 1989) as a simple injection of labeled ligand with a lower specific activity. This approach does not need to take into account the unlabeled ligand kinetics, and only particular equations including different specific activities have to be used. However, such an approach is not suitable for simulating a displacement experiment (injection of pure unlabeled ligand).

Parameter identification requires knowledge of the model input function $C_a^*(t)$, which usually reflects the nonmetabolized labeled ligand concentration in the plasma. The arterial unlabeled ligand concentration $C_a(t)$ is simulated from $C_a^*(t)$ in the assumption that the unlabeled ligand kinetics are similar to those of the labeled ligand. The input function is usually obtained from arterial blood samples, but in some favorable cases (heart studies) it can be estimated from vascular PET ROIs.

This model contains between five and eight parameters which have to be identified from PET data. However, when the number of parameters is too large in comparison with the experimental data, the uncertainties of parameters may be so great that the identified values are meaningless. Either the model has to be simplified by a reduction in the number of parameters or the experimental protocol has to be further elaborated in order to obtain more experimental information.

IV. Modeling Using Simplified Models

The simplification of the model has several advantages since, if this simplification is valid, it can lead to easier estimation of the parameters. For example, some authors consider that the PET data are not sensitive enough to detect a possible nonspecific binding reaction with association–dissociation kinetic rate constants much larger than the other compartmental rate constants. Such nonspecific binding is then located in the free compartment (Perlmutter et al. 1986; Mintun et al. 1984).

Other authors have used a simplified model assuming that the tracer occupies a negligible fraction of the available receptors (Farde et al. 1986; Mintun et al. 1984; Perlmutter et al. 1986; Wong et al. 1986a,b; Logan et al. 1987). The model then becomes linear but neither the receptor density B'_{max} nor the equilibrium dissociation constant K_d can be separately measured. The rate constant k_3 [equal to the product $(k_{+1}/V_R)B'_{max}$] gives only an indication of the "binding potential" that reflects the capacity of a given tissue to bind a labeled molecule (Mintun et al. 1984; Perlmutter et al. 1986).

The equations also can be further simplified if steady-state conditions between blood and free ligand compartment are assumed and if the ligand is supposed to bind irreversibly to the receptor sites ($k_{-1} = 0$). When both assumptions are made, a graphic method can then be used (Patlak et al. 1983; Wong et al. 1986a,b). This simplified method is very fruitful as it provides a simple way of estimating the receptor concentration variations. However, the hypotheses which are at the basis of this simplified method have to be validated, which can be difficult. In the absence of any validation the use of this simplified method can lead to doubtful results. As an example, it has been possible to show that the slope of the Patlak plot obtained with a ligand such as methylquinuclidinyl benzilate (MQNB) (Fig. 7) is not related to the binding of the free ligand (parameter k_3) but reflects the input from the blood compartment to the free compartment (parameter k_1) (Delforge et al. 1990). In this case, the simplified graphic method does not allow estimation of the receptor concentration variation since the PET images obtained after a single injection of high-affinity MQNB are primarily related not to receptor binding but to local blood flows (in the heart).

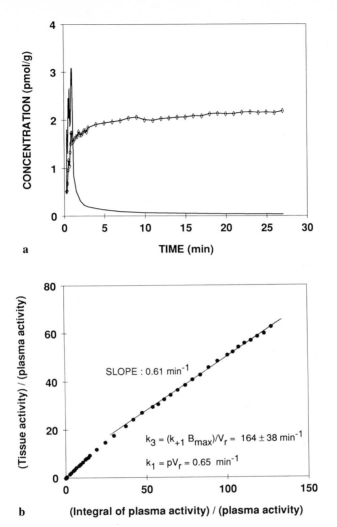

Fig. 7 a,b. Example of normalized graphic plot used in analysis of myocardial tissue data obtained after intravenous injection of [^{11}C]MQNB. **a** Kinetic curves of the concentration of the labeled ligand in the blood (*solid line*) and in the tissue (*symbols*). **b** Plot of the ratio of tissue to plasma activity versus the "normalized time" defined as the integral of plasma activity from time 0 to t divided by plasma activity at time t, according to the method first proposed by Patlak. The asymptotic slope of this curve (shown with a *straight line*) allows estimation of $(k_1 k_3)/(k + k_3)$. This slope is often used to estimate the magnitude of the binding probability (k_3). However, in the case of MQNB, comparison with the model parameters, obtained using the multi-injection approach, showed that this slope corresponds to the order of magnitude of the transfer probability from the arterial compartment to the free ligand compartment (k_1). This result demonstrates that the PET images obtained after injection of a trace amount of [^{11}C]MQNB reflect the blood flow more than the receptor density or affinity

V. Modeling Using the Multi-injection Approach

When an estimation of the receptor concentration is needed, a usual method consists in identifying all the model parameters even if the interest of some parameters is weak. In this case, when a large number of parameters have to be estimated from the data registered during a single PET experiment, a multi-injection approach is mandatory. Such an approach implies the use of an experimental protocol including at least two injections, one of which should induce occupation of a significant percentage of receptor sites.

The first example of such a multi-injection approach can be found in the study of [11C]MQNB binding to muscarinic receptors in dog heart (Delforge et al. 1990b). In this study, the initial attempt led to disappointing numerical results, most of the parameters having to be considered unidentifiable. To improve the parameter estimation, a new experimental design consisting of a first tracer injection followed 30 min later by an injection of the cold ligand (displacement experiment) was investigated. This second protocol led to two very different numerical solutions. To determine the only biologically valid solution, a third protocol including both a displacement and a coinjection was proposed. Finally, it appeared that a fourth injection (a sizeable load of unlabeled ligand) made it possible to identify and to estimate irreversible and nonspecific binding.

This multi-injection approach has been successfully used both in heart (Delforge et al. 1990b, 1991a) and in brain studies (Delforge et al. 1991b, 1993).

These complex protocols, though often unusable in clinical investigation, are nevertheless mandatory to set up and validate simplified clinical models. Theoretical studies using experimentally designed protocols (Delforge et al. 1989) have shown that the more appropriate protocol in human studies consists in a tracer injection followed by a coinjection of labeled and unlabeled ligand (the mass of unlabeled ligand having to be calculated in such a way that it will occupy about half the available receptors). Such a protocol has been successfully used in the clinical investigations of the status of β-adrenergic and muscarinic receptors in heart diseases using respectively [11C]CGP 12177 and [11C]MQNB (Merlet et al. 1991; Delforge et al. 1991c) as specific ligands.

H. Conclusion

The previous examples reviewed in this article have shown that it is possible to tackle in vivo with PET the three basic approaches of tissue drug pharmacokinetic studies: the descriptive approach (how the absorption, the distribution, and elimination take place), the mathematical approach (calculation of rate constants), and the analytical approach (relation between the generated data and pharmacological information).

All three approaches are based on the measurements of concentrations in body fluid and tissues of the unchanged drug and of its metabolites. However, PET methodology does not allow us to separately measure each of these radiolabeled compounds. Usually the metabolism of the radio-labeled drug is primarily studied in animals. Therefore the value of a human PET pharmacokinetic study can be heavily dependent on the accuracy of the extrapolation to humans of this animal metabolic study.

Positron emission tomography methodology has already been proved to be a useful tool for following the kinetics of drug actions in the living human brain. PET allows close analysis of the relationship between receptor occupancy and the onset of desired pharmacological effects and unwanted side-effects. The pursuit of such studies is likely to lead to a greater understanding of the relationship between drug pharmacokinetic properties (receptor occupancy) and therapeutic effects. The possibility of labeling drugs or precursors or metabolites by a radioisotope ethically administrable to humans opens up entirely new prospects. PET has opened a new era in human biochemistry and promises to have important applications in pharmacokinetic studies, clinical pharmacology, and drug development.

References

Baron J-C, Roeda D, Crouzel C, Chodkiewicz JP, Comar D (1983) Brain regional pharmacodynamics of ^{11}C-labeled diphenylhydantoin: positron emission tomography in humans. Neurology (NY) 33:580–585

Beck JV, Arnold KJ (1977) Parameter estimation in engineering and science. Wiley, New York

Blin J, Pappata S, Kiyosawa M, Crouzel C, Baron J-C (1988) (^{18}F)Setoperone: a new high affinity ligand for positron emission tomography study of the serotonin-2 receptors in baboon brain in vivo. Eur J Pharmacol 147:73–82

Blin J, Sette G, Fiorelli M, Bletry O, Elghozi J-L, Crouzel C, Baron J-C (1990) A method for the in vivo investigation of the serotoninergic S2 receptors in the human cerebral cortex using positron emission tomography and ^{18}F-labeled setoperone. J Neurochem 54:1744–1754

Blomqvist G, Pauli S, Farde L, Eriksson L, Persson A, Halldin C (1990) Maps of receptor binding parameters in the human brain – a kinetic analysis of PET measurements. Eur J Nucl Med 16:257–265

Bottlaender M, Brouillet E, Varastet M, Lebreton C, Schmid L, Sitbon R, Crouzel C, Mazière M (1993) In vivo high intrinsic efficacy of Triazolam: a positron emission tomography study in non-human primates. J Neurochem (in press)

Brouillet E, Chavoix C, Hantraye P, Kunimoto M, Khalili-Varastet M, Chevalier P, Frydman A, Gaillot J, Prenant C, Crouzel M, Mazière B, Mazière M (1990) Interaction of suriclone with central type benzodiazepine receptors in living baboons. Eur J Pharmacol 175:49–55

Cambon H, Baron J-C, Boulenger J-P, Loc'h C, Zarifian E, Mazière B (1987) In vivo assays for neuroleptic receptor binding in the striatum. Positron emission tomography in humans. Br J Psychiatry 151:824–830

Carson ER (1986) Parameter estimation in PET, positron emission tomography and autoradiography. In: Phelps ME, Mazziotta J, Schelbert HR (eds) Principles and application of PET for the brain and heart. Raven, New York, pp 347–390

Charbonneau P, Syrota A, Crouzel C, Valois J-M, Prenant C, Crouzel M (1986) Peripheral-type benzodiazepine receptors in the living heart characterized by positron emission tomography. Circulation 73:476–483

Cobelli C, DiStefano J III (1980) Parameters and structural identifiability concepts and ambiguities: a critical review and analysis. Am J Physiol 239:R7–R24

Comar D, Zarifian E, Verhas M, Soussaline F, Mazière M, Berger G, Loo H, Cuche H, Kellershohn C, Denicker P (1979) Brain distribution and kinetics of ^{11}C-chlorpromazine in schizophrenics: positron emission tomography studies. Psychiatry Res 1:23–29

Comar D, Berridge M, Mazière B, Crouzel C (1982) Radiopharmaceuticals labelled with positron-emitting radioisotopes. In: Ell PJ, Holman BL (eds) Computed emission tomography. Oxford University Press, Oxford, pp 42–90

Crawley JC, Smith T, Veall N, Zanelli GD (1984) Distribution, retention and radiation dosimetry of ^{77}Br-p-bromospiperone. Radiat Protect Dosimetry 8: 147–153

Crouzel C, Mestelan G, Kraus E, Lecomte J-M, Comar D (1980) Synthesis of a ^{11}C-labelled neuroleptic drug: pimozide. Int J Appl Radiat Isot 31:545–548

Crouzel C, Clark J, Brihaye C, Langstrom B, Lemaire C, Meyer GJ, Nebeling B, Stone-Elander S (1993) Radiochemistry automation for PET. In: Stöcklin G, Pike VW (eds) Radiopharmaceuticals for positron emission tomography. Methodological aspects. Kluwer, Dordrecht, pp 45–90

Dannals RF, Langstrom B, Ravert HT, Wilson AA, Wagner HN (1988) Synthesis of radiotracers for studying muscarinic cholinergic receptors in the living human brain using positron emission tomography: (^{11}C)dexetimide and (^{11}C)levetimide. Appl Radiat Isot 39:291–295

Delforge J, Syrota A, Mazoyer B (1989) Experimental design optimization: theory and application to estimation of receptor model parameters using dynamic positron emission tomography. Phys Med Biol 34:419–435

Delforge J, Syrota A, Mazoyer BM (1990a) Identifiability analysis and parameter identification of an in-vivo receptor model PET data. IEEE Trans Biomed Eng 37:653–662

Delforge J, Janier M, Syrota A, Crouzel C, Vallois JM, Cayla J, Lancon JP, Mazoyer B (1990b) Noninvasive quantification of muscarinic receptors in vivo with positron emission tomography in the dog heart. Circulation 82:1494–1504

Delforge J, Syrota A, Lancon JP, Nakajima K, Loc'h C, Janier M, Vallois JP, Cayla J, Crouzel C (1991a) Cardiac beta-adrenergic receptor density measured in vivo using PET, CGP 12177 and a new graphical method. J Nucl Med 32:739–748

Delforge J, Loc'h C, Hantraye P, Stulzaft O, Khalili-Varasteh M, Mazière M, Syrota A, Mazière B (1991b) Kinetic analysis of central ^{76}Br-bromolisuride binding to dopamine D2 receptors studied by PET. J Cereb Blood Flow Metab 11:914–925

Delforge J, Le Guludec D, Syrota A, Crouzel C, Merlet P (1991c) In vivo quantification of myocardial muscarinic receptors in human by PET. Circulation 84:II-423

Delforge J, Syrota A, Bottlaender M, Varastet M, Bendriem B, Crouzel C, Brouillet E, Mazière M (1993) Modeling analysis of ^{11}C-flumazenil kinetic studied by PET: application to a critical study of the equilibrium approaches. J Cereb Blood Flow Metab 13:454–468

Derlon JM, Bourdet C, Bustany P, Chatel M, Therson J, Darcel F, Syrota A (1989) [^{11}C]L-methionine uptake in gliomas. Neurosurgery 25:720–728

Dewey SL, Macgregor RR, Brodie JD, Bendriem B, King PT, Volkow ND, Schlyer DJ, Fowler JS, Wolf AP, Gatley J, Hitzamann R (1990) Mapping muscarinic receptors in human and baboon brain using [N-^{11}C-methyl]-benztropine. Synapse 5:213–223

Evkhoff P (1974) System identification. Parameter and state estimation. Wiley, New York

Farde L, Hall H, Ehrin E, Sedvall G (1986) Quantitative analysis of D2 dopamine receptor binding in the living human brain by PET. Science 231:258–261

Farde L, Pauli S, Hall H, Eriksson L, Halldin C, Hogberg T, Nilsson L, Sjogren I, Stone-Elander S (1988) Stereoselective binding of ^{11}C-raclopride in the living human brain – a search for extrastriatal central D2 dopamine receptors by PET. Psychopharmacology (Berlin) 94:471–478

Farde L, Eriksson L, Blomquist G, Halldin C (1989) Kinetic analysis of ^{11}C-raclopride binding to D2 dopamine receptors studied by PET – a comparison to equilibrium analysis. J Cereb Blood Flow Metab 9:696–708

Farde L, Nordstrom A-L, Wiesel F-A, Pauli S, Halldin C, Sedvall G (1992) Positron emission tomographic analysis of central D1 and D2 dopamine receptor occupancy in patients with classical neuroleptics and clozapine. Arch Gen Psychiatry 49:538–544

Fischman AJ, Livni E, Babich J, Alpert NM, Liu YY, Thom E, Cleeland R, Prosser BL, Callahan RJ, Correia JA, Strauss HW, Rubin RH (1992) Pharmacokinetics of F-18-labeled fleroxacin in rabbits with *Escherichia coli* infections, studied with positron emission tomography. Antimicrob Agents Chemother 36:2286–2292

Fowler JS, MacGregor RR, Wolf AP, Arnett CD, Dewley SL, Schlyer D, Christman D, Logan J, Smith M, Sachs H, Aquilonius SM, Bjurling P, Halldin C, Hartvig P, Leenders KL, Lundqvist H, Oreland L, Stalvacke CG, Langstrom B (1987) Mapping human brain monoamine oxydase A and B with ^{11}C-labelled suicide inactivators and PET. Science 235:481–485

Frey KA, Hichwa RD, Ehrenkaufer RLE, Agranoff BW (1985) Quantitative in vivo receptor binding. III. Tracer kinetic modeling of muscarinic cholinergic receptor binding. Proc Natl Acad Sci USA 82:6711–6715

Frey KA, Koeppe RA, Mulholland GK, Jewett DM, Hichwa RD, Agranoff BW, Kuhl DE (1988) Muscarinic receptor imaging in human brain using (^{11}C)scopolamine and positron emission tomography. J Nucl Med 29:808

Frost JJ, Wagner HN, Dannals RF, Ravert HT, Wilson AA, Links JM, Rosenbaum AE, Trifiletti RR, Snyder SH (1986) Imaging benzodiazepine receptors in man with (^{11}C)suriclone by positron emission tomography. Eur J Pharmacol 122:381–383

Frost JJ, Mayberg HS, Douglas KH, Fischer R, Pearlson G, Ross C, Dannals RF, Links JM, Snyder H, Wagner HN (1987) Alteration of cerebral mu opiate receptors in the temporal lobe epilepsy and following electroconvulsive therapy. J Cereb Blood Flow Metab 7 (Suppl 1):421

Gjedde A (1988) A exchange diffusion of large neutral amino acids between blood and brain. In: Rakic L, Begley DJ, Dawson H, Zlovic BV (eds) Peptide and amino acid transport mechanisms in the central nervous system. Macmillan, London, pp 209–217

Hantraye P, Kaijima M, Prenant C, Guibert B, Sastre J, Crouzel M, Naquet R, Comar D, Mazière M (1984) Central type benzodiazepine binding sites: a positron emission tomography study in the baboon's brain. Neurosci Lett 48:115–120

Hantraye P, Chavoix C, Guibert B, Fukuda H, Broouillet E, Dodd RH, Prenant C, Crouzel M, Naquet R, Mazière M (1988) Benzodiazepine receptors studied in living primates by positron emission tomography: antagonist interactions. Eur J Pharmacol 153:25–32

Harvey J, Firnau G, Garnett ES (1985) Estimation of the radiation dose in man due to 6-[18F]fluoro-L-dopa. J Nucl Med 26:931–935

Herzog H, Coenen HH, Kuwert T, Langen KJ, Feinendegen LE (1990) Quantification of the whole-body distribution of PET radiopharmaceuticals, applied to 3-N-([^{18}F]fluoroethyl)spiperone. Eur J Nucl Med 16:77–83

Hoffman JM, Melega WP, Hawk TC, Grafton SC, Luxen A, Mahoney DK, Barrio JR, Huang S-C, Mazziotta JC, Phelps ME, (1992) The effects of carbidopa on 6-[^{18}F]fluoro-L-dopa kinetics in positron emission tomography. J Nucl Med 33:1472–1477

Huang S-C, Barrio JR, Phelps ME (1986) Neuroreceptor assay with positron emission tomography: equilibrium versus dynamic approaches. J Cereb Blood Flow Metab 6:515

Huang S-C, Bahn M, Barrio JR, Hoffman JM, Satyamurthy N, Hawkins NA, Mazziotta JC, Phelps ME (1989) A double injection technique for in vivo measurement of dopamine D2 receptor density in monkey with 3-N-2'-^{18}F-fluoroethylspiperone and dynamic positron emission tomography. J Cereb Blood Flow Metab 9:850–858

Jones AKP, Luthra SK, Mazière B, Pike VW, Loc'h C, Crouzel C, Syrota A, Jones T (1988) Regional cerebral opioid receptor studies with (^{11}C)diprenorphine in normal volunteers. J Neurosci Methods 23:121–129

Jones T, Tisley DW, Wilson BJ, Lammertsma AA, Brown G, Brady F, Price PM (1992) Positron emission tomography for tumor assessment. NMR Biomed 5:265–269

Kagiwada HH (1974) System identification. Methods and applications. Addison-Wesley, Reading

Kilbourn MR, Carey JE, Koeppe RA, Haka MS, Hutchins GD, Sherman PS, Kuhl D (1989) Biodistribution, dosimetry, metabolism and monkey PET studies of ^{18}F-GBR 13119. Imaging the dopamine uptake system in vivo. Nucl Med Biol 6:569–576

Koeppe RA, Shulkin BL, Rosenspire KC, Shaw LA, Betz AL, Mangner T, Price JC, Agranoff BW (1991) Effect of aspartame-derived phenylalanine on neutral amino acid uptake in human brain: a positron emission tomography study. J Neurochem 56:1526–1535

Le Bars D, Thivolle P, Bojkowski C, Chazot G, Arendt J, Frackowiak R, Claustrat B (1991) PET and pharmacokinetic studies after bolus intravenous administration of [^{11}C]melatonin in humans. Nucl Med Biol 18:357–362

Lee MC, Wagner HN, Tanada S, Frost JJ, Bice AN, Dannals RF (1988) Duration of occupancy of opiate receptors by naltrexone. J Nucl Med 29:1207–1211

Leenders KL, Poewe WH, Palmer A, Brenton DP, Frackowiac RSJ (1986) Inhibition of fluorodopa uptake into human brain by amino acids demonstrated by positron emission tomography. Ann Neurol 20:258–262

leskinen-Kallio S, Huovinen R, Nagren K, Lehikoinen P, Ruotsalainen U, Treas M, Joensuu H (1992) [^{11}C]methionine quantitation in cancer PET studies. J Comput Assist Tomogr 16:468–474

Logan J, Wolf AP, Shiue C-Y, Fowler JS (1987) Kinetic modelling of receptor-ligand binding applied to positron emission tomographic studies with neuroleptic tracers. J Neurochem 48:73–83

Martinot J-L, Paillére-Martinot ML, Loc'h C, Péron Magnan P, Mazoyer B, Lecrubier Y, Hardy P, Beaufils B, Alilaire JF, Mazière B, Syrota A (1990) Central D2 receptor blockade and antipsychotic effects of neuroleptics. Preliminary study with positron emission tomography. Psychiatr Psychobiol 5: 231–240

Mathias CJ, Welch MJ, Katznellenbogen JA, Brodack JW, Kilbourn MR, Carlson KE, Kiesewetter DO (1987) Characterization of the uptake of 16α-([^{18}F]fluoro)-17-estradiol in DEMBA-induced mammary tumors. Nucl Med Biol 14:15–25

Mazière B, Mazière M (1991) Positron emission tomography studies of brain receptors. Fundam Clin Pharmacol 5:61–91

Mazière B, Loc'h C, Hantraye P, Guillon R, Duquesnoy N, Soussaline F, Naquet R, Comar D, Mazière M (1984) [76]Br-bromospiroperidol: a new tool for quantitative in-vivo imaging of neuroleptic receptors. Life Sci 35:1349–1356

Mazière B, Loc'h C, Baron J-C, Sgouropoulos P, Duquesnoy N, D'Antona R, Cambon H (1985) In vivo imaging of dopamine receptors in human brain using positron emission tomography and [76]Br-bromospiperone. Eur J Pharmacol 114:267–272

Mazière B, Loc'h C, Stulzaft O, Hantraye P, Ottaviani M, Comar D, Mazière M (1986) [76]Br-bromolisuride: a new tool for quantitative in vivo imaging of D2 dopamine receptors. Eur J Pharmacol 127:239–247

Mazière M, Todd-Pokropek AE, Berger G, Comar D (1977) Carbon-11 labelled compounds in dynamic imaging studies of the brain. In: Medical radionuclide imaging, vol 2. IAAE, Vienna, pp 203–212 (SM 210/155)

Mazière M, Prenant C, Sastre J, Crouzel M, Comar D, Hantraye P, Kajima M, Guibert B, Naquet R (1983) ^{11}C-RO-15-1788 et ^{11}C-flunitrazepam, deux coordinats pour l'étude par tomographie par positrons des sites de liaison des benzodiazépines. C R Acad Sci (III) 296:871–876

Mazière M, Hantraye P, Kaijima M, Dodd R, Guibert B, Prenant C, Sastre J, Crouzel M, Comar D, Naquet R (1985) Visualization by positron emission tomography of the apparent regional heterogeneity of central type benzodiazepine receptors in the brain of living baboons. Life Sci 36:1609–1616

Mazziotta JC, Phelps ME (1986) Positron emission tomography studies in the brain. In: Phelps ME, Mazziotta J, Schelbert HR (eds) Principles and application of PET for the brain and heart. Raven, New York, pp 493–580

Meltzer C, Bryan R, Holcomb H, Kimball A, Mayberg H, Sadzot B, Leal H, Wagner HN, Frost JJ (1990) Anatomical localization for PET using MR imaging. J Comput Assist Tomogr 14:418–422

Merlet P, Delforge J, Dubois Rande JL, Benvenuti C, Crouzel C, Valette H, Fournier D, Castaigne A, Syrota A (1991) Decreased beta-adrenergic receptor concentration in idiopathic cardiomyopathy assessed by positron emission tomography. Circulation 84:II-423

Mintun MA, Raichle ME, Kilbourn MR et al. (1984) A quantitative model for the in vivo assessment of drug binding sites with positron emission tomography. Ann Neurol 15:217–227

Pappata S, Samson Y, Chavoix C, Prenant C, Mazière M, Baron J-C (1988) Regional specific binding of [^{11}C]RO 15 1788 to central type benzodiazepine receptors in human brain: quantitative evaluation by PET. J Cereb Blood Flow Metab 8:304–313

Patlak CS, Blasberg RG (1985) Graphical evaluation of blood-to-brain transfer constants from multiple-time uptake data Generalizations. J Cereb Blood Flow Metab 5:584

Patlak CS, Blasberg RG, Fensternmacher JD (1983) Graphical evaluation of blood-to-brain transfer constants in multiple-time uptake data. J Cereb Blood Flow Metab 3:1–7

Perlmutter J, Larson KB, Raichle ME, Markham J, Mintun MA, Kilbourn MR, Welch MJ (1986) Strategies for in vivo measurement of receptor binding using positron emission tomography. J Cereb Blood Flow Metab 6:154–169

Persson A, Ehrin E, Eriksson L, Farde L, Hedstrom CG, Litton JE, Mindus P, Gedvall G (1985) Imaging of ^{11}C-labelled Ro 15 188 binding to benzodiazepine receptors in the human brain by positron emission tomography. J Psychiatry Res 19:609–622

Pert CB, Danks JA, Channing MA, Eckelman WE, Larson SM, Bennet JM, Burke TR, Rice KC (1984) 3-[^{18}F]Acetylcyclofoxy: a useful probe for the visualization of opiate receptors in living animals. FEBS Lett 177:281–286

Phelps ME, Huang SC, Hoffman EJ, Selin C, Sokoloff L, Kuhl DE (1979) Tomographic measurement of local cerebral glucose metabolic rate in humans with (F-18-2-fluoro-2-deoxy-D-glucose): validation of the method. Ann Neurol 6: 371–388

Samson Y, Hantraye P, Baron J-C, Soussaline F, Comar D, Mazière M (1985) Kinetics and displacement of (^{11}C)RO 15 1788, a benzodiazepine antagonist, studied in vivo in human brain by positron tomography. Eur J Pharmacol 110:247–251

Sato K, Kameyama M, Ishiwata K, Hatazawa J, Katakura R (1992) Dynamic study of methionine uptake in glioma using positron emission tomography. Eur J Nucl Med 19:426–430

Schelbert HR, Schwaiger M (1986) PET studies in the heart. ^{14}C-deoxyglucose method for the measurement of local cerebral glucose utilization: theory, procedure and normal values in the conscious and anesthetized albino rat. In: Phelps ME, Mazziotta J, Schelbert HR (eds) Principles and application of PET for the brain and heart. Raven, New York, pp 581–662

Sokoloff L, Reivich M, Kennedy C, des Rosiers MH, Patlack CS (1977) The [^{14}C]deoxyglucose method for the measurement of local glucose utilization: theory, procedure, and normal values in the conscious and anesthesized albino rat. J Neurochem 28:897–916

Syrota A (1989) In vivo investigation of myocardial perfusion, metabolism and receptors by positron emission tomography. Int J Microcirc Clin Exp 8:411–422

Syrota A, Paillotin G, Davy JM, et Aumont M-C (1984) Kinetics of in vivo binding of antagonist to muscarinic cholinergic receptor in the human heart studied by positron emission tomography. Life Sci 35:937–945

Tyler JL, Yamamoto YL, Diksic M, Théron J, Villemure JG, Worthington C, Evans A, Feindel W (1986) Pharmacokinetics of superselective intra-arterial and in-travenous [^{11}C]BCNU evaluated by PET. J Nucl Med 27:775–780

Wagner HN, Burns HD, Dannals RF, Wong DF, Langstrom B, Duelfer T, Frost JJ, Ravert HT, Links JM, Rosenbloom SB, Lukas SE, Kramer AV, Kuhar MJ (1983) Imaging dopamine receptors in the human brain by positron emission tomography. Science 221:1264–1266

Wollmer P, Pride NB, Rhodes C, Sanders A, Pike VW, Palmer AJ, Silvester DJ, Liss RH (1982) Measurement of pulmonary erythromycin, concentration in patients with lobar pneumonia by means of positron tomography. Lancet 2: 1361–1364

Wong DF, Gjedde A, Wagner HN Jr (1986a) Quantification of neuroreceptors in living human brain. I. Irreversible binding of ligands. J Cereb Blood Flow Metab 6:137–146

Wong DF, Gjedde A, Wagner HN, Dannals RF, Douglass KH, Links JM, Kuhar MI (1986b) Quantification of neuroreceptors in living human brain. II. Inhibition studies of receptor density and affinity. J Cereb Blood Flow Metab 6:147–153

Wong DF, Lever JR, Hartig PR, Dannals RF, Villemagne V, Hoffman BJ, Wilson AA, Ravert HT, Links JM, Scheffel U, Wagner HN (1987) Localization of serotonin 5-HT2 receptors in living human brain by positron emission tomography using N1(^{11}C-methyl)-2-Br-LSD. Synapse 1:393–398

CHAPTER 17
In Vivo Imaging in Drug Discovery and Design

A.J. FISCHMAN, R.H. RUBIN, and H.W. STRAUSS

A. Introduction

Over the past decade advances in membrane and molecular biology, receptor biochemistry, and molecular modeling have radically altered the
process of drug development. Currently the drug design/discovery process
relies more on the application of basic molecular and biological principles
than on screening large numbers of samples of soil or toxins as was common
in the past.

The introduction of a new drug into clinical practice usually proceeds in
a five-step process: (a) chemical synthesis and in vitro screening of a series
of compounds designed to achieve a particular biochemical objective; (b)
studies in animal models to determine the pharmacokinetic and pharmacodynamic profile of the drug; (c) validation of safety and efficacy in animal
trials; (d) determination of pharmacokinetic and pharmacodynamic profile in man; and (e) assessment of clinical effects and side-effects in well-
controlled, multicenter studies involving large numbers of patients. The
challenge to the clinician-pharmacologist has been to translate the detailed
measurements that can be made in animal models to the effective treatment
of human disease, despite the lesser data base that can be gathered in man.
Issues of dosing schedules, determination of tissue concentration, assessment of pharmacodynamic effects, and the influence of the drug on normal
and abnormal cell function are less easily assessed in man because of the
need for noninvasive testing. Frequently, the results of studies in animals
cannot be directly extrapolated to man and what has long been needed is a
noninvasive technology for studying the pharmacokinetics and pharmacodynamics of novel therapies in man.

In recent years, advances in single-photon imaging [planar and single-
photon emission computed tomography (SPECT)], positron emission tomography (PET), and magnetic resonance imaging and spectroscopy (MRI and
NMRS) have created a new technology for making precise physiological and
pharmacological measurements. Due to the noninvasive nature of these approaches, repetitive and/or continuous measurements are possible. Although
these techniques have thus far been primarily used for diagnostic purposes,
experience suggests that in the future, a major use of these methodologies
will be in the evaluation of new drug therapies. The high-quality information

that these techniques provide can be extremely useful since a cornerstone of evaluating a new drug is the quality of the measurements made to assess the patient prior to study entrance and the quality of the measurements that can be made to assess the drug effects.

Physiological measurements with new imaging technologies, when combined with classical pharmacological methods, provide a powerful new tool for evaluating innovative therapies. This approach should be particularly useful in the early phases of drug evaluation both in animals and in humans (phase I and II), where issues such as dosing schedules, pharmacodynamic effects, tissue delivery, comparative efficacy, and nonidiosyncratic adverse effects are of particular concern. In this chapter we will define those areas in which imaging techniques may be particularly useful in drug evaluation and development.

B. Pharmacokinetics

Radioactive tracer techniques have numerous roles in drug development and evaluation, ranging from defining static and time-dependent distributions of drug in tissue, to the identification of metabolites and routes of excretion. In general, tracer methods are preferred to chemical determinations because of their intrinsic sensitivity, i.e., their ability to detect picogram and even femtogram quantities of drug. In most cases, initial pharmacokinetic studies are performed with drugs that are labeled with beta-emitting nuclides [tritium (^{3}H) and carbon (^{14}C)], because radiolabeling does not alter biological behavior of the drug. Since both these radionuclides have long half-lives compared to the interval of interest for tracing drug behavior, processes requiring hours to days for completion can be readily evaluated. A disadvantage of these tracers is the inability to determine their distribution by external imaging.

The simplest type of tracer analysis relies on isotope dilution techniques. With these methods the size of various distribution "compartments" can be determined. By repetitive sampling of bodily fluids such as blood, urine, bile, or gastric juice or expired air, the relative rate of entry and loss of the drug or its metabolites from various organs can be determined. When these measurements are combined with chemical assay techniques or performed with a drug that is labeled with both ^{3}H and ^{14}C, metabolism can be evaluated. Using conventional assays, the label should be associated with a specific chemical species, while the dual-label approach assumes a constant relative concentration of labels in specimens where the drug remains unmetabolized; a decrease in the relative abundance of one tracer signifies catabolism of the drug.

Simple tracer dilution techniques can yield substantial information about the kinetics of drug distribution, but provide little detail about where the agent is accumulated or metabolized. This information can be obtained by high-resolution autoradiography of either tissue specimens or sections of the whole body of the animal (HUMPHREY et al. 1985). Under experimental conditions, where film exposure is in the linear portion of the Heulich and Dryle scale and aliquots containing known amounts of radioactivity are exposed in parallel with the tissue samples, the grain density of the autoradiographs can be quantified to yield absolute concentrations of drug in small volumes of tissue (YONEKURA et al. 1983; SOM et al. 1983; MORELL et al. 1989; SCHNITZER et al. 1987). To define the kinetics of a drug several animals have to be examined at each point in time.

Although autoradiography is very useful, a major difficulty is that the destructive nature of the technique permits only a single time point to be assessed in each animal. Determining the temporal sequence of drug behavior requires large numbers of animals and is frequently subject to significant errors, particularly if the experimental conditions under investigation are difficult to reproduce.

With external imaging, the temporal sequence of drug distribution can be determined in a single animal if the drug is labeled with a gamma-emitting nuclide. Serial imaging following a single injection permits simultaneous measurements in multiple organs over time. This approach markedly reduces the sample size required for pharmacokinetic measurements. From these observations, measures of blood clearance, organ uptake, binding, and excretion can be calculated. The imaging approach offers the advantage of following not only the natural course of drug distribution but also the changes that are brought about by an intervention – such as a change in blood pressure, renal function, or cardiac output. In some cases, it may be possible to label a drug at more than one site with γ-emitting radionuclides of different energies. Under these circumstances, it is possible to perform detailed studies of drug metabolism by dual-photon imaging. Taken together, these properties allow the imaging approach to provide information on drug distribution, kinetics, and metabolism in human subjects under a variety of physiological and pathological conditions.

If a drug contains iodine, fluorine, gold, cobalt, or any of a large number of other atoms with radionuclides that have convenient half-lives and gamma emissions, labeling is a simple matter of substitution. The behavior of the drug can be traced in similar fashion to a ^{14}C- or ^{3}H-labeled compound except serial images of the distribution of drug can be obtained. If the molecule does not contain a readily exchangeable atom with a convenient radionuclide for imaging, more innovative approaches to radiolabeling are required.

When the drug to be studied has a high molecular weight (proteins such as growth hormone, antibodies, interleukin-2, etc.), radiolabeling can be accomplished by derivatization with a small functional group that can be labeled. Since the molecular weight of the labeling group is significantly lower than that of the molecule to be labeled, derivatization represents a minor structural perturbation and the biological behavior of the derivative can be assumed to closely approximate that of the native drug. Although this assumption is generally true, bioequivalence must always be validated. For example, if derivatization modifies a part of the drug that is critical for receptor binding, biological activity can be totally lost and biodistribution radically altered. Many functional groups have been described for this purpose, including Bolton-Hunter reagent for iodination, diethylenetriamine penta-acetic acid (DTPA) for indium labeling, and the hydrazino nicatinamide group for technetium labeling (BOLTON and HUNTER 1973; KREJCAREK and TUCKER 1977; ABRAMS et al. 1990). In general, the choice of radionuclide for labeling is dictated by the time frame over which the drug is to be studied.

When the drug under investigation has a low molecular weight, the approaches used for protein labeling are generally unusable. Under these circumstances the molecule may be labeled with the positron-emitting nuclides: ^{11}C (20.4-min half-life) or ^{13}N (10.0-min half-life). These nuclides are useful under circumstances where a rapid synthesis of the molecule is possible and the process(es) of interest occur rapidly. With these radionuclides, imaging can be performed using PET. Compared to conventional single-photon gamma camera imaging, PET has several advantages: higher resolution, greater sensitivity, and the possibility for absolute quantitation. A disadvantage of ^{11}C- and ^{13}N-labeled drugs is the limited time frame over which biological processes can be studied. The very latest time points at which useful data can be obtained with ^{11}C- and ^{13}N-labeled drugs are 90 and 45 min respectively (about 4.5 physical half-lives; typically measurements are limited to about 3 half-lives). When it is not possible to design a synthesis for the rapid incorporation of ^{11}C or ^{13}N in the native structure of a drug it may be necessary to synthesize an analog of the drug. With low-molecular-weight drugs, analogs that are minor perturbations of the native structure can be prepared by fluorination, methylation, and amidation. Although analogs are acceptable from an imaging perspective, the behavior of the analog relative to the native molecule must be well understood for the measurements to provide the desired information.

In addition to radionuclide imaging, drug metabolism can also be studied in vivo by MRI or NMRS. With these techniques, it is possible to simultaneously evaluate the time dependence of concentrations of drug and metabolites. The most promising nuclides for these studies are ^{19}F and to a lesser extent ^{13}C. Unfortunately, the low intrinsic sensitivity of this technique ($\sim 10^{6}$–10^{9} lower than radionuclide methods) limits applications to drugs that are administered in very high doses (Table 1).

Imaging methods have been used to study the in vivo pharmacokinetics of a large variety of drugs including antibiotics, antineoplastic agents, neuroleptics, opiates, enzyme inhibitors, and hormones. The following is a summary of some representative examples.

Table 1. Characteristics of PET, SPECT, NMRS, and MRI for in vivo drug evaluation

	PET	SPECT	NMRS	MRI
Sensitivity	pM-fM	μM-pM	mM-μM	mM
Labeling flexibility	+++++	+++	++	+
Quantitation	Absolute	Relative	Difficult	Very difficult
Time scale	≤6 h	Days	Unlimited	Unlimited
Simultaneous measurements	No	+++	+++++	++
Sequential measurements	+++++	+++	+++++	+++++
Invasiveness	++	++	Minimal	Minimal
Resolution	~5 mm	10–15 mm	1–10 cm	1 mm
Cost	+++++	+++	++++	++++

I. Antimicrobial Agents

Successful antimicrobial therapy depends on the delivery of concentrations of active drug to the site of infection that exceed the level necessary to inhibit the growth or kill the invading microorganism. Although levels of drug may be measured serially in blood and urine without difficulty, other bodily fluids such as cerebrospinal fluid and bile and most tissues are not easily sampled in man. Therefore, prior to trials in patients with active infection, dosing schedule determinations are usually based on animal tissue data and human blood and urine data. Unfortunately, there is an incomplete relationship between drug levels in blood and urine and concentrations achieved in such tissues as brain, liver, prostate, and bone. Therefore, approaches in which traditional blood and urine measurements can be correlated with tissue concentrations determined by imaging techniques hold great promise for defining appropriate dosage schedules and speeding up drug development.

1. Erythromycin

Erythromycin was the first antimicrobial agent to be studied by PET. The molecule was labeled at the dimethylamino group of the D-desosamine portion of the molecule by reductive methylation of N-demethylerythromycin with ^{11}C-formaldehyde and was shown to be identical to authentic erythromycin (PIKE et al. 1982). After intravenous injection in human subjects, local concentrations of the antibiotic were measured by PET. In patients with pneumonia, the time course of uptake of drug was measured in normal and pneumonic lung (WOLLMER et al. 1982). During the first hour after injection, the extravascular concentration of drug was similar in normal and infected tissue ($6.6 \pm 2.2 \mu g/g$ vs $5.5 \pm 2.2 \mu g/g$). These concentrations were achieved within 10 min after injection and were maintained throughout the 60 min of observation.

This study was successful because the rapid equilibration of erythromycin in tissues made ^{11}C with its 20-min physical half-life appropriate for labeling, i.e., the label and the process were well matched. Unfortunately, many antibiotics require hours to days to equilibrate in tissue, thereby requiring radionuclides with longer physical half-lives to permit sufficient time for observation.

2. Fluconazole

Several antimicrobial agents contain fluorine atoms in their native structure and can be studied over a longer time interval by substitution of the native ^{19}F with radioactive [18]F. The antifungal agent fluconazole is an example of this class of drug. Recently, we developed a method for preparing [^{18}F]fluconazole which is identical chemically and microbiologically to the authentic drug (LIVNI et al. 1992). This reagent was used to measure the pharmacokinetics of fluconazole in rabbits by PET. When [^{18}F]fluconazole was coinjected with a pharmacological dose of unlabeled drug there was rapid equilibration to a relatively uniform distribution of radioactivity in most organs of the rabbit. When [^{18}F]fluconazole was injected alone ("carrier-free"), blood clearance was accelerated, spleen, muscle, and heart accumulation was decreased, and liver accumulation was increased. These observations illustrate an important point. Since "pharmacokinetics" are under investigation, rather than the behavior of the carrier-free compound, it is important to administer the drug in amounts known to be pharmacologically active, to avoid misleading results. Quantitative analysis of the images demonstrated that concentrations of $\geqslant 15\,\mu g/g$ tissue were present at 2 h after administering a dose of 5 mg/kg. Based on in vitro and animal model experiences, one would predict that this level of drug would be necessary for a therapeutic effect, and that lower doses would be more problematic. It is of interest that clinical experience with different dosage schedules has led to similar conclusions. Even more reassuring is the observation that the drug concentrated more rapidly at sites of infection than in normal tissue (Fig. 1).

A mathematical model was used to summarize the kinetics of fluconazole in normal and infected muscle (FISCHMAN et al. 1991). The model hypothesizes that fluconazole is compartmentalized in blood and tissue, with rate constants describing the transition between compartments. An example of the fit of the model to drug concentrations measured by PET is illustrated in Fig. 2. Direct measurement of the partition coefficient of [4-^{18}F]fluconazole in normal and infected muscle was in close agreement with the predictions of the kinetic model, suggesting that fluconazole enters tissue via a passive transport mechanism. Transport rates of fluconazole, into (K_{in}) and out of tissue (k_{out}), were increased in infected compared to normal muscle (K_{in}: 0.064 ± 0.001 vs 0.0270 ± 0.0002, $P < 0.0001$; k_{out}: 0.063 ± 0.002 vs 0.035 ± 0.001, $P < 0.0001$). The model also indicates that there is increased blood volume in the infected tissue (0.123 ± 0.0192 vs 0.0625 ± 0.0168, $P = $ NS).

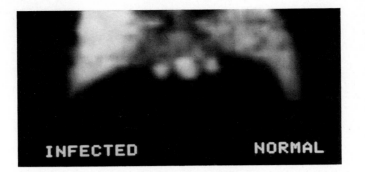

Fig. 1. PET image (coronal reconstruction) of the lower extremities of a rabbit 2 h after injection of 1.0 mCi [4-^{18}F]fluconazole. The right thigh was infected with *Candida albicans* 24 h earlier

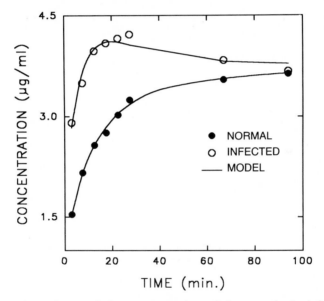

Fig. 2. Time dependence of the concentration of fluconazole in infected (*open circles*) and normal thigh muscle (*filled circles*) of a rabbit measured by PET. The *solid curves* indicate the least-squares fit of the data to the proposed kinetic model. The animals were infected 24 h prior to injection

These studies illustrate the power of a noninvasive technique that will permit the determination of the effect of infection, inflammation, congestive heart failure, renal failure, metabolic factors, etc. on the delivery of effective concentrations of an antimicrobial agent to clinically important sites of infection. Figure 3 is an example of a PET image and corresponding CT slice of the brain of a normal volunteer injected with [^{18}F]fluconazole.

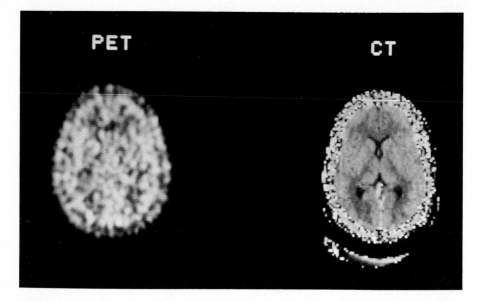

Fig. 3. PET and CT images of the brain of a normal volunteer injected with [^{18}F]fluconazole

II. Antineoplastic Agents

Antineoplastic drug therapy is a highly complex undertaking in which potentially toxic compounds are administered to severely ill patients in the hope of achieving objective regression of the cancer and increased survival. With radionuclide techniques candidate drugs can be radiolabeled with radionuclides suitable for external imaging and uptake of the drug by the tumor (a necessary step for therapeutic benefit) can be evaluated. Also, the determination of drug concentrations in normal tissues such as liver, kidney, and bone marrow can have important implications for potential toxicity.

1. Platinum Compounds

The platinum complexes, *cis*-dichlorodiammine platinum (II), *cis-trans*-dichlorodihydroxy-bis-isopropylamine platinum (IV), *cis*-dichloro-bis-cyclopropylamine platinum (II), and *cis*-diamino 1,1-cylobutanedicarboxylate platinum (II) have been radiolabeled with ^{191}Pt and serial in vivo images acquired in patients with malignant disease (OWENS et al. 1985). The pharmacokinetics of uptake and clearance in liver and kidney were shown to be similar for all four drugs. Unfortunately, unequivocal evidence of tumor accumulation was not found for any of the agents.

2. 5-Fluorouracil

In a recent report, patients with colorectal tumors were injected with [^{18}F]5-fluorouracil (5FU) and radioactivity in normal liver and metastasis was monitored for 2 h by PET (PORT et al. 1989). A kinetic model was developed to calculate the concentration of 5FU and its metabolites. It is possible that in the future, this model can be used to help predict therapeutic response and permit evaluation of the kinetic effects of different methods of drug delivery.

III. Neuroleptics

Cognitive function is the area in which humans are most strikingly different from other species. There are few reliable animal models of human psychiatric disease. Thus, the development of effective neuroleptic agents is in many ways the most complex area of modern drug development. Not only must a drug cross the blood-brain barrier in sufficient quantity to be pharmacologically effective but its regional cerebral distribution must coincide with the distribution of receptors to which it is directed. The observation that binding to neurotransmitter receptors can be used as a predictor of clinical potency of neuroleptic drugs of diverse chemical structure adds a rational basis to drug development (CREESE et al. 1976). External imaging of radiolabeled drugs is the only potentially reliable method of studying these processes in humans and could become an important tool in early phase I drug development.

Studies with the drug, raclopride, can be considered to be prototypes for methods that can be applied to studying neuroleptic drugs in humans (FARDE et al. 1988, 1989, 1990). The rate of uptake and equilibration of this drug in the CNS is sufficiently rapid to use ^{11}C as a tracer. Also, as with most drugs of this class of compounds, the presence of substitutable alkyl groups makes radiolabeling with ^{11}C relatively straightforward. Not only has it been possible to measure the regional CNS distribution of drug by PET, but by in vivo saturation analysis D_2 dopamine receptor density (B_{max}) and affinity (K_d) could be determined. These methods could be extremely useful in screening new neuroleptic drugs. By measuring the displacement of radiolabeled raclopride by a candidate drug, interaction of the drug with D_2 receptors can be evaluated. Also, to define possible side-effects, the receptor specificity of new drugs can be determined by using other radiolabeled ligands that interact with different receptor systems.

IV. Angiotensin-Converting Enzyme Inhibitors

Angiotensin-converting enzyme inhibitors (ACEIs) have become important drugs for the treatment of hypertension and congestive heart failure. With the synthesis and in vitro testing of numerous new analogs, it has become apparent that different tissues have different ACEs that are more or less affected by different ACEIs. A question that remains to be answered is whether these in vitro differences are clinically important; for example, currently available ACEIs cannot be safely used in patients with renovascular hypertension because of their effects on afferent arteriolar pressures. Newer ACEIs are more renal sparing (in terms of their effects on renal ACE) and may be safer in this circumstance. The ability to study these effects in man in vivo, particularly combining measurements of drug–enzyme interaction with measurements of the hemodynamic effects of the drug (see below), should greatly facilitate the evaluation of new compounds.

In a recent report, an ^{18}F-labeled analog of captopril was synthesized and its biodistribution was measured (HWANG et al. 1991). At 30 min after injection there was high uptake in organs known to have high concentrations of ACE: lung, kidney, and aorta. Faster clearance was observed for lung and kidney compared to aorta. When the radiolabeled drug was coadministered with unlabeled captopril, uptake in lung and kidney was blocked. These observations establish the feasibility of studying the pharmacokinetics of ACEIs in vivo using PET.

V. Nuclear Magnetic Resonance

Applications of NMR to the study of in vivo pharmacokinetics are slowly beginning to emerge. Due to the low intrinsic sensitivity of the method it is unlikely to be generally applicable to drug studies. However, in those situations in which it can be applied, unique information about the details of drug metabolism can be obtained.

Fluorine-19 NMRS has been used to study the pharmacokinetics of 5-FU in tumors in both animal models and human subjects (STEVENS et al. 1984; WOLF et al. 1987, 1990). The results of these studies indicate that free 5-FU is trapped in some tumors after intravenous administration (600 mg/m^2) and there is a correlation between uptake and response to therapy. While only a limited number of patients have been studied, the technique has great promise. As stated in one of the articles, "The key observation is that it is now possible to measure the time course of a therapeutic agent (as an unequivocal chemical species) in its intended target site in humans" (WOLF et al. 1990).

In another study, one-dimensional ^{19}F chemical shift imaging of the neuroleptic, fluphenazine, was used to determine the distribution of drug and metabolites in rat brain in vivo (NAKADA and KWEE 1989). The results showed the expected distribution and verified that the primary fluorinated species in brain is intact drug. Also, an unidentified fluorinated metabolite was detected in subcutaneous tissue.

One therapeutic area in which NMR methods could be particularly useful is in the study of the fluoroquinolones, perhaps the most rapidly growing class of antimicrobial agents. Not only are such issues as therapeutic tissue concentrations important with these agents, but also the possible relationship between tissue concentrations and toxicity is of critical import-ance. In particular, neurological side-effects such as seizures have been of major concern, especially in elderly patients receiving theophylline and those with pre-existing epileptogenic foci. The presence of fluorine in the native structure of these drugs makes NMR an ideal technique for studying the uptake and metabolism of fluoroquinolone analogs in the brain. In vivo NMR data could greatly facilitate the development of new compounds that are less toxic than currently available members of this class of drugs. Recently, an NMR study of the in vivo pharmacokinetics of the fluoro-quinolone, fleroxacin, in liver and muscle of humans was reported (JYNGE et al. 1990). Unfortunately, the low signal-to-noise ratio of the spectra signi-ficantly limited the precision of derived pharmacokinetic parameters.

Clearly, the combined use of NMRS and PET could have profound implications for studying drug pharmacokinetics and metabolism. Due to its high sensitivity and quantitation, PET can provide detailed kinetic data on total radiolabeled drug plus metabolites while the molecular resolution of NMRS can yield information on the distribution of label in specific meta-bolites. In the future, NMRS measurements will almost certainly be used to provide the molecular information that is required for detailed kinetic modeling of PET data, just as conventional MRI imparts the anatomical substrate for interpreting PET images.

C. Pharmacodynamics

The influence of a drug on organ function or metabolism can be readily determined by radionuclide imaging techniques. Table 2 lists some measure-ments of organ function that can be performed with existing equipment and procedures following either intravenous administration or inhalation of the tracer material.

Reviewing specific procedures and their application in the evaluation of a hypothetical drug may help clarify specific applications.

I. Cardiovascular

1. Ventricular Function

The gated blood pool scan can be used to measure the size, shape, and contractile function of the heart before and after administration of a drug. To record this information the patient's red blood cells or plasma proteins are radiolabeled. Blood pool labeling is most commonly accomplished with ^{99m}Tc, but other nuclides such as ionic ^{113}In or ^{68}Ga (which bind to the β-globulin transferrin), or [^{11}C]carbon monoxide (which binds to hemoglobin) can be used. Following blood pool labeling, data are recorded by "gating"

Table 2. Common tracer procedures and their application

Procedure	Application	Radiopharmaceutical	Nature Single	Continuous
Gated scan	Cardiac function	^{99m}Tc-labeled red blood cells		✓
Perfusion	Tissue flow	^{201}Tl, ^{133}Xe, ^{82}Rb	✓	
DTPA scan	Renal function	^{99m}Tc-DTPA		✓
IgG scan	Inflammation	^{111}In-IgG	✓	
C^{15}O$_2$ inhalation	Perfusion/ ventilation	C^{15}O$_2$	✓	
MAA perfusion	R/L shunt, lung perfusion	^{99m}Tc-MAA	✓	
Ventilation	Gas exchange	^{133}Xe	✓	
FDG scan	Glucose metabolism	^{18}F[FDG]	✓	
Bone scan	New bone formation	^{99m}Tc-MDP	✓	
Bone density	Mineral mass	None	✓	
Reticuloendothelial system scan	Liver/spleen function	^{99m}Tc-labeled colloid	✓	
VEST	Cardiac function	^{99m}Tc-labeled red blood cells		✓
Renal monitor	Renal function	^{99m}Tc-DTPA		✓
Gastric emptying	GI transit time	^{99m}Tc-labeled food		✓
Biliary scan	Bile production	^{99m}Tc-DISIDA	✓	

DTPA, diethylenetriamine penta-acetic acid; MAA, macroaggregated albumin; FDG, fluorodeoxyglucose; MDP, methylene diphosphonate; DISIDA, diisopropyl-iminodiacetic acid

the scintillation camera/computer to record data in synchrony with the cardiac cycle, using the R wave of the electrocardiogram as the physiological trigger. Data are usually recorded over an interval of about 8–10 min/view to provide a series of images with sufficient resolution to permit analysis of global and regional cardiac function. The strength of this technique is derived from the linear relationship between counts recorded over the cardiac chambers and the volume of blood in the chambers. Although absolute calibration can be achieved to within ~25 ml of the chamber volume, relative changes can be determined with far greater precision. Analyzing serial acquisitions recorded after a single injection permits monitoring of relative left and right ventricular volumes, cardiac output, and ejection fraction. These measurements can be made with the subject at rest or during graded exercise to determine the reserve function of the heart. In addition to global function, the images can be assessed for regional wall motion. This information can be of great value in determining the impact of a drug on zones of the myocardium prone to ischemia or subject to contractile dysfunction secondary to myopathy.

Standard blood pool imaging averages cardiac function over multiple cardiac cycles. In patients with arrhythmias, sudden onset of severe ischemia, or dynamic outflow obstruction, marked changes in function may occur over a few beats. To evaluate these changes in function, data must be recorded on a beat-by-beat basis. This measurement can be performed with a radionuclide detector fixed over the left ventricular blood pool. One such instrument, the VEST, consists of a single radionuclide detector interfaced to a modified Holter recorder and mounted in a vest-like garment (WILSON et al. 1983). With this device the time-activity curve of the left ventricle is continuously monitored (for up to 24h) to provide a beat-by-beat measure of cardiac performance in concert with the patient's EKG (Fig. 4). The combined measurement is particularly useful to characterize episodes of ischemia. Previous work has demonstrated a striking incidence of painless episodes of decreased ejection fraction in patients following acute myocardial infarction (KAYDEN et al. 1990). Subjects demonstrating this behavior had a high incidence of severe recurrent cardiac events in the year following recovery from their initial infarct. Defining the influence of a specific therapy, such as a calcium channel blocker or β-blocking drug on these episodes would be helpful in establishing the drug's efficacy.

A major thrust of cardiovascular drug development in recent years has been the development of long-acting preparations of drugs that have long

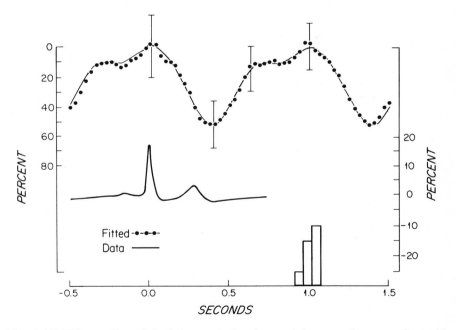

Fig. 4. VEST recording of the left ventricular time-activity curve from a patient with sinus rhythm (*upper curve*). The *middle trace* is the patient's EKG and the *lower trace* is the R-R histogram

been in clinical use, but have required multiple dose regimens. Single long-acting preparations of calcium channel blockers, antiarrhythmic agents, etc. are coming into clinical use. The ambulatory ventricular function monitor provides an ideal way of proving the comparability of long-acting drugs to traditional agents. While the patient is maintained on the conventional treatment regimen, cardiovascular function can be monitored over a 24-h period both at rest and during standardized exercise testing. The patient can then be switched to the new formulation and the monitoring repeated under the identical conditions a few days later. Thus, functional and pharmaco-dynamic comparability of the two regimens could be demonstrated. Since each patient serves as his own control, useful data could be obtained from studying a limited number of subjects and evaluation of new candidate compounds could be greatly facilitated.

2. Blood Volume

Redistribution of blood volume into or out of the central circulation can have marked effects on exercise performance. The sequence of changes in blood volume with graduated physical exertion can define the mechanisms employed to increase central volume to maintain cardiac performance with increased demand. The influence of drugs on arterial and/or venous tone can be monitored by measuring the regional changes in blood volume in the lower extremities, abdomen, and lungs during rest and physical exertion in a control state and after administration of a drug. These measurements can be made using a large field of view gamma camera to monitor the thoracic and abdominal blood volume and a camera collimated with a pinhole placed about 2 m away to image the whole body. When this information is com-bined with data from the VEST and/or measurements of pulmonary func-tion, the influence of the drug on the physiological redistribution of blood volume is well characterized. Changes in pulmonary blood volume are useful indicators of preload, for example, while reduction in splenic blood volume correlates with changes in peripheral hematocrit, white blood cell count, and platelet count.

Recently the feasibility of making these measurements in normal sub-jects was validated (FLAMM et al. 1990). After injection of ^{99m}Tc-labeled autologous red blood cells, measurements were made at rest, zero-load cycling, and at 50%, 75%, and 100% of maximum oxygen uptake. In going from rest to zero-load cycling, leg blood volume decreased (32% $\pm$ 2%), end-diastolic volume increased (9.6% $\pm$ 1.2%), and lung blood volume in-creased (18% $\pm$ 2%). With increasing workload, leg blood volume stabilized, blood volume in the abdominal organs decreased (spleen: 46% $\pm$ 2%; kidney: 24% $\pm$ 4%; liver: 18% $\pm$ 4%), and lung blood volume increased (50% $\pm$ 4%). Representative images demonstrating the effect of graded exercise on the blood volume of the abdominal organs are shown in Fig. 5.

Clearly, these types of measurements (with or without exercise) could be useful in evaluating the effects of a variety of drugs, including calcium channel blockers, ACEIs, ionotropic agents, and rheological agents.

3. Cardiac Output

The distribution of cardiac output may be altered by drugs. Since a number of radiopharmaceuticals distribute in proportion to cardiac output, whole-body images of these tracers provide a picture of the relative partitioning of perfusion to the muscles of the extremities, bowel, liver, kidneys, and myocardium. Previous work with ^{201}Tl demonstrated the changes in cardiac output distribution in patients with mitral and aortic valve disease (SVENSSON et al. 1982). Similar studies can be performed before and after drug administration in both healthy volunteers and patients with significant heart disease to demonstrate the ability to effectively mobilize cardiac output after drug administration.

II. Renal Perfusion and Function

A decrease in arterial pressure can reduce renal perfusion, especially in patients with preexisting renal artery stenosis. Renal perfusion can be measured on a relative basis using a number of different radiopharmaceuticals, including ^{43}K and ^{201}Tl, and imaging with a conventional gamma camera. When absolute quantitation is desired the measurements can be performed with ^{82}Rb or $H_2^{15}O$ and positron tomography. Recently a report from our laboratory demonstrated the use of PET with ^{82}Rb for measuring the effect of captopril on renal blood flow in dogs with experimental renal artery stenosis (TAMAKI et al. 1988). In this study, the sequence and magnitude of acute changes in renal blood flow following injection of captopril were measured by PET. Data were recorded in nine dogs under baseline conditions, during renal artery stenosis and during stenosis when captopril was administered intravenously. In the affected kidney, stenosis resulted in

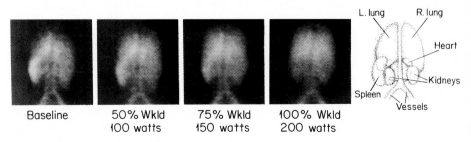

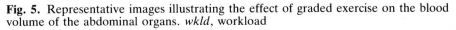

Fig. 5. Representative images illustrating the effect of graded exercise on the blood volume of the abdominal organs. *wkld*, workload

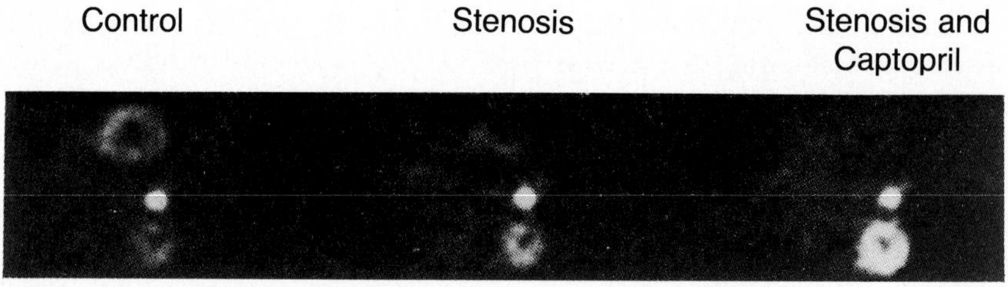

Control   Stenosis   Stenosis and
                                                      Captopril

Fig. 6. Representative PET images of both kidneys of a dog during control period, stenosis (upper kidney in figure), and stenosis plus captopril. (From TAMAKI et al. 1988)

a ~75% decrease in blood flow which was not significantly affected by administration of captopril. In five dogs, stenosis was associated with reduced flow to the contralateral kidney; however, following administration of captopril contralateral perfusion increased and exceeded baseline flow (Fig. 6). In three dogs, stenosis with or without captopril did not have a significant effect on blood flow to the contralateral kidney. In one dog, contralateral flow was reduced during stenosis and further reduced after captopril infusion.

Clearly, similar studies can be performed in humans and could be extremely important in evaluating new ACEIs. In fact, due to the larger size of the human kidney it might be possible to quantify regional renal blood flow.

In many clinical situations, the evaluation of renal perfusion may not be as important as the measurement of function. Global and regional renal function can be determined by imaging the kidneys following intravenous injection of ^{99m}Tc-DTPA, an agent that is excreted by glomerular filtration. When more precise regional quantitation is required, PET with ^{68}Ga-DTPA can be used. To determine overall renal function, a device similar to the VEST, but modified to measure clearance from the extracellular fluid space of the arm, can be used to monitor glomerular filtration rate over several hours. These measurements could be particularly helpful in defining the effect of specific interventions on renal function in extremely ill, hypotensive, patients who are being treated in intensive care units.

III. Antineoplastic Agents

Positron emission tomography using reagents such as [^{18}F]fluorodeoxyglucose (FDG) (a glucose analog), ^{11}C-methionine (the radiolabeled form of the amino acid), and $^{15}O_2$ (the radiolabeled form of molecular oxygen) can provide sensitive measures of the metabolic activity of both normal and abnormal tissue. In many cases metabolic changes connoting drug effect can be detected significantly before changes in the size of a tumor mass can be appreciated. Similarly, metabolic changes in normal tissues could presage

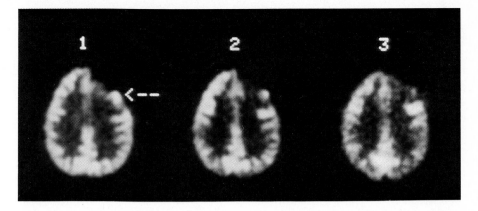

Fig. 7. Effect of chemotherapy on the [¹⁸F]FDG PET images of a patient with grade 3/4 glioma. *Arrow* indicates lesion. *1*, Pretherapy; *2*, 1 month posttherapy; *3*, 3 months posttherapy

significant toxicity. Figure 7 shows sequential [¹⁸F]FDG PET images of the brain of a patient with a grade 3/4 glioma who was being treated with chemotherapy. At all imaging times, changes in glucose metabolism preceded changes in tumor size detected by anatomical imaging.

IV. Liver Function

The liver is the primary site of metabolism of many drugs. Similarly, many drugs can alter liver function. Hepatic parenchymal cell function can be assessed by the rate of uptake and clearance of ^{99m}Tc-labeled iminoacetic acid derivatives. These agents are concentrated in the hepatic parenchyma and excreted via the biliary tree. Prolongation of hepatic transit time can serve as an indicator of liver injury as a result of drug administration.

V. Intestinal Function

Drugs useful for treating bowel dysmotility can be readily evaluated with a variety of tracer-labeled meals. Transit through the esophagus, stomach, small bowel, and large bowel can be assessed separately for the liquid, solid, and fatty portions of a test meal.

An additional application of imaging technology is evaluating the site of dissolution of orally administered capsules or tablets in the gastrointestinal tract. Labeling the drug and recording sequential images following its administration (with or without an accompanying test meal) allows the site of absorption to be identified by observing activity outside the gastrointestinal tract while noting the location of the residual ingested activity in the gut.

VI. Antimicrobial Agents

Antibiotic preparations should reduce the degree of inflammation at a site of infection as the lesion is treated effectively. The use of ^{111}In-IgG for imaging focal sites of infection has been extensively validated in both animals and man (RUBIN et al. 1989a,b; FISCHMAN et al. 1988). Recently, we demonstrated that the rate of regression of inflammation can be monitored using serial injections of radiolabeled IgG (WILKINSON et al. 1989). This technique can be employed to assess the relative efficacy of a therapy for the treatment of focal infection. Following infection of a group of animals, one untreated subgroup would define the natural history of the lesion, another subgroup treated with the clinically favored therapy would define the expected rate of improvement, and a third subgroup treated with the new drug would complete the comparison. Objective evaluation of the relative tracer intensity at the site of the lesion by a region of interest analysis permits assessment of the change in the degree of inflammation as a function of the therapy.

Clinically, inflammation scanning can be very useful in defining the response to therapy. For example, serial ^{111}In-IgG scans have shown that when therapy is incomplete, inflammation will persist, and the patient will promptly relapse if antibiotics are discontinued at this point even if such traditional clinical markers as fever and peripheral white blood cell count have returned to normal. Such "proof of cure" studies are particularly useful in evaluating the efficacy of therapy in such difficult to treat infections as osteomyelitis, prosthetic joint infections, postoperative infections, and intravascular infections.

VII. Nuclear Magnetic Resonance

In recent years, NMR techniques have begun to be applied to the study of pharmacodynamics. These applications can be divided into two categories: proton imaging and spectroscopy and tracer studies (^{19}F or ^{13}C).

When the effect of a drug can be monitored by proton imaging or spectroscopic techniques, the problem of low intrinsic sensitivity of NMR is reduced. Under these circumstances, the exquisite spatial resolution of conventional MRI and the ability to image individual molecular species by chemical shift imaging can provide in vivo data that are not available by any other method. An interesting application of MRI to drug evaluation is its use to study the effect of aldose reductase inhibitors on the water content of peripheral nerves in diabetics. In a recent study, the water content of the sural nerve was compared in a group of patients ($n = 39$) comprising symptomatic diabetics with sensory neuropathy, symptomatic diabetics with sensory neuropathy treated with an aldose reductase inhibitor, neurologically asymptomatic diabetics, and normal controls (GRIFFEY et al. 1988). Significant increase in water content was detected in more than half the symptomatic diabetics. In 2 of 11 neurologically asymptomatic diabetics increased hydration was detected, suggesting presymptomatic alteration. All symptomatic diabetics treated with aldose reductase inhibitor had normal nerve water content. These results suggest that MRI may be a useful technique for detecting early complications of diabetes and for monitoring response to drug therapy. Clearly, the technique can be extended to monitor the effect of any drug on water content. With chemical shift imaging other substances can be monitored.

Recently, MRI techniques which can be used to evaluate cerebral hemodynamic changes between rest and activated cognitive states have been developed (BELLIVEAU et al. 1991; ROSEN et al. 1991). With this methodology it is possible to record functional images at the time scale of neural activation. In the future, these procedures will undoubtedly have significant applications for studying some classes of drugs.

The use of NMR tracer techniques to monitor response to drug treatment is more limited, but can provide unique and useful information. An interesting application of NMR is the use of ^{19}F NMRS to monitor the effect of the aldose reductase inhibitor, sorbinil, on in vivo metabolism of 3-fluoro-3-deoxy-D-glucose (3-FDG) in rat brain (KWEE et al. 1987). Following intravenous infusion of 3-FDG, four resonances were detected and assigned to: the alpha and beta anomers of 3-FDG, 3-fluoro-3-deoxy-D-sorbitol, and 3-fluoro-3-deoxy-D-fructose. After oral administration of sorbinil, there was reduced flux of 3-FDG into the aldose reductase sorbitol pathway. The use of 3-FDG to evaluate the aldose reductase sorbitol pathway has been extended to imaging studies. In a recent report, selective excitation ^{19}F MRI was used to obtain individual images of 3-FDG and its metabolites in the head of a rabbit (Fig. 8) (NAKADA et al. 1988). Images of 3-fluoro-3-deonxy-D-sorbitol showed the distribution of aldose reductase activity. Since 3-FDG has extremely low toxicity, it is possible that in the future similar studies will be performed in humans (HALAMA et al. 1984).

D. Summary

The noninvasive physiological, biochemical, and anatomical measurements that can be performed in humans with modern imaging techniques offer great promise for defining the exact state of a patients disease and its response to therapy. Although the primary application of this technology thus far has been for diagnostic purposes, it is already clear that these methods will greatly facilitate the evaluation of new therapies. In general, there are two critical points in drug development where such innovative techniques are likely to be most useful: (a) in preclinical studies, where a new drug can be precisely compared to standard therapies or where one compound from a series of analogs is being chosen for further development on the basis of performance in an appropriate animal model; (b) in phase

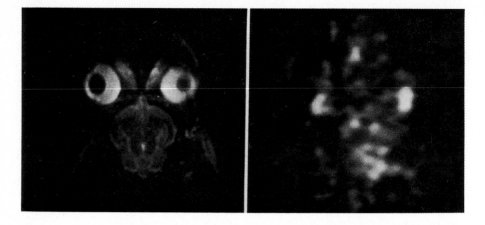

Fig. 8. Image of 3-fluoro-3-deoxy-D-sorbitol distribution in the head of a rabbit (*left*). The corresponding proton image is shown on the *right*. (From Kwee et al. 1987)

I–II human studies, where classic pharmacokinetic measurements can be coupled with imaging measurements to define the proper dosing schedule and the potential utility of interventions in particular clinical situations and to formulate the design of phase III studies that are crucial for drug licensure. In general, the types of measurements that should be possible can be grouped into the following categories:

1. In situations where the drug can be radiolabeled, the time course of tissue delivery can be determined noninvasively in vivo in health and disease. Ligand-receptor binding can be assessed in vivo in two ways. Radiolabeled drug can be used to directly assess the distribution and time course of binding. Alternatively, the ability of the drug to displace standard radiolabeled ligands from its receptors can be measured. These measurements are particularly useful for studying compounds acting on the CNS and cardiovascular systems. Such information should be most useful for determining dosing schedules, establishing efficacy, and predicting possible toxicity.
2. Measurements of tissue metabolism are useful for determining the effects of therapies aimed at particular metabolic abnormalities (e.g., aldose reductase inhibition at particular anatomical sites).
3. The effects of drugs on the heart, kidneys, liver, brain, or gastrointestinal tract can be measured exquisitely with a variety of tracer and magnetic resonance techniques.

We would suggest that the joining of classical clinical pharmacology to exquisite imaging measurements will help form the basis for clinical drug development in the future.

References

Abrams MJ, Juweid M, tenKate CI, Schwartz DA, Hauser MM, Gaul FE, Fuccello AJ, Rubin RH, Strauss HW, Fischman AJ (1990) ^{99m}Tc human polyclonal IgG radiolabeled via the hydrazino nicatinamide derivative for imaging focal sites of infection in rats. J Nucl Med 31:2022–2028

Belliveau JW, Kennedy DN, McKinstry RC, Buchbinder BR, Weisskoff RM, Cohen MS, Vevea JM, Brady TJ, Rosen BR (1991) Functional mapping of the human visual cortex by magnetic resonance imaging. Science 254:716–719

Bolton AE, Hunter WM (1973) The labeling to high specific radioactivities by conjugation to a ^{125}I-containing alkylating agent. Biochem J 133:529–539

Creese I, Burt DR, Snyder SH (1976) Dopamine receptor binding predicts clinical and pharmacological potencies of anti-schizophrenic drugs. Science 192:481–483

Farde L, Wiesel FA, Jannson P, Uppfeldt G, Wahlen A, Sedvall G (1988) An open label trial of raclopride in acute schizophrenia. Confirmation of D2-dopamine receptor occupancy by PET. Psychopharmacology 94:1–7

Farde L, Ericksson L, Blomquist G, Halldin C (1989) Kinetic analysis of central [^{11}C]raclopride binding to D_2-dopamine receptors studied by PET – a comparison to the equilibrium analysis. J Cereb Blood Flow Metab 9:696–708

Farde L, Wiesel FA, Stone-Elander S, Halldin C, Nordstrom AL, Hall H, Sedvalle G (1990) D_2 dopamine receptors in neuroleptic-native schizophrenic patients. Arch Gen Psychiatry 47:213–219

Fischman AJ, Rubin RH, Khaw BA, Callahan RJ, Wilkinson R, Keech F, Dragotakes S, Kramer P, LaMuraglia GM, Lind S, Strauss HW (1988) Detection of acute inflammation with ^{111}In-labeled non-specific polyclonal IgG. Semin Nucl Med 18:335–344

Fischman AJ, Alpert NM, Livni E, Ray S, Sinclair I, Elmaleh DR, Weiss S, Correia JA, Webb D, Liss R, Strauss HW, Rubin RH (1991) Pharmacokinetics of ^{18}F-labeled fluconazole in rabbits with candidal infections studied with positron emission tomography. J Pharmacol Exp Ther 259(3):1351–1359

Flamm SD, Taki J, Moore R, Lewis SF, Keech F, Maltais F, Ahmad M, Callahan R, Dragotakes S, Alpert N, Strauss HW (1990) Redistribution of regional organ blood volume and effect on cardiac function in relation to upright exercise intensity in healthy human subjects. Circulation 81:1550–1559

Griffey RH, Eaton RP, Sibbitt RR, Sibbitt WL, Bicknell JM (1988) Diabetic neuropathy. Structural analysis of nerve hydration by magnetic resonance spectroscopy. JAMA 260:2872–2878

Halama JR, Gatley SJ, DeGrado TR, Bernstein DR, Ng CK, Holden JE (1984) Validation of 3-deoxy-3-fluoro-D-glucose as a glucose transport analog in rat heart. Am J Physiol 247:H754–759

Humphrey MJ, Jevons S, Tarbit MH (1985) Pharmacokinetic evaluation of UK-49,858, a metabolically stable triazole antifungal drug, in animals and humans. Antimicrob Agents Chemother 28:648–653

Hwang DR, Eckelman WC, Mathias CJ, Petrillo EW, Lloyd J, Welch MJ (1991) Positron-labeled angiotensin-converting enzyme (ACE) inhibitor: fluorine-18-fluorocaptopril. Probing the ACE activity in vivo by positron emission tomography. J Nucl Med 33:1730–1737

Jynge P, Skjetne T, Gribbestad I, Kleinbloesem CH, Hoogkamer FW, Antonsen O, Krane J, Bakoy OE, Furuheim KM, Nilsen OG (1990) In vivo tissue pharmacokinetics by fluorine magnetic resonance spectroscopy: a study of liver and muscle disposition of fleroxacin in humans. Clin Pharmacol Ther 48:481–489

Kayden DS, Wackers FJ, Zaret BJ (1990) Silent left ventricular dysfunction during routine activity after thrombolytic therapy for acute myocardial infarction. J Am Coll Cardiol 15:1500–1507

Krejcarek GE, Tucker KL (1977) Covalent attachment of chelating groups to macromolecules. Biochem Biophys Res Commun 77:581–585

Kwee IL, Nakada T, Card PJ (1987) Noninvasive demonstration of in vivo 3-fluoro-3-deoxy-D-glucose metabolism in rat brain by ^{19}F nuclear magnetic resonance spectroscopy: suitable probe for monitoring cerebral aldose reductase activities. J Neurochem 49:428–433

Livni E, Fischman AJ, Ray S, Sinclair I, Elmaleh DR, Alpert NM, Weiss S, Correia JA, Webb D, Dahl R, Robeson W, Margouleff D, Liss R, Strauss HW, Rubin RH (1992) Synthesis of ^{18}F-labeled fluconazole and positron emission tomography studies in rabbits. Int J Appl Radiat Isot [B] 19(2):191–199

Morrell EM, Tompkins RG, Fischman AJ, Strauss HW, Rubin RH, Wilkinson RA, Yarmush MY (1989) An autoradiographic method for quantitation of radiolabeled proteins in tissue using indium-111. J Nucl Med 30:1538–1545

Nakada T, Kwee IL (1989) One-dimensional chemical shift imaging of fluorinated neuroleptics in rat brain in vivo by ^{19}F NMR rotating frame zeumatography. Magn Reson Imaging 7:543–545

Nakada T, Kwee IL, Griffey BV, Griffey RH (1988) F-19 MR imaging of glucose metabolism in the rabbit. Radiology 168:823–825

Owens SE, Thatcher N, Sharma H, Adam N, Harrison R, Smith A, Zaki A, Baer JC, McAuliffe CA, Crowther D (1985) In vivo distribution studies of radioactively labelled platinum complexes; cis-dichlorodiammine platinum(II), cis-trans-dichlorodihydroxy-bis-isopropylamine platinum(IV), cis-dichloro-bis-cyclopropylamine platinum(II), and cis-diamino 1,1-cyclobutanedicarboxylate platinum (II). Cancer Chemother Pharmacol 14:253–257

Pike VW, Palmer AJ, Horlock, Perun TJ, Freiberg LA, Dunnigan DA, Liss RH (1982) Preparation of carbon-11 labeled antibiotic-erythromycin lactobionate. J Chem Soc Chem Commun 173–174.

Port RE, Strauss LG, Clorius JH (1989) Positron emission tomography after brief infusion of 5-[^{18}F] uracil: linear model for the kinetics of ^{18}F radioactivity in tumors. Onkologia 12:51–52

Rosen BR, Belliveau JW, Aronen HJ, Kennedy D, Buchbinder BR, Fischman AJ, Gruber M, Glass J, Weisskoff RM, Cohen MS, Hochberg FH, Brady TJ (1991) Susceptibility contrast imaging of cerebral blood volume: human experience. Magn Reson Med 22(2):293–299

Rubin RH, Fischman AJ, Callahan RJ, Khaw BA, Keech F, Ahmad M, Wilkinson RA, Strauss HW (1989a) The utility of ^{111}In-labeled nonspecific immunoglobulin scanning in the detection of focal inflammation. N Engl J Med 321:935–940

Rubin RH, Fischman AJ, Nedelman M, Wilkinson R, Callahan RJ, Khaw BA, Hansen WP, Kramer P, Strauss HW (1989b) The use of radiolabeled, nonspecific polyclonal human immunoglobulin in the detection of focal inflammation by scintigraphy: comparison with gallium-67 citrate and technetium-99m labeled albumin. J Nucl Med 30:385–389

Schnitzer JJ, Morell EM, Colton CK, Smith KA, Stemerman MB (1987) Absolute quantitative autoradiography of low concentrations of ^{125}I-labeled proteins in arterial tissue. J Histochem Cytochem 35:1439–1450

Som P, Yonekura Y, Oster ZH, Meyer MA, Pelletteri ML, Fowler JS, MacGregor RR, Russell JA, Wolf AP, Fand I, McNally, Brill AB (1983) Quantitative autoradiography with radiopharmaceuticals, Part 2: Application in radiopharmaceutical research: concise communication. J Nucl Med 24:238–244

Stevens AN, Morris PG, Iles RA, Sheldon PW, Martino R (1984) 5-Fluorouracil metabolism monitored by in vivo ^{19}F NMR. Br J Cancer 50:113–117

Svensson SE, Lomsky M, Olsson L, Persson S, Strauss HW, Westling H (1982) Noninvasive determination of the distribution of cardiac output in man at rest and during exercise. Clin Physiol 2:467–477

Tamaki N, Alpert NA, Rabito CA, Barlai-Kovach M, Correia JA, Strauss HW (1988) The effect of captopril on renal blood flow in renal artery stenosis assessed by positron tomography with rubidium-82. Hypertension 11:217–222

Wilkinson RA, Fischman AJ, Rubin RH, Strauss HW (1989) Monitoring response to antimicrobial therapy with ^{111}In-labeled polyclonal IgG. J Nucl Med 30:P890

Wilson RA, Sullivan PJ, Moore RH, Zielonka JS, Alpert NM, Boucher CA, McKusick KA, Strauss HW (1983) An ambulatory ventricular function monitor: validation and preliminary clinical results. Am J Cardiol 52:601–606

Wolf W, Albright MJ, Silver MS, Weber H, Reichardt U, Sauer R (1987) Fluorine-19 NMR spectroscopic studies of the metabolism of 5-fluorouracil in the liver of patients undergoing chemotherapy. Magn Res Imaging 5:165–169

Wolf W, Presant CA, Servis KL, El-Tahtawy A, Albright MJ, Barker PB, Ring R, Atkinson D, Ong R, King M, Singh M, Ray M, Wiseman C, Balayney D, Shani J (1990) Tumor trapping of 5-fluorouracil: in vivo ^{19}F NMR spectroscopic pharmacokinetics in tumor-bearing humans and rabbits. Proc Natl Acad Sci USA 87:492–496

Wollmer P, Rhodes CG, Pike VW, Silvester DJ, Pride NB, Sanders A, Palmer AJ, Liss RH (1982) Measurement of pulmonary erythromycin concentration in patients with lobar pneumonia by means of positron emission tomography. Lancet 2:1361–1364

Yonekura Y, Brill AB, Som P, Bennett GW, Fand I (1983) Quantitative autoradiography with radiopharmaceuticals: 1. Digital film-analysis system by videodensitometry: concise communication. J Nucl Med 24:231–237

G. Appendix

CHAPTER 18

Considerations on Data Analysis Using Computer Methods and Currently Available Software for Personal Computers

M. GEX-FABRY and L.P. BALANT

A. Introduction

The early stages of computer science in the 1940s, before it started to interfere more or less obviously with everybody's life, were relatively discreet. The 1980s were marked by the first personal computers (PCs), which subsequently have gained access to an increasing number of offices and homes. During the same period, education in computer use and programming became increasingly popular so that few domains now remain untouched by the computer phenomenon.

As stated by BERMAN et al. in 1962, scientists realized rapidly that "physical and mathematical models provide a useful technique for the study of biological systems," but that estimation of parameters "can be a considerable task even for a relatively simple model, and only through the use of high speed computers has it become possible to treat more complex models." Computer programs have evolved together with the computer technology, from the early batch programs developed for large mainframe computers to the current user-friendly software for PCs (BALANT and GARRETT 1983). Many of the earlier programs, such as SAAM/CONSAM and NONLIN, have been adapted over the years and have kept a number of faithful users. Others have appeared on the market more recently, trying to satisfy an increasing demand for programs dedicated to the specific problems encountered in the pharmaceutical industry rather than to more general modeling purposes.

The aim of the present appendix is to describe features and requirements of presently available programs for pharmacokinetic data analysis. It is intended to help potential new users to better define their specific needs and orientate them through a number of products available on the market. It may also help experienced users to appraise the various possibilities offered by competing programs.

As we have not performed any benchmark testing, we do not provide any kind of rating of the various software packages. The first part of this chapter covers the different stages involved in pharmacokinetic data analysis, from data entry to printing and plotting results, with emphasis on features that are believed to be a requirement and a short description of more sophisticated possibilities. This view does not pretend to be objective but rather reflects the beliefs and experience of the authors.

In the second part, more than 40 different software packages are briefly described and practical information on how to obtain them is provided. Only products available for IBM-compatible and Macintosh personal computers are reviewed, excluding work stations and larger systems. This information was collected through a two-stage survey. Potential users at drug companies, universities, and government agencies were first asked about the software currently in use in their offices and laboratories. Software developers were then contacted for more detailed information about their products. This survey does not pretend to be exhaustive or representative and the authors apologize in advance for omission of products that they have not been informed of.

B. Program Features and Requirements

When starting an analysis, the pharmacokineticist is generally faced with one or more data sets, often concentrations measured at various time intervals and/or amounts excreted versus time. The various stages involved in computer-aided data interpretation are as follows: data entry, specification of a pharmacokinetic model, definition of an error model, parameter estimation per se, judging the quality of estimates, measuring the goodness of fit, and printing and plotting results. This sequence is generally recursive: results often reveal inadequacies of the model and the process is then repeated several times. Each of the stages mentioned above is now described, with emphasis on the different possibilities offered by PC software packages.

I. Data Entry

Data entry can be a very tedious task as soon as more than one individual data set is to be analyzed. Features to facilitate it are thus worthy of attention. Some programs, such as SIPHAR, integrate a very complete spreadsheet-like system with the possibility of identifying several subjects, treatment groups, and formulations. The pharmacokinetic database can be associated with a clinical database, including biological as well as sociodemographic characteristics.

Alternatively, some programs, such as MINSQ and MKMODEL, offer the possibility of importing data from a large number of software packages, including spreadsheets such as EXCEL or LOTUS, or database systems such as dBASE. Others, like HOEREP-PC, provide an interface to the SAS statistical package, while those running under the Windows environment allow one to cut and paste pieces of data from other programs. However, many pharmacokinetic systems only provide a two-column matrix to enter time and concentration values, with a possible third column for individual weights. Finally, other software packages simply rely on external text editors to provide them with the data.

In general, data and models are stored in independent files in order to avoid inadvertent change of model specifications when modifying data. However, a few programs regrettably combine data and model definition in a single file.

II. Pharmacokinetic Model Specification

Pharmacokinetic models are of various kinds. A first family of models used to describe concentration versus time data are compartmental models. Parameters of interest may be coefficients and exponents of exponential functions, rate constants between compartments, or clearances and volumes of distribution; the philosophical issue behind these different ways of thought is beyond the scope of the present chapter (DI STEFANO and LANDAW 1984).

Other categories of models include noncompartmental evaluations, based on estimation of the area under the concentration versus time plot, pharmacodynamic models, and specific techniques developed to analyze absorption kinetics or to study kinetics of cumulative renal excretion.

Finally, two areas of increasing interest will be briefly discussed: population data analysis and optimization of dosage regimen.

1. Compartmental Models

Assuming the pharmacokineticist is interested in analyzing a single concentration versus time curve for a given volunteer or patient, he probably expects his pharmacokinetic software to provide him with a library of classical one- and two-compartment models, with input functions such as intravenous bolus, constant rate infusion, and extravascular administration. Most programs offer such predefined models but some do not. They require the user to define each model explicitly, using mathematical formulation of the concentration versus time function or differential equations. This is the case for some powerful general-purpose modeling software packages, as well as for some mathematically oriented parameter estimation software packages.

Multiple dosing schedules for one- and two-compartment models are generally also predefined, but sometimes for simulation purposes only. EDFAST allows definition of extremely complex dosing schedules through the concept of universal elementary dosage regimen (SEBALDT and KREEFT 1987).

Time lags or delays may be incorporated in the models. The user should be aware of the different ways of specifying them. As an example, for the Bateman function, the time lag may appear as $(t-t_0)$ in the exponents or as two different coefficients for the absorption and elimination terms.

As metabolite kinetics become more and more frequently required, definition of more complex models and simultaneous fit of two or more curves are important for a number of users. However, the facility to develop models varies greatly between software packages. As an example, PH/ EDSIM offers a very nice graphic editor for creation and modification of compartmental models under the Microsoft Windows environment, making it very attractive for educational purposes. Other software packages require knowledge of programming languages to write and compile new models. Large models of physiological, biochemical, and pharmacological systems probably remain the favorite application area of software packages such as SAAM, MLAB, and SCoP.

In addition, models incorporating capacity-limited processes may be available: TOPFIT includes 16 different predefined models with Michaelis-Menten kinetics.

2. Noncompartmental Approach

This approach, sometimes inappropriately called model independent, is based on the calculation of the area under a concentration versus time curve (AUC), or area under the moment curve (AUMC). These areas are generally approximated by trapezoidal or log-linear trapezoidal rule, and extrapolated to time of administration and infinity. Total clearance, apparent volume of distribution, and mean residence time are derived from these values.

Since this approach has become very popular, several software packages dedicated to pharmacokinetics incorporate such a calculation, either as a default output or in a module separate from classical curve-fitting methods. The program AUC-RPP concentrates on this type of noncompartmental approach.

3. Pharmacodynamic Models

When analyzing the time course of drug effects in relation to concentration, assuming effects are directly and reversibly related to concentrations, three stages should be considered: (a) specification of a pharmacokinetic model to describe plasma concentration versus time data; (b) a link model to define a time-dependent relationship between plasma concentration and concentration at the target organ or receptor; (c) a pharmacodynamic model, generally time independent, for prediction of pharmacological response from concentrations at the effect site (Holford and Sheiner 1982). Mathematical models based on receptor theory are used to describe concentration–effect relationships. A majority of software packages dedicated to pharmacokinetic data analysis incorporate such predefined models: a large choice is offered by TOPFIT, with a library of 20 different concentration–effect functions.

Whereas pharmacokinetic models have been applied extensively and often successfully, a number of difficulties may be encountered when combining them with pharmacodynamic models for in vivo studies. As described by Oosterhuis and Van Boxtel (1988), the relationship between effect site and plasma concentrations may be difficult to establish. Certain effects may be difficult to quantify. Different types of receptors or target tissues may be involved. The presence of endogenous agonists may play a role, as well as physiological homeostatic response or development of drug tolerance. Adequate weighting is another difficulty. Accordingly, pharmacodynamic models should often be viewed as empirical descriptions of the observed effect and parameter estimates should be interpreted with caution.

4. Absorption Kinetics and Bioavailability Studies

Problems encountered when trying to characterize absorption kinetics from fitting model parameters to concentration versus time data have prompted many investigators to seek better methods of analysis. Traditional methods such as the Wagner-Nelson and Loo-Riegelmann methods are based on the construction and evaluation of percent absorbed versus time plots, for one-compartment and multicompartment models respectively. However, deconvolution methods, which do not require any assumption about a specific model, seem to be becoming a standard in pharmacokinetics, so that an increasing number of users may require them. Such techniques are also increasingly recommended by regulatory authorities for the evaluation of controlled-release products. In such cases, knowledge of the disposition kinetics is usually derived from a reference experiment with an oral solution or suspension (SKELLY 1990).

The number of software packages to choose from drastically decreases if these techniques are needed, a small number of programs dedicated to pharmacokinetics incorporating them in their menu. For users who frequently deal with absorption kinetics and specific statistical tests on bioequivalence, two packages are worth citing: KINBES, which is a supplement to MW/PHARM, and BIOPAK, which is a comprehensive package for such studies.

5. Urinary Data Analysis

Analysis of the cumulative amount of drug excreted in the urine often proceeds according to one of the following graphic methods: the rate method, which uses a semilogarithmic plot of the excretion rate versus time, and the sigma-minus method, which considers the amount of drug remaining to be excreted. Renal clearance can also be estimated from excretion rate versus concentration plots. These simple approaches are often useful before simultaneous fitting of plasma and urine data is performed. However, a limited number of software packages allow such initial calculations to be performed without the need to recode the data.

6. Population Pharmacokinetics

The aim of population pharmacokinetics is to describe the relationship of physiological parameters to pharmacokinetic parameters in addition to estimating the average drug behavior in a population. NONMEM is the most often cited program in this field (Sheiner and Beal 1984). Alternatively, packages such as ATS (alternative two-stage method), MLG (maximum likelihood gradient method), and MULTI2 (BAYES) have been developed more recently in Japan (Amisaki and Tatsuhara 1988). Finally, USC*PACK incorporates a module that performs population kinetics through nonparametric expectation maximization (NPEM). It must be emphasized that all the programs cited here are intended for experienced users of population pharmacokinetic theory.

7. Calculation of Individual Dosage Regimen

Optimization of dosage regimen in individual patients is closely related to population pharmacokinetics. The Bayesian method proposed by Sheiner and Beal (1982) integrates already available information regarding population behavior of the drug with information from observed drug concentrations in individual patients. Since posology adjustment is of particular concern for the clinical pharmacologist, the hospital pharmacist, or interested therapists, a number of software packages have been developed for this purpose. In addition to a Bayesian module, several of them include a library of population parameters for a number of drugs known to have a narrow therapeutic range (DATAKINETICS, DRUGCALC, KINETIDEX, MW-PHARM, SIMKIN, TDMS, USC*PACK). The French program APIS allows dynamic dosage adjustments by means of Bayesian estimation, with real-time monitoring and control of drug concentrations for patients whose parameters vary over time.

III. Error Model Specification

Any type of experimental data is subject to random measurement error or noise. Time is generally assumed to be known precisely. The errors in the dependent variables (i.e., concentrations, amount excreted, pharmacodynamic response) are assumed to consist of independent, zero mean random variables, the variances of which are known at least up to a proportionality constant. If several independent replicates can be obtained at the different time intervals, direct estimation of the error variance may be possible. However, this is generally not the case in pharmacokinetic experiments. It is thus common to postulate a model for the error variance, such as:

$$s_i^2 = a + by_i^c, \tag{1}$$

where y_i are measured values, and a, b, and c are coefficients. With $a = 0$ and $c = 0$, the error variance is constant over time (homoscedasticity). With $a = 0$ and $c = 1$, the error variance increases linearly with measured values, while $a = 0$ and $c = 2$ correspond to a constant coefficient of variation.

Parameters of the error model may also be estimated together with pharmacokinetic parameters (see below).

In any case, correct specification of the error variance structure is important for two reasons: (a) precision of the parameter estimates is optimal if weights are inversely proportional to the actual variance of the error (i.e., $w_i = 1/s_i^2$), and (b) correct summary of the statistics of the estimates depends on knowledge of the data error structure (LANDAW and DI STEFANO 1984). In addition, an improper weighting scheme may lead to aberrant parameter estimates, some data being virtually ignored if given insufficient weight. Adequate weighting becomes even more difficult for cumulative urinary excretion (BOXENBAUM et al. 1974) or when analyzing parent compound and metabolites, with concentrations varying by an order of magnitude or more. Most software packages distributed for pharmacokinetic data analysis incorporate the different weighting schemes mentioned above.

IV. Parameter Estimation

Given a set of observations, e.g., N concentration measurements y_i at different time points t_i, one would like to summarize the data by a small number of parameters such as half-life, volume of distribution, or absorption rate. The hypothesis is that observations can be adequately described by a model, the parameters of which are to be estimated.

The basic approach is to define a function that measures the agreement between the data and the model. Parameters are then adjusted in order to optimize (generally minimize) that function. Besides obtaining parameter estimates, we need to assess whether or not the model is appropriate through a statistical measure of goodness of fit. In addition, we also want to know the accuracy of the parameter estimation from the data.

These aspects of pharmacokinetic data analysis are often hardly mentioned in classical textbooks and the interested reader is generally referred to literature which supposes a sufficient background in mathematics. However, a minimum understanding of the principles of parameter estimation is believed to be a requirement for judicious and successful use of pharmacokinetic software packages. Techniques are thus summarized below, trying to point out the basic concept of each method and to avoid unnecessary mathematical developments.

1. Least-Squares and Maximum Likelihood Estimators

Suppose a model $y(t) = y(t; p_1 \ldots p_M)$ where p_j are the parameters to be estimated.

The familiar least-squares estimator (LS) attempts to minimize the following sum of squares (SS):

$$\text{SS} = \sum_{i=1}^{N} [y_i - y(t_i; p_1 \ldots p_M)]^2, \tag{2}$$

where y_i are measured values. Least-squares fitting leads to maximum likelihood estimates of the parameters, if measurement errors are independent and normally distributed with constant standard deviation. This is often not the case in practice.

If the different data points y_i have different standard deviations s_i, weighted least-squares (WLS) fitting is performed by minimizing the following weighted sum of squares (WSS):

$$\text{WSS} = \sum_{i=1}^{N} w_i [y_i - y(t_i; p_1 \ldots p_M)]^2, \tag{3}$$

where weights w_i are defined as $1/s_i^2$. Since the error variance s_i^2 is generally unknown, the error model described by Eq. 1 is often postulated. WLS is the most common estimator in pharmacokinetics and most software packages offer it as a default option.

Extended least squares (ELS) is a further generalization to the case of an error model, the parameters of which are to be estimated together with parameters of the pharmacokinetic model. The objective function (OF) to be minimized becomes:

$$\text{OF} = \sum_{i=1}^{N} \left[\frac{y_i - y(t_i; p_1 \ldots p_M)}{s_i} \right]^2 + \ln s_i^2. \tag{4}$$

If the error model described by Eq. 1 is postulated, coefficients a, b, and c enter Eq. 4 to be optimized. Although ELS sounds attractive and allows one to avoid the burden of specifying error model parameters, it has an inherent drawback: it allows the error structure to change from one set of data to another, which is generally not desirable. Furthermore, three additional parameters need to be estimated from the data.

2. Linear Equations

In the present section, linear equations are understood as "linear with respect to the parameters to be estimated." They include equations that can be linearized, such as concentration following an intravenous bolus for a one-compartment open body model, since $\log y(t) = \log C_o - k_e t$ is linear.

In this case, parameters can be estimated in a straightforward manner, using linear regression methods. Two different techniques may be used: normal equations and singular value decomposition. The latter method is particularly useful when normal equations are close to singular, i.e., when data do not allow distinction between two or more solutions.

3. Nonlinear Equations

When equations are nonlinear with respect to parameters, minimization must proceed iteratively, that is, given initial values of the parameters, a strategy is followed that aims at finding new values until a minimum is found. Two types of methods, briefly described below, may be used. Direct methods only need evaluations of the function to be minimized; they include the downhill simplex method and Powell's method. The others are called gradient methods and require calculation of the derivatives of that function with respect to parameters. More detailed information about all these techniques can be found in the excellent books by KENNEDY and GENTLE (1980) and PRESS et al. (1986). In any case, some information should be provided about the method(s) offered by each software package, at least in the documentation, if not on the screen.

a) Choice of Initial Estimates

The importance of initial estimates is often neglected when using numerical methods of parameter estimation. Methods are designed to converge, providing there is a minimum in the vicinity of the initial estimates. In general, many local minima may exist in addition to the global minimum. Inadequate initial estimates may thus lead any otherwise powerful computational method to get trapped into a local minimum and to provide a solution very different from that corresponding to the true global minimum. This problem is particularly delicate when dealing with complicated (too complicated?) models. If such a problem is suspected, it might be a good idea to perturb parameters from a local minimum and see whether the optimization procedure returns to the same values or not. Another strategy is to repeat the optimization process, starting from very different initial values, and eventually selecting the smallest of the local minima.

The stripping method, sometimes called the peeling method or the method of residuals, is often used in pharmacokinetics to obtain initial parameter estimates. The basic idea is to describe part of a concentration versus time curve by a monoexponential function, subtract that function from the data, fit another portion of the data by a second exponential, and so on. Simple linear regression is performed each time. CSTRIP and PKCALC are programs that concentrate on polyexponential stripping, but many software packages include it among other methods.

Two other features are of interest when developing complex models. One is the possibility to specify constraints on some parameters, such as $k_{ij} > 0$ or $k_{12} > k_{21}$. The other is to "freeze," or fix, the values of some parameters, while adjusting some others. In that case, the fitting procedure has to be repeated with all parameters adjustable, to ascertain a minimum has been found for the whole model. These features are found in general-purpose modeling packages such as SAAM and MLAB but less frequently in other pharmacokinetic packages.

b) Direct Methods

Several software packages provide one direct method of optimization, in addition to one or more gradient methods, generally believed to be more competitive in terms of rate of convergence and overall efficiency. The following two methods have been cited in our survey.

The downhill simplex method (or Nelder and Mead method) considers a geometrical figure in the space of parameters. The function to be minimized is evaluated at each point and the figure is modified in order to "escape" from points where the function is the largest. The method is not very efficient but it is robust. It is a valuable choice when initial parameters are not easy to determine. One important drawback is that it does not provide statistics of the estimated parameters.

Powell's method is based on consecutive one-dimensional minimizations along directions chosen so as not to interfere with each other. These directions in the space of parameters are updated so that preceding minimizations are not "spoiled" by subsequent ones.

c) Gradient Methods

Among the methods which require derivatives with respect to the parameters, the Gauss–Newton method is the most classical and is very often implemented in pharmacokinetic software packages. It proceeds through linear approximation of the nonlinear function to be minimized, each iteration requiring a system of linear equations to be solved. It is very powerful when initial estimates are quite good and thus the iteration proceeds in the vicinity of the minimum. Unfortunately, it may lack dependability in some applications since it is relatively sensitive to initial values.

The steepest descent method is complementary to the Gauss–Newton method since it becomes slow as the minimum is approached. The underlying principle is to adjust parameters in order to follow the direction of the local gradient.

The Marquardt-Levenberg method is based on the idea of a continuous transition from the steepest descent method to a Gauss–Newton or similar method as the minimum is approached. This technique seems to work very well in practice and has become a standard in many nonlinear least-squares software packages. This is the technique most often cited in our survey of pharmacokinetic packages.

More recent techniques include quasi-Newton methods. The most frequently cited methods are the Davidon-Fletcher-Powell (DFP), Broyden-Fletcher-Goldfarb-Shanno (BFGS) and Beal modified Gauss–Newton (BMGN). The matrix of second-order derivatives with respect to the parameters is approximated. Large amounts of computer memory are thus needed for sizable models. Experience has shown that quasi-Newton methods are among the best, when initial estimates are reasonably good. A few software packages provide one of them in their menu.

Conjugate gradient methods, such as the Fletcher-Reeves method, may be considered as refinements of the steepest descent method. The basic idea is to proceed along independent descent directions, constructed to account for previous ones, thus reducing the number of steps to reach a minimum. The conjugate gradient methods are not very demanding in terms of computer memory and can be used for extremely complex models.

When model parameters are subject to constraints, specific methods are needed. Constrained optimization techniques are beyond the scope of this appendix but are implemented in some of the most powerful modeling packages.

V. Confidence Limits on Estimated Parameters

Assuming that a given model and a set of *"true" parameters* allow a certain type of experiment to be described, different data sets may nevertheless be obtained due to experimental error. Each of these data sets would provide a somewhat different set of *parameter estimates*. The pharmacokineticist does not have the possibility of performing multiple experiments to assess the variability of parameter estimates, but is interested in characterizing their distribution with respect to true parameters. Two types of values are needed, the standard deviations of the estimates and the correlation coefficients between them. When minimization is performed through gradient methods, the required covariance matrix is derived from the matrix of partial derivatives in a straightforward manner. However, as mentioned above, it can only be interpreted correctly if the measurement errors are actually normally distributed.

In practice, a large standard deviation for one parameter indicates that a slightly different data set may produce a very different estimate, i.e., the data do not allow the parameter to be estimated accurately. A large correlation coefficient between two parameters means that they might both vary together if the experiment were to be duplicated, suggesting that the data are not adequate to distinguish between them. Such problems can occur when two exponentials exhibit nearly indistinguishable exponents. However, similar results are common when fitting a model with too many parameters or when sampling times do not allow description of the full dynamic range of the model (LANDAW and DI STEFANO 1984).

In any case, careful examination of both standard deviations and correlation coefficients is an important step in data modeling. It is thus regrettable that a few software packages dedicated to pharmacokinetics do not include this type of statistical information.

VI. Statistical Measures of Goodness of Fit

Measures of goodness of fit are another important issue in data modeling. The pharmacokineticist needs a means of assessing whether or not his model is appropriate and of selecting one model among several possible candidates which all appear to describe his data adequately. The function used in the minimization procedure obviously provides such a measure since it decreases as the difference between measured and model predicted values decreases. Such functions include simple sum of squares, weighted sum of squares, and objective function as defined above. Their main drawback is that they generally lead to disregard simple models and favor complex ones, since they decrease as the number of parameters in the model increases. However, they can be used in an F-test to check whether a larger model is significantly better than a simpler submodel (Landaw and Di Stefano 1984).

Akaike and Schwartz criteria incorporate a penalty function proportional to the number of parameters in the model in order to take into account the principle of parsimony, i.e., selection of the model with the fewest parameters that fits the data (Landaw and Di Stefano 1984). Akaike suggested selection of the model with the smallest value of:

$$AC = -2\log \text{ likelihood} + 2P, \qquad (5)$$

where P is the number of parameters to be estimated. Schwartz proposed use of the following criterion:

$$SC = -2\log \text{ likelihood} + P\ln N, \qquad (6)$$

where N is the number of observations. The log likelihood term is derived from the sum of squares, weighted sum of squares or objective function entering the minimization procedure. Many general-purpose modeling packages do not include such criteria, while those dedicated to pharmacokinetics generally include at least one of them.

VII. Solving Systems of Differential Equations

In many cases, the pharmacokineticist is interested in simple one- or two-compartment linear models. At this point, linearity is understood in a pharmacokinetic sense, i.e., as rate constants being independent of concentration or dose. The concentration versus time function for each compartment can then be written explicitly and can be found in a number of textbooks. In other cases, however, the model can only be described as a system of differential equations that cannot be solved analytically. This is the case for complex user-defined models and for models which incorporate nonlinearities such as Michaelis-Menten kinetics. Before optimization is performed, numerical techniques are required to integrate the differential equations and calculate the predicted values $y(t_i, p_1 \ldots p_M)$ which enter the function to be minimized. In addition to the equations themselves, initial values at $t = 0$ are needed for each compartment in the model.

Whereas a number of simple pharmacokinetic software packages are limited to models that can be solved analytically, many allow the user to define his own possibly nonlinear models and incorporate one or several methods of numerical integration. The most often cited methods are briefly described below. More detailed description of each technique can be found in the book by Press et al. (1986).

The most classical methods of numerical integration are the Runge-Kutta techniques. The fourth-order Runge-Kutta method with a fixed stepsize has limited accuracy. Adaptive stepsize control is a requirement for more efficient computation, leading to fifth-order methods such as Runge-Kutta-Fehlberg and others.

The Burlisch-Stoer method is often recommended as a very accurate method but is restricted to relatively smooth functions. It is based on extrapolating calculated values to values obtained with smaller and smaller substeps.

Unlike the approaches mentioned above, which only use the value of the function at the beginning of a time interval to calculate the next value, predictor–corrector methods record previous values and extrapolate them to achieve a rough estimate of the new value. This value is used to calculate derivatives which are in turn used to correct the initial estimate. The most popular methods are Adams-Bashforth-Moulton schemes.

One problem that may arise in pharmacokinetics is the presence of a *stiff* system of equations. Stiffness occurs when kinetics combines very rapid and very slow variations with time. The Gear method is particularly designed to deal with such problems and has been implemented in a few software packages.

VIII. Graphic Display of Results

A pharmacokinetic analysis cannot be complete until the fit of the model to the data has been displayed and examined. Plots of observed values and model predictions, generally as a function of time, are a requirement in both linear and semilogarithmic coordinates. They often reveal systematic deviations and lead to reconsideration of the specification of the pharmacokinetic model. The pharmacokineticist is also interested in obtaining the average concentration versus time curve, together with error bars, for a population of patients or volunteers.

A plot of the differences between observed and predicted values versus time, or versus predicted values, is another simple way of detecting nonrandom deviations between data and model. Ideally, these residuals should be spread randomly above and below zero. Nonrandomness of the errors can be formally tested by the runs test. It frequently occurs when a low-order model (e.g., one compartment) is fit to data for which a higher-order model (e.g., two compartments or more) is appropriate.

Additional information is gained by plotting weighted residuals, i.e., $w_i^{1/2} [y_i - y(t_i; p_1 \ldots p_M)]$ versus time. If the error model is correctly specified, a uniformly wide band of randomly scattered points should be observed. Moreover, a plot of the logarithm of squared residuals versus the logarithm of predicted or measured values should be a straight line with slope equal to c under the general error model in Eq. 1, and assuming $a = 0$ (LANDAW and DI STEFANO 1984).

A majority of software packages provide graphic display of concentration versus time curves, although quality may differ as well as possibilities to change dimensions, titles, or labels of the graphics. The number of programs which provide plots of the residuals is much lower, but many of them do print residuals and some include a runs test of randomness (MW-PHARM). More sophisticated analysis of residuals can be found in MINSQ and RSTRIP, which print weighted residuals and provide a heteroscedasticity measure of the correlation between the magnitude of the residuals and the magnitude of observed values.

IX. Printing and Plotting Results

Once a final model has been retained and a satisfactory fit to the data has been obtained, the pharmacokineticist generally expects the printout to reflect his efforts. Raw data should be printed, together with subject identification, drug name, and dosing schedule. The selected pharmacokinetic as well as error models should be clearly specified, with parameters easily identifiable. Initial estimates should be provided. The printout should include the method chosen for optimization, the number of iterations, and goodness of fit criteria. Parameter estimates should be given together with standard deviations or coefficients of variation, and correlation matrix. Whatever the parameters used in the model specification and the optimization procedure, pharmacokinetic parameters such as clearance, half-life, volume of distribution, predicted AUC, MRT, T_{max}, and C_{max} should be derived and included in the printout. SIPHAR, TOPFIT, and MICROPHARM are a few software packages that produce complete report-quality printouts.

The importance of good-quality plots also needs to be emphasized. The user of pharmacokinetic software would like to include them in reports or publications without having to redraw them or transfer them to another graphics software for refinements. All too often, the quality of graphic output is not up to the level of other parts of pharmacokinetic software packages.

X. User Interface and Documentation

Unlike first-generation batch programs, currently distributed PC software is expected to provide the user with an easy-to-use interface and to require little mathematics, at least for the most classical techniques. The purpose of such a user-friendly interface is not only to look nice on the screen, but to facilitate the modeling process and guide the user through the various steps involved. Several softwares surveyed are menu driven, while a few products are simply available as portable source code. Help functions are not frequently found, while on-screen tutorials are virtually absent from these products. The quality of the manuals is thus of utmost importance as a complement to the information on screen. Many manuals include full analysis of examples, with data files provided together with the software.

Since the Microsoft Windows graphic environment is tending to become a standard for PCs, some users may appreciate packages taking advantage of that environment, such as APIS, DRUGCALC, SIPHAR and PH/EDSIM. New versions of MICROPHARM and MW/PHARM are currently under development under the Windows environment.

Although it is probable that no software can replace a full course in pharmacokinetics, computer-aided data analysis may be a valuable complement for teaching in that domain. MAXSIM is a simulation package developed specifically for educational purposes at the University of Uppsala, Sweden.

XI. Hardware and Software Requirements

Before deciding to purchase a given product a final thought should be given to the compatibility between its hardware and software requirements and the computer environment already available. Most software can be used on 286-type machines. The necessary disk space greatly varies, some of the most complete products asking for 2 to 4 megabytes. Mathematical coprocessor may also be recommended. Presence of adequate printer and plotter drivers may be another point to ascertain, in order to obtain high-quality printouts and graphics.

Software requirements may include FORTRAN, PASCAL, BASIC, or C compilers for some programs, while Microsoft Windows is needed for those taking advantage of that environment.

C. Directory of Surveyed Software

In the present section, all software mentioned to the authors in their survey is listed, independently of features and performances. Again, the survey did not pretend to be exhaustive or representative, and the authors apologize in advance for omission of products that they have not been informed of.

Software	Short description	Contact address	Phone/Fax
ABSPLOTS	A Lotus 123 spreadsheet which calculates drug absorption rates in multicompartment systems through Wagner-Nelson method	Dr. Robert C. Shumaker Wallace Laboratories 301B College Rd. East Princeton, NJ 08540 USA	Phone: (1) 609-951-2013 Fax: (1) 609-951-2116
ADAPT II	Mathematics software for pharmacokinetic/ pharmacodynamic system analysis, including design of optimal sampling schedule	Dr. David Z. D'Argenio Biomedical Simulations Resource USC, Olin Hall of Engineering 500 Los Angeles, CA 90089-1451 USA	Phone: (1) 213-740-0834 Fax: (1) 213-740-0343

Software	Short description	Contact address	Phone/Fax
APIS	User-friendly software under Microsoft Windows graphics environment, with special emphasis on Bayesian estimation, optimal sampling and dosage regimen	Mr. M. Iliadis or Mr. M. Laplane MIIPS 19-21 Rue Brandis F-13005 Marseille France	Phone: (33) 91-25-89-77 Fax: (33) 91-80-14-91
ATS	Nonlinear least squares estimation. Program provided as Fortran source code	Dr. Takashi Amisaki Shimane University 1060 Nishikawatsu Matsue 690 Japan	Phone: (81) 852-21-7100 Fax: (81) 852-31-0812
AUC-RPP	Noncompartmental evaluation of pharmacokinetic parameters	Prof. W.A. Ritschel University of Cincinnati College of Pharmacy, Bldg 401 3223 Eden Ave. Cincinnati, OH 45267 USA	Phone: (1) 513-558-0726 Fax: (1) 513-558-4372
BIOPAK	Statistical analysis of bioavailability/bioequivalence studies, including noncompartmental evaluation of parameters	Mrs. Bonnie L. Ward SCI Software (Clin Trials Inc.) South Creek Office Park 2365 Harrodsburg Rd, Suite A-290 Lexington, KY 40504-3399 USA	Phone: (1) 606-224-2438 Fax: (1) 606-224-2430
BOOMER	General purpose nonlinear regression program for models defined as integrated or differential equations. Improved version of MULTI-FORTE for Macintosh and IBM compatible computers	Dr. David Bourne University of Oklahoma College of Pharmacy P.O. Box 26901 Oklahoma City, OK 73190-5040 USA	Phone: (1) 405-271-6471 Fax: (1) 405-271-3830
CSTRIP	Polyexponential stripping program	Dr. John G. Wagner 2142 Spruceway Lane Newport West Ann Arbor, MI 48103 USA	Phone: (1) 313-662-7861
DATAKINETICS	Drug monitoring software system intended primarily for hospital pharmacists	Dr. Kathleen A. Neugebauer Am. Soc. of Hospital Pharmacists 7272 Wisconsin Ave. Bethesda, MD 20814 USA	Phone: (1) 301-657-3000 Ext. 211 Fax: (1) 301-657-8817
DIFFEQ	Menu-driven program for solving ordinary differential equations numerically. Includes parameter estimation	Mr. Robin Kemker Micromath Scientific Software P.O. Box 21550 Salt Lake City, UT 84121-550 USA	Phone: (1) 801-943-0290 or 800-942-6284 Fax: (1) 801-943-0299
DRUGCALC	Focus on optimization of drug therapy through Bayesian forecasting. Microsoft Windows version available	Dr. Dennis Mungall MEDIFORE 573 Pacific Parkway Lansing, MI 48910 USA	Phone: (1) 517-372-5862 Fax: (1) 517-372-5862
EASYFIT	Analysis of compartmental models with graphics interface for Macintosh computers	Dr. Maurizio Rocchetti Mario Negri Institute Biomathematic Unit Via Eritrea 62 I-Milano 20157 Italy	Phone: (39) 2-390-141 Fax: (39) 2-354-6277
EDFAST	"Exact Disposition Fitter and Simulator of Linear Pharmacokinetic Models" allowing extremely complex dosage regimens	Mr. J. Lamble BIOSOFT 22 Hills Road Cambridge CB2 1JP UK	Phone: (44) 223-68622 Fax: (44) 223-312873

Software	Short description	Contact address	Phone/Fax
FRENDLIFIT	A series of files with predefined pharmacokinetic models for the Microsoft Excel spreadsheet under Windows environment	Dr. Porchet ARES SERONO 2 Chemin des Mines Case Postale 54 1202 Geneva 20 Switzerland	Phone: (41) 22-7388000 Fax: (41) 22-7312179
HOEREP-PC	Interactive or batch program for noncompartmental and compartmental analysis of pharmacokinetic data	Dr. Dierk Brockmeier HOECHST AG Clinical Research H 840 PO Box 80 03 20 6230 Frankfurt am main 80 Germany	Phone: (49) 69-305-3863 Fax: (49) 69-359-386
I THINK	General modeling language for systems dynamics on Macintosh computers. Allows simulation of pharmacokinetic/ pharmacodynamic systems	Dr. Michel Karsky KBS 340 Rue St. Jacques 75005 Paris France	Phone: (33) 1-4354-4796 Fax: (33) 1-4407-0059
KINETIDEX	Therapeutic drug monitoring system for therapy individualization, taking into account age, renal dysfunction and liver disease	Mrs. Cynthia Gilman MICROMEDEX Inc. 600 Grant Street Denver, CO 80203-3527 USA	Phone: (1) 800-525-9083 Ext. 6522 Fax: (1) 303-837-1717
LAPLACE	Definition of pharmacokinetic models through Laplace transforms. Curve fitting and parameter estimation	Mr. Robin Kemker Micromath Scientific Software PO Box 21550 Salt Lake City, UT 84121-550 USA	Phone: (1) 801-943-0290 or 800-942-6284 Fax: (1) 801-943-0299
MAXSIM	Simulation package developed mainly for education in pharmacokinetics and pharmacodynamics	Dr. Johan Gabrielsson Dept of Pharmacokinetics, B54:3 KABI Pharmacia Therapeutics AB 11287 Stockholm Sweden	Phone: (46) 8-6959378 Fax: (46) 8-137678
MICROPHARM	Analysis of pharmacokinetic data, including a rich library of binding and tissue extraction models	Dr. Saïk Urien Lab. de Pharmacologie Faculté de Médecine 8 Rue du Général Sarrail 94010 Creteil France	Phone: (33) 1-49813671
MINSQ	Menu-driven nonlinear curve fitting and model development program. A pharmacokinetic library of over 25 predefined models can be purchased	Mr. Robin Kemker Micromath Scientific Software PO Box 21550 Salt Lake City, UT 84121-550 USA	Phone: (1) 801-943-0290 or 800-942-6284 Fax: (1) 801-943-0299
MKMODEL	Comprehensive extended least squares modeling program, including pharmacokinetic, pharmacodynamic, and binding models	Dr. Nick Holford University of Auckland Dept. of Pharmacology Private Bag Auckland New Zealand	Phone: (64) 9-379-730 Fax: (64) 9-770-956
MLAB	Powerful program for interactive mathematical modeling and data analysis. Includes a large library of functions in mathematics and statistics. Aimed at "all mathematically literate people"	Dr. Gary Knott Civilized Software, Inc. 7735 Old Georgetown Road # 410 Bethesda, MD 20814 USA	Phone: (1) 301-652-4714

Software	Short description	Contact address	Phone/Fax
MLG	Compact "NONMEM like" programs for population pharmacokinetic analysis. Provided as Fortran or C source code	Dr. Takashi Amisaki Shimane University 1060 Nishikawatsu Matsue 690 Japan	Phone: (81) 852-21-7100 Fax: (81) 852-31-0812
MLTIDOSE	A multiple dose simulation program for any combination of intravenous and extravascular doses	Dr. Gary A. Thompson Procter & Gamble Company Clinical Investigations Department 11370 Reed Hartman Highway Cincinnati, OH 45241-2422 USA	Phone: (1) 513-626-2058 Fax: (1) 513-626-1860
MODFIT	Comprehensive PK/PD program "soon" available for IBM compatible computers	Dr. Graham D. Allen SMITHKLINE BEECHAM The Frythe, Welwyn Hertfordshire AL69AR UK	Phone: (44) 0438-782593
MULTI(FILT) MULTI(RUNGE) MULTI2(BAYES)	Nonlinear least squares analysis programs based on equations in Laplace domain, on ordinary differential equations and Bayesian optimization, respectively	Dr. Kiyoshi Yamaoka Faculty of Pharmaceutical Sciences Kyoto University Sakyo-ku, Kyoto Kyoto 606 Japan	Phone: (81) 75-753-4531 Fax: (81) 75-753-4578
MULTI-FORTE	Expanded version of the MULTI non linear fitting programs for the Macintosh computer	Dr. David Bourne University of Oklahoma College of Pharmacy P.O. Box 26901 Oklahoma City, OK 73190-5040 USA	Phone: (1) 405-271-6471 Fax: (1) 405-271-3830
MW/PHARM	Primarily aimed at clinical pharmacists. Includes individual parameter estimation and Bayesian optimization of dosage regimen. Additional module KINBES for bioavailability studies	Mr. N.C. Punt MediWare BV Zernike Park 2 Groningen 9747 AN The Netherlands	Phone: (31) 50-745707 Fax: (31) 50-634556
NONMEM	Nonlinear mixed effect model developed primarily for analysis of population data and assessing factors responsible for between subjects variability. Available as portable Fortran code	Dr. Stuart Beal University of California Department of Laboratory Medicine Room C-255, Box 0626 San Francisco, CA 94143 USA	Phone: (1) 415-426-1949
PCNONLIN	Nonlinear modeling program which benefits from over 20 years of mainframe and microcomputer development. Includes a library of about 20 predefined 1 to 3 compartment models	Mrs. Bonnie L. Ward SCI Software (Clin Trials Inc.) South Creek Office Park 2365 Harrodsburg Rd, Suite A-290 Lexington, KY 40504-3399 USA	Phone: (1) 606-224-2438 Fax: (1) 606-224-2430
PH/EDSIM	Easy to use software for simulation and analysis of compartmental models under the Microsoft Windows environment. Very suitable for educational purposes	Mr. N.C. Punt MediWare BV Zernike Park 2 Groningen 9747 AN The Netherlands	Phone: (31) 50-745707 Fax: (31) 50-634556
PKCALC	Descriptive statistics of multisubject data and initial estimates of parameters by peeling method	Dr. Robert C. Shumaker Wallace Laboratories 301B College Rd East Princeton, NJ 08540 USA	Phone: (1) 609-951-2013 Fax: (1) 609-951-2116

Software	Short description	Contact address	Phone/Fax
RSTRIP	Menu-driven, easy-to-use program for polyexponential stripping and least squares optimization of parameters	Mr. Robin Kemker Micromath Scientific Software P.O. Box 21550 Salt Lake City, UT 84121-550 USA	Phone: (1) 801-943-0290 or 800-942-6284 Fax: (1) 801-943-0299
SAAM & CONSAM	General purpose interactive environment for simulation, analysis and modeling in biomedical research	Dr. Loren A. Zech Lab. of Mathematical Biology NIH, National Cancer Institute Building 10, Room 4B56 Bethesda, MD 20892 USA	Phone: (1) 301-496-8914 or 301-496-8915 Fax: (1) 301-480-2871
SCoP	High-level environment for generating menu-driven model solvers, including optimizer, graphics and statistics	Mrs. J. Mailen Kootsey Simulation Resources, Inc. 300 S. Bluff Street Berrien Springs, MI 49103 USA	Phone: (1) 616-473-3234 Fax: (1) 616-473-4436
SIMKIN	System designed for physicians and clinical pharmacists to help interpretation of therapeutic drug monitoring data and customization of dosage regimens	Mrs. Barbara Orler SIMKIN, Inc. 408 W. University Ave., Suite 301 Gainesville, FL 32601 USA	Phone: (1) 904-372-8531 Fax: (1) 904-372-5873
SIPHAR	Integrated system dedicated to pharmacokinetics. Incorporates most classical models and techniques. Available for Macintosh and PCs under DOS or Windows	Dr. Roberto Gomeni SIMED 9-11 rue G. Enesco 94008 Creteil Cedex France	Phone: (33) 1-43990479 Fax: (33) 1-43990588
TDMS	Clinically oriented package for therapeutic drug monitoring	Dr. Jenn Ting HEALTHWARE Inc. P.O. Box 33483 San Diego, CA 92163 USA	Phone: (1) 619-452-0297
TOPFIT	Comprehensive pharmacokinetic software. Predefined models include sophisticated input functions and complex pharmacodynamic and drug binding models	Dr. Günther Heinzel Dr. Karl Thomae GmbH Abteilung Biochemie Postfach 1755 7950 Biberach/Riss Germany	Fax: (49) 7351-542168
TRIOMPHE	Model-dependent and -independent analysis of plasma and urine kinetics. Simulation	Dr. Philippe D'Athis Laboratoire d'Informatique Médicale 2 Bd Maréchal de Lattre de Tassigny 21034 Dijon France	Phone: (33) 16-80293462 Fax: (33) 16-80293421
USC*PACK	Includes BOXES for definition of compartmental models, ADAPT1 for parameter identification, NPEM for non parametric population modeling and AC for adaptative control of dosage regimen	Dr. Roger W. Jelliffe Lab. of Applied Pharmacokinetics USC School of Medicine 2250 Alcazar Street, CSC 134B Los Angeles, CA 90033 USA	Phone: (1) 213-342-1300 Fax: (1) 213-342-1302

D. Conclusion

The first part of the present appendix describes the different stages involved in computer-aided analysis of pharmacokinetic data. In the second part, a number of software packages are listed, in order to help potential users to identify which of the currently available products is most appropriate to their needs. The ease of data entry, the number of predefined models, the facility to develop more complex models, the sophistication of the algorithms, and the quality of display and printouts are some elements that play a role in this respect. However, other factors have to be taken into account, including validation of the techniques implemented, maintenance of the software over the years, support to users, and price. Personal characteristics of the user, for example experience in mathematics and computer science, general policies of the company, for example one full-time experienced user versus several part-time users, and research focus in academic institutes, for example purely pharmacokinetic versus more general modeling interests, are other points to be borne in mind. In other words, "the best" software is hardly likely to be found unless specific needs and wishes are carefully examined.

Acknowledgements. The authors would like to thank the users and developers of pharmacokinetic software who kindly answered to their survey. They are also grateful to Dr. Silvia Pace, Sigma-Tau SpA, Pomezia, Italy, for her participation in reviewing the information and for her useful comments.

References

Amisaki T, Tatsuhara T (1988) An alternative two stage method via the EM-algorithm for the estimation of population pharmacokinetic parameters. J Pharmacobiodyn 11:335–348

Balant LP, Garrett ER (1983) Computer use in pharmacokinetics. In: Garrett ER, Hirtz JL (eds) Drug fate and metabolism. Dekker, New York, pp 1–150

Berman M, Shahn E, Weiss MF (1962) The routine fitting of kinetic data to models: a mathematical formalism for digital computers. Biophys J 2:275–287

Boxenbaum HG, Riegelman S, Elashoff RM (1974) Statistical estimations in pharmacokinetics. J Pharmacokinet Biopharm 2:123–148

Di Stefano JJ, Landaw EM (1984) Multiexponential, multicompartmental, and noncompartmental modeling: I. Methodological limitations and physiological interpretations. Am J Physiol 246:R651–R664

Holford NHG, Sheiner LB (1982) Kinetics of pharmacologic response. Pharmacol Ther 16:143–166

Kennedy WJ, Gentle JE (1980) Statistical computing. Dekker, New York

Landaw EM, Di Stefano JJ (1984) Multiexponential, multicompartmental, and noncompartmental modeling: II. Data analysis and statistical considerations. Am J Physiol 246:R665–R677

Oosterhuis B, Van Boxtel CJ (1988) Kinetics of drug effect in man. Ther Drug Monit 10:121–132

Press WH, Flannery BP, Teukolsky SAS, Vetterling WT (1986) Numerical recipes. The art of scientific computing. Cambridge University Press, Cambridge

Sebaldt RJ, Kreeft JH (1987) Efficient pharmacokinetic modeling of complex clinical dosing regimens: the universal elementary dosing regimen and computer algorithm EDFAST. J Pharm Sci 76:93–100

Sheiner LB, Beal SL (1982) Bayesian individualization of pharmacokinetics: simple implementation and comparison with non-bayesian methods. J Pharm Sci 71: 1344–1348

Sheiner LB, Beal SL (1984) Estimation of altered kinetics in populations. In: Benet LZ et al. (eds) Pharmacokinetic basis for drug treatment. Raven, New York, pp 357–365

Skelly J (1990) Regulatory recommendations in USA on investigation and evaluation of oral controlled release products. In: Gundert-Remy U, Möller H (eds) Oral controlled release products: therapeutic and biopharmaceutic assessment. Wissenschaftliche Verlagsgesellschaft, Stuttgart, pp 175–193

Subject Index

Printing: Saladruck, Berlin
Binding: Buchbinderei Lüderitz & Bauer, Berlin